Improving Functional Outcomes in Physical Rehabilitation

Improving Functional Outcomes in Physical Rehabilitation

SUSAN B. O'SULLIVAN, PT, EdD
Professor
Department of Physical Therapy
School of Health and Environment
University of Massachusetts Lowell
Lowell, Massachusetts

THOMAS J. SCHMITZ, PT, PhD
Professor
Division of Physical Therapy
School of Health Professions
Long Island University
Brooklyn Campus
Brooklyn, New York

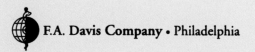
F.A. Davis Company • Philadelphia

F. A. Davis Company
1915 Arch Street
Philadelphia, PA 19103
www.fadavis.com

Printed in the United States of America

Last digit indicates print number: 10 9 8 7 6 5 4

Acquisitions Editor: Melissa A. Duffield
Developmental Editor: Yvonne N. Gillam
Publisher: Margaret M. Biblis
Manager of Content Development: George W. Lang
Art and Design Manager: Carolyn O'Brien

As new scientific information becomes available through basic and clinical research, recommended treatments and drug therapies undergo changes. The author(s) and publisher have done everything possible to make this book accurate, up to date, and in accord with accepted standards at the time of publication. The author(s), editors, and publisher are not responsible for errors or omissions or for consequences from application of the book, and make no warranty, expressed or implied, in regard to the contents of the book. Any practice described in this book should be applied by the reader in accordance with professional standards of care used in regard to the unique circumstances that may apply in each situation. The reader is advised always to check product information (package inserts) for changes and new information regarding dose and contraindications before administering any drug. Caution is especially urged when using new or infrequently ordered drugs.

Library of Congress Cataloging-in-Publication Data

O'Sullivan, Susan B.
  Improving functional outcomes in physical rehabilitation / Susan B. O'Sullivan, Thomas J. Schmitz.
    p. ; cm.
  ISBN-13: 978-0-8036-2218-0
  ISBN-10: 0-8036-2218-X
  1. Physical therapy—Case studies. I. Schmitz, Thomas J. II. Title.
  [DNLM: 1. Rehabilitation—Case Reports. 2. Activities of Daily Living—Case Reports. 3. Motor Activity—Case Reports. 4. Treatment Outcome—Case Reports. WB 320 O85i 2010]
  RM701.O88 2010
  615.8'2—dc22

                                                                          2009037800

PREFACE

We are heartened by the reception given to our earlier text, *Physical Rehabilitation Laboratory Manual: Focus on Functional Training*. In response to reviewer, faculty, and student feedback, we have so substantially revised and expanded the original work that it developed into the current text and is newly titled *Improving Functional Outcomes in Physical Rehabilitation*.

Given the frequency with which physical therapists apply their movement expertise to improving functional outcomes, our goal was to present an integrated model applicable to a wide spectrum of adult patients engaged in physical rehabilitation.

Part I, *Promoting Function: Conceptual Elements*, addresses the foundations of clinical decision-making and provides a conceptual framework for improving functional outcomes. The organization of content provides the student a logical learning progression of the strategies and interventions used to improve motor function, including task-specific, neuromotor, and compensatory approaches. Integration of motor control and motor learning strategies assists the student in acquiring a comprehensive approach to developing a plan of care.

Part II, *Interventions to Improve Function*, presents strategies and interventions to promote functional independence in a number of different functional skills (Chapters 3 to 10). Each chapter includes a description of the general characteristics of the posture and activity (e.g., base of support provided, location of center of mass, impact of gravity and body weight, and so forth) accompanied by a description of required lead-up skills, appropriate techniques, and progressions. Also provided are a description of patient outcomes consistent with the American Physical Therapy Association's *Guide to Physical Therapist Practice*, together with clinical applications and patient examples.

Our contributing chapter authors significantly enhanced Part II. Gutman and Mortera address interventions to improve upper extremity function from the unique perspective of the occupational therapist. Fulk provides distinctive insights for developing and implementing a plan of care designed to improve transfers and wheelchair skills. Lastly, Morris and Taub provide their distinguished perspectives on the history, treatment elements, and substantial potential of constraint-induced movement therapy.

The interventions presented address many types of impairments and activity limitations that patients may exhibit across practice patterns. They should not be considered as practice pattern-specific but as specific to the physical therapy *diagnosis* and *plan of care*. Our goal was to provide useful, practical examples of interventions that can be used to enhance functional performance.

Part III is titled *Case Studies*. This portion of the work provided us with the distinct privilege of bringing together a group of outstanding clinicians from across the country to contribute case studies in both written (Part III) and video format (accompanying DVD). The case studies present examples of patient management strategies based on effective clinical decision-making for patients with a variety of diagnoses (e.g., traumatic brain injury, stroke, spinal cord injury, peripheral vestibular dysfunction, and Parkinson's disease). The guiding questions included with each case study are designed to enhance clinical decision-making and to challenge the student to address the unique needs of the individual patients presented. The DVD captures each patient at three critical points within the episode of care: (1) at the initial examination, (2) during a treatment session, and (3) near discharge from physical therapy intervention. Our hope is that the case studies will facilitate meaningful dialogue between and among physical therapy students and teachers.

The text includes numerous pedagogical applications. Important information has been emphasized using boxes and tables. The designation "Red Flag" alerts the student to precautions or preventative safety measures. The term "Clinical Note" provides additional insights based on clinical observations. Each chapter includes numerous figures illustrating the interventions discussed. Included also are student practice activities designed to enhance learning.

The text recognizes the continuing growth of the profession and the importance of basic and applied clinical research in guiding and informing evidence-based practice. It also integrates terminology and interventions presented in the *Guide to Physical Therapist Practice*.

Without question, the text has benefited enormously from our talented group of contributors. We are honored by their participation in the project. The breadth and scope of their professional knowledge and expertise are well reflected in their contributions.

Our greatest hope is that the text will enhance the understanding of strategies to improve functional outcomes that lead to independence and ultimately an improved quality of life for our patients.

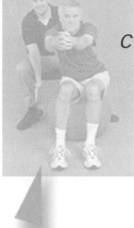

CONTRIBUTING AUTHORS

Paula Ackerman, MS, OTR/L
Shepherd Center, Inc.
Atlanta, Georgia

Elizabeth Ardolino, PT, MS
Magee Rehabilitation Center
Philadelphia, Pennsylvania

Myrtice Atrice, BS, PT
Shepherd Center, Inc.
Atlanta, Georgia

Jason Barbas, PT, MPT, NCS
Outpatient Rehabilitation
Rehabilitation Institute of Chicago
Chicago, Illinois

Andrea L. Behrman, PT, PhD
Associate Professor
College of Public Health and Health Professions
University of Florida
Department of Physical Therapy
Gainesville, Florida

Edward William Bezkor, PT, DPT, MTC
Clinical Specialist, Outpatient Physical Therapy
NYU Langone Medical Center
Rusk Institute of Rehabilitation Medicine
New York, New York

Temple T. Cowden, PT, MPT
Adult Brain Injury Service
Rancho Los Amigos National Rehabilitation Center
Downey, California

Teresa Foy, BS, OTR/L
Shepherd Center, Inc.
Atlanta, Georgia

George D. Fulk, PT, PhD
Assistant Professor
Department of Physical Therapy
Clarkson University
Potsdam, New York

Sharon A. Gutman, PhD, OTR
Associate Professor
Columbia University
Programs in Occupational Therapy
New York, New York

Susan Harkema, PhD
Associate Professor
Department of Neurological Surgery
University of Louisville
Louisville, Kentucky
Owsley B. Frazier Chair in Neurological Rehabilitation
Louisville, Kentucky
Rehabilitation Research Director
Kentucky Spinal Cord Injury Research Center
Louisville, Kentucky
Research Director
Frazier Rehab Institute
Louisville, Kentucky
Director of the NeuroRecovery Network
Louisville, Kentucky

Polly Hopkins, MOTR/L
Shepherd Center, Inc.
Atlanta, Georgia

Shari McDowell, BS, PT
Shepherd Center, Inc.
Atlanta, Georgia

JoAnn Moriarty-Baron, PT, DPT
Southern New Hampshire Rehabilitation Center
Nashua, New Hampshire

David M. Morris, PT, PhD
Associate Professor
Department of Physical Therapy
University of Alabama at Birmingham
Birmingham, Alabama

Sarah Morrison, BS, PT
SCI Program Director
Shepherd Center, Inc.
Atlanta, Georgia

Marianne H. Mortera, PhD, OTR
Assistant Professor
Columbia University
Programs in Occupational Therapy
New York, New York

Darrell Musick, PT
Director of Physical Therapy
Craig Hospital
Englewood, Colorado

Susan B. O'Sullivan, PT, EdD
Professor
Department of Physical Therapy
School of Health and Environment
University of Massachusetts Lowell
Lowell, Massachusetts

Sonya L. Pearson, PT, DPT
University of Alabama at Birmingham
Birmingham, Alabama

Heidi Roth, PT, MSPT, NCS
Research and Clinical Physical Therapist
Rehabilitation Institute of Chicago
Chicago, Illinois

Mary Schmidt-Read, PT, DPT, MS
Magee Rehabilitation Center
Philadelphia, Pennsylvania

Thomas J. Schmitz, PT, PhD
Professor
Division of Physical Therapy
School of Health Professions
Long Island University
Brooklyn Campus
Brooklyn, New York

Lauren Snowdon, PT, DPT
Clinical Manager, Inpatient Physical Therapy
Kessler Institute for Rehabilitation
West Orange, New Jersey

Edward Taub, PhD
Professor
Director CI Therapy Research Group and Taub Training Clinic
Department of Psychology
University of Alabama at Birmingham
Birmingham, Alabama

Elizabeth Watson, PT, DPT, NCS
Magee Rehabilitation Center
Philadelphia, Pennsylvania

Laura S. Wehrli, PT, DPT, ATP
Craig Hospital
Englewood, Colorado

Lynn Wong, PT, DPT, MS, GCS
Caritas Home Care
Methuen, Massachusetts

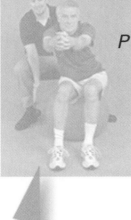

PROPOSAL REVIEWERS

Bill Andrews, PT, MS, EdD, NCS
Assistant Professor
Elon University
Department of Physical Therapy Education
Elon, North Carolina

Pamela R. Bosch, PT, PhD
Associate Professor
A. T. Still University
The Arizona School of Health Sciences
Physical Therapy Department
Mesa, Arizona

Karen Jones, PT
Instructor
Herkimer County Community College
Physical Therapy Department
Herkimer, New York

Toby Sternheimer, PT, MEd
Cuyahoga Community College
Physical Therapist Assistant Program
Cleveland, Ohio

Shannon Williams, PT, MEd, FAAOMPT
Clinic Director
Texas State University–San Marcos
Physical Therapy Department
San Marcos, Texas

ACKNOWLEDGMENTS

Improving Functional Outcomes in Physical Rehabilitation is a product of our combined years of experience in clinical practice and in teaching physical therapy students. From the outset, it has been a collaborative venture, bringing together a talented group of contributing authors from both academic and clinical practice settings. Their willingness to share their expertise as well as their interest in the professional development of physical therapy students was continually evident throughout project development. We extend heartfelt gratitude to our outstanding chapter contributors and the expert clinicians and educators who contributed case studies.

The authors express sincere appreciation to the individuals who reviewed the manuscript at different points during development. Their constructive comments substantially enhanced the content and order of presentation. For her content expertise and insightful suggestions, particular thanks are extended to Cristiana Kahl Collins, PT, MA, NCS, Associate Director, Division of Physical Therapy, School of Health Professions, Long Island University, Brooklyn, New York. As always, thanks are extended to Ivaldo Costa, MSW, and Stacy Jaffee Gopack, PT, PhD, Associate Professor and Director, Division of Physical Therapy, School of Health Professions, Long Island University, Brooklyn, New York.

Our gratitude is conveyed to the following individuals who contributed their exceptional photography skills to create the numerous figures used throughout the text: Paul Coppens, Director of Media Services, University of Massachusetts Lowell, Lowell, Massachusetts; Christopher F. Lenney, University Photographer, Clarkson University, Potsdam, New York; and Mark Lozier Photography, Cherry Hill, New Jersey.

We are indebted to the generous individuals who cordially posed for photographs. For their gracious time commitment, belief in the importance of the project, and unfailing patience, we recognize Natasha Chevalier-Richards, Sally Healy, Karen Kubicina, Joel Lindstrom, Philomena (Mini) G. Mungiole, Whitney Odle, Natalie Pieczynski, Robert Margeson Sr., Khushbu Shah, Whitney Sippl, and J. Anthony Tomaszewski. For his kind assistance with locating photography subjects, we gratefully acknowledge Stephen Carp, PT, PhD, GCS, Director of Admissions and Outcomes Assessment, Doctor of Physical Therapy Program, College of Health Professions, Temple University, Philadelphia, Pennsylvania. For their kind assistance in locating needed equipment for the photographs, we offer thanks to Robin Dole, PT, EdD, PCS, Associate Professor, Associate Dean and Program Director, Institute for Physical Therapy Education, Widener University, Chester, Pennsylvania; and Tom Weis, Media Arts Department, Long Island University, Brooklyn, New York.

For her patience and competent attention to detail, gratitude is extended to Marsha Hall, Project Manager, Progressive Publishing Alternatives, Emigsville, Pennsylvania. Our thanks also go to those who contributed to the production and editing of the case study DVD that accompanies the text: Mitchell Shuldman, EdD, Librarian and Head, Division of Media Services, University of Massachusetts Lowell, Lowell, Massachusetts; and Beholder Productions, Inc., Horsham, Pennsylvania.

Our appreciation is extended to the dedicated professionals at F. A. Davis Company, Philadelphia, Pennsylvania: Margaret M. Biblis, Publisher; Melissa A. Duffield, Acquisitions Editor; George W. Lang, Manager of Content Development; Yvonne N. Gillam, Developmental Editor; Kirk Pedrick, Manager of Electronic Product Development; Carolyn O'Brien, Art and Design Manager; and Stephanie A. Casey, Departmental Associate, Health Professions and Medicine. Their continued support, encouragement, and unwavering commitment to excellence have contributed significantly to the development of this text as well as to the expansion of the physical therapy literature. Our appreciation is considerable.

Last, although hardly least, we wish to thank our students and patients who continually challenge us to improve our teaching and clinical skills. It is our sincere hope that this text will prove a valuable resource in the development of clinical decision-making and practice skills of aspiring professionals.

Susan B. O'Sullivan
Thomas J. Schmitz

TABLE OF CONTENTS

PART I

Promoting Function: Conceptual Elements 1

CHAPTER 1

Framework for Clinical Decision-Making 3
SUSAN B. O'SULLIVAN, PT, EdD

CHAPTER 2

Interventions to Improve Motor Control and Motor Learning 12
SUSAN B. O'SULLIVAN, PT, EdD

PART II

Interventions to Improve Function 43

CHAPTER 3

Interventions to Improve Bed Mobility and Early Trunk Control 45
THOMAS J. SCHMITZ, PT, PhD

CHAPTER 4

Interventions to Improve Sitting and Sitting Balance Skills 97
SUSAN B. O'SULLIVAN, PT, EdD

CHAPTER 5

Interventions to Improve Kneeling and Half-Kneeling Control 120
THOMAS J. SCHMITZ, PT, PhD

CHAPTER 6

Interventions to Improve Transfers and Wheelchair Skills 138
GEORGE D. FULK, PT, PhD

CHAPTER 7

Interventions to Improve Standing Control and Standing Balance Skills 163
SUSAN B. O'SULLIVAN, PT, EdD

CHAPTER 8

Interventions to Improve Locomotor Skills 194
THOMAS J. SCHMITZ, PT, PhD

CHAPTER 9

Interventions to Improve Upper Extremity Skills 216
SHARON A. GUTMAN, PhD, OTR
MARIANNE H. MORTERA, PhD, OTR

CHAPTER 10

Constraint-Induced Movement Therapy 232
DAVID M. MORRIS, PT, PhD
EDWARD TAUB, PhD

PART III

Case Studies 247

CASE STUDY 1

Traumatic Brain Injury 251
TEMPLE T. COWDEN, PT, MPT

CASE STUDY 2

Traumatic Brain Injury: Balance and Locomotor Training 257
HEIDI ROTH, PT, MSPT, NCS
JASON BARBAS, PT, MPT, NCS

CASE STUDY 3

Spinal Cord Injury: Locomotor Training 262
ELIZABETH ARDOLINO, PT, MS
ELIZABETH WATSON, PT, DPT, NCS
ANDREA L. BEHRMAN, PT, PhD
SUSAN HARKEMA, PhD
MARY SCHMIDT-READ, PT, DPT, MS

CASE STUDY 4

Spinal Cord Injury 274
DARRELL MUSICK, PT
LAURA S. WEHRLI, PT, DPT, ATP

CASE STUDY 5

Peripheral Vestibular Dysfunction 278
JOANN MORIARTY-BARON, PT, DPT

CASE STUDY 6

Parkinson's Disease 281
EDWARD W. BEZKOR, PT, DPT, MTC

CASE STUDY 7

Spinal Cord Injury 287

PAULA ACKERMAN, MS, OTR/L
MYRTICE ATRICE, PT, BS
TERESA FOY, BS, OTR/L
SARAH MORRISON, PT, BS
POLLY HOPKINS, MOTR/L
SHARI McDOWELL, PT, BS

CASE STUDY 8

Stroke: Home Care Rehabilitation 293

LYNN WONG, PT, DPT, MS, GCS

CASE STUDY 9

Stroke: Constraint-Induced Movement Therapy 296

DAVID M. MORRIS, PT, PhD
SONYA L. PEARSON, PT, DPT
EDWARD TAUB, PhD

CASE STUDY 10

Stroke 318

LAUREN SNOWDON, PT, DPT, ATP

APPENDIX A

Outcome Measures Organized by the *International Classification of Functioning, Disability, and Health (ICF)* Categories 324

INDEX 330

Promoting Function: Conceptual Elements

Part I, *Promoting Function: Conceptual Elements*, is comprised of two chapters. Chapter 1, *Framework for Clinical Decision-Making,* provides the foundational context for clinical decision-making. It addresses the *International Classification of Functioning, Disability, and Health (ICF)* model as the basis for planning. Theories of motor control and motor learning are examined, and strategies to promote enhanced motor function and motor recovery are considered. The chapter is organized around the characteristics of three critical elements: the *task*, the *individual*, and the *environment*. The major focus of Chapter 2, *Interventions to Improve Motor Control and Motor Learning*, is to assist the learner in acquiring a conceptual framework for developing a comprehensive plan of care (POC) to improve functional outcomes. It directs attention to the components of task analysis and progresses to a discussion of task-oriented, activity-based strategies as the foundation of intervention. Motor learning strategies are organized and discussed according to stages of motor learning. Conventional neuromotor approaches and strategies are also presented, including Proprioceptive Neuromuscular Facilitation (PNF), Neuro-Developmental Treatment (NDT), and sensory stimulation techniques. Finally, compensatory strategies are examined as a component of the continuum of available strategies to improve functional outcomes.

Framework for Clinical Decision-Making

SUSAN B. O'SULLIVAN, PT, EdD

Optimal functional recovery is the primary goal of all rehabilitation professionals. Although individuals have traditionally been identified or categorized by their disease or medical condition (e.g., spinal cord injury [SCI]), the World Health Organization's (WHO) *International Classification of Functioning, Disability, and Health (ICF)* model,[1] provides an important framework for examining and treating the patient by clearly defining health condition, impairment, activity limitation, and participation restriction. Thus the patient with SCI presents with paralysis; sensory loss; autonomic dysfunction (impairments); loss of independent function in bed mobility, dressing, bathing, and locomotor ability (activity limitations); and an inability to work or go to school (participation restrictions). Physical therapist practice intervenes primarily at the level of impairments, activity limitations, and participation restrictions. Effective clinical decision-making is based on an understanding of the *ICF* model and related contextual factors (environmental and personal factors) in order to arrive at effective choices for intervention. In addition, clinicians must understand factors that improve quality of life, prevention, wellness, and fitness. An effective plan of care (POC) clarifies risk factors and seeks to fully involve the patient in determining meaningful functional goals. This text focuses on improving motor function (motor control and motor learning) and muscle performance (strength, power, and endurance) through activities and exercises that optimize functional outcomes. Definitions of disablity terminology are presented in Box 1.1.

An effective POC is based on the concept that normal motor function emerges from the practice of tasks that are activity based. A POC uses a logical, sequential progression in terms of increasing difficulty. In general, the patient learns to control increasingly larger segments of the body simultaneously with gradual increases in the effects of gravity and body weight. Thus, during the progression of activities, the base of support (BOS) is gradually narrowed while the center of mass (COM) is elevated, placing increased demands on postural control and balance. Activity-based training helps the patient develop motor skills using synergistic patterns of muscles with movements that occur in multiple axes and planes of movement. Different types and combinations of muscle contractions (concentric, eccentric, isometric) are utilized. The types and variations of contractions used more closely represent the work muscles typically do during the execution of daily activities as compared to those trained using other methods such as progressive resistance exercise. Somatosensory, vestibular, and

---

BOX 1.1 Terminology: Functioning, Disability, and Health

From World Health Organization's (WHO) *International Classification of Functioning, Disability, and Health (ICF)*[1]
Health condition is an umbrella term for disease, disorder, injury or trauma and may also include other circumstances, such as aging, stress, congenital anomaly, or genetic predisposition. It may also include information about pathogeneses and/or etiology.
Body functions are physiological functions of body systems (including psychological functions).
Body structures are anatomical parts of the body such as organs, limbs, and their components.
Impairments are the problems in body function or structure such as a significant deviation or loss.
Activity is the execution of a task or action by an individual.
Participation is involvement in a life situation.
Activity limitations are difficulties an individual may have in executing activities.

Participation restrictions are problems an individual may experience in involvement in life situations.
Contextual factors represent the entire background of an individual's life and living situation.

- **Environmental factors** make up the physical, social, and attitudinal environment in which people live and conduct their lives, including social attitudes, architectural characteristics, and legal and social structures.
- **Personal factors** are the particular background of an individual's life, including gender, age, coping styles, social background, education, profession, past and current experience, overall behavior pattern, character, and other factors that influence how disability is experienced by an individual.

(box continues on page 4)

> **BOX 1.1** Terminology: Functioning, Disability, and Health (continued)
>
> **Performance** describes what an individual does in his or her current environment.
>
> **Capacity** describes an individual's ability to execute a task or an action (highest probable level of functioning in a given domain at a given moment).
>
> (In June 2008, the American Physical Therapy Association [APTA] joined the WHO, the World Confederation for Physical Therapy, the American Therapeutic Recreation Association, and other international organizations in endorsing the ICF.)
>
> From *Guide to Physical Therapist Practice,* ed 2[2]
>
> **Pathology/pathophysiology (disease, disorder, condition)** describes an abnormality characterized by a particular cluster of signs and symptoms and recognized by either the patient/client or the practitioner as abnormal. It is primarily identified at the cellular level.
>
> **Impairment** is the loss or abnormality of anatomical, physiological, mental, or psychological structure or function.
>
> **Functional limitation** is the restriction of the ability to perform, at the level of the whole person, a physical action, task, or activity in an efficient, typically expected, or competent manner.
>
> **Disability** is the inability to perform or a limitation in the performance of actions, tasks, and activities usually expected in specific social roles that are customary for the individual or expected for the person's status or role in a specific sociocultural context and physical environment. Categories are self-care, home management, work (job/school/play), and community/leisure.
>
> **Health status** describes the state or status of the conditions that constitute good health.

visual inputs from the body assist in movement control and balance. Owing to the inherent use of body weight and gravity, enhanced demands for postural control are placed on the trunk and limb segments during performance. Activity-based training activities are complex movements in which the primary focus is coordinated action, not isolated muscle or joint control.

The key to successful intervention is a thorough understanding of its basic elements: the task, the individual's performance capabilities, and the environment (Fig. 1.1). Each will be discussed in this chapter.

The foundational underlying theories on which motor function is based include: *motor control theory (systems and motor program theories)* and *motor learning theory*. *Systems theory* describes motor function as the result of a series of interacting systems that contribute to different aspects of control. For example, the musculoskeletal system, the sensory system, and the neural control systems (synergistic control, coordination, and balance) all contribute to the movements produced. *Motor programming theory* is based on the concept of a *motor program,* which is defined as an abstract code that, when initiated, results in the production of a coordinated movement sequence. Thus movement patterns are stored and can be initiated using pre-programmed instructions without peripheral inputs or feedback information (termed an *open-loop system*). Movement

TASK ⇔	**INDIVIDUAL** ⇔	**ENVIRONMENT**
Functions: BADL, IADL	Arousal, Attention	Physical Environment
Attributes:	Cognition, Motivation	Variability
Mobility	Sensory-Perceptual Integrity	Regulatory Features
Stability	Muscle Strength, Motor Function	Psychosocial Factors
Controlled Mobility	Posture, ROM, Flexibility	
Skill	Gait, Locomotion, Balance	
Characteristics:	Aerobic Capacity/Endurance	
Velocity	Co-morbidities, Complications	
Amplitude	Activity Limitations	
	Disability	
	Overall Health Status	

MOTOR FUNCTION

FIGURE 1.1 Motor function emerges from interactions among the task, the individual, and the environment.
Abbreviations: BADL, basic activities of daily living; IADL, instrumental activities of daily living; ROM, range of motion.

patterns can also be initiated and modified using sensory inputs and feedback information (termed a *closed-loop system*). In a closed-loop system, feedback is used for error detection and modification of the movement responses, as seen when learning a new skill. *Motor learning theory* is based on concepts of feedback and practice that are used to influence the type and degree of learning and lead to relatively permanent changes in performance capabilities. Use of appropriate motor learning strategies (discussed in Chapter 2) enhances motor skill acquisition. Organized practice schedules and appropriate feedback delivery are essential elements. Additional terminology is presented in Box 1.2. For a thorough review of these concepts, the reader is referred to the excellent works of Schmidt and Lee[3] and Shumway-Cook and Woollacott.[4]

The acquisition of motor skills in infants and children that are critical to independent function (such as rolling over, sitting up, sitting, crawling, kneeling, standing up, standing, walking, and eye-hand coordination) is a function of neuromuscular maturation and practice. These activities, sometimes termed *developmental skills* or *developmental sequence skills,* form the basis of a set of skills needed for life-long independent function. The development of motor control in the infant and child is marked by *motor milestones* that emerge at somewhat predictable ages. Development generally progresses from head to foot (cephalo-caudal) and proximal to distal. In infants and children the development of motor function is

viewed as a spiral progression with considerable variability, not as a strict linear progression. Primitive and static attitudinal reflexes are believed to become integrated as the central nervous system (CNS) matures and higher-level postural reflexes (righting and equilibrium reactions) emerge *(reflex hierarchical theory).* Systems theory helps to better define both the adaptive capacity and the modifiability of responses seen during normal development. Emerging motor behaviors are dependent on the maturation and function of different system components during critical stages in development. The emergence of postural development and control is a good example of this.

In the adult, the motor skills acquired early in life are maintained and remain relatively stable across the life span. Skills such as rolling over and sitting up are used every day as a normal part of life. However, these movement patterns are responsive to change and can be modified by a number of different factors. Primary factors include genetic predisposition and changes associated with aging causing a decline in overall function of the CNS, including sensory decline in visual, somatosensory, and vestibular functions; changes in synergistic control of movement and timing; and a decline in balance. Secondary and potentially modifiable factors include changing body dimensions (changes in body weight, body shape and topography, and posture), level of physical activity (changes in muscle strength, flexibility, and range of motion [ROM] associated with inactivity), nutrition, and environmental factors. The physically frail older adult and

---

BOX 1.2 Terminology: Motor Control

Degrees of freedom: The number of separate independent dimensions of movement in a system that must be controlled.[4(p463)]

Degrees of freedom problem: The difficulty in explaining the simultaneous control of multiple, independently moving body parts.

Motor control: The underlying substrates of neural, physical, and behavioral aspects of movement.

- **Reactive motor control:** Movements are adapted in response to ongoing feedback (e.g., muscle stretch causes an increase in muscle contraction in response to a forward weight shift).
- **Proactive (anticipatory) motor control:** Movements are adapted in advance of ongoing movements via feedforward mechanisms (e.g., the postural adjustments made in preparation for catching a heavy, large ball).

Motor program: An abstract representation that, when initiated, results in the production of a coordinated movement sequence.[3(p466)]

Motor learning: A set of internal processes associated with feedback or practice leading to relatively permanent changes in the capability for motor skill.[3(p466)]

Motor recovery: The reacquisition of movement skills lost through injury.

Schema: A set of rules, concepts, or relationships formed on the basis of experience[3(p467)]; schema serve to provide a basis for movement decisions and are stored in memory for the reproduction of movement.

- **Recall schema:** The relationship among past parameters, past initial conditions, and the movement outcomes produced by these combinations.
- **Recognition schema:** The relationship among past initial conditions, past movement outcomes, and the sensory consequences produced by these combinations.

Task analysis: A process of determining the underlying abilities and structure of a task or occupation.[3(p468)]

Task organization: How the components of a task are interrelated or interdependent.

- **Low organization:** Task components are relatively independent.
- **High organization:** Task components are highly interrelated.

the physically dependent individual will likely demonstrate the greatest changes in basic motor skills. This adaptability or change is evidence of the CNS's ability for ongoing reorganization of motor skills, which is life-long. As in infants and children, there is no one predictable pattern of movement to accomplish functional goals that characterizes all adults or all older adults.

In the adult patient with activity limitations and participation restrictions, motor skills are modified in the presence of integumentary, musculoskeletal, neuromuscular, or cardiorespiratory impairments. *Motor recovery,* the reacquisition of movement skills lost through injury, is highly variable and individualized. Complete recovery, in which the performance of reacquired skills is identical in every way to preinjury performance, may not be possible. Rather it is likely that the preinjury skills are modified in some way. For example, the patient with stroke regains walking ability but now walks with a slowed gait and increased hip and knee flexion on the more affected side. *Compensation* is defined as behavioral substitution—that is, the adoption of alternative behavioral strategies to complete a task. For example, the patient with stroke learns to dress independently using the less affected upper extremity (UE). Or the patient with a complete T1 SCI learns to roll using both UEs and momentum. *Spontaneous recovery* refers to the initial neural repair processes that occur immediately after injury. For example, the patient with stroke regains some UE motor function approximately 2 to 3 weeks after insult as cerebral edema resolves. *Function-induced recovery* (use-dependent cortical reorganization) refers to the ability of the nervous system to modify itself in response to activity and environmental stimulation. Stimulation early after injury is important to prevent *learned nonuse.* For example, the patient with stroke who undergoes limited rehabilitation learns to use the less affected extremities to achieve functional goals and fails to use the more affected extremities. In order for later rehabilitation to be successful, these faulty patterns must be unlearned while correct patterns are learned. Early exposure to training can prevent this learned nonuse and the development of faulty or poor motor patterns. There is ample evidence that training is also effective for patients with chronic disability. For example, patients with stroke for more than 1 year respond positively to functional task-oriented training using constraint-induced (CI) movement therapy (discussed in Chapter 10 and Case Study 9). Locomotor training using partial body weight support (BWS), a treadmill, and early assisted limb movements has also been shown to promote function-induced recovery (discussed in Chapter 8 and Case Study 3). The elements essential for success with these interventions are that (1) practice is task-specific and (2) practice is intense with steady increases in duration and frequency. For example, with CI therapy, the patient with stroke practices grasping and manipulating objects during daily tasks using the more affected UE 4 to 6 hours per day, every day. The less affected UE may be constrained with a mitt or sling, thereby preventing all attempts for compensatory movements.

Understanding the Task

Tasks are classified according to motor functions: mobility, stability, controlled mobility, and skill. Each function is discussed in turn.

Mobility

Mobility is the ability to move from one position to another independently and safely. Early mobility often involves discrete movements of the limbs or trunk (e.g., the patient reaches across the body and rolls toward sidelying) with limited postural or antigravity control. Movements may be poorly sustained or controlled. Later function is characterized by more controlled movements of the body superimposed on postural control (e.g., the patient stands up and walks across the room).

Deficits in mobility control range from failure to initiate or sustain movement to poorly controlled movements. Limited or varying degrees of postural control are evident, and movement outcomes may be limited.

Stability

Stability (also known as *static postural control*) is the ability to maintain a position with the body at rest with orientation of the COM over the BOS. A steady posture can be maintained with minimum sway, no loss of balance, and no external stabilization support. Prolonged holding (an endurance function) is an integral part of stability control. Stability comes largely from tonic muscle activity and control of proximal segments and trunk. Increasing antigravity stability control is evident with the acquisition and maintenance of more upright postures (e.g., sitting to kneeling to standing).

Deficits in stability control range from widened BOS or lowered COM, increased sway, handhold or leg support, to loss of balance and falls.

Controlled Mobility

Controlled mobility (dynamic postural control) is the ability to maintain postural stability and orientation of the COM over the BOS while parts of the body are in motion. An individual is able to move in a posture without losing postural control (e.g., the patient maintains a sitting position while shifting weight back and forth or side to side). The distal segments (feet and buttocks) are fixed while the trunk is moving. Movement control normally develops through increments of range (small to large). Movement through decrements of range (large to small) can be used in treatment for progression to stability control for patients with hyperkinetic disorders such as cerebellar ataxia. Full ROM and easy controlled reversals of direction are expected in normal controlled mobility function.

The ability to shift weight onto one side and free the opposite limb for non-weightbearing dynamic activity is also evidence of controlled mobility function (sometimes called *static-dynamic control*). The initial weight shift and redistributed weightbearing place increased demands on support segments while the dynamic limb challenges control. For example, a patient with traumatic brain injury (TBI) is positioned in quadruped (all fours) and is able to lift first one UE, then the other, or opposite upper and lower extremities. Or in sitting, the patient is able to reach forward and sideward in all directions without losing sitting stability.

Deficits in controlled mobility range from postural instability and falls to poorly controlled and limited dynamic limb movements. A major distinguishing factor between normal and abnormal controlled mobility function is the degree to which core muscles (trunk and proximal limbs) can stabilize effectively during the limb movements.

Skill

A *skill* is an action that has a specific goal and requires a coordinated movement sequence to achieve the goal. Several characteristics are common to skilled movements. Skills have a specific purpose such as investigation and interaction with the physical and social environment (e.g., grasp and manipulation of objects or walking). Skills require voluntary control; thus reflexes or involuntary movements cannot be considered skilled movements. The term *skill* also designates quality of performance. Thus skilled movements are characterized by consistency, fluency, precise timing, and economy of effort in achieving the target goal (e.g., how well an individual accomplishes the action). Skills require coordinated

actions of body and limb segments. Thus the trunk and proximal segments stabilize while the distal limbs complete the skilled action (e.g., eating with a knife and fork or dressing). Skills are learned and task specific. Acquisition is the direct result of practice and experience. Skill in one task does not necessarily carry over to another task without additional practice and experience. *Adaptation* refers to the ability to modify a skill in response to changing task and environmental demands. Thus a learned skill such as a transfer from bed to wheelchair is adapted to permit an individual to transfer successfully from wheelchair to toilet or wheelchair to car. It is important to distinguish ability from skill. *Motor ability* is the general capacity of an individual to perform a skill or task and is based on stable characteristics or traits that are genetically defined and not influenced by practice. For example, a professional athlete demonstrates a high degree of abilities (e.g., eye-hand coordination and neuromuscular control) required to successfully play a competitive sport.

Motor skills are varied and serve a large variety of action goals. Classification systems have been developed to organize motor skills into general categories based on components, goals, and contexts in which they must be performed. The terms may serve as anchor points along a continuum (e.g., open skill versus closed skill). It is important to remember that skills can fall anywhere along that continuum, not just at either end. Box 1.3 provides general definitions for the different classifications of motor skills.

Motor skill performance also has been defined by the timing of movement. *Reaction time* (RT) is the interval of time between the onset of the initial stimulus to move and the initiation of a movement response. *Movement time* (MT)

BOX 1.3 TERMINOLOGY: MOTOR SKILLS

Ability: A genetically predetermined characteristic or trait of an individual that underlies performance of certain motor skills.

Motor skill: An action or task that has a goal to achieve; acquisition of skill is dependent on practice and experience and is not genetically defined. *Alternative definition*: an indicator of the quality of performance.

- **Gross motor skills:** Motor skills that involve large musculature and a goal where precision of movement is not important to the successful execution of the skill (e.g., running or jumping).
- **Fine motor skills:** Motor skills that require control of small muscles of the body to achieve the goal of skill; this type of task (e.g., writing, typing, or buttoning a shirt) typically requires a high level of eye-hand coordination.
- **Closed motor skill:** A skill performed in a stable or predictable environment (e.g., walking in a quiet hall).
- **Open motor skill:** A skill performed in a variable or unpredictable environment (e.g., walking across a busy gym).

- **Discrete motor skills:** Skills that have distinct beginning and end points defined by the task itself (e.g., locking the brake on a wheelchair).
- **Serial motor skills:** Skills that are discrete or individual skills put together in a series. (e.g., the highly individual steps required to transfer from a bed to a wheelchair).
- **Continuous motor skills:** Skills that have arbitrary beginning and end points defined by the performer or some external agents (e.g., swimming, running).
- **Simple motor skills:** Movements that involve a single motor program that produces an individual movement response (e.g., kicking a ball while sitting in a chair).
- **Complex motor skills:** Movements that involve multiple actions and motor programs combined to produce a coordinated movement response (e.g., running and kicking a soccer ball during a game).
- **Dual-task skills:** Movements that involve simultaneous actions (motor programs) performed together (e.g., walking and carrying a tray, walking and talking).

is the interval of time between the initiation of movement and the completion of movement. The sum of both is called *response time,* which can be expected to improve as skill learning progresses as evidenced by a decrease in overall time. *Speed-accuracy trade-off* is a principle of motor skill performance that defines the influence of the speed of performance by movement accuracy demands. The trade-off is that increasing speed decreases accuracy, while decreasing speed improves accuracy. Speed-accuracy demands are task specific. In tasks with high accuracy requirements such as aiming tasks (e.g., throwing a football), speed must be kept within reasonable limits to permit accuracy. Speed-accuracy trade-off typically affects older adults. For example, with declining postural and balance abilities, movements such as walking are slowed in order to permit accurate and safe progression. When the older adult tries to walk fast, the result may be a loss of control and a fall.

Deficits in skilled function range from poorly coordinated movements, including deficits in movement composition (dyssynergia), movement accuracy and timing (dysmetria), and ability to rapidly reverse movements (dysdiadochokinesia), to deficits in fixation or limb holding and postural stability (equilibrium). Delayed reaction times and slowed movement times are also evident.

Table 1.1 presents a classification of tasks according to movement function.

Lead-Up Skills

Learning a motor skill is a complex process. For patients with motor dysfunction, whole-task training may not be initially possible. For example, the patient with poor head and trunk control following TBI cannot learn head control first in unsupported standing. There are simply too many body segments to control in order to be successful. This has been referred to as a *degrees of freedom problem.* In these situations the therapist is challenged to make critical decisions about how to break the task down into its component parts (*lead-up skills* or simple motor skills) within a functionally relevant context. Each lead-up skill represents a component of a larger functional task, referred to as the *criterion skill.* A single lead-up skill may involve a number of criterion skills. For example, lower trunk rotation is an important lead-up skill to upright stepping as well as rolling and scooting. *Parts-to-whole training* addresses mastery of individual component skills with progression to a criterion skill. It also has the positive benefit of reducing fear and desensitizing patients who might be quite fearful of performing certain movements. For example, bridging activities can be used to prepare patients for sit-to-stand tranfers. Hip extensor control is enhanced while the degrees of freedom problem and fear are reduced. Skills with highly independent parts (e.g., bed-to-wheelchair transfer) can usually be successfully trained using this strategy. Parts-to-whole transfer

TABLE 1.1 Classification of Tasks According to Movement Function[a]

Categories	Characteristics	Examples	Deficits
Mobility	Ability to move from one position to another	Rolling; supine-to-sit; sit-to-stand; transfers	Failure to initiate or sustain movements through the range; poorly controlled movements
Stability (Static postural control)	Ability to maintain postural stability and orientation with the COM over the BOS with the body not in motion	Holding in antigravity postures: prone-on-elbows, quadruped, sitting, kneeling, half-kneeling, plantigrade, or standing	Failure to maintain a steady body position; excessive postural sway; wide BOS; high guard arm position or UE support; loss of balance
Controlled Mobility (Dynamic postural control)	Ability to maintain postural stability and orientation with the COM over the BOS while parts of the body are in motion	Weight shifting, or limb movements (lifting, reaching, stepping) in the above antigravity postures	Failure to control posture during weight shifting or limb movements with increased sway or loss of balance
Skill	Ability to consistently perform coordinated movement sequences for the purposes of investigation and interaction with the physical and social environment	Reach and manipulation; bipedal ambulation	Poorly coordinated movements; lack of precision, control, consistency, and economy of effort; inability to achieve a task goal

Abbreviations: COM, center of mass; BOS, base of support.
[a]From O'Sullivan and Schmitz,[5] Table 13.2 Motor Skills (with permission).

is generally less successful with skills that have highly integrated parts, such as walking. In this situation, it is generally better to implement practice of the criterion skill (whole-task training) as soon as possible. The successes therapists have had with locomotor training using body weight support and a motorized treadmill (discussed in Chapter 8 and Case Study 3) illustrates this point.

Clinical Note: It is important to remember that prolonged practice of lead-up skills without accompanying practice of the criterion skill can lead to limited motor transfer. Thus the patient is able to perform lead-up skills but cannot demonstrate the required criterion skill. Some patients are unable to make the transfer due to CNS dysfunction (e.g., the patient with severe stroke). These patients may develop *splinter skills,* defined as skills that are not adaptable or easily modified to other skills or to other environments.

Understanding the Individual

The first step in the treatment planning process is an accurate examination of the patient. This includes taking a history, performing systems review, and conducting definitive tests and measures as indicated. Evaluation of the data permits the therapist to identify impairments and activity limitations upon which the POC is based. For example, impairments in muscle strength and motor function, joint flexibility and ROM, sensory and perceptual integrity, cognition and attention, and endurance will all influence the selection of interventions and activities. Some of these impairments will need to be resolved before progressing to advanced skills such as walking. For example, the patient will be unable to practice sit-to-stand activities if hip joint ROM is limited and hip flexion contractures are present. Some impairments can be successfully addressed during activity-based training. For example, hip extensor weakness can be strengthened using bridging activities.

Activity-based training focuses on skills that allow the patient to achieve independence in *basic activities of daily living (BADL),* such as feeding, dressing, hygiene, and *functional mobility* (rolling, supine to sit, sit to stand, walking). In addition, training focuses on helping the individual achieve independence in varying environmental contexts such as home management *(instrumental or IADL),* work (job/school/play), and community and leisure settings. In selecting activities and interventions, the therapist must accurately identify those activities that are meaningful for the patient and that the patient is capable of achieving. Overall goals focus on increasing levels of activity, reducing activity limitations and participation restrictions, and improving quality of life.

The skilled clinician is also able to recognize *environmental risk factors,* defined as the behaviors, attributes, or environmental influences that increase the chances of developing impairments, functional limitations, or disability. The development of an *asset list* is also an important part of the clinical decision-making process. Assets include the patient's strengths, abilities, and positive behaviors or helping strategies that can be reinforced and emphasized during therapy. This gives the therapist an opportunity to provide positive reinforcement and allows the patient to experience success. Improved motivation and adherence are the natural outcomes of reinforcement of patient assets and successes.

Understanding the Environment

Environmental factors influence motor function and functional recovery and include the physical, attitudinal (psychosocial), and social environments in which the patient functions and lives. They can have a positive effect on rehabilitation, enabling successful motor learning and performance. Or they can have a negative effect, limiting motor learning and performance. They can also significantly affect disability and overall quality of life.

Physical Environment

An accurate examination of the patient's ability to perform within the clinic, home, and community environments is essential in developing a POC that successfully restores function and returns the patient to his or her habitual environment. The reader is referred to Chapter 12 in O'Sullivan and Schmitz[5] for a thorough discussion of this topic.

The environment in which individuals normally function is not static, but rather is variable and changing. Training in *complex activities* in which the patient performs in changing and real-world environments is therefore critical to ensuring independent function. Many patients are able to develop skills such as walking in a stable clinic environment but fail miserably when asked to walk outside in the community where they are faced with a changing environment. The therapist assists in this transition by gradually modifying the practice environment to include varying environmental demands. For example, the patient practices walking in a quiet clinic hallway with few interruptions. Progression is to walking in the busy clinic gym or hospital lobby with an increasing level of distractions and then to walking on variable surfaces such as carpets or outside on sidewalks and grass.

The environment in which individuals normally function also includes varying levels of regulatory features. *Anticipation-timing* (time-to-contact) refers to the ability to time movements to a target or an event (e.g., doorway threshold) in the environment, requiring precise control of movements. It is a function of dynamic processing of visual information. Moving through a stationary target—for example, a doorway—is easier than intercepting a moving target. For example, walking through a revolving door or onto a moving walkway requires that the individual match the speed of movements to the speed of the objects in order to safely progress. The term *visual proprioception* refers to the ability to perceive movements and positions of the body in space and in the environment during movement. Thus vision is critical in interpreting environmental cues and adapting our actions.

Box 1.4 provides definitions of terms related to motor function and the environment.

Attitudinal (Psychosocial) Factors

A number of attitudinal (psychosocial) factors can influence an individual's ability to successfully participate in rehabilitation, including motivation, personality factors, emotional state, spirituality, life roles, and educational level. Preexisting psychiatric and psychosocial conditions can have a marked impact on rehabilitation training and outcomes. It is important to remember that psychosocial adaptation to disability and chronic illness is an ongoing and evolving process. At any point in an episode of care, patients can exhibit grief, mourning, anxiety, denial, depression, anger, acknowledgment, or adjustment. Coping style is also an important variable. Patients with effective coping strategies are able to participate in rehabilitation better, seeking the information they need and demonstrating effective problem-solving skills. They are also able to better utilize social supports and are likely to have more positive outcomes. Patients with maladaptive coping skills are likely to fix blame and are less able to participate effectively in rehabilitation. Avoidance and escape along with substance abuse are examples of maladaptive behaviors.

Social Environment

Adequate social support is critical in helping patients achieve favorable outcomes. Spouses, family, and significant others can offer considerable help in the form of emotional support, financial support, and physical assistance. Rehabilitation outcomes and quality of life are dramatically improved in patients who have strong social support over individuals who do not have anyone able to provide assistance. Social isolation is a frequent outcome of lack of social support.

The reader is referred to Chapter 2 in O'Sullivan and Schmitz[5] for a thorough discussion of these topics. The therapist needs to be able to accurately identify and understand the impact of these factors on the patient undergoing rehabilitation in order to plan successful interventions. Empowering patients and their families is key to ensuring successful outcomes. Patients need to be helped to develop goals based on their needs, values, and level of functioning.

The successful plan will optimize patient and family/caregiver involvement. This includes involvement in goal setting, selection of activities, as well as ongoing evaluation of progress. Patients need to be encouraged to solve their own problems as movement challenges are presented. They also need to be challenged to critique their own movements with questions like: *"How did you do that time?"* and *"How can you improve your next attempt?"* Complex training activities can be difficult and frustrating; for example, practicing sit-to-stand transitions challenges control of large segments of the body and balance through activities that decrease BOS and elevate COM. These are skills that not only are important to patients but also were previously performed with little effort or conscious thought. It is important to motivate and support patients. For example, the therapist can begin a training session with those functional skills that the patient can master or almost master, thereby letting the patient experience success. The therapist can then challenge skill development by having the patient practice a number of more difficult task variations. It is equally important to end treatment sessions with a relatively easy task so that the patient leaves the session with a renewed feeling of success and motivation to continue rehabilitation.

BOX 1.4 Terminology: Motor Function and the Environment

Skill movements are shaped to the specific environments in which they occur.

Anticipation-timing (time-to-contact): The ability to time movements to a target or an event (e.g., an obstacle) in the environment, requiring precise control of movements (e.g., running to kick a soccer ball).

Regulatory conditions: Those features of the environment to which movement must be molded in order to be successful (e.g., stepping on a moving walkway or into a revolving door).

- **Closed skills:** Movements performed in a stable or fixed environment (e.g., activities practiced in a quiet room).
- **Open skills:** Movements performed in a changing or variable environment (e.g., activities practiced in a busy gym).

- **Self-paced skills:** Movements that are initiated at will and whose timing is controlled or modified by the individual (e.g., walking).
- **Externally paced skills:** Movements that are initiated and paced by dictates of the external environment (e.g., walking in time with a metronome).

Visual proprioception: Gibson's concept that vision can serve as a strong basis for perception of the movements and positions of the body in space.[3(p469)]

SUMMARY

This chapter has presented an overview of clinical decision-making and the components that must be considered in developing an effective POC. Successful intervention is based on an understanding of motor function and consideration of three basic elements: the task, the individual's performance capabilities, and the environment.

REFERENCES

1. The World Health Organization. International Classification of Functioning, Disability, and Health Resources (ICF). World Health Organization, Geneva, Switzerland, 2002.
2. American Physical Therapy Association. Guide to Physical Therapist Practice, ed 2. Phys Ther 81:1, 2001.
3. Schmidt, R, and Lee, T. Motor Control and Learning—A Behavioral Emphasis, ed 4. Human Kinetics, Champaign, IL, 2005.
4. Shumway-Cook, A, and Woollacott, M. Motor Control—Translating Research into Clinical Practice, ed 3. Lippincott Williams & Wilkins, Philadelphia, 2007.
5. O'Sullivan, SB, and Schmitz, TJ. Physical Rehabilitation, ed 5. FA Davis, Philadelphia, 2007.

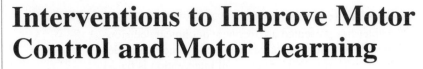

CHAPTER 2

Interventions to Improve Motor Control and Motor Learning

Susan B. O'Sullivan, PT, EdD

areful examination and evaluation of impairments, activity limitations, and participation restrictions enables the therapist to identify movement deficiencies that will be targeted for training. Functional training, defined as an *activity-based, task-oriented intervention,* frequently forms the basis of the physical rehabilitation plan of care (POC). In order to be most effective, task-oriented training should be intensive and shaped to the patient's capabilities as well as integrate active learning strategies using motor learning principles. Some patients with limited motor function who are unable to perform voluntary movements may benefit from augmented training strategies during early recovery. This can take the form of guided, assisted, or facilitated movements. Neuromotor approaches such as *Proprioceptive Neuromuscular Facilitation (PNF)* and *Neuro-Developmental Treatment (NDT)* incorporate a number of these strategies that can serve as a bridge to later active functional movements. Patients with severe impairments and limited recovery potential (e.g., the patient with complete spinal cord injury) benefit from *compensatory training* designed to promote optimal function using altered strategies and intact body segments. The successful therapist understands the full continuum of intervention strategies available to aid patients with movement

deficiencies (Fig. 2.1). Equally important is an understanding of their indications and contraindications.

Task Analysis

Activity-based task analysis is the process of breaking an activity down into its component parts to understand and evaluate the demands of a task. It begins with an understanding of normal movements and normal kinesiology associated with the task. The therapist examines and evaluates the patient's performance and analyzes the differences compared to "typical" or expected performance. Critical skills in this process include: accurate observation, recognition and interpretation of movement deficiencies, determination of how underlying impairments relate to the movements, and determination of how the environment affects the movements observed. The therapist evaluates what needs to be altered and determines how (i.e., what are the blocks or obstacles to moving in the correct pattern and how can they be changed). For example, the patient who is unable to transfer from bed to wheelchair may lack postural trunk support (stability), adequate lower extremity (LE) extensor

NEUROMOTOR/ AUGMENTED TRAINING STRATEGIES	ACTIVITY-BASED, TASK-ORIENTED TRAINING STRATEGIES	MOTOR LEARNING TRAINING STRATEGIES	COMPENSATORY TRAINING STRATEGIES
PNF	Task Training	Feedback: KP, KR, Schedule	Substitution
NDT	Whole Task Practice	Practice: Order, Schedule	Adaptation
Guided Movements	Part-to-Whole Practice	Transfer Training	Assistive/Supportive
Facilitated Movements	Environmental Structure	Environmental Context	Devices
Somatosensory Training	Behavioral Shaping	Problem Solving	

INTERVENTIONS

FIGURE 2.1 Training to improve motor function: intervention approaches and strategies. Abbreviations: KP, Knowledge of Performance; KR, Knowledge of Results; NDT, Neuro-Developmental Treatment; PNF, Proprioceptive Neuromuscular Facilitation.

control (strength), and rotational control of the trunk (controlled mobility). In addition, the patient who is recovering from traumatic brain injury (TBI) may be highly distractible and demonstrate severely limited attention. The busy clinic environment in which the activity is performed renders this patient incapable of listening to instructions or concentrating on the activity. Sociocultural influences must also be considered in gaining understanding of the patient's performance. For example, in some cultures close hands-on assistance may be viewed as a violation of the patient's personal space or inappropriate if the therapist is of the opposite gender.

Categories of activities include *basic activities of daily living* or *BADL* (self-care tasks such as dressing, feeding, and bathing) and *instrumental ADL* or *IADL* (home management tasks such as cooking, cleaning, shopping, and managing a checkbook). *Functional mobility skills (FMS)* are defined as those skills involved in moving by changing body position or location. Examples of FMS include rolling, supine-to-sit, sit-to-stand, transfers, stepping, walking, and running. The term *activity demands* refers to the requirements imbedded in each

step of the activity. The term *environmental demands* refers to the physical characteristics of the environment required for successful performance. Questions posed in Box 2.1 can be used as a guide for qualitative task analysis.

Filming performance is a useful tool to examine patients with marked movement disturbances (e.g., the patient with pronounced ataxia or dyskinesias). Filming allows the therapist to review performance repeatedly without unnecessarily tiring the patient. Filmed motor tasks can also serve as a useful training strategy to aid patients in understanding their movement deficiencies.

Activity-Based, Task-Oriented Intervention

Activity-based, task-oriented intervention is guided by evaluation of functional status and activity level data. The therapist selects activities and modifies task demands to determine an appropriate POC. Extensive practice and appropriate patient feedback are essential to enhance the reacquisition of skills

---

BOX 2.1 Functional Activity Analysis[a]

A. What are the normal requirements of the functional activity being observed?
1. What is the overall movement sequence (motor plan)?
2. What are the initial conditions required? Starting position and initial alignment?
3. How and where is the movement initiated?
4. How is the movement performed?
5. What are the musculoskeletal and biomechanical components required for successful completion of the task? Cognitive and sensory/perceptual components?
6. Is this a *mobility, stability, controlled mobility* or *skill* activity?
7. What are the requirements for timing, force, and direction of movements?
8. What are the requirements for postural control and balance?
9. How is the movement terminated?
10. What are the environmental constraints that must be considered?

B. How successful is the patient's overall movement in terms of outcome?
1. Was the overall movement sequence completed (successful outcome)?
2. What components of the patient's movements are normal? Almost normal?
3. What components of the patient's movements are abnormal?
4. What components of the patient's movements are missing? Delayed?

5. If abnormal, are the movements compensatory and functional or noncompensatory and nonfunctional?
6. What are the underlying impairments that constrain or impair the movements?
7. Do the movement errors increase over time? Is fatigue a constraining factor?
8. Is this a mobility level activity? Are the requirements met?
9. Is this a stability level activity? Are the requirements met?
10. Is this a controlled mobility level activity? Are the requirements met?
11. Is this a skill level activity? Are the requirements met?
12. Are the requirements for postural control and balance met? Is patient safety maintained throughout the activity?
13. What environmental factors constrain or impair the movements?
14. Can the patient adapt to changing environmental demands?
15. What difficulties do you expect this patient will have in other environments?
16. Can the patient effectively analyze his or her own movements and adapt to changing activity or task demands?
17. What difficulties do you expect this patient will have with other functional activities?
18. Are there any sociocultural factors that might influence performance?

---

[a]Adapted from *A Compendium for Teaching Professional Level Neurologic Content,* Neurology Section, American Physical Therapy Association, 2000.

and recovery. For example, training the patient with stroke focuses on use of the more involved extremities during daily tasks, while use of the less involved extremities is minimized (e.g., constraint-induced [CI] movement therapy).[1-4] Initial tasks are selected to ensure patient success and motivation (e.g., grasp and release of a cup, forward reach for upper extremity [UE] dressing).

Using partial body weight support and a motorized treadmill provides a means of early locomotor training for patients with stroke or incomplete spinal cord injury.[5-9] Tasks are continually altered to increase the level of difficulty. Motor learning strategies are utilized, including *behavioral shaping techniques* that use reinforcement and reward to promote skill development. This approach represents a shift away from the traditional neuromotor approaches that utilize an extensive hands-on approach (e.g., guided or facilitated movements). While initial movements can be assisted, active movements are the overall goal in functional training. The therapist's role is one of coach, structuring practice and providing appropriate feedback while encouraging the patient. Box 2.2 presents a summary of task-oriented training strategies to promote function-induced recovery.

Clinical Note: Activity-based, task-oriented training effectively counteracts the effects of immobility and the development of indirect impairments such as

muscle weakness and loss of flexibility. It prevents *learned nonuse* of the more involved segments while stimulating recovery of the central nervous system, or CNS (neuroplasticity).

The selection and use of activities depend on the movement potential, degree of recovery, and severity of motor deficits the patient exhibits. Patients who are not able to participate in task-oriented training include those who lack initial voluntary control or have limited cognitive function. The patient with TBI who is in the early recovery stages has limited potential to participate in training that involves complex activities. Similarly, patients with stroke who experience profound UE paralysis would not be eligible for activity training emphasizing the UE. One of the consistent exclusion criteria for CI therapy has been the inability to perform voluntary wrist and finger extension of the involved hand. Thus *threshold abilities* to perform the basic components of the task need to be identified. The therapist needs to answer the question: What can the patient do or almost do? Careful analysis of underlying impairments with a focus on intervention (e.g., strength, range of motion [ROM]) complements activity-based, task-oriented training. For example, during locomotor training using body weight support (BWS) and a motorized treadmill (TM), stepping and pelvic motions are guided into an efficient motor pattern. Patients need to demonstrate

---

BOX 2.2 Activity/Task-Oriented Intervention Strategies to Promote Function-Induced Recovery[a]

Focus on early activity as soon as possible after injury or insult to utilize specific windows of opportunity, challenge brain functions, and avoid *learned nonuse:* "Use it or lose it."
Consider the individual's past history, health status, age, and experience in designing appropriate, interesting, and stimulating functional activities.
Involve the patient in goal setting and decision-making, thereby enhancing motivation and promoting active commitment to recovery and functional training.
Structure practice utilizing activity-based, task-oriented interventions.
- Select tasks important for independent function; include tasks that are important to the patient.
- Identify the patient's abilities/strengths and level of recovery/learning; choose tasks that have potential for patient success.
- Target active movements involving affected body segments; constrain or limit use of less involved segments.
- Avoid activities that are too difficult and result in compensatory strategies or abnormal, stereotypical movements.
- Provide adequate repetition and extensive practice as appropriate.
- Assist (guide) the patient to successfully carry out initial movements as needed; reduce assistance in favor of active movements as quickly as possible.

- Provide explicit verbal feedback to improve movement accuracy and learning and correct errors; promote the patient's own error detection and correction abilities.
- Provide verbal rewards for small improvements in task performance to maintain motivation.
- Provide modeling (demonstrations) of ideal task performance as needed.
- Increase the level of difficulty over time.
- Promote practice of task variations to promote adaptation of skills.
- Maximize practice: include both supervised and unsupervised practice; use an activity log to document practice outside of scheduled therapy sessions.
Structure context-specific practice.
- Promote initial practice in a supportive environment, free of distracters to enhance attention and concentration.
- Progress to variable practice in real-world environments.
Maintain focus on therapist's role as *coach* while minimizing hands-on therapy.
Continue to monitor recovery closely and document progress using valid and reliable functional outcome measures.
Be cautious about timetables and predictions, as recovery and successful outcomes may take longer than expected.

[a]Adapted from O'Sullivan and Schmitz.[10]

essential prerequisites of basic head and trunk stability during upright positioning to be considered appropriate candidates for this type of training.

The therapist also needs to consider the postures in which training occurs. As postures progress in difficulty by elevating the center of mass (COM) and decreasing the base of support (BOS), more and more body segments must becoordinated (presenting a *degrees of freedom problem*). Patients are likely to demonstrate increasing problems in synergistic control, posture, and balance. Thus the patient with TBI and significant movement deficiencies (e.g., pronounced ataxia) may need to begin activity training in more stable postures such as quadruped or modified plantigrade. With recovery,

progression in training is then to more upright postures such as sitting and standing. Box 2.3 identifies the potential treatment benefits of different postures and activities.

Impairments

Identifying and correcting impairments (e.g., limited range of motion, decreased strength) are essential elements in improving functional performance. The therapist must accurately identify those impairments that are linked to deficits in functional performance. An inability to stand up or climb stairs may be linked to weakness of hip and knee extensors. A strengthening program that addresses these impairments can be

---

BOX 2.3 Postures: Primary Focus, Potential Treatment Benefits, and Activities[a]

Posture/Description	Primary Focus/Benefits/Activities
Prone on elbows Prone, weightbearing on elbows Stable posture Wide BOS Low COM	• Focus on improving upper trunk, UE, and neck/head control • Improve ROM in hip extension • Improve shoulder stabilizers • Lead-up for I bed mobility, quadruped activities, floor-to-stand transfers • Activities in posture: holding, weight shifting, UE reaching, assumption of posture • Modified prone on elbows can also be achieved in sitting and plantigrade (modified standing) positions
Quadruped All fours position (hands and knees) Weightbearing at knees, through extended elbows and hands Stable posture Wide BOS Low COM	• Focus on improving trunk, LE, UE, and neck/head control • Improve trunk, hip, shoulder, and elbow stabilizers • Decrease extensor tone at knees by prolonged weightbearing • Decrease flexor tone at elbows, wrists, and hands by prolonged weightbearing • Promote extensor ROM at elbows, wrists, and fingers • Lead up for I plantigrade activities, floor-to-standing transfers, antigravity balance control • Activities in posture: holding, weight shifting, UE reaching, LE lifts, assumption of posture, locomotion on all fours
Bridging Weightbearing at feet and ankles, upper trunk Stable posture Wide BOS Low COM	• Focus on improving lower trunk and LE control • Improve hip and ankle stabilizers • Weightbearing at feet and ankles • Lead-up for bed mobility, sit-to-stand transfers, standing, and stair climbing • Activities in posture: holding, weight shifting, assumption of posture, LE lifts
Sitting Weightbearing through trunk and at buttocks, feet Can include weightbearing through extended elbows and on hands Intermediate BOS Intermediate height COM	• Focus on improving upper trunk, lower trunk, LE, and head/neck control • Important for upright balance control • Lead-up for UE ADL skills; wheelchair locomotion • Activities in posture: holding, weight shifting, UE reaching, assumption of posture

(box continues on page 16)

BOX 2.3 Postures: Primary Focus, Potential Treatment Benefits, and Activities^a (continued)

Posture/Description	Primary Focus/Benefits/Activities
Kneeling and half-kneeling Weightbearing at knees and through hips, trunk Weightbearing through forward ankle in half-kneeling Upright, antigravity position Intermediate height of COM Narrow BOS, kneeling Wide BOS, half-kneeling	• Focus on improving head/neck, upper trunk, lower trunk, and LE control • Weightbearing through hips and at knees; upright, antigravity position • Decrease extensor tone at knees by prolonged weightbearing • Improve hip and trunk stabilizers • Weightbearing through ankle in half-kneeling • Lead-up for upright balance control, standing and stepping, floor-to-standing transfers • Activities in posture: holding, weight shifting, UE reaching, assumption of posture, knee walking
Modified plantigrade Standing with weightbearing on hands through extended elbows (on support surface) and through trunk, LEs Modified upright antigravity position Stable posture Wide BOS High COM	• Focus on improving head/neck, trunk, and UE/LE control in supported, modified upright posture • Decrease tone in elbow, wrist, and finger flexors by prolonged weightbearing • Increase extensor ROM at elbows, wrists, and fingers • Hips flexed, COM forward of weight bearing line creating an extension moment at the knee • Increased safety for early standing (four-limb posture) • Lead-up for upright balance control, standing and stepping; standing UE ADL tasks • Activities in posture: holding, weight shifting, UE reaching, LE stepping, assumption of posture
Standing Weightbearing through trunk and LEs Full upright, antigravity position Narrow BOS High COM	• Focus on improving head/neck, trunk, and LE control in fully upright posture • Hips and knees fully extended • Lead-up for upright balance control, stepping, locomotion, stair climbing; standing UE ADL skills • Activities in posture: holding, weight shifting, UE reaching, LE stepping, assumption of posture

Abbreviations: ADL, activities of daily living; BOS, base of support; COM, center of mass; I, independent; LE, lower extremity; UE, upper extremity; ROM, range of motion.

^aAdapted from O'Sullivan and Schmitz.[10]

expected to improve function. Interventions can include traditional muscle-strengthening techniques (e.g., progressive resistance training utilizing weights and open-chain exercises). Task-specific, functional training activities can also be utilized. For example, the patient who is unable to stand up independently can practice sit-to-stand training first from a high seat; as control improves, the seat is gradually lowered to standard height. The patient with difficulty in stair climbing can first practice step-ups using a low, 4-inch step; as control improves, the height of the step can be increased to standard height. The activity modification reduces the overall range in which muscles must perform, making it possible for the patient to successfully complete the activity. These examples illustrate an important training principle—that is, *specificity of training*. The physiological adaptations to exercise training are highly specific to the type of training utilized. Transfer effects to improved function in sit-to-stand or stair climbing can be expected to be greater when the muscle performance and neuromuscular adaptation requirements during the functional training tasks closely approximate the desired skill.

Guided Movement

During initial training, the therapist may provide manual assistance during *early* movement attempts. This can take the form of passive movements quickly progressing to active-assistive movements. Guidance (hands-on assistance) is used to help the learner gain an initial understanding of task requirements. During early assisted practice, the therapist can substitute for the missing elements, stabilize posture or parts of a limb, constrain unwanted movements, and guide the patient toward correct movements. For example, constraining or holding the patient to ensure an upright sitting posture and shoulder stabilization in a position of function (70 degrees of shoulder flexion) allows the patient to focus on and control early hand-to-mouth movements. This reduces the number of body segments the patient must effectively control, thereby reducing the degrees of freedom. Guided movement also allows the learner to experience the tactile and kinesthetic inputs inherent in the movements—that is, to learn the *sensation of movement.* The supportive use of hands can allay fears and instill confidence while ensuring safety. For example, the patient recovering from stroke with impaired sensation and perception can be manually guided through early weight shifts and sit-to-stand transfers. The therapist must anticipate the patient's needs and how best to provide assistance. As the need for manual guidance decreases, the patient assumes active control of movements. The overall goal of training is active movement control and trial-and-error discovery learning.

Verbal Instructions and Cueing

Verbal instructions prepare the patient for correct movement and assist the patient in learning "what to do." The therapist needs to help the patient focus on critical task elements in order to maximize early movement success. Timing cues assist the patient in premovement preparatory adjustments that focus on learning "when to move." For example, during sit-to-stand transfers the therapist instructs the patient: *"On three, I want you to shift your weight forward over your feet and stand up. One, two, three."* Verbal cueing during practice is used to provide feedback and assist the patient in modifying and correcting movements. Normally the cerebellum drives motor learning and adaptation through the use of intrinsic sensory feedback information (somatosensory, visual, and vestibular inputs). In the absence of intrinsic feedback or with an inability to correctly use intrinsic feedback, verbal cues (augmented feedback) may be necessary. The therapist needs to select critical cues and refocus the patient on recognizing intrinsic error signals associated with movement or coming from the environment. Once the movement is completed, the patient should be asked to evaluate performance *("How did you do?")* and then to recommend corrections *("What do you need to do differently next time to ensure success?").* This helps to keep the focus on active movement control and trial-and-error discovery learning. Box 2.4 poses relevant questions for the therapist to consider for anticipating patient needs.

Clinical Note: The key to success in using guided movements is to promote active practice as soon as possible, providing only as much assistance as needed and removing assistance as soon as possible. As manual guidance is reduced, verbal cueing can substitute. Guidance is most effective for slow postural responses (positioning tasks) and less effective during rapid or ballistic tasks.

BOX 2.4 Guided Movements: Questions to Consider for Anticipating Patient Needs[a]

- What are the critical elements of the task necessary for movement success?
- How can I help the patient focus on these critical elements?
- How much assistance is needed to ensure successful performance?
- When are the demands for my assistance the greatest? The least?
- How should I position my body to assist the patient effectively during the movement without interfering with the movement?
- When and how can I reduce the level of my assistance?
- What verbal cues are needed to ensure successful performance?
- When and how can I reduce the level of my verbal cues?
- At what point is the patient ready to assume active control of the movement?
- How can I foster independent practice and critical decision-making skills that allow for adaptability of skills?

[a]Adapted from O'Sullivan and Schmitz.[1]

Red Flag: Overuse of manually guided movements or verbal cueing is likely to result in dependence on the therapist for assistance, thus becoming a "crutch." It is important not to persist in excessive levels of assistance long after the patient needs such support. This may result in the patient becoming overly dependent on the therapist (the *"my therapist syndrome"*). In this situation, the patient responds to the efforts of assistance from someone new with comments such as, *"You're not doing it correctly, my therapist does it this way."* This is strong evidence of an overdependence on the original therapist and the assistance being given.

Parts-to-Whole Practice

Some complex motor skills can be effectively broken down into component parts for practice. Practice of the component parts is followed closely by practice of the integrated whole task. For example, during initial wheelchair transfer training, the transfer steps are practiced (e.g., locking the brakes, lifting the foot pedals, moving forward in the chair, standing up, pivoting, and sitting down). During the same therapy session, the transfer is also practiced as a whole. Delaying practice of the integrated whole can interfere with learning of the whole task.

Clinical Note: Parts-to-whole practice is most effective with discrete or serial motor tasks that have highly independent parts (e.g., transfers). Parts-to-whole practice is less effective for continuous movement tasks (e.g., walking) and for complex tasks with highly integrated parts (e.g., fine motor hand skills). Both require a high degree of coordination with spatial and temporal sequencing of elements. For these tasks, emphasis on the practice of the integrated whole is desirable.

Motor Learning Strategies

Motor learning is defined as "a set of internal processes associated with practice or experience leading to relatively permanent changes in the capability for skilled behavior."[11(p466)] Learning a motor skill is a complex process that requires spatial, temporal, and hierarchical organization of the CNS. Changes in the CNS are not directly observable but rather are inferred from changes in motor behavior.

Measures of Motor Learning

Performance changes result from practice or experience and are a frequently used measure of learning. For example, with practice an individual is able to develop appropriate sequencing of movement components with improved timing and reduced effort and concentration. Performance, however, is not always an accurate reflection of learning. It is possible to practice enough to temporarily improve performance but not retain the learning. Conversely, factors such as fatigue, anxiety, poor motivation, and medications may cause performance to deteriorate, although learning may still occur. Because performance can be affected by a number of factors, it may reflect a temporary change in motor behavior seen during practice sessions. *Retention* is an important measure of learning. It is the ability of the learner to demonstrate the skill over time and after a period of no practice *(retention interval)*. A *retention test* looks at performance after a retention interval and compares it to the performance observed during the original learning trial. Performance can be expected to decrease slightly, but it should return to original levels after relatively few practice trials (termed *warm-up decrement*). For example, riding a bike is a well-learned skill that is generally retained even though an individual may not have ridden for years. The ability to apply a learned skill to the learning of other similar tasks is termed *adaptability* or *generalizability* and is another important measure of learning. A *transfer test* looks at the ability of the individual to perform variations of the original skill (e.g., performing step-ups to climbing stairs and curbs). The time and effort required to organize and perform these new skill variations efficiently are reduced if learning the original skill was adequate. Finally, *resistance to contextual change* is another measure of learning. This is the adaptability required to perform a motor task in altered environmental situations. Thus, an individual who has learned a skill (e.g., walking with a cane on indoor level surfaces) should be able to apply that learning to new and variable situations (e.g., walking outdoors or walking on a busy sidewalk). Box 2.5 defines measures of motor learning.[11]

Stages of Motor Learning

The process of motor learning has been described by Fitts and Posner[12] as occurring in relatively distinct stages, termed *cognitive, associative,* and *autonomous.* These stages provide

---

BOX 2.5 Measures of Motor Learning

- **Performance test:** An examination of observable improvements with attention to the quality of movements and the success of movement outcomes after a period of skill practice.
- **Retention:** The ability of the learner to demonstrate a learned skill over time and after a period of no practice (termed a *retention interval*).
- **Retention test:** An examination of a learned skill administered after a period of no practice (*retention interval*).
- **Generalizability (adaptability of skills):** The ability to apply a learned skill to the performance of other similar or related skills.
- **Resistance to contextual change (adaptability of context):** The ability to perform a learned skill in altered environmental situations.
- **Transfer test:** An examination of performance of similar or related skills compared to a previously learned skill.

---

a useful framework for describing the learning process and for organizing intervention strategies.

Cognitive Stage

During the initial *cognitive stage* of learning, the major task is to develop an overall understanding of the skill, called the *cognitive map* or cognitive plan. This decision-making phase of "what to do" requires a high level of cognitive processing as the learner performs successive approximations of the task, discarding strategies that are not successful and retaining those that are. The resulting *trial-and-error practice* initially yields uneven performance with frequent errors. Processing of sensory cues and perceptual-motor organization eventually leads to the selection of a motor strategy that proves reasonably successful. Because the learner progresses from an initially disorganized and often clumsy pattern to more organized movements, improvements in performance can be readily observed during this acquisition phase. The learner relies heavily on vision to guide early learning and movement.

Strategies to Enhance Learning

The overall goal during the early cognitive stage of learning is to facilitate task understanding and organize early practice. The learner's knowledge of the skill and its critical task elements must be ascertained. The therapist should highlight the purpose of the skill in a functionally relevant context. The task should seem important, desirable, and realistic to learn. The therapist should demonstrate the task exactly as it should be done (i.e., coordinated action with smooth timing and ideal performance speed). This helps the learner develop an internal cognitive map or *reference of correctness*. Attention should be directed to the desired outcome and critical task elements. The therapist should point out similarities to other learned tasks so that subroutines that are part of other motor programs can be retrieved from memory.

Highly skilled individuals who have been successfully discharged from rehabilitation can be *expert models* for demonstration. Their success in functioning in the "real world" will also have a positive effect in motivating patients new to rehabilitation. For example, it is very difficult for a therapist with full use of muscles to accurately demonstrate appropriate transfer skills to an individual with C6 complete tetraplegia (American Spinal Injury Association [ASIA] Impairment Scale designation of A). A former patient with a similar level of injury can accurately demonstrate how the skill should be performed. Demonstration has also been shown to be effective in producing learning even with unskilled patient models. In this situation the learner/patient benefits from the cognitive processing and problem-solving as he or she watches the unskilled model and evaluates the performance, identifying errors, and generating corrections. Demonstrations can also be filmed. Developing a visual library of demonstrations of skilled former patients is a useful strategy to ensure the availability of effective models. The learner's initial performance trials can also be recorded for later viewing and analysis.

During initial practice, the therapist should give clear and concise verbal instructions and not overload the learner with excessive or wordy instructions. The overall goal is to prepare the patient for movement and reduce uncertainty. It is important to reinforce correct performance with appropriate feedback and intervene when movement errors become consistent or when safety is an issue. The therapist should *not* attempt to correct all the numerous errors that characterize this stage but rather allow for trial-and-error learning during practice. Feedback, particularly visual feedback, is important during early learning. Thus the learner should be directed to "look at the movement" closely. Practice should allow for adequate rest periods and focus on repeated practice of the skill in an environment conducive to learning. This is generally one that is free of distractions (closed environment) because the cognitive demands are high during this phase of learning.

Associative Stage

During the middle or *associative stage* of learning, motor strategies are refined through continued practice. Spatial and temporal aspects become organized as the movement develops into a coordinated pattern. As performance improves, there is greater consistency and fewer errors and extraneous movements. The learner is now concentrating on "how to do" the movement rather than on "what to do." Proprioceptive cues become increasingly important, while dependence on visual cues decreases. Thus the learner learns to experience the correct "feel of the movement." Learning takes varying lengths of time depending on a number of factors, such as the nature of the task, prior experience and motivation of the learner, available feedback, and organization of practice.

Strategies to Enhance Learning

During this middle stage of learning, the therapist continues to provide feedback, intervening as movement errors become consistent. The learner is directed toward an appreciation of proprioceptive inputs associated with the movement (e.g., *"How did that feel?"*). The learner is encouraged to

self-assess motor performance and recognize intrinsically (naturally) occurring feedback during the movement. Practice should be varied, encouraging practice of variations of the skill and gradually varying the environment. For example, the learner practices bed-to-wheelchair transfers, wheelchair-to-mat transfers, wheelchair-to-toilet transfers, and finally wheelchair-to-car transfers. The therapist reduces hands-on assistance, which is generally counterproductive by this stage. The focus should be on the learner's active control and active decision-making in modifying skills in this stage of learning.

Autonomous Stage

The final or *autonomous stage* of learning is characterized by motor performance that, after considerable practice, is largely automatic. There is only a minimal level of cognitive monitoring, with motor programs so refined they can almost "run themselves." The spatial and temporal components of movement are becoming highly organized, and the learner is capable of coordinated movement patterns. The learner is now free to concentrate on other aspects of performance, such as "how to succeed" in difficult environments or at competitive sports. Movements are largely error-free with little interference from environmental distractions. Thus the learner can perform equally well in a stable, predictable environment and in a changing, unpredictable environment. Many patients undergoing active rehabilitation are discharged before achieving this final stage of learning. For these patients, refinement of skills comes only after continued practice in home and community environments. The patient with TBI and significant cognitive impairment may never achieve this level of independent function, continuing to need structure and assistance for the rest of his or her life.

Strategies to Enhance Learning

Training strategies begun during associative learning are continued in this final phase. The therapist continues to promote practice. By this stage, movements should be largely automatic. The therapist can provide distractions to challenge the learner. If the learner is successful at this stage, the distractions will do little to deteriorate the movements. The therapist can also incorporate *dual-task training,* in which the learner is required to perform two separate tasks at one time. For example, the patient is required to walk and carry on a conversation (*Walkie-Talkie test*) or to walk while carrying a tray with a glass of water on it. The learner should be equally successful at both tasks performed simultaneously. Only occasional feedback is needed from the therapist, focusing on key errors. Massed practice (rest time is much less than practice time) can be used while promoting varying task demands in environments that promote open skills. The learner should be confident and accomplished in decision-making from repeated challenges to movement skills that have been posed by the therapist. The outcome of this stage of learning is successful preparation to meet the multitask challenges of home, community, and work/play environments. Table 2.1 presents a summary of the stages of motor learning and training strategies.

Feedback

Feedback is a critical factor in promoting motor learning. Feedback can be *intrinsic,* occurring as a natural result of the movement, or *extrinsic,* sensory cueing not normally received during the movement task. Proprioceptive, visual, vestibular, and cutaneous signals are types of intrinsic feedback, while visual, auditory, and tactile cueing are forms of extrinsic feedback (e.g., verbal cues, tactile cues, manual contacts, and biofeedback devices). During therapy, both intrinsic and extrinsic feedback is manipulated to enhance motor learning. *Concurrent feedback* is given during task performance, and *terminal feedback* is given at the end of task performance. Augmented feedback about the end result or overall outcome of the movement is termed *knowledge of results (KR).* Augmented feedback about the nature or quality of the movement pattern produced is termed *knowledge of performance (KP).* The relative importance of KP and KR varies according to the skill being learned and the availability of feedback from intrinsic sources. For example, tracking tasks (e.g., trace a star task) are highly dependent on intrinsic visual and kinesthetic feedback (KP), while KR has less influence on the accuracy of the movements. KR provides key information about how to shape the overall movements for the next attempt. Performance cues (KP) that focus on task elements and error identification are not useful without KR.

Questions that guide and inform clinical decisions about feedback include:

- What type of feedback should be employed *(mode)*?
- How much feedback should be used *(intensity)*?
- When should feedback be given *(scheduling)*?

Choices about the type of feedback involve the selection of which intrinsic sensory systems to highlight, what type of augmented feedback to use, and how to pair extrinsic feedback with intrinsic feedback. The selection of sensory systems depends on specific examination findings of sensory integrity. The sensory systems selected must provide accurate and usable information. If an intrinsic sensory system is impaired and provides distorted or incomplete information (e.g., impaired proprioception with diabetic neuropathy), then the use of alternative sensory systems (e.g., vision) should be emphasized. Supplemental augmented feedback can also be used to enhance learning. Decisions are also based on the stage of learning. Early in learning, visual feedback is easily brought to conscious attention and is important. Less consciously accessible sensory information such as proprioception becomes more useful during the middle and final stages of learning.

Decisions about frequency and scheduling of feedback (when and how much) must be reached. Constant feedback (e.g., given after every trial) quickly guides the learner to the correct performance but slows retention. Conversely, feedback that is varied (not given after every trial) slows the initial acquisition of performance skills but improves retention. This is most likely due to the increased depth of cognitive processing that accompanies the variable presentation of feedback. Feedback schedules are presented in Box 2.6.

BOX 2.6 Feedback Schedules to Enhance Motor Learning

- **Constant feedback:** Feedback is given after every practice trial.
- **Summed feedback:** Feedback is given after a set number of trials; for example, feedback is given after every other practice trial or every third trial.
- **Faded feedback:** Feedback is given at first after every trial and then less frequently; for example, feedback is given after every second trial, progressing to every fifth trial.
- **Bandwidth feedback:** Feedback is given only when performance is outside a given error range; for example, feedback is given if performance (gait) is too slow or too fast but not if it falls within a predetermined range.
- **Delayed feedback:** Feedback is given after a brief time delay; for example, feedback is given after a 3-second delay.

It is important to provide the learner with the opportunity and time for introspection and self-assessment. If the therapist bombards the patient with augmented feedback during or immediately after task completion, this will likely prove excessive and preclude active information processing by the learner. The patient's own decision-making skills are minimized, while the therapist's verbal feedback dominates. This may well explain why the patient who is undergoing training may show minimal carryover and limited retention of newly acquired motor skills. The withdrawal of augmented feedback should be gradual and carefully paired with the patient's efforts to correctly utilize intrinsic feedback systems.

Feedback in the form of positive reinforcement and rewards is an important motivational tool to shape behavior. Helping the patient recognize and attend to successes in training goes a long way toward reducing anxiety and depression. The institutional environment and the nature of the disability contribute to feelings of *learned helplessness.* Therapists play a major role in counteracting these feelings and ensuring that the patient is motivated to succeed. This includes making sure that the patient is an active participant in all phases of the treatment planning process, including goal setting. For task-related training to succeed, it must have meaning and relevance for the patient.

Practice

A second major factor that influences motor learning is *practice.* In general, the more practice that is built into the training schedule, the greater the learning. For example, the patient who practices daily in both supervised (clinic) and unsupervised settings (home or hospital unit) will demonstrate increased learning over the patient who is seen once a week in an outpatient clinic without the benefit of any additional practice incorporated into the hospital stay or home exercise program (HEP). The therapist's role is to ensure that the patient practices the correct movements. Practice of incorrect movement patterns can lead to *negative learning,* in which faulty habits and postures must be unlearned before the correct movements can be mastered. This sometimes occurs when a patient goes home for an extended period before participating in active rehabilitation. The organization of practice depends on several factors, including the patient's motivation, attention span, concentration, endurance, and the type of task. Additional factors include the frequency of allowable therapy sessions, which is often dependent on hospital scheduling, and the availability of services and payment (socioeconomic factors). For outpatients, practice at home is highly dependent on motivation, family support, and suitable environment as well as a well-constructed HEP.

Questions that guide and inform clinical decisions about practice include:

- How should practice periods and rest periods be spaced *(distribution of practice)*?
- What tasks and task variations should be practiced *(variability of practice)*?
- How should the tasks be sequenced *(practice order)*?
- How should the environment be structured *(closed vs. open)*?

Massed practice refers to a sequence of practice and rest intervals in which the rest time is *much less* than the practice time. Fatigue, decreased performance, and risk of injury are factors that must be considered when using massed practice. *Distributed practice* refers to spaced practice intervals in which the practice time is *equal to or less* than the rest time. Although learning occurs with both, distributed practice results in the most learning per training time, although the total training time is increased. It is the preferred mode for many patients undergoing active rehabilitation who demonstrate limited performance capabilities and endurance. With adequate rest periods, performance can be improved without the interfering effects of fatigue or increasing safety issues. Distributed practice is also beneficial if motivation is low or if the learner has a short attention span, poor concentration, or motor planning deficits (e.g., the patient with dyspraxia). Distributed practice should also be considered if the task itself is complex, is long, or has a high energy cost. Massed practice can be considered when motivation and skill levels are high and when the patient has adequate endurance, attention, and concentration. For example, the patient with spinal cord injury (SCI) in the final stages of rehabilitation may spend long practice sessions acquiring the wheelchair skills needed for independent community mobility.

Blocked practice refers to a practice sequence organized around one task *performed repeatedly*, uninterrupted by the practice of any other task. *Random practice* refers to a practice sequence in which a variety of tasks are *ordered randomly* across trials. While both allow for motor skill acquisition, random practice has been shown to have superior long-term retention effects. For example, a variety of different transfers (e.g., bed-to-wheelchair, wheelchair-to-toilet, wheelchair-to-tub seat) can be practiced, all within the same therapy session. Although skilled performance of individual tasks may be initially delayed, improved

retention of transfer skills can be expected. The constant challenge of varying the task demands provides high *contextual interference* and increases the depth of cognitive processing through retrieval practice from memory stores. The acquired skills can then be applied more easily to other task variations or environments (promoting *adaptability*). Blocked practice will result in superior initial performance due to low contextual interference and may be required in certain situations (e.g., the patient with TBI who requires a high degree of structure and consistency for learning).

Practice order refers to the sequence in which tasks are practiced. *Blocked order* is the repeated practice of a single task or group of tasks in order with a specified number of trials (three trials of task 1, three trials of task 2, three trials of task 3: 111222333). *Serial order* is a predictable and repeating order (practicing multiple tasks in the following order: 123123123). *Random order* is a nonrepeating and nonpredictable practice order (123321312). Although skill acquisition can be achieved with all three orders, differences have been found. Blocked order produces improved early acquisition and performance of skills, while serial and random orders produce better retention and adaptability of skills. This is again due to contextual interference and increased depth of cognitive processing. The key element here is the degree to which the learner is actively involved in memory retrieval. For example, a treatment session can be organized to include practice of a number of different tasks (e.g., forward-, backward-, and side-stepping, and stair climbing). Random ordering of the tasks may initially delay acquisition of the desired stepping movements but over the long-term will result in improved retention and adaptability of skills.

Mental practice is a practice strategy in which performance of the motor task is imagined or visualized without overt physical practice. Beneficial effects result from the cognitive rehearsal of task elements. It is theorized that underlying motor programs for movement are activated but with subthreshold motor activity. Mental practice has been found to promote the acquisition of motor skills. It should be considered for patients who fatigue easily and are unable to sustain physical practice. Mental practice is also effective in alleviating anxiety associated with initial practice by previewing the upcoming movement experience. Patients who combine mental practice with physical practice can increase the accuracy and efficiency of movements at significantly faster rates than subjects who used physical practice alone. Box 2.7 defines practice schedules that can be used to enhance motor learning.

Clinical Note: When using mental practice, the therapist must ensure that the patient understands the task and is actively rehearsing the correct movements. This can be assured by having the patient verbalize aloud the steps he or she is rehearsing.

Red Flag: Mental practice is generally contraindicated in patients with cognitive, communication, and/or perceptual deficits. These patients typically have difficulty understanding the idea of the task.

BOX 2.7 Practice Schedules Used to Enhance Motor Learning[a]

- **Massed practice:** A sequence of practice and rest times in which the rest time is much less than the practice time; for example, practice is for 1 hour with a 10-minute rest.
- **Distributed practice:** A sequence of practice and rest periods in which the practice time is often equal to or less than the rest time; for example, practice is for 10 minutes with a 10-minute rest.
- **Blocked practice:** A practice sequence organized around one task performed repeatedly, uninterrupted by practice on any other task; low contextual interference. For example, three trials of task 1 are practiced (111); other tasks practiced that session are also blocked: three trials of task 2 (222), three trials of task 3 (333), and so on.
- **Serial practice:** A predictable and repeating order of practice of multiple tasks; for example, three tasks are practiced in repeating order: 123123123.
- **Random practice:** A practice sequence in which the tasks being practiced are ordered (quasi-) randomly across trials; high contextual interference. For example, three tasks are practiced in random order: 123321312.
- **Mental practice:** A practice method in which performance of the motor task is imagined or visualized without overt physical practice. For example, an individual cognitively rehearses the steps of a stair climbing sequence using an assistive device before physically practicing the skill (the sound LE leads up and the cane and affected LE follow).

[a]From Schmidt, pp. 562–566.[11]

Unsupervised Practice

Regularly scheduled therapy time typically does not provide the substantial amount of practice time required for skill learning. The hours the patient spends outside of therapy either on the hospital unit or at home are generally times of limited activity. The therapist needs to engage the patient and family to use this time efficiently for meaningful practice. Patient and family training in the activities to be performed on the unit or at home (HEP) is essential. Instructions should be clear, concise, and in writing. Activities should be first demonstrated and practiced in a supervised setting. The patient should be instructed to document unsupervised practice using an *activity log* in which the patient records the activity practiced, the duration (number of repetitions) of practice, and comments as needed (e.g., level of pain, dizziness, or discomfort). The therapist should evaluate activity log recordings on a regular basis. The environment should be chosen or organized to ensure success in unsupervised practice. Patient safety and adequate rest periods are critical elements. For example, standing balance exercises are often performed in the home at the kitchen counter because of safety issues—hence the name "kitchen sink exercises."

Transfer of Learning

Transfer of learning refers to the gain (or loss) in the capability of task performance as a result of practice or experience on some other task.[1] Learning can be promoted through practice using contralateral extremities, termed *bilateral transfer.* For example, the patient with stroke first practices the desired movement pattern using the less affected extremity. This initial practice enhances the formation or recall of the necessary motor program, which can then be applied to the opposite, more involved extremity. This method cannot, however, substitute for lack of movement potential of the affected extremities (e.g., a flaccid limb on the hemiplegic side). Transfer effects are optimal when the tasks (e.g., components and actions) and environments are similar. For example, optimal transfer can be expected with practice of an UE flexion pattern first on one side and then with an identical pattern on the other side. Practice of dissimilar activities can lead to negative transfer or loss in the capability to perform the criterion task.

Lead-up activities (subskills) are commonly used in physical therapy. Lead-up activities are simpler task versions or component parts of a larger, more complex task. Lead-up activities are practiced typically in easier postures with significantly reduced postural demands and degrees of freedom. Anxiety is also reduced and safety is ensured. For example, initial upright postural control of the trunk and hips can be practiced in kneeling, half-kneeling, and plantigrade before standing. The patient develops the required hip extension/abduction stabilization control required for upright stance but without the demands of the standing position or fear of falling. The more closely the lead-up activities resemble the requirements of the final task, the better the transfer to the criterion task.

Structuring the Environment

Environmental context is an important consideration in structuring practice sessions. Early learning benefits from practice in a stable or predictable *closed environment.* As learning progresses, the environment should be varied to incorporate more variable features consistent with real-world, *open environments.* Practicing walking only inside the physical therapy clinic might lead to successful performance in that setting *(context-specific learning)* but does little to prepare the patient for ambulation at home or in the community. The therapist should begin to gradually modify the environment as soon as performance begins to become consistent. It is important to remember that some patients (e.g., the patient with severe TBI and limited recovery) may never be able to function in anything but a highly structured environment.

The social benefits of working in an enriched or group environment should not be underestimated. Patients admitted for rehabilitation often have difficulty working in unfamiliar and unstimulating environments. Depression and lack of motivation are the natural outcomes. Therapists should encourage patients to socially interact with others and promote participation in group classes whenever possible. An active, engaged patient is also a motivated one.

TABLE 2.1 Characteristics of Stages of Motor Learning and Training Strategies^a

Cognitive Stage Characteristics	Training Strategies
The learner develops an understanding of task, *cognitive mapping:* assesses abilities, task demands; identifies stimuli, contacts memory; selects response; performs initial approximations of task; structures motor program; modifies initial responses *"What to do"* decision	Highlight purpose of task in functionally relevant terms. Demonstrate ideal performance of task to establish a *reference of correctness*. Have patient verbalize task components and requirements. Point out similarities to other learned tasks. Direct attention to critical task elements. Select appropriate feedback. **Emphasize intact sensory systems, intrinsic feedback systems.** • Carefully pair extrinsic feedback with intrinsic feedback. • High dependence on vision: have patient watch movement. • Provide *Knowledge of Performance (KP):* focus on errors as they become consistent; do not cue on large number of random errors. • Provide *Knowledge of Results (KR):* focus on success of movement outcome. Ask learner to evaluate performance, outcomes; identify problems, solutions. Use reinforcements (praise) for correct performance and continuing motivation. **Organize feedback schedule.** • Feedback after every trial improves performance during early learning. • *Variable feedback* (summed, fading, bandwidth) increases depth of cognitive processing, improves retention; may decrease performance initially. **Organize practice.** • Stress controlled movement to minimize errors. • Provide adequate rest periods using *distributed practice* if task is complex, long, or energy costly or if learner fatigues easily, has short attention, or has poor concentration. • Use manual guidance to assist as appropriate. • Break complex tasks down into component parts; teach both parts and integrated whole. • Utilize *bilateral transfer* as appropriate. • Use *blocked practice* of same task to improve performance. • Use *variable practice* (serial or random practice order) of related skills to increase depth of cognitive processing and retention; may decrease performance initially. • Use *mental practice* to improve performance and learning; reduce anxiety. **Assess and modify arousal levels as appropriate.** • High or low arousal impairs performance and learning. • Avoid stressors, mental fatigue. **Structure environment.** • Reduce extraneous environmental stimuli and distracters to ensure attention, concentration. • Emphasize closed skills initially, gradually progressing to open skills.
Associated Stage Characteristics	**Training Strategies**
The learner practices movements, refines motor program, spatial and temporal organization; decreases errors, extraneous movements	**Select appropriate feedback.** • Continue to provide KP; intervene when errors become consistent. • Emphasize proprioceptive feedback, "feel of movement" to assist in establishing an internal reference of correctness. • Continue to provide KR; stress relevance of functional outcomes. • Assist learner to improve self-evaluation and decision-making skills. • Facilitation techniques; guided movements are counterproductive during this stage of learning.

(table continues on page 24)

TABLE 2.1 Characteristics of Stages of Motor Learning and Training Strategies[a] *(continued)*

Associated Stage Characteristics	Training Strategies
Dependence on visual feedback decreases, increases for use of proprioceptive feedback; cognitive monitoring decreases ***"How to do"*** decision	**Organize feedback schedule.** • Continue to provide feedback for continuing motivation; encourage patient to self-assess achievements. • Avoid excessive augmented feedback. • Focus on use of variable feedback (summed, fading, bandwidth) designs to improve retention. **Organize practice.** • Encourage consistency of performance. • Focus on variable practice order (serial or random) of related skills to improve retention. **Structure environment.** • Progress toward open, changing environment. • Prepare the learner for home, community, work environments.
Autonomous Stage Characteristics	**Training Strategies**
The learner practices movements and continues to refine motor responses; spatial and temporal highly organized, movements are largely error-free; minimal level of cognitive monitoring ***"How to succeed"*** decision	Assess need for conscious attention, automaticity of movements. **Select appropriate feedback.** • Learner demonstrates appropriate self-evaluation and decision-making skills. • Provide occasional feedback (KP, KR) when errors are evident. **Organize practice.** • Stress consistency of performance in variable environments, variations of tasks (open skills). • High levels of practice (massed practice) are appropriate. **Structure environment.** • Vary environments to challenge learner. • Ready the learner for home, community, and work environments. Focus on competitive aspects of skills as appropriate, e.g., wheelchair sports.

[a]From O'Sullivan and Schmitz,[10] Table 13.1 Characteristics of Motor Learning Stages and Training Strategies (with permission).

Enhancing Patient Decision-Making

As learning progresses, the patient should be actively involved in self-monitoring, analysis, and self-correction of movements. The therapist can prompt the learner in early decision-making by posing the key questions listed in Box 2.8.

The therapist should confirm the accuracy of the patient's responses. If errors are consistent, the patient's efforts can be redirected. For example, the patient recovering from stroke with pusher syndrome (ipsilateral pushing) consistently pushes to the affected side and will likely fall if not guarded. The therapist can pose the questions: *"What direction do you feel you will fall?"* and *"What do you need to do to correct this problem?"* The therapist can also use augmented cues (e.g., tapping or light resistance) to assist the patient in correcting postural responses and in moving toward a more symmetrical

BOX 2.8 Guiding Questions to Promote Decision-Making Skills

Key questions include:

• "What is the intended functional outcome of the movement?"
• "How well did you do in achieving the intended functional outcome?"
• "What problems did you have during the movement?"
• "What do you need to do differently to correct the problems in order to achieve success?"

If a complex task is practiced, the patient can be asked:

• "What are the necessary components or steps of the task?"
• "How should the components be sequenced?"
• "How well did you do in sequencing the steps and in achieving the intended functional outcome?"

posture. The development of independent decision-making skills is critical in ensuring learning and adaptability required for community living.

Neuromotor Training Approaches and Neuromuscular Facilitation Techinques

An understanding of how the brain regulates movement is essential to making sound clinical decisions in selecting interventions. The diversity of problems experienced by patients with disordered motor function negates the idea that any one approach or training strategy can be successful for all patients. As patients recover, their functional abilities and needs change. During early recovery, patients with limited voluntary control typically benefit from a more hands-on approach to training. This can consist of guided or facilitated movements using neuromuscular facilitation techniques to promote voluntary control. Two popular neuromotor approaches in current use are *Proprioceptive Neuromuscular Facilitation* and *Neuro-Developmental Treatment*. Both are discussed in this section.

Clinical Note: Patients who demonstrate sufficient recovery and consistent voluntary movement control would not benefit from an intensive hands-on approach. Rather, these patients are candidates for functional task-oriented training that emphasizes active control. Patients who demonstrate severely limited recovery and multiple comorbidities and impairments (e.g., the patient with stroke who also demonstrates severe cardiac and respiratory compromise or memory deficits associated with Alzheimer's disease) are typically not good candidates either. Rather, *compensatory intervention strategies* in which the early resumption of functional skills using the uninvolved or less involved segments for function can be emphasized (discussed in the next section). All three major areas of interventions (outlined in Fig. 1.1) are important in the rehabilitation process.

Clinical Note: Interventions organized around a behavioral goal are the best way to promote functional recovery and retention rather than interventions that specifically target remediation of an impairment (e.g., spasticity). The remediation of specific impairments can be built into a functional training activity. For example, in hooklying, lower trunk rotation in which the knees move from side to side (knee rocks) can increase the strength of hip extensors and abductors while reducing LE extensor tone. Functionally it promotes independent bed mobility.

Neuromuscular facilitation techniques and approaches are important treatment choices for a group of patients involved in rehabilitation. For example, patients with stroke or TBI who are early in recovery and have limited voluntary movement abilities are good candidates. These interventions may help the patient bridge the gap between absent or severely disordered movements and active movements. Thus they are used to "jump start" recovery.

Red Flag: Once the patient develops adequate voluntary control, these interventions are generally counterproductive and should be discontinued.

Proprioceptive Neuromuscular Facilitation

Motor function can be improved using *Proprioceptive Neuromuscular Facilitation (PNF)*, an approach initially developed by Dr. Herman Kabat and Maggie Knott (a physical therapist).[13] Synergistic patterns of movement were identified as components of normal movement. A developmental (functional) task emphasis was added later by Dorothy Voss to include practice in various different activities and postures (rolling, prone on elbows, quadruped, kneeling, half-kneeling, modified plantigrade, standing, and gait). Extremity patterns of movement are rotational and diagonal in nature rather than straight plane movements. Coordination within and between patterns is stressed. For example, the technique of *dynamic reversals* is used to establish smooth linkages between agonist and antagonist actions during reversing patterns. Patterns can be unilateral or bilateral and combined with various trunk patterns and postures. A number of different facilitation techniques, largely proprioceptive, are utilized to facilitate movement (e.g., stretch, resistance, traction, approximation, and so forth). Precise manual contacts are used to provide important directional cues and enhance the function of underlying muscles. PNF also incorporates a number of important motor learning strategies (e.g., practice, repetition, visual guidance of movement, verbal cues, and so forth). PNF is directed at improving functional performance and coordinated patterns of movement and has been used effectively to treat patients with both neuromuscular and musculoskeletal deficits.[13,14] PNF is taught today in recognized courses.

PNF Patterns

Normal motor activity occurs in synergistic and functional patterns of movement. PNF patterns are "spiral and diagonal" in character and combine motion in all three planes: flexion/extension, abduction/adduction, and transverse rotation. They closely resemble patterns used in normal functional activities and sports. Extremity patterns are named for the action occurring at the proximal joint or by the diagonal (antagonist pairs of patterns make up the diagonal). Patterns are varied by changing the action of the intermediate joint (i.e., elbow or knee) or by changing the position of the patient (e.g., supine, sitting, or standing). Patterns can be unilateral or bilateral; bilateral patterns can be symmetrical, asymmetrical, or reciprocal.[13] PNF patterns are presented in Box 2.9, PNF basic procedures for facilitation are presented in Box 2.10, and PNF techniques are presented in Box 2.11.

(text continues on page 36)

BOX 2.9 PNF Patterns[a]

Upper Extremity Patterns
Terminology:

• *Flexion-adduction-external rotation,* or *diagonal 1 flexion (D1F), supine* (Fig. 2.2): The hand closes with wrist and finger flexion; the upper limb externally rotates and pulls up and across the face, moving into shoulder adduction and flexion. The elbow remains straight. Verbal cue: *"Squeeze my hand, turn, and pull up and across your face."*

• *Extension-abduction-internal rotation,* or *diagonal 1 extension (D1E), supine* (Fig. 2.3): The hand opens with wrist and finger extension; the upper limb internally rotates and pushes down and out, moving into shoulder abduction and extension. The elbow remains straight. Verbal cue: *"Open your hand, turn, and push down and out toward me."*

• *Flexion-abduction-external rotation,* or *diagonal 2 flexion (D2F), supine* (Fig. 2.4): The hand opens with wrist and finger extension; the upper limb externally rotates and lifts up and out, moving into shoulder abduction and flexion. The elbow remains straight. Verbal cue: *"Open your hand, turn, and lift it up and out toward me."*

• *Extension-adduction-internal rotation,* or *diagonal 2 extension (D2E), supine* (Fig. 2.5): The hand closes with wrist and finger flexion; the upper limb internally rotates and pulls down and across the body, moving into shoulder adduction and extension. The elbow remains straight. Verbal cue: *"Squeeze my hand, turn, and pull down and across your body."*

Note: The terms *proximal* and *distal hand* refer to the location of the therapist's hands placed on the patient.

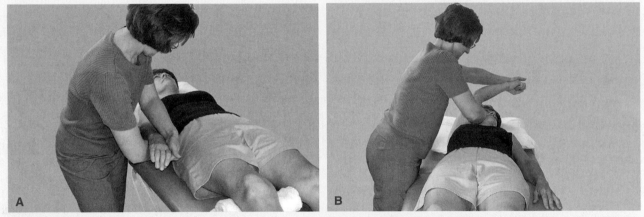

FIGURE 2.2 PNF pattern: supine, UE D1F (flexion-adduction-external rotation), with elbow straight. **(A)** (start of pattern) The therapist's distal hand is placed in the patient's palm; the proximal hand grips the patient's arm from underneath. The therapist applies initial stretch and resistance to shoulder flexors, adductors, and external rotators (proximal hand) and wrist and finger flexors (distal hand). Resistance is maintained as the UE moves through the range to the end position **(B).**

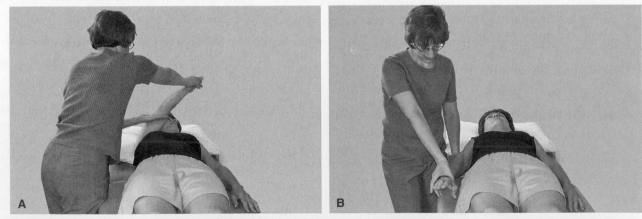

FIGURE 2.3 PNF pattern: supine, UE D1E (extension-abduction-internal rotation), with elbow straight. **(A)** (start of pattern) The therapist's distal hand grips the dorsal-ulnar surface of the patient's hand; the proximal hand applies pressure to the posterior-lateral surface of the patient's arm. The therapist applies initial stretch and resistance to shoulder extensors, abductors, and internal rotators (proximal hand) and wrist and finger extensors (distal hand). Resistance is maintained as the UE moves through the range to the end position **(B).**

BOX 2.9 PNF Patterns[a] (continued)

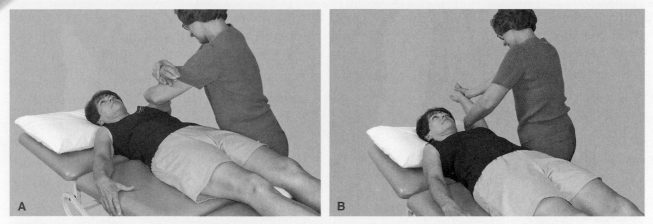

FIGURE 2.4 PNF pattern: supine, UE D2F (flexion-abduction-external rotation), with elbow straight. **(A)** (start of pattern) The therapist's distal hand grips the dorsal-radial surface of the patient's hand; the proximal hand applies pressure over the anterior-lateral surface of the patient's arm. The therapist applies initial stretch and resistance to shoulder flexors, abductors, and external rotators (proximal hand) and wrist and finger extensors (distal hand). Resistance is maintained as the UE moves through the range to the end position **(B).**

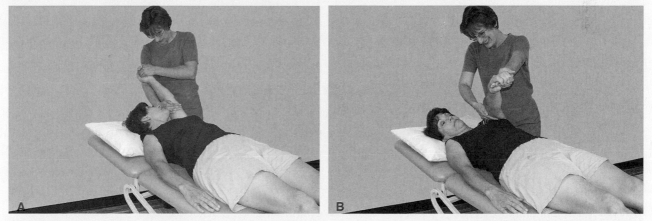

FIGURE 2.5 PNF pattern: supine, UE D2 E (extension-adduction-internal rotation), with elbow straight. **(A)** (start of pattern) The therapist's distal hand is placed in the palm of the patient's hand; the proximal hand provides pressure to the posterior-medial surface of the patient's arm. The therapist applies initial stretch and resistance to shoulder extensors, adductors, and internal rotators (proximal hand) and wrist and finger flexors (distal hand). Resistance is maintained as the UE moves through the range to the end position **(B).**

Lower Extremity Patterns
Terminology: *Lower extremity (LE) patterns* are named for motions occurring at the proximal joint (hip). The intermediate joint (knee) may be extended (straight leg pattern) or moving into flexion or extension (intermediate pivot).

- *Flexion-adduction-external rotation,* or *diagonal 1 flexion (D1F), supine* (Fig. 2.6): The foot dorsiflexes and inverts; the lower limb externally rotates and pulls up and across the body, moving into hip adduction and flexion. The knee remains straight. Verbal cue: *"Pull your foot up, turn your heel in, and pull your leg up and across your body."*
- *Extension-abduction-internal rotation,* or *diagonal 1 extension (D1E), supine* (Fig. 2.7): The foot plantarflexes and everts; the lower limb internally rotates and pushes down and out, moving into hip abduction and

extension. The knee remains straight. Verbal cue: *"Push your foot down, turn your heel out, and push down and out toward me."*
- *Intermediate joint action* (Fig. 2.8): LE D1F with knee extension, sitting. Verbal cue: *"Foot up, heel in, now kick up and across your body."*
- *Intermediate joint action* (Fig. 2.9): LE D1E with knee flexion, sitting. Verbal cue: *"Push your foot down, now bend your knee down and out toward me."*
- *Flexion-abduction-internal rotation,* or *diagonal 2 flexion (D2F), supine* (Fig. 2.10): The foot dorsiflexes and everts; the lower limb internally rotates and lifts up and out, moving into hip abduction and flexion. The knee remains straight. Verbal cue: *"Foot up, turn and lift your leg up and out toward me."*

(box continues on page 28)

BOX 2.9 PNF Patterns[a] (continued)

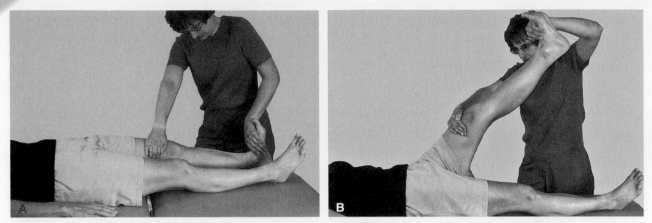

FIGURE 2.6 PNF pattern: supine, LE D1F (flexion-adduction-external rotation), with knee straight. **(A)** (start of pattern) The therapist's distal hand grips the patient's dorsal-medial foot; the proximal hand applies pressure on the anterior-medial surface of the patient's thigh just proximal to the knee. The therapist applies initial stretch and resistance to hip flexors, adductors, and external rotators (proximal hand) and ankle dorsiflexors and invertors (distal hand). Resistance is maintained as the LE moves through the range to the end position **(B).**

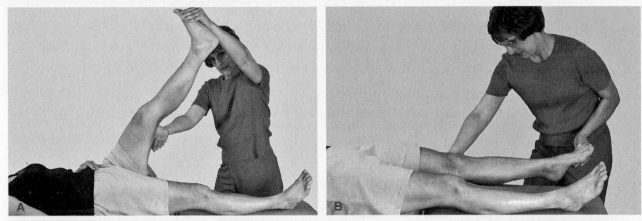

FIGURE 2.7 PNF pattern: supine, LE D1E (extension-abduction-internal rotation), with knee straight. **(A)** (start of pattern) The therapist's distal hand grips the plantar-lateral surface of the patient's foot; the proximal hand applies pressure on the patient's posterior-lateral thigh. The therapist applies stretch and resistance to hip extensors, abductors, and internal rotators (proximal hand) and ankle plantarflexors and evertors (distal hand). Resistance is maintained as the LE moves through the range to the end position **(B).**

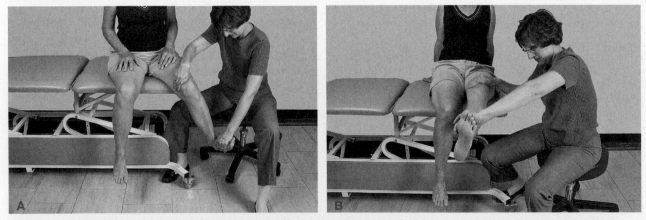

FIGURE 2.8 PNF pattern: sitting, LE D1F (flexion-adduction-external rotation) with knee extension. **(A)** (start of position) The therapist's distal hand grips the patient's dorsal medial foot. The proximal hand applies pressure over the patient's anterior-medial thigh. The therapist applies stretch and resistance to knee extensors and ankle dorsiflexors (distal hand). Resistance is maintained as the LE moves through the range to the end position of full knee extension with hip flexion-adduction-external rotation **(B).**

BOX 2.9 PNF Patterns^a (continued)

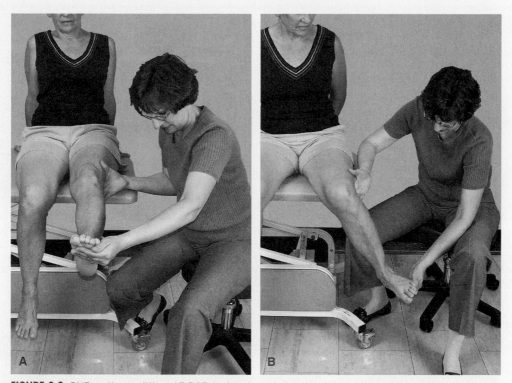

FIGURE 2.9 PNF pattern: sitting, LE D1E (extension-abduction-internal rotation), with knee flexion. **(A)** (start of pattern) The therapist's distal hand grips the plantar-lateral surface of the patient's foot. The proximal hand applies pressure on the patient's posterior-lateral thigh. The therapist applies stretch to knee flexors and ankle plantarflexors (distal hand). Resistance is provided as the LE moves through the range to the end position of full knee flexion with hip abduction and ankle plantarflexion **(B).**

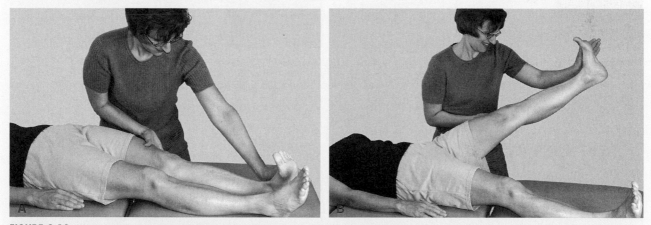

FIGURE 2.10 PNF pattern: supine, LE D2F (flexion-abduction-internal rotation), with knee straight. **(A)** (start of pattern) The therapist's distal hand grips the patient's dorso-lateral foot; the proximal hand applies pressure on the patient's anterior-lateral thigh. The therapist applies stretch and traction to hip flexors, abductors, and internal rotators (proximal hand) and ankle dorsiflexors and evertors (distal hand). Resistance is provided as the LE moves through the range to the end position **(B).**

- *Extension-adduction-external rotation,* or *diagonal 2 extension (D2E),* supine (Fig. 2.11): The foot plantarflexes and inverts; the lower limb externally rotates and pushes down and in, moving into hip adduction and extension. The knee remains straight. Verbal cue: *"Foot down, turn and push your leg down and across your body."*

- *Intermediate joint action* (Fig. 2.12): *D2F with knee flexion,* supine. Verbal cue: *"Foot up, now bend your knee and lift up and out toward me."*
- *Intermediate joint action* (Fig. 2.13): *D2E with knee extension,* supine. Verbal cue: *"Push your foot down, now push down and in, straighten your knee."*

(box continues on page 30)

BOX 2.9 PNF Patterns[a] (continued)

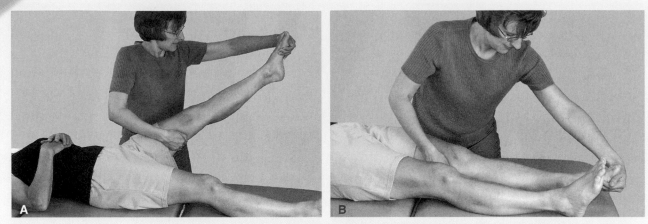

FIGURE 2.11 PNF pattern: supine LE D2E (extension-adduction-external rotation), with knee straight. **(A)** (start of pattern) The therapist's distal hand grips the medial-plantar surface of the patient's foot; the proximal hand applies pressure over the posterior-medial aspect of the patient's thigh. The therapist applies stretch and resistance to hip extensors, adductors, and external rotators (proximal hand) and ankle plantarflexors and invertors (distal hand). Resistance is maintained as the LE moves through the range to the end position **(B).**

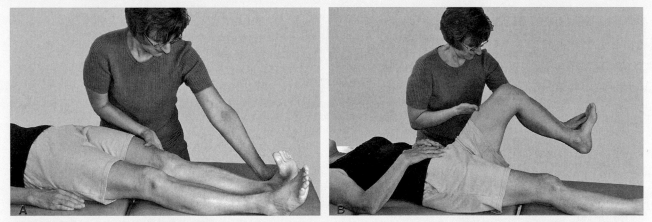

FIGURE 2.12 PNF pattern: supine, LE D2F (flexion-abduction-internal rotation), with knee flexion. **(A)** (start of pattern) The therapist's distal hand grips the patient's dorsal-lateral foot; the proximal hand applies pressure on the patient's anterior-lateral thigh. The therapist applies stretch to hip flexors, abductors, and internal rotators (proximal hand) and knee flexors, ankle dorsiflexors, and evertors (distal hand). Resistance is provided as the knee flexes and the LE moves through the range to the end position **(B).**

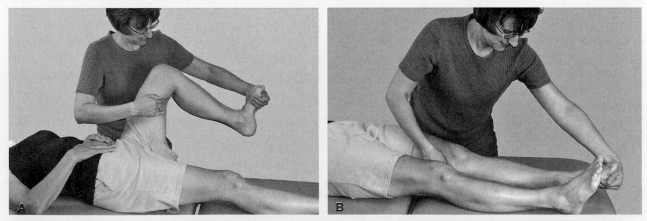

FIGURE 2.13 PNF pattern: supine, LE D2E with knee extending. **(A)** (start of pattern) The therapist's distal hand grips the medial-plantar surface of the patient's foot; the proximal hand applies pressure over the posterior-medial aspect of the patient's thigh. The therapist applies stretch and resistance to hip extensors, adductors, and external rotators (proximal hand) and knee extensors, ankle plantarflexors, and invertors (distal hand). Resistance is maintained as the knee extends and the LE moves through the range to the end position **(B).**

BOX 2.9 PNF Patterns^a (continued)

- *Intermediate joint action* (Fig. 2.14): *D2F with knee extension, sitting.* Verbal cue: *"Foot up and out, now kick your leg up and out toward me."*

Head and Trunk Patterns
Note: Head and trunk patterns combine trunk flexion or extension with rotation.

- *Chop (bilateral asymmetrical UE extension with flexion and rotation to right or left)* (Fig. 2.15): The lead arm moves in D1E; the assist arm holds on from the top of the wrist; the elbows are straight. The head and trunk flex and rotate to the right or left. Both elbows are straight. Verbal cue: *"Push your arms down and toward me, turn and look down at your hands. Reach down toward your knee."*
- *Reverse chop in the opposite direction of chop (bilateral asymmetrical UE flexion with neck extension and rotation to right or left)* (Fig. 2.16). Verbal cue: *"Squeeze my hand, turn and pull your arms up and*

across your face, turn and look up at your hands. Reach up and around."
- *Lift (bilateral asymmetrical UE flexion with neck extension and rotation to right or left)* (Fig. 2.17): The lead arm moves in D2F; the assist arm holds on from underneath the wrist; the elbows are straight. The head and trunk extend and rotate to the right or left. Both elbows are straight. Verbal cue: *"Lift your arms up and out toward me, turn and look up at your hands. Reach up and around."*
- *Reverse lift (bilateral asymmetrical UE extension with neck flexion and rotation to right or left) in the opposite direction of lift* (Fig. 2.18). Verbal cue: *"Squeeze my hand, turn, and pull your arms down and across your body. Lift and turn your head. Reach down and across."*
- *Bilateral LE flexion with knee flexion for lower trunk rotation to left (or right)* (Fig. 2.19): The hips flex; the legs pull up and across the body toward one side; the knees are typically flexed. Verbal cue: *"Feet up, now bend both knees and swing your feet up and toward me."*

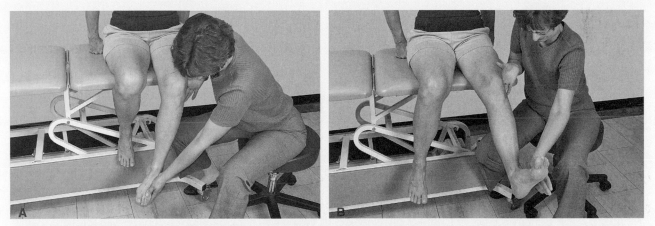

FIGURE 2.14 PNF pattern: sitting, LE D2F with knee extending. **(A)** (start of pattern) The therapist's distal hand grips the patient's dorso-lateral foot; the proximal hand applies pressure on the patient's anterior-lateral thigh. The therapist applies stretch and resistance to knee extensors and ankle dorsiflexors and evertors (distal hand). Resistance is maintained as the knee extends and the LE moves through the range to the end position **(B).**

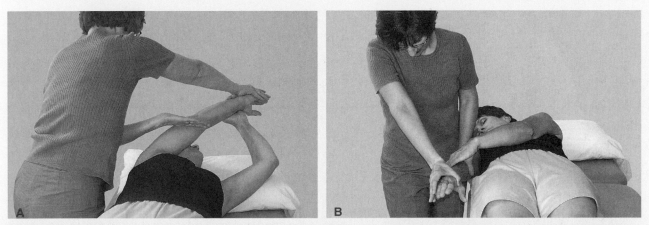

FIGURE 2.15 PNF pattern: supine, chop (bilateral asymmetrical UE extension with neck and trunk flexion with rotation). **(A)** (start of pattern) The therapist's distal hand grips the patient's right hand (lead arm), dorsal-ulnar aspect. The proximal hand applies pressure to the patient's lateral-posterior arm. The therapist applies stretch and resistance to the lead arm, shoulder extensors, abductors, and internal rotators (proximal hand) and wrist and finger extensors (distal hand) as both UEs move through the range to the end position; the head and trunk flex and rotate **(B).**

(box continues on page 32)

BOX 2.9 PNF Patterns^a (continued)

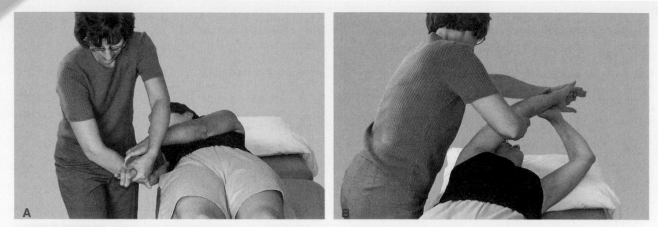

FIGURE 2.16 PNF pattern: supine, reverse chop. **(A)** (start of pattern) The therapist's distal hand is placed in the patient's right palm (lead arm); the proximal hand grips the patient's arm from underneath. The therapist applies stretch and resistance to shoulder flexors, adductors, and external rotators (proximal hand) and wrist and finger flexors (distal hand) as both UEs move through the range to the end position; the head and trunk extend and rotate **(B).**

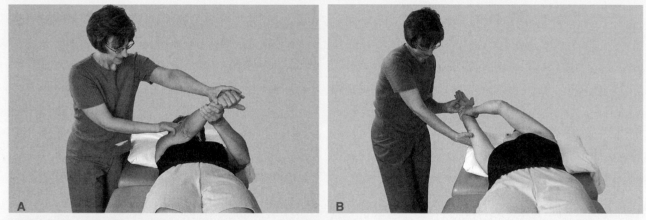

FIGURE 2.17 PNF pattern: supine, lift (bilateral asymmetrical UE flexion with neck and trunk extension with rotation). **(A)** (start of pattern) The therapist's distal hand grips the patient's right hand (lead hand); the proximal hand provides pressure to the patient's anterior-lateral arm. The therapist applies stretch and resistance to the lead arm, shoulder flexors, abductors, and external rotators (proximal hand) and wrist and finger extensors (distal hand) as both UEs move through the range to the end position; the head and trunk extend and rotate **(B).**

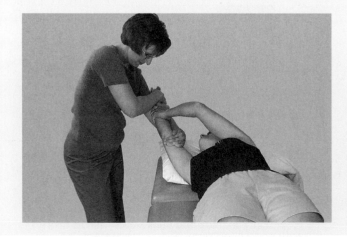

FIGURE 2.18 PNF pattern: supine, reverse lift. (start of pattern) The therapist's distal hand is placed in the palm of the patient's right hand (lead arm); the proximal hand provides pressure to the posterior-medial surface of the patient's arm. The therapist applies stretch and resistance to the lead arm, shoulder extension, adduction, and internal rotation (proximal hand) and wrist and finger flexion (distal hand) as both UEs move through the range to the end position; the head and trunk extend and rotate (not shown).

BOX 2.9 PNF Patterns[a] (continued)

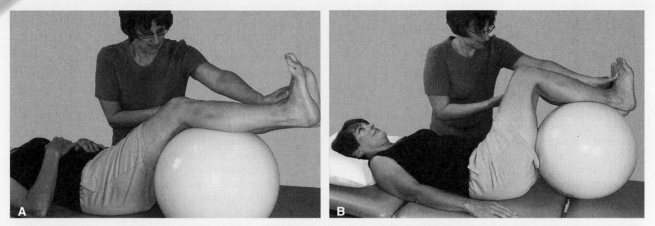

FIGURE 2.19 PNF pattern: supine, bilateral LE flexion, with knee flexion for lower trunk flexion (left), feet on ball. **(A)** (start of pattern) The therapist's distal hand provides pressure to both of the patient's feet on the dorsal-lateral surfaces; the proximal hand applies pressure to the patient's anterior-lateral thighs. The therapist applies stretch and resistance to both feet, ankle dorsiflexors (distal hand), and both thighs (proximal hand) as the patient bends both hips and knees and swings the feet up and toward the therapist (**B** end position).

[a]Adapted from Voss et al.[13]

BOX 2.10 Foundational PNF Procedures for Facilitation[a]

- **Timing:** Normal timing ensures smooth, coordinated movement. In PNF patterns, normal timing is from distal to proximal. Distal segments (hand/wrist or foot/ankle) move first, followed closely by more proximal components. Rotation occurs throughout the pattern, from beginning to end.
- **Timing for emphasis (TE):** Maximum resistance is used to elicit a strong contraction and allow overflow to occur from strong to weak components within a synergistic pattern; the strong muscles are resisted isometrically ("locking in") while motion is allowed in the weaker muscles. *Indications:* Weakness and/or poor coordination.
- **Resistance:** Resistance facilitates muscle contraction. Both intrafusal and extrafusal muscle fibers contract, resulting in recruitment of motor units and improved strength of contraction. Resistance is applied manually and functionally through the use of gravity to all types of contractions (isotonic—concentric and eccentric; isometric). *Tracking* or *light resistance* applied to weak muscles is facilitatory and is usually applied in combination with light stretch. *Maximal resistance* is used to generate maximal effort and adjusted to ensure smooth, coordinated movement; maximal resistance varies according to the individual patient. *Indications:* Facilitate weak muscles to contract; enhance kinesthetic awareness of motion; increase strength; increase motor control and motor learning.
- **Overflow or irradiation:** Overflow or irradiation is the spread of muscle response from stronger muscles in a synergistic pattern to weaker muscles; maximal resistance is the main mechanism for securing overflow or irradiation. Stronger patterns can also be used to reinforce weaker patterns through mechanisms

of overflow or irradiation from one extremity to the other, or from extremity to trunk. *Indications:* Enhance synergistic actions of muscles; increase strength.
- **Manual contacts (MC):** Precise manual contacts (hand placements) are used to provide pressure to tactile and pressure receptors overlying muscles to facilitate contraction and guide direction of movements; pressure is applied opposite the direction of the desired motion. *Indications:* Enhance contraction and synergistic patterns.
- **Positioning:** Muscle positioning at optimal range of function allows for optimal responses of muscles *(length-tension relationship).* The greatest muscle tension is generated in mid-ranges; weak contractile force *(active insufficiency)* occurs in the shortened ranges. The lengthened range provides optimal stretch for muscle spindle support of contraction, while the shortened range with muscle spindle unloading provides the least amount of muscle spindle support for contraction. *Indication:* Enhance weak contraction.
- **Therapist position and body mechanics:** The therapist is positioned directly *in line* with the desired motion (facing the direction of the movement) in order to optimize the direction of resistance that is applied. *Indications:* Enhance therapist's control of the patient's movements; reduce therapist fatigue through effective use of body weight and position.
- **Verbal cues (VC):** Verbal cues allow for the use of well-timed words and appropriate volume to direct the patient's movements. *Preparatory verbal cues* ready the patient for movement (what to do). They should be clear and concise and are optimally accompanied by demonstration and/or guided movement. *Action verbal cues* guide the patient through the movement

(box continues on page 34)

BOX 2.10 Foundational PNF Procedures for Facilitation[a] (continued)

(when and how to move). Strong, dynamic action verbal cues are used when maximal stimulation of movement is the goal; soft action verbal cues are used when relaxation is the goal. Timing is critical to coordinate the patient's actions with the therapist's VCs, resistance, and MCs. *Corrective verbal cues* provide augmented feedback to help the patient modify movements. *Indications:* Verbal stimulation enhances strength of muscle contraction and guides the synergistic actions in patterns of movement; verbal corrections provide augmented feedback to enhance motor learning.

- **Visual guidance:** Vision is used to guide the patient's movements and enhance muscle contractions and synergistic patterns of movement. The patient is instructed to look at the movements as they are occurring. *Indications:* Enhance initial motor control and motor learning.
- **Stretch (STR):** The elongated position (lengthened range) and the stretch reflex are used to facilitate muscle contraction. All muscles in the pattern are elongated to optimize the effects of stretch. Verbal cues for voluntary movement are always synchronized with

stretch to enhance the response. *Repeated stretch* can be applied throughout the range to reinforce contraction in weak muscles that are fading out. *Indications:* Enhance strength of muscle contraction and synergistic patterns of movement.

- **Approximation (AP):** Approximation (compressing the joint surfaces) is used to facilitate extensor/stabilizing muscle contraction and stability. It can be applied manually, functionally through the use of gravity acting on the body during upright positions, or mechanically using weights or weighted vests or belts. Approximation is applied manually during upright, weightbearing positions and in PNF extensor patterns. *Indications:* Weakness, inability of extensor muscle to function in weightbearing for stabilization control.
- **Traction (TR):** A distraction force (separating the joint surfaces) is used to facilitate muscle contraction and motion, especially in flexion patterns or pulling motions. Force is applied manually during PNF flexor patterns. Gentle distraction is also useful in reducing joint pain. *Indications:* Weakness, inability of flexor muscles to function in mobilizing patterns.

[a]Adapted from Voss et al.[13]

BOX 2.11 PNF Techniques[a]

- **Rhythmic initiation (RI):** The patient is instructed to relax (*"Relax, let me move you"*). The therapist moves the patient passively through the range, establishing appropriate speed and rhythm using verbal cues. Movements are then progressed to active-assisted (*"Now, help me move you"*). Finally movements are lightly resisted (*"Now, push up"*). Light tracking resistance is used during the resistive phase to enhance movement. At the end, the patient is asked to move independently (*"Now, move up on your own"*). *General goals:* Promote initiation of movement, teach the movement, improve coordination, promote relaxation, and promote independent movement. *Indications:* Inability to relax, hypertonicity (e.g., spasticity and rigidity); difficulty initiating movement; uncoordinated movement; motor planning or motor learning deficits (e.g., apraxia or dyspraxia); communication deficits (e.g., aphasia).
- **Reversals of antagonists:** A group of techniques that allow for agonist contraction followed by antagonist contraction without pause or relaxation.
  - **Dynamic reversals (DR) (slow reversals):** Dynamic reversals use isotonic contractions of first agonists, then antagonists performed against resistance. First, the therapist resists contraction of one pattern (e.g., D1F, *"Now, pull up and across your body"*); at the end of the desired range a preparatory command is given to reverse direction, and the therapist's hands are switched to resist the opposite pattern. The patient is then instructed to move in the opposite

direction (e.g., action command for D1E: *"Now, push down and out toward me"*). Reversals are repeated as often as necessary. If an imbalance exists, the stronger pattern is selected first, with progression to the weaker pattern. Modifications include working in a particular part of the range, progressing to full ROM *(increments of ROM)*. ROM can be decreased in each direction, progressing to holding steady *(decrements of ROM)*. The patient can also be asked to hold steady at any point in the range or the endpoint of ROM, typically the end range *(slow reversals, hold)*. An initial stretch is used to initiate the movement response. *General goals:* Improve coordination (smooth reversals of antagonists, rate of movement), strength, active range of motion, endurance; reduce fatigue. *Indications:* Impaired strength, range, and coordination; inability to easily reverse directions between agonist and antagonist; fatigue.

- **Stabilizing reversals:** Stabilizing reversals use alternating isotonic contractions of first agonists (*"Don't let me push you backward"*) and then antagonists (*"Now, don't let me push you forward"*) against resistance, allowing only very limited movement. The technique progresses to stabilizing holds *(alternating isometrics)* until the patient is holding steady in the position. Before hands are moved, a preparatory command is given (*"Now"*) before the patient is asked to reverse directions. If an imbalance exists, the stronger pattern is selected

BOX 2.11 PNF Techniques[a] (continued)

first, with progression to the weaker pattern. *General goals:* Improve stability, strength, coordination, endurance, range of motion. *Indications:* Impaired strength, stability and balance, coordination.

- **Rhythmic stabilization (RS):** Rhythmic stabilization uses isometric contractions of antagonist patterns, focusing on co-contraction of muscles. RS of the trunk utilizes resistance applied to one segment (e.g., on the anterior shoulder, the therapist's right hand pushes backward) while applying resistance to the other segment (e.g., on posterior pelvis, the therapist's left hand pulls forward). The therapist builds the resistance up slowly; no movement is allowed. Verbal cues include *"Hold, don't let me move you, hold, hold."* The therapist then shifts hands and applies resistance in the opposite direction, keeping each hand on the same section of the trunk (e.g., the therapist's right hand pulls forward on the shoulder while the left hand pushes backward on the pelvis). Verbal cues include *"Now, don't let me move you the other way, hold, hold."* An alternative command is *"Don't let me twist you, hold, hold."* Upper trunk flexors and rotators are resisted at the same time as lower trunk extensors and rotators. *General goals:* Improve stability (co-contraction of antagonists), strength, endurance, ROM, and coordination; promote relaxation and decrease pain. *Indications:* Impaired strength and coordination, limitations in ROM; impaired stabilization control and balance.

- **Repeated stretch (repeated contractions):** Repeated isotonic contractions are performed, directed to the agonist muscles, initiated by a quick stretch and enhanced by resistance. The stretch can be performed from the beginning of the range (lengthened range) or throughout the range at a point of weakness. The therapist gives a preparatory command *("Now")* while providing quick stretch of the muscles working in the pattern. An action command *("Pull up and across")* follows. The technique can be repeated (three or four stretches) during one pattern *("Again, pull up and across")* or until contraction weakens. *General goals:* Enhance initiation of motion, motor learning; increase agonist strength, endurance, coordination, ROM; reduce fatigue. *Indications:* Impaired strength, difficulty initiating movement, fatigue, and limitations in active ROM. The technique should not be applied in the presence of joint instability, pain, or injured muscle.

- **Combination of isotonics (agonist reversals):** Resisted concentric contraction of agonist muscles moving through the range is followed by a stabilizing contraction (holding in the position) and then eccentric, lengthening contraction, moving slowly back to the start position; there is no relaxation between the types of contractions. Verbal cues are directed toward each phase of the movement *("Push up." "Now, hold." "Now, go down slowly")*. The technique is typically used in antigravity activities and assumption of postures (e.g., bridging and sit-to-stand transitions). *General goals:* Improve motor learning and coordination; increase strength; promote stability and eccentric control. *Indications:* Weak postural muscles,

inability to eccentrically control body weight during movement transitions, poor dynamic postural control.

- **Contract-relax (CR):** This relaxation technique is usually performed at a point of limitation of ROM in the agonist pattern *("Pull your foot up, turn your leg out, and lift up and out")*. The therapist then asks for a strong isotonic contraction of the range-restricting muscles (antagonists) with emphasis on the rotation *("Now, turn your leg in and hold")*. The contraction is held for 5 to 8 seconds and is then followed by voluntary relaxation and active movement into the new range of the agonist pattern *("Relax, now turn and lift your leg up and out")*. This can be repeated until no additional range is obtained. Improvements in range are obtained through the combined effects of both reciprocal inhibition and autogenic inhibition. The technique can be followed with repeated contractions of the agonist muscles in order to enhance gains in range. *General goals:* Improve ROM. *Indications:* Limitations in ROM.

- **Hold-relax (HR):** This relaxation technique is usually performed in a position of comfort and below a level that causes pain. The patient moves the limb to the end of pain-free ROM. A strong isometric contraction of the restricting muscles (antagonists) is resisted (providing autogenic inhibition), followed by voluntary relaxation and passive movement into the newly gained range of the agonist pattern. The therapist instructs the patient to pattern: *"Hold, don't let me move you."* This is followed by a command to *"Relax, now, let me move your leg up and out."*

- **Hold-relax-active contraction (HRAC):** This is similar to HR except movement into the newly gained range of the agonist pattern is active, not passive. Active contraction is always desirable as it serves to maintain the inhibitory influence through effects of reciprocal inhibition. *General goals:* Improve ROM and decrease pain. *Indications:* Limitations in passive ROM (PROM) with pain.

- **Replication (hold-relax-active motion):** The patient is positioned in the end position (shortened range) of a movement and is told: *"Hold, don't let me move you."* The isometric contraction is resisted, followed by voluntary relaxation and passive movement into the lengthened range *("Relax, now let me move you back")*. The therapist then instructs the patient: *"Now, push back"* into the end position again. Stretch and tracking resistance are applied to facilitate the isotonic contraction. For each repetition, increasing ROM is desired. *General goals:* Promote motor learning, improve coordination and control in the shortened range. *Indications:* Marked weakness; inability to sustain a contraction in the shortened range.

- **Resisted progression (RP):** Stretch, approximation, and tracking resistance are applied manually to facilitate lower trunk/pelvic motion and progression during locomotion (walking or crawling); the level of resistance is light so as to not disrupt the patient's momentum, coordination, and velocity. RP can also be applied using an elastic resistance band. Verbal cues include: *"On three, I want you to step forward with*

(box continues on page 36)

> **BOX 2.11** PNF Techniques[a] (continued)
>
> your right foot. One, two, three, and step, step, step." *General goals:* Improve coordination and timing of lower trunk/pelvis during locomotion. *Indications:* Impaired timing and control of lower trunk/pelvic segments during locomotion, impaired endurance.
>
> • **Rhythmic rotation (RRo):** Relaxation is achieved using slow, repeated rotations of a limb or body segment. Rotations can be passive or active. Verbal cues include: *"Relax, let me move you, back and forth, back and*
>
> *forth"* (passive movements) or *"Relax, roll your legs outward, now roll them inward"* (active movements). The rotations are continued until muscle tension relaxes. Movements are slow and gently progress through increased range. *General goals:* Promote relaxation and increased range in muscles restricted by excess tone. *Indications:* Relaxation of hypertonia (spasticity, rigidity) combined with passive or active ROM of the range-limiting muscles.

[a]Adapted from Voss et al[13] and Adler, Beckers, and Buck.[14]

Recent modifications in the terminology for PNF techniques have occurred. A comparison of new and traditional terminology is presented in Table 2.2.

Neuro-Developmental Treatment

Neuro-Developmental Treatment (NDT) is an approach developed in the late 1940s and early 1950s by Dr. Karel Bobath, an English physician, and Berta Bobath, a physiotherapist.[15] Their work focused on patients with neurological dysfunction (cerebral palsy and stroke). The essential problems of these patient groups were identified as a release of abnormal tone (spasticity) and abnormal postural reflexes (primitive spinal cord and brainstem reflexes) from higher center CNS control with resulting loss of the normal postural reflex mechanism (righting, equilibrium, and protective extension reactions) and normal movements. The role of sensory feedback was viewed as critical in inhibiting abnormal reactions and facilitating more normal movement patterns.

Current NDT has realigned itself with newer theories of motor control (systems theory and a distributed model of CNS control). Many different factors are recognized as contributing to loss of motor function in patients with neurological dysfunction, including the full spectrum of sensory and

motor deficits (weakness, limited ROM, and impaired tone and coordination). Emphasis is on the use of both feedback and feedforward mechanisms to support postural control. Postural control is viewed as the foundation for all skill learning. Normal development in children and normal movement patterns in all patients are stressed. The patient learns to control posture and movement through a sequence of progressively more challenging postures and activities. NDT uses physical *handling techniques* and *key points of control* (e.g., shoulders, pelvis, hands, and feet) directed at supporting body segments and assisting the patient in achieving active control. Sensory stimulation (facilitation and inhibition via primarily proprioceptive and tactile inputs) is used during treatment. Postural alignment and stability are facilitated, while excessive tone and abnormal movements are inhibited. For example, in the patient with stroke, abnormal obligatory synergy movements are restricted, while out-of-synergy movements are facilitated. Activities are selected that are functionally relevant and varied in terms of difficulty and environmental context. Compensatory training strategies (use of the less involved segments) are avoided. Carryover is promoted through a strong emphasis on patient, family, and caregiver education. NDT is taught today in recognized training courses.[16] Foundational NDT principles are presented in Box 2.12; NDT intervention strategies and techniques are presented in Box 2.13.

Facilitated Movements (Neuromuscular Facilitation/Sensory Stimulation)

A number of therapeutic techniques can be used to facilitate, activate, or inhibit muscle contraction. These have been collectively called *facilitation techniques,* although this term is a misnomer because they also include techniques used for inhibition. The term *facilitation* refers to the enhanced capacity to initiate a movement response through increased neuronal activity and altered synaptic potential. An applied stimulus may lower the synaptic threshold of the alpha motor neuron but may not be sufficient to produce an observable movement response. *Activation,* on the other hand, refers to the actual production of a movement response and implies reaching a critical threshold level for neuronal firing. *Inhibition* refers to the decreased capacity to initiate a movement response through altered synaptic potential. The

TABLE 2.2 PNF Techniques: Comparison of New and Traditional Terminology	
New	**Traditional**
Combination of Isotonics	Agonist Reversals
Dynamic Reversals	Slow Reversals
Replication	Hold-Relax-Active-Motion
Rhythmic Initiation (no change)	Rhythmic Initiation
Rhythmic Stabilization (no change)	Rhythmic Stabilization
Stabilizing Reversals	Alternating Isometrics

> **BOX 2.12** NDT Foundational Principles[a]

- NDT is based on an ongoing analysis of sensorimotor function and carefully planned interventions designed to improve function. Principles of motor control, motor learning, and motor development guide the planning process.
- Interventions focus on the client's strengths and competencies while at the same time addressing impairments, activity limitations, and participation restrictions. Negative signs (weakness, impaired postural control, and paucity of movement) are equally important to address in treatment as positive signs (spasticity, hyperactive reflexes).
- The plan of care is developed in partnership with the patient, family, and interdisciplinary team.
- Treatment focuses on the relationship between sensory input and motor output.
- Therapeutic handling is the primary NDT intervention strategy. Facilitatory and/or inhibitory inputs are provided to influence the quality of motor responses.

- Training is focused on specific task goals and functional skills. The task and/or environment are modified as needed to enhance function.
- Active participation by the patient is a goal and an expectation of treatment.
- A major role of the therapist is completing an accurate analysis of motor problems and development of effective solutions.
- Motor learning principles are adhered to in the therapeutic setting, including: verbal reinforcement, repetition, facilitation of error awareness (trial-and-error practice), and an environment conducive to learning, engaging the patient/client/family, and ensuring motivation.
- Direct teaching of the patient/client/family/caregiver to ensure carryover of functional activities in the home and community setting is an important component of NDT.

[a]Adapted from Howle.[10]

> **BOX 2.13** NDT Treatment Strategies and Interventions

Therapeutic handling: Therapeutic handling is used to influence the quality of the motor response and is carefully matched to the patient's abilities to use sensory information and adapt movements. It includes neuromuscular facilitation, inhibition, or frequently a combination of the two. Manual contacts are used to:

- Direct, regulate, and organize tactile, proprioceptive, and vestibular input.
- Direct the client's initiation of movement more efficiently and with more effective muscle synergies.
- Support or change alignment of the body in relation to the BOS and with respect to the force of gravity prior to and during movement sequences.
- Decrease the amount of force the client uses to stabilize body segments.
- Guide or redirect the direction, force, speed, and timing of muscle activation for successful task completion.
- Either constrain or increase the flexibility in the degrees of freedom needed to stabilize or move body segments in a functional activity.
- Sense the response of the client to sensory input and the movement outcome and provide nonverbal feedback for reference of correction.
- Recognize when the client can become independent of the therapist's assistance and take over control of posture and movement.
- Direct the client's attention to meaningful aspects of the motor task.[16(p259)]

  Key points of control: Key points are parts of the body recommended as optimal to control (inhibit or facilitate) postures and movement.

- *Proximal key points* include the shoulders and pelvis and are used to influence proximal segments and trunk.

- *Distal key points* include the head and upper and lower extremities (typically the hands and feet).

  Key points of control are also used to provide inhibition of abnormal tone and postures. Examples include:

- Head and trunk flexion decreases shoulder retraction, trunk and limb extension (key points of control: head and trunk).
- Shoulder external rotation and abduction with elbow extension decrease flexion tone of the UE (key point of control: humerus).
- Thumb abduction and extension with forearm supination decrease flexion tone of the wrist and fingers (key point of control: the thumb).
- Hip external rotation and abduction decrease extensor/adductor tone of the LE (key point of control: hip).

  Note: Components of posture and movement that are essential for successful functional task performance are **facilitated** through therapeutic handling and key points of control.

  Components of posture and movement that are atypical and prevent development of desired motor patterns are inhibited. While originally this term referred strictly to the reduction of tone and abnormal reflexes, in current NDT practice it refers to *reduction of any underlying impairment that interferes with functional performance.*
  Inhibition can be used to:

- Prevent or redirect those components of a movement that are unnecessary and interfere with intentional, coordinated movement.
- Constrain the degrees of freedom, to decrease the amount of force the client uses to stabilize posture.
- Balance antagonistic muscle groups.

(box continues on page 38)

BOX 2.13 NDT Treatment Strategies and Interventions (continued)

- Reduce spasticity or excessive muscle stiffness that interferes with moving specific segments of the body.[16(p 261)]

    Rhythmic rotation (RRo): Relaxation is achieved using slow, repeated rotations of a limb or body segment. Range is typically limited by tight, spastic muscles. The patient is instructed: *"Relax, let me move you, back and forth, back and forth."* The rotations are continued until the muscles relax. Movements are slow and gently progress through increased range. For example, the patient is positioned in hooklying and the knees are gently rocked side to side to relax LE extensor tone. Or the arm is gently rotated back and forth while moving the elbow into extension to relax UE flexor tone. The limb is then positioned in extension, abduction, and external rotation with the hand open (fingers extended) and weightbearing. The patient can also be instructed to use active movements (voluntary effort) for RRo.

    Tapping: Tapping is used to stabilize muscle tone and facilitate muscle actions. Types of tapping include the following:

- **Inhibitory tapping:** Tapping applied to muscles that have previously been inhibited to raise tone to normal levels. Caution must be used to not restore muscle to its hypertonic state.

- **Sweep tapping:** Strong tapping applied with a sweeping motion over muscles in the direction of a movement.
- **Alternate tapping:** Alternate tapping is applied to agonist and antagonist muscles to promote reciprocal actions.
- **Pressure tapping:** Uses both weightbearing and joint compression to facilitate action of stabilizing muscles and postural tone and to reinforce desired postural alignment.

    Resistance: Resistance is used to activate movements and improve direction and timing.

    Placing and holding: Body segments are assisted into correct alignment for functional movements; the patient is asked to hold in the position and then to practice moving out of and back into the position.

[a]Adapted from Howle.[16]

synaptic threshold is raised, making it more difficult for the neuron to fire and produce movement. The combination of spinal inputs and supraspinal inputs acting on the alpha motor neuron (final common pathway) will determine whether a muscle response is facilitated, activated, or inhibited.

Several general guidelines are important. Facilitative techniques can be *additive.* For example, several inputs applied simultaneously, such as quick stretch, resistance, and verbal cues, are commonly combined during the use of PNF patterns. These stimuli collectively can produce the desired motor response, whereas the use of a single stimulus may not. This demonstrates the property of *spatial summation* within the CNS. *Repeated stimulation* (e.g., repeated quick stretches) may also produce the desired motor response owing to *temporal summation* within the CNS, whereas a single stimulus does not. Thus, stretch is used repeatedly to ensure that the patient with a weak muscle is able to move from the lengthened to the shortened range. The response to stimulation or inhibition is unique to each patient and depends on a number of different factors, including level of intactness of the CNS, arousal, and the specific level of activity of the motoneurons in question. For example, a patient who is depressed and hypoactive or taking CNS suppressant drugs may require large amounts of stimulation to achieve the desired response. Stimulation is generally contraindicated for the patient with hyperactivity, while inhibition/relaxation techniques are of benefit. The intensity, duration,

and frequency of simulation need to be adjusted to meet individual patient needs. Unpredicted responses can result from inappropriate application of techniques. For example, stretch applied to a spastic muscle may increase spasticity and negatively affect voluntary movement. Facilitation techniques are *not* appropriate for patients who demonstrate adequate voluntary control. They should be viewed primarily as a bridge to voluntary movement control during preactivity training.

The term *neuromuscular technique* refers to the facilitation or inhibition of muscle contraction or motor responses. The term *sensory stimulation* refers to the structured presentation of stimuli to improve (1) alertness, attention, and arousal; (2) sensory discrimination; or (3) initiation of muscle activity and improvement of movement control. Effects are immediate and specific to the current state of the nervous system. Additional practice using inherent or naturally occurring inputs and feedback is necessary for meaningful and lasting functional change to occur. Variable perceptions exist among patients. For example, decreased sensitivity to stimulation may be evident in some older adults and in some patients with neurological conditions such as stroke or TBI.

Box 2.14 presents a review of proprioceptive facilitation techniques. These techniques are important elements of interventions that may be used with patients with poor voluntary motor function. These interventions may serve as a bridge to later function in these more severely affected

BOX 2.14 Proprioceptive Facilitation Techniques

Quick Stretch

Stimulus: Brief stretch applied to a muscle.

Activates muscle spindles (facilitates Ia endings); sensitive to velocity and length changes. Has both segmental (spinal cord) and suprasegmental (CNS higher centers) effects.

Response: Stretch reflex: facilitates or enhances agonist muscle contraction; phasic.

Additional peripheral reflex effects: Inhibits antagonists, facilitates synergists (reciprocal innervation effects). Influences perception of effort.

Techniques: Quick stretch; more effective when applied in the lengthened range (e.g., PNF patterns); tapping over muscle belly or tendon.

Comments: A low-threshold response, relatively short-lived; can add resistance to maintain contraction.

Adverse effects: May increase spasticity when applied to spastic muscles.

Prolonged Stretch

Stimulus: Slow, maintained stretch, applied at maximum available lengthened range.

Activates muscle spindles (higher threshold response, primarily II), golgi tendon organs (Ib endings); sensitive to length changes; has both segmental (spinal cord) and suprasegmental (CNS higher centers) effects.

Response: Inhibits or dampens muscle contraction and tone due largely to peripheral reflex effects *(stretch-protection reflex).*

Techniques: Positioning; alternate applications include inhibitory casting and mechanical low-load weights using traction.

Comments: Higher threshold response; may be more effective in extensor muscles than flexors due to the added effects of II inhibition. To maintain inhibitory effects, follow with activation of antagonist muscles *(reciprocal inhibition effects).*

Resistance

Stimulus: A force exerted to muscle.

Activates muscle spindles (Ia and II endings) and golgi tendon organs (Ib endings); sensitive to velocity and length changes. Has both segmental (spinal cord) and suprasegmental (CNS higher centers) effects.

Response: Facilitates or enhances muscle contraction owing to: (1) peripheral reflex effects: muscle spindle effects via reciprocal innervation (facilitates agonist, inhibits antagonists, facilitates synergists); golgi tendon effects via autogenic inhibition: dampens or smoothes out the force of contraction; and (2) suprasegmental effects: recruits both alpha and gamma motoneurons, additional motor units. Hypertrophies extrafusal muscle fibers; enhances kinesthetic awareness.

Techniques: Manual resistance is carefully graded for optimal muscle function.

Use of body weight and gravity provides resistance in upright positions.

Alternate applications include mechanical resistance provided by use of weights, elastic resistance bands, cuffs, or vests; isokinetic resistance applied to a muscle contracting at a constant rate.

Comments: Tracking (light manual) resistance is used to facilitate and accommodate to very weak muscles. With weak hypotonic muscles, eccentric and isometric contractions are used before concentric (enhances muscle spindle support of contraction with less spindle unloading). Maximal resistance may produce overflow from strong to weak muscles within the same muscle pattern (synergy) or to contralateral extremities.

Precautions: Too much resistance can easily overpower weak, hypotonic muscles and prevent voluntary movement, encouraging substitution. May possibly increase spasticity in spastic muscles, especially if strong.

Joint Approximation

Stimulus: Compression of joint surfaces.

Activates joint receptors, primarily static, type I receptors. Has both segmental (spinal cord) and suprasegmental (CNS higher centers) effects.

Response: Facilitates postural extensors and stabilizing responses (co-contraction); enhances joint awareness.

Techniques: Manual joint compression. Alternate applications include weighted harness, vest, or belt; elastic tubing with compression of joints; and bouncing while sitting on a therapy ball.

Comments: Used in PNF extensor extremity patterns, pushing actions.

Approximation applied to top of shoulders or pelvis in upright weightbearing positions facilities postural extensors and stability (e.g., sitting, kneeling, or standing).

Precautions: Contraindicated with inflamed, painful joints.

Joint Traction

Stimulus: Distraction of joint surfaces.

Activates joint receptors, possibly phasic, type II. Has both segmental (spinal cord) and suprasegmental (CNS higher centers) effects.

Response: Facilitates joint motion; enhances joint awareness.

Techniques: Manual distraction.

Comments: Used in PNF flexor extremity patterns, pulling actions. Joint mobilization uses slow, sustained traction to improve mobility, relieve muscle spasm, and reduce pain.

Precautions: Contraindicated in hypermobile or unstable joints.

Inhibitory Pressure

Stimulus: Deep, maintained pressure applied across the longitudinal axis of tendons; prolonged positioning in extreme lengthened range.

Activates muscle receptors (golgi tendon organs) and tactile receptors (Pacinian corpuscles). Has both segmental (spinal cord) and suprasegmental (CNS higher centers) effects.

Response: Inhibition, dampens muscle tone.

Techniques: Firm, maintained pressure applied manually or with positioning.

(box continues on page 40)

BOX 2.14 Proprioceptive Facilitation Techniques (continued)

Clinical Note: Pressure from prolonged weightbearing on knees (e.g., quadruped or kneeling) dampens extensor tone/spasticity. Pressure from prolonged weightbearing on extended arm, wrist, and fingers dampens flexor tone/spasticity (e.g., sitting with weightbearing on an extended arm and hand, modified plantigrade). Pressure over calcaneus dampens plantarflexor tone. Alternate applications include firm objects (cones) in hand and inhibitory splints or casts (e.g., wrist, lower leg).

Comments: Inhibitory effects can be enhanced by combining them with other relaxation techniques (e.g., deep-breathing techniques, mental imaging).

Precaution: Sustained positioning may dampen muscle contraction enough to affect functional performance (e.g., difficulty walking after prolonged kneeling).

patients who may not benefit from activity-based, task-oriented interventions. Numerous examples of commonly used applications are presented in Part II, *Interventions to Improve Function.* Exteroceptive, vestibular, visual, and auditory stimulation may be used for a smaller group of select patients with sensory deficits who are candidates for sensory retraining (e.g., the patient with stroke) or sensory stimulation for improving arousal (e.g., the patient with TBI who is minimally conscious). The reader is referred to Chapter 13 of O'Sullivan and Schmitz[10] for a thorough discussion of these techniques.

Compensatory Intervention Strategies

Compensatory intervention strategies focus on the early resumption of function by using the less involved (sound) body segments for function. For example, a patient with left hemiplegia is taught to dress using the right UE; a patient with a complete T1-level spinal cord lesion is taught to roll using UEs, head/upper trunk, and momentum. Central to this approach is the concept of *substitution.* Changes are made in the patient's overall approach to functional tasks. A second central tenet of this approach is modification of the environment *(adaptation)* to facilitate relearning of skills, ease of movement, and optimal performance. For example, the patient with unilateral neglect is assisted in dressing by color coding of the shoes (red tape on the left shoe, yellow tape on the right shoe). The wheelchair brake toggle is extended and color coded to allow easy identification by the patient.

A compensatory approach may be the only realistic approach possible when improvement is limited and reaches an early plateau or the patient presents with severe impairments and functional losses with little or no expectation for additional recovery. Examples include the patient with complete SCI and the patient recovering from stroke with severe sensorimotor deficits and extensive comorbidities (e.g., severe cardiac and respiratory compromise). The latter example suggests severe limitations in the ability to actively move and participate in rehabilitation and to relearn motor skills. Box 2.15 presents basic principles and strategies of compensatory intervention.

BOX 2.15 Compensatory Intervention: Basic Principles and Strategies[a]

- The patient is made aware of movement deficiencies.
- Alternative ways to accomplish a task are considered, simplified, and adopted.
- The patient is taught to use the segments that are intact to compensate for those that have been lost.
- The patient practices and relearns the task; repeated practice results in consistency and habitual use of the new pattern.
- The patient practices the functional skill in environments in which function is expected to occur.
- Energy conservation techniques are taught to ensure that the patient can complete all daily tasks.
- The patient's environment is adapted to facilitate practice and learning of skills, ease of movement, and optimal performance.
- Assistive devices are incorporated as needed.

[a]Adapted from O'Sullivan and Schmitz.[10]

Red Flags: Several important precautions should be noted with use of compensatory intervention strategies. Focus on the uninvolved segments to accomplish daily tasks may suppress recovery and contribute to learned nonuse of the impaired segments. For example, the patient with stroke may fail to learn to use the involved extremities.

In addition, focus on task-specific learning of component skills may result in the development of *splinter skills* in some patients with brain damage. *Splinter skills* are skills that cannot easily be generalized to other environments or variations of the same task (poor adaptability).

SUMMARY

As patients recover, their functional abilities and needs change. Therapists must be attuned to the patient's changing status and recognize that anticipated goals and expected outcomes may change along with the interventions likely to be most effective. Interventions to improve functional skills and motor learning also need to promote adaptability of skills for function in real-world environments. Goals and functional activities practiced must be meaningful and worthwhile to

BOX 2.16 Examples of Anticipated Goals and Expected Outcomes for Patients with Disorders of Motor Function[a]

Impact of pathology/pathophysiology is reduced.
- Risk of recurrence of condition is reduced.
- Risk of secondary impairment is reduced.
- Intensity of care is decreased.

Impact of impairments is reduced.
- Alertness, attention, and memory are improved.
- Joint integrity and mobility are improved.
- Sensory awareness and discrimination are improved.
- Motor function (motor control and motor learning) is improved.
- Muscle performance (strength, power, and endurance) is improved.
- Postural control and balance are improved.
- Gait and locomotion are improved.
- Endurance is increased.

Ability to perform physical actions, tasks, or activities is improved.
- Functional independence in activities of daily living (ADL) and instrumental activities of daily living (IADL) is increased.
- Functional mobility skills are improved.
- Level of supervision for task performance is decreased.

- Tolerance of positions and activities is increased.
- Flexibility for varied tasks and environments is improved.
- Decision-making skills are improved.
- Safety of patient/client, family, and caregivers is improved.

Disability associated with acute or chronic illness is reduced.
- Activity participation is improved (home, community, leisure).

Ability to assume/resume self-care, home management, and work (job/school/play) is improved.

Health status is improved.
- Sense of well-being is increased.
- Insight, self-confidence, and self-image are improved.
- Health, wellness, and fitness are improved.

Satisfaction, access, availability, and services are acceptable to patient/client.

Patient/client, family, and caregiver knowledge and awareness of the diagnosis, prognosis, anticipated goals/expected outcomes, and interventions are increased.

[a]Adapted from *Guide to Physical Therapist Practice.*[17]

the patient. Collaborating with the patient, the therapist must select those activities that have the greatest chance of success. The choice of interventions must also take into consideration a host of other factors, including the availability of care, cost-effectiveness in terms of length of stay and number of allotted physical therapy visits, age of the patient and number of comorbidities, social support, and potential discharge placement. Examples of anticipated goals and expected outcomes for improving motor function are presented in Box 2.16.

REFERENCES

1. Taub, E, Uswatte, G, and Pidikiti, R. Constraint-induced movement therapy: A new family of techniques with broad application to physical rehabilitation: A clinical review. J Rehabil Res Dev 36:237, 1999.
2. Hakkennes, S, and Keating, J. Constraint-induced movement therapy following stroke: A systematic review of randomised controlled trials. Aust J Physiother 51:221, 2005.
3. Page, S, and Levine, P. Modified constraint-induced therapy in patients with chronic stroke exhibiting minimal movement ability in the affected arm. Phys Ther 87:872, 2007.
4. Taub, E, Uswatte, G, King, DK, A placebo-controlled trial of constraint-induced movement therapy for upper extremity after stroke. Stroke 37:1045, 2006.
5. Richards, C, Malouin, F, Wood-Dauphinee, S, et al: Task-specific physical therapy for optimization of gait recovery in acute stroke patients. Arch Phys Med Rehabil 74:612, 1993.
6. Visitin, M, Hugues, B, Korner-Bitensky, N, et al. A new approach to retrain gait in stroke patients through body weight support and treadmill stimulation. Stroke 29:1122, 1998.
7. Behrman, A, Lawless-Dixon, AR, Davis, SB, et al. Locomotor training progression and outcomes after incomplete spinal cord injury. Phys Ther 85:1356, 2005.
8. Barbeau, H, Nadeau, S, and Garneau, C. Physical determinants, emerging concepts, and training approaches in gait of individuals with spinal cord injury. J Neurotrauma 23 (2–4):571 (Review), 2006.
9. Sullivan, K, et al: Effects of task-specific locomotor and strength training in adults who were ambulatory after stroke: Results of the STEPS Randomized Clinical Trial. Phys Ther 87:1580, 2007.
10. O'Sullivan, SB, and Schmitz, TJ. Physical Rehabilitation, ed 5. FA Davis, Philadelphia, 2007.
11. Schmidt, R, and Lee, T. Motor Control and Learning, ed 4. Human Kinetics, Champaign, IL, 2005.
12. Fitts, P, and Posner, M. Human Performance. Brooks/Cole, Belmont, CA, 1967.
13. Voss, D, Ionta, MK, Myers, BJ, et al. Proprioceptive Neuromuscular Facilitation: Patterns and Techniques, ed 3. Harper & Row, Philadelphia, 1985.
14. Adler, S, Beckers, D, and Buck, M. PNF in Practice, ed 3. Springer-Verlag, New York, 2008.
15. Bobath, B. The treatment of neuromuscular disorders by improving patterns of coordination. Physiotherapy 55:1, 1969.
16. Howle, J. Neuro-Developmental Treatment Approach. Neuro-Developmental Treatment Association, Laguna Beach CA, 2002.
17. American Physical Therapy Association. Guide to Physical Therapist Practice, ed 2. Phys Ther 81:1, 2001.

Interventions to Improve Function

Part II presents strategies and interventions to promote enhanced motor function and independence in key functional skills. The interventions presented in each chapter include a description of the general characteristics of each activity (e.g., base of support provided, location of center of mass, impact of gravity and body weight, and so forth) together with a description of required lead-up skills, appropriate techniques, and progressions. Patient outcomes consistent with the *Guide to Physical Therapist Practice*[1] are described as well as clinical applications and patient examples. Practice activities to enhance student learning are provided.

The chapters are organized around a broad range of postures and activities required for normal human function (e.g., functional mobility skills, basic and instrumental activities of daily living). Postures and activities such as rolling and sidelying are presented first, with progression through upright standing and locomotion. Although the content is presented as a sequence from dependent to independent postures and activities, it should not be viewed as a "lock-step" progression. This means there are no absolute requirements for how the activities are sequenced or integrated into an individual plan of care. This has several implications for clinical practice:

- It will be the exception, rather than the norm, that an individual patient will require or benefit from the entire sequence of interventions presented.
- Evaluation of examination data will guide selection and sequencing of interventions for an individual patient.
- Interventions may be organized in a different sequence, used concurrently, expanded, or eliminated (i.e., deemed inappropriate) when developing a plan of care.
- The content should be viewed and used as a source of treatment ideas based on the desired functional outcome—and not as a prescribed sequence. For example, if a patient requires improved core (trunk) strength or increased ankle range of motion, consideration is given to those strategies and interventions designed to address the specific impairments.

(text continues on page 44)

PART

II

• The interventions include suggested therapist *positioning* and *hand placements*. These suggestions reflect an effective strategy for the application of resistance and maintenance of appropriate and safe body mechanics. Again, these are not intended to be prescriptive. There are multiple factors that influence selection of hand placements and therapist positioning. Although not an inclusive list of factors, several examples include: specific movement components at which the intervention is directed, height and size of the treatment surface, desired outcomes, type and severity of impairments and activity limitations, characteristics of the patient (e.g., height, weight, and size of individual body segments), and the physical therapist's body size and type.

Finally, the interventions address many types of impairments and activity limitations across practice patterns. They should not be considered practice pattern–specific but rather specific to the physical therapy *diagnosis* and *plan of care.*

Interventions to Improve Bed Mobility and Early Trunk Control

THOMAS J SCHMITZ, PT, PHD

This chapter focuses on bed mobility and interventions to improve skills in rolling and positional changes. It also describes activities and strategies to improve control in prone on elbows, quadruped (all fours), hooklying, and bridging. A description of the general characteristics of each posture or activity is provided. Interventions are organized by specific motor control goals: acquisition of *mobility*, *stability*, and *controlled mobility* functions. Patient outcomes consistent with the *Guide to Physical Therapist Practice*[1] are described together with clinical applications and patient examples.

Interventions to Improve Control in Bed Skills

Bed skills involve rolling from supine to sidelying or prone positions, moving in bed (scooting), and moving from supine to sit and sit to supine. Normal adults utilize a variety of strategies and patterns to roll, all characterized by smooth transitions between postures. Patients with neurological involvement or extensive weakness (e.g., musculoskeletal trauma) often demonstrate difficulty with transitions and antigravity control.

Rolling

General Characteristics

Rolling is typically begun from supine, which provides a large base of support (BOS) and low center of mass (COM). Thus, the initial posture is very stable. Supine weightbearing occurs through large body segments with minimal antigravity control requirements. Transitions from supine to sidelying are minimally *resisted* by gravity, and transitions from sidelying to prone are minimally *assisted* by gravity.

Rolling allows for positional changes in bed. The movement pattern typically requires a rotatory component of the trunk combined with movements of the upper and/or lower extremities (UEs/LEs). Most individuals roll using a segmental rolling pattern characterized by the shoulder/upper trunk segment leading the activity while the pelvis/lower trunk segment follows, or vice versa. In contrast, some individuals use a logrolling pattern with the trunk rolling as a whole (both shoulders/upper trunk and pelvis/lower trunk

move together). Head/neck motions are typically combined with upper trunk rotation as normal components of movement. Head/neck rotation with flexion and upper trunk rotation assist in rolling from supine to sidelying, while head/neck rotation with extension and upper trunk rotation assist in transitions from prone to sidelying. Patterns may vary based on the direction of rolling, general fitness level, body weight, and level of motor control. Patients with neurological involvement and activity limitations often demonstrate difficulty with initiating the rolling movement and moving smoothly through the full range.

In the presence of trunk weakness, rolling can be assisted by movements of the limbs and momentum to propel the body through the roll. Common strategies for generating momentum include lifting the upper or LEs up and across the body in the direction of the roll movement (e.g., for rolling to the right, the left UE and/or left LE is lifted up and across the midline of body to the right). An alternative strategy involves positioning one LE in approximately 60 degrees of hip and knee flexion with the foot flat on supporting surface (a modified hooklying position) to push the body into sidelying and then further into prone. This is referred to as a *modified* hooklying position because only one LE is flexed; normal hooklying involves bilateral hip and knee flexion to approximately 60 degrees from a supine position. From prone to supine, shoulder abduction and elbow flexion with a fisted or open hand placed on the mat can be used to help push the body into sidelying.

Clinical Note: Normal postural reactions contribute to rolling. Patients who present with excessive (hyperactive) symmetrical or asymmetrical tonic reflex activity (Box 3.1) coupled with excess tone may demonstrate difficulty with rolling and, in particular, segmental trunk patterns. Normal postural reactions that contribute to rolling in young children include body-on-body righting reactions and neck righting reactions; these are normally integrated in the postural responses of healthy adults. In addition, supine or prone positions may be difficult or contraindicated for patients with cardiopulmonary involvement such as chronic obstructive pulmonary disease (COPD) or congestive heart failure (CHF) or with recent surgical procedures involving the trunk.

BOX 3.1 Tonic Reflexes: Impact on the Acquisition of Functional Rolling

Symmetrical tonic labyrinthine reflex (STLR): The STLR causes fluctuations in tone in infants and some patients with brain injury that are influenced by *body position* (prone versus supine). In the prone position, there is an increase in flexor tone; in supine, there is increased extensor tone. Excess extension or flexion tone impedes rolling motions. The therapist may consider initial sidelying rolling to eliminate prone or supine reflex influences.

Asymmetrical tonic neck reflex (ATNR): The ATNR causes fluctuations in tone in infants and some patients with brain injury that are influenced by *right or left neck rotation*. Rotation of the neck to one side results in extension of the UE on the side the head is rotated toward (chin side) and flexion of the opposite UE (skull side). The extended UE position that accompanies head turning to that side effectively blocks rolling. Normal head/neck (neutral) alignment should be maintained and the patient prevented from turning the head toward the side of the roll.

Symmetrical tonic neck reflex (STNR): The STNR causes fluctuations in tone in infants and some patients with brain injury that are influenced by *flexion or extension of the head/neck*. Head/neck flexion produces flexion of the UEs and extension of the LEs; extension of the head/neck causes extension of the UEs and flexion of the LEs. Normal head/neck (neutral) alignment should be maintained, and strategies to promote rolling that involve head/neck flexion or extension should be avoided.

Treatment Strategies and Considerations to Improve Rolling

- Interventions to improve rolling may begin in supine or sidelying (see the following section) and progress from small ranges to larger ranges (increments in range of motion [ROM]), and finally to full ROM—for example, from a sidelying position, rolling first one-quarter turn forward, then backward, to one-half turns, to a full turn moving from sidelying to supine, or to prone.
- Limb movements and momentum can be used to assist rolling when trunk muscles are weak.
  - UEs or LEs or both can flex up and across the body to facilitate rolling from supine to sidelying position.
  - The addition of weights to the UEs (wrist cuffs) can assist in developing momentum to facilitate movement (Fig. 3.1). For example, patients with complete tetraplegia or high-level paraplegia often benefit from the use of cuff weights when initially learning momentum strategies for rolling. The patient is instructed to swing the UEs up and across the body. The UEs are swung several times across the body to create momentum, and on the count of three, the roll is initiated. Momentum is key; the slower the movement, the greater the effort required to roll. Progression is from heavier cuff weights (3 pounds [1.36 kg]) to lighter weights (e.g., 1 to 2 pounds [0.45 to 0.90 kg]) to finally no weights.

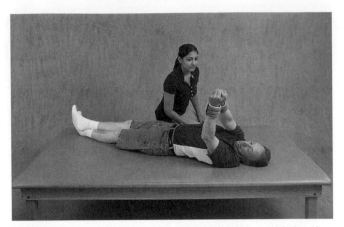

FIGURE 3.1 Weights (wrist cuffs) can be used to assist development of momentum during initial rolling.

- Prepositioning the limbs (before movement begins) can also be used to promote rolling.
  - UEs: From sidelying or supine, the lowermost UE (the one closest to the direction of the roll) can be flexed overhead to avoid getting it "trapped" under the body; if shoulder ROM is limited, the shoulder may be adducted and the hand tucked under the hips close to the body.
  - LEs:
    - Prepositioning the LEs with the ankles crossed (described below) or positioning the hips on a pillow creating a one-quarter turn is a useful initial strategy. As the patient progresses, the pillow can be removed and the LEs uncrossed.
    - From supine, the uppermost LE, or the one opposite the direction of the roll (e.g., the right LE if rolling toward the left), can be positioned in modified hooklying position (Fig. 3.2) to initially propel the roll (e.g., the patient with stroke). This LE positioning can also be used for rolling from a sidelying position. Alternatively, from a supine position, the LE can be extended with the foot crossed over the other (e.g., the patient with tetraplegia). When one foot is crossed over the other, the uppermost foot is placed in the direction of

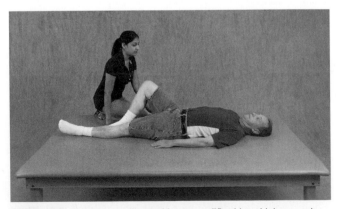

FIGURE 3.2 Patient positioned in a modified hooklying position. The right LE is in approximately 60 degrees of hip and knee flexion with the foot flat on the supporting surface in preparation for rolling to the left.

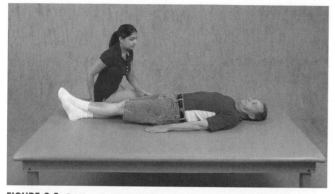

FIGURE 3.3 Patient positioned in supine with the knees extended and the left foot crossed over the right in preparation for rolling toward the right.

the roll (Fig. 3.3). For example, in rolling toward the right, the left foot is crossed over the right.

- The therapist's position and movements should not restrict or limit the patient's ease of movement. The therapist is positioned behind or in front of the patient to assist movements as needed. Patients with communication deficits (e.g., aphasia) or those who depend heavily on visual or verbal cueing benefit from being able to see the therapist positioned in front.

- Optimal use of momentum will decrease the effort required to accomplish the roll.

- The therapist should provide instructions and verbal cueing to focus the patient's attention on key task elements and improve overall awareness of task demands. Examples of instructions follow.

  - *"On the count of three, I want you to lift your head and shoulder up and over toward me and roll onto your side. One, two, three."*

  - *"On the count of three, I want you to lift your arm (or leg) up and over toward me and roll onto your side. One, two, three."*

  - *"On the count of three, I want you to push down on your foot (from modified hooklying) and lift your arm up and over toward me and roll onto your side. One, two, three."*

Clinical Note: Patients recovering from stroke will require practice in rolling to both sides: over onto the *more affected side* and over onto the *less affected side* (the more difficult activity). The more involved UE can be effectively supported to keep the shoulder forward by having the patient clasp the hands together with fingers intertwined, both elbows extended, and shoulders flexed (hands-clasped position).

Rolling: Prerequisite Requirements

Because rolling often serves as the initial start point of interventions to improve function for patients with significant motor deficits, prerequisite requirements are not extensive. Although not considered a lead-up activity, initiation of rolling requires functional ROM in the proximal and intermediate joints (e.g., spine, neck, shoulder, elbows, pelvis/hip, and knees). Thus, the focus of early interventions is on acquisition of initial mobility

and development of component skills that will later become parts of larger functional tasks. Application of Proprioceptive Neuromuscular Facilitation (PNF) extremity patterns to assist rolling also carries the prerequisite requirement of functional ROM.

Task Analysis Guidelines

Task analysis informs the therapist about the link between abnormal movement (patient-selected movement strategies) and underlying impairments. The information helps identify the need for additional examination procedures and directs and guides selection of intervention strategies. Critical to performing a task analysis is knowledge of normal movement and the ability to deconstruct a task into its component skills.

An analysis of rolling requires the therapist to address questions related to understanding *the task of rolling, characteristics of the individual patient*, and *the impact of the environment* on motor control strategies. Inherent to each of these components of task analysis are questions to be

---

BOX 3.2 Rolling: Components of Task Analysis

Understanding the Task of Rolling: Questions to Consider/Answer
- What individual component skills are needed to accomplish rolling in an intact subject?
- How is rolling *initiated* (initial conditions, start position, quality of initiation, alignment), *executed* (musculoskeletal requirements; timing, force, direction of movement), and *terminated*?
- What motor control strategies are required for rolling (i.e., mobility, stability [static postural control], and dynamic balance [dynamic postural control])?

Characteristics of the Individual Patient: Questions to Consider/Answer
- What impairments exist (i.e., any loss or abnormality of anatomical, physiological, mental, or psychological structure or function[1])?
- Do underlying impairments constrain or diminish the quality of movement?
- Can the task be completed?
- How does the patient initiate, execute, and terminate rolling?
- What movement components are normal or close to normal?
- What movement components are abnormal, missing, or delayed?
- If abnormal, are the movement's components compensatory (using the uninvolved or less involved segments) or functional (reacquiring skill and enhancing recovery of involved segments)?

Impact of the Environment: Questions to Consider/Answer
- How does the environment affect the selection of movement strategies?
- What features of the environment constrain or promote movement?
- Can adaptations be made to change environmental demands (e.g., closed *versus* open environment)?

considered and answered by the therapist (Box 3.2). Task analysis further informs development of the physical therapy plan of care (POC). See Box 3.3 Student Practice Activity to guide the task analysis of rolling.

Rolling: Interventions, Outcomes, and Management Strategies

Position and Activity: Rolling Into Sidelying on Elbow Position

From supine, the patient turns and lifts the head and trunk up, moving into the sidelying on elbow position. The therapist can promote elevation and rotation of the upper trunk by manually assisting the trunk using both hands on the patient's upper trunk under the axillae (Fig. 3.4). The patient's lowermost UE is prepositioned with the elbow in 90 degrees of flexion. The patient's uppermost UE is prepositioned with the elbow extended and the hand placed on the therapist's shoulder for support. This positioning helps guide movement and further promote upper trunk rotation.

> **Clinical Note:** Patients recovering from stroke may tilt or slump laterally toward the more involved side when sitting in a chair or may demonstrate spasticity in the trunk. This contributes to a loss of trunk flexibility and poor sitting posture. Rolling into the sidelying on elbow position is an important activity to promote early weight-bearing on the more involved elbow and shoulder with same-side elongation of the trunk.

Position and Activity: Sidelying, Logrolling, and Segmental Rolling

The patient is positioned in sidelying with the LEs extended in midposition or in slight flexion; the UEs are positioned to avoid interference with the roll. The patient's UEs may be flexed bilaterally at the shoulder and positioned overhead (Fig. 3.5). Alternatively, the upper limbs may be placed asymmetrically, with the lowermost flexed overhead and the uppermost at the side of the trunk, with the hand resting on the pelvis. The therapist is positioned in front or behind the patient. During *logrolling,* the upper trunk/shoulder moves

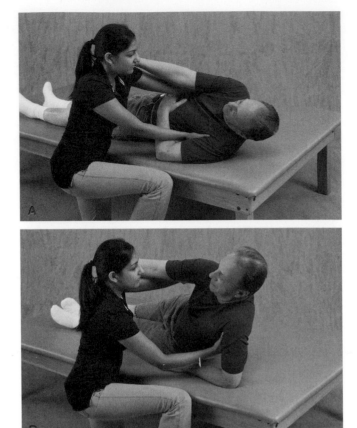

FIGURE 3.4 Therapist manually assists patient into the sidelying on elbow position. **(A)** The patient turns and begins to lift the head and upper trunk. Note that the left UE (closest to the mat) is prepositioned in approximately 90 degrees of elbow flexion. **(B)** The patient then brings the elbow under the shoulder into a weightbearing position.

BOX 3.3 STUDENT PRACTICE ACTIVITY: ROLLING TASK ANALYSIS

OBJECTIVE: To analyze rolling movements of healthy individuals.

PROCEDURE: Work in groups of two or three. Begin by having each person in the group roll on the mat from supine to prone and prone to supine several times in a row at normal speeds. Then have each person slow the movement down and speed the movement up, rolling in each direction.

OBSERVE AND DOCUMENT: Using the following questions to guide your analysis, observe and record the variations and similarities among the different rolling patterns represented in your group.

▲ How and where is the movement initiated? Terminated?

▲ How is the movement executed?
  • Segmental roll pattern? Log roll pattern? Other?
  • Role of the trunk?
  • Use of extremity movements?
  • Is the pattern changed (or altered) with change of direction?
  • Is the pattern changed (or altered) with change of speed?
▲ How does rolling differ among the group members?
▲ What types of pathology/impairments might affect a patient's ability to roll?
▲ What compensatory strategies might be necessary?
▲ What environmental factors might constrain or impair rolling movements?
▲ What modifications are needed?

as one unit together with the lower trunk/pelvis (see Fig. 3.5). During *segmental rolling,* the upper trunk/shoulder moves first, followed by the lower trunk/pelvis, or vice versa (Fig. 3.6).

TECHNIQUES AND VERBAL CUES (TO IMPROVE TRUNK CONTROL AND ROLLING)

Rhythmic Initiation Rhythmic initiation can be used to instruct the patient in the desired movement, to facilitate the initiation of movement, and to promote relaxation. Movements are first passive, then active-assistive, and then appropriately resisted (passive → active-assistive → resisted).[2] Finally, the patient performs the movement independently. Progression to each phase of movement is dependent on the patient's ability to relax and participate in the movements.

For the application of rhythmic initiation in sidelying, the therapist is heel-sitting behind the patient (Fig. 3.7). Manual contacts are on the trunk (under the axilla and on the pelvis). The patient is instructed to relax. The therapist first moves the patient passively through the desired movement, rolling either toward supine or toward prone and back into sidelying. The patient is then instructed to begin active participation in the movement while the therapist assists

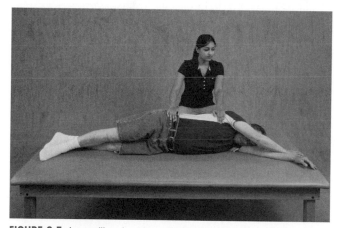

FIGURE 3.5 Logrolling involves the shoulder/upper trunk and pelvis/lower trunk body segments moving together as a whole unit.

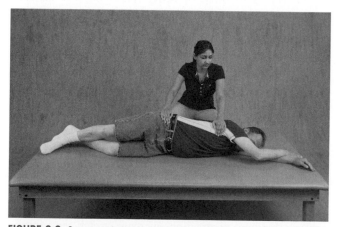

FIGURE 3.6 Segmental rolling is characterized by either upper trunk/shoulder leading (as shown here) or lower trunk/pelvis leading; the opposite segment follows.

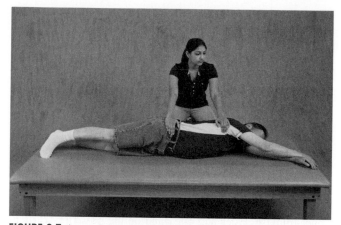

FIGURE 3.7 Logrolling using rhythmic initiation with manual contacts under the axilla and on the pelvis. Movements are first passive, next active-assistive, and then resisted (using graded increments of appropriate levels of resistance).

(active-assistive movement) and continues to provide passive return to sidelying. This sequence is repeated with gradual increments of appropriate levels of resistance (typically beginning with light facilitative resistance). If necessary, quick stretch can be used to facilitate the initiation of movement in the desired direction.

Verbal Cues for Rhythmic Initiation in Sidelying
Verbal cues (VCs) are timed with passive movements: *"Relax, let me move you back (patient is moved toward supine) and forward (return to sidelying)"* or *"Relax, let me move you forward (toward prone) and back (return to sidelying)."* VCs are timed with active-assistive movements: *"Now move forward (or backward) with me, and let me bring you back (to sidelying)."* VCs are timed with resisted movements: *"Now pull forward (or push backward) while I resist, and let me move you back."* VCs should be soothing, slow, rhythmic, and well timed with movements. Resistance is used to facilitate muscle contraction. If optional quick stretches are used to promote movement, they should be well timed with VCs. To avoid dependence on external stimuli, quick stretches should be used only if required to improve motor output.

Clinical Note: Slow sidelying passive rolling (rocking) movements provide slow vestibular input that promotes relaxation, which is beneficial for patients with spasticity or rigidity. Rhythmic initiation is also a valuable technique for the patient with stroke who is unable to initiate rolling (apraxia) and for the patient who demonstrates impaired cognition and motor learning (e.g., traumatic brain injury [TBI]). The initial passive and active-assisted movements also assist in teaching the patient the desired movement.

Dynamic Reversals Dynamic reversals promote active concentric movement in one direction followed by active concentric movement in the reverse direction without relaxation.[2] The technique involves continuous resisted movement in opposing directions, with VCs used to mark the initiation of movement in the opposite direction (continuous movement ↔ resistance ↔ VCs). Resistance is typically applied first in the stronger direction of movement. Dynamic reversals are used to increase strength and active ROM as well as to promote normal transitions between opposing muscle groups. A smooth reversal of motion is the goal.

For using dynamic reversals in sidelying, the therapist is heel-sitting behind the patient. Manual contacts for application of resistance are selected to allow smooth transitions between opposing directions of movement. For example, using dynamic reversals in sidelying for a patient with stronger trunk extensors, the therapist first places one hand on the posterior upper trunk/shoulder and one hand on the posterior pelvis to resist extension (movement toward supine) (Fig. 3.8). The therapist's hands then move (hand contact is maintained) to the anterior upper trunk/shoulder and anterior pelvis.

Verbal Cues for Dynamic Reversals in Sidelying

"Pull forward" (the patient is moving toward prone); *"now push back"* (the patient is moving toward supine). When the patient is ready to move in the new direction, a preparatory cue of *"Now, reverse"* is used to direct the patient's attention to the new movement. At the same time as the VC to change directions, the therapist repositions the hands to resist the new direction of motion. If a hold (isometric contraction) is added to dynamic reversals, the VC is *"Pull forward and hold; and now reverse, push back and hold."*

Comments

- Movements begin with small-range control (e.g., one-quarter turn forward to one-quarter turn backward) and progress through increasing ROM (increments of ROM) to full-range control (from full prone to full supine position).

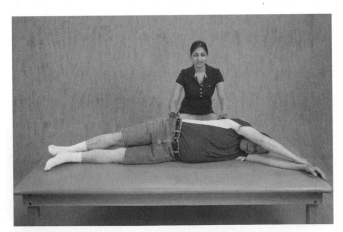

FIGURE 3.8 Application of dynamic reversals in sidelying. Continuous resistance is applied to active concentric movement in both directions (toward prone *and* toward supine) without relaxation. In this example, manual contacts are on the posterior upper trunk/shoulder and the posterior pelvis to resist movement toward supine (manual contacts are then positioned on the opposite surfaces to resist movement toward prone).

- Initially, movements are slow and controlled with emphasis on careful grading of resistance; progression is to increase speed of movement while maintaining control.
- An isometric hold may be added in the shortened range or at any point of weakness within the range. The hold is a momentary pause for one count (the patient is instructed to *"Hold"*); the antagonist movement pattern is then facilitated. The hold can be added in one direction only or in both directions.
- Careful attention must be directed to providing the patient a preparatory VC (such as *"Now, reverse"*) to indicate that a change in movement direction is about to take place.

Indications Dynamic reversals using carefully controlled VCs and manual resistance can be used to improve coordination and timing (e.g., patients with ataxia) and increase strength and active ROM.

Replication Replication is a unidirectional technique, emphasizing movement in one direction.[2] It is used to teach the end result of a movement as well as to improve coordination and control. The patient is passively moved to the end of the desired motion or available range (agonists are in shortened range) and asked to hold against resistance (isometric contraction); the patient then relaxes and is moved passively through a small range in the opposite direction; and finally the patient actively returns (concentric contraction) to the initial end range position. Movement is through increments of range until full range is achieved (passive movement to end range → active hold against resistance → relaxation → passive movement in opposite direction → active return to initial end range).

For using replication to promote rolling, the therapist is positioned in heel-sitting behind the patient. Depending on the direction of movement, hand placements are on either the *anterior* or *posterior* surface of the upper trunk/shoulder and lower trunk/pelvis. From a neutral sidelying position (start position), the patient is passively moved forward (toward prone) through one-quarter of range (shortened range for abdominals) and asked to hold the position against resistance for several counts. This is followed by active relaxation. The therapist then passively moves the trunk backward (toward supine) one-quarter of the range past neutral and asks the patient to contract actively through the range back to the original start position (Fig. 3.9).

Verbal Cues for Replication in Sidelying

"Let me move you (forward or backward), now hold this position, don't let me move you, hold, hold, hold. Now relax and let me move you (forward or backward). Now pull/push (forward or backward) to the starting position."

Comments

- Resistance to the isometric hold is built up gradually; isometric (holding) contractions increase stretch sensitivity (gamma bias) and enhance muscle response to stretch.

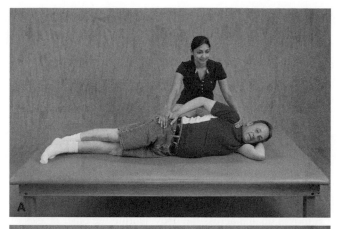

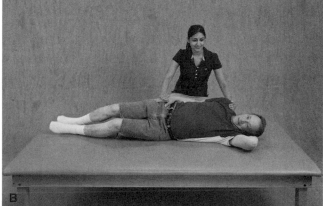

FIGURE 3.9 Application of replication to rolling in sidelying position. **(A)** The patient is passively moved forward (toward prone) through a partial ROM (e.g., one-quarter of range) and asked to hold; this is followed by active relaxation. **(B)** The therapist then passively moves the trunk backward (toward supine) one-quarter of the range past neutral. *Not shown:* Finally, the patient actively returns to the original starting position. Note the alternative positioning of the patient's UEs. The lowermost UE (left) is flexed at the shoulder and elbow and supports the head. The uppermost UE (right) is resting on the trunk with the distal segment fixed by the therapist (this is particularly useful for patients with significant loss of UE control).

- Active relaxation is important; the patient should not be passively moved in the opposite direction until the contraction is completely released (relaxation is achieved).
- If needed, a quick stretch can be applied in the lengthened range to facilitate the return movement.
- With successive replication of movement, the range is gradually increased until full range is accomplished.
- Replication is a unidirectional technique, emphasizing movement in one direction. The hold is built up slowly over several counts. The patient is moved back through the range once relaxation is achieved.

Indications Sidelying promotes rolling in the presence of muscle weakness and hypotonia and instructs the patient in the end result (outcome) of the movement.

Position and Activity: Rolling, Application of PNF Extremity Patterns
TECHNIQUES AND VERBAL CUES (TO IMPROVE TRUNK CONTROL AND ROLLING)
Upper Extremity Flexion/Adduction/External Rotation Pattern; Diagonal 1 Flexion (UE D1F), Rhythmic Initiation Application of the UE D1F pattern to rolling assumes the prerequisite requirement of UE function. This technique utilizes overflow of stronger limb movements to weaker trunk muscles. The patient is positioned in supine or one-quarter turn toward sidelying using a pillow for support. The LE is in a modified hooklying position, with one foot flat on the support surface. The therapist is heel-sitting or positioned in half-kneeling at the side of the patient's trunk. One of the therapist's hands assists (initial learning) or resists the UE pattern; the other hand is on the posterior trunk and helps the patient roll onto the sidelying position (Fig. 3.10). In order to provide assistance with the roll, these manual contacts represent a modification of typical hand placements used for the application of UE D1F (typically on the palmar surface of the patient's hand and the radial side of the distal forearm).

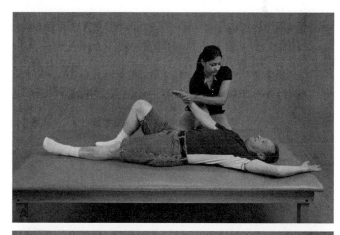

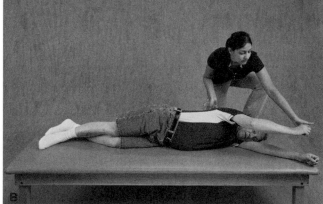

FIGURE 3.10 Application of upper extremity D1F pattern to rolling from supine to sidelying using rhythmic initiation. **(A)** Approaching midrange of pattern; note that the patient is in a modified hooklying position to push into the roll using the right LE. The left shoulder is abducted overhead with the limb resting on the mat to prevent interference with rolling movement. **(B)** End range of pattern; note that in this example, UE D1F hand placements are modified to provide assistance with the roll.

With rhythmic initiation, movements are first passive, then active-assistive, and finally resisted (passive → active-assistive → resisted). The therapist provides the return motion. Progression to each phase of movement is dependent on the patient's ability to relax and participate in the movements (recruit motor unit activity). Movement can also be resisted using dynamic reversals.

Verbal Cues for UE D1F Pattern, Rhythmic Initiation in Sidelying

Passive phase: *"Relax, let me move your arm up and across your face. Turn your head and watch your hand."* Active-assistive phase: *"Now begin moving with me, up and across. I will bring you back."* Resistive phase: *"Continue to move as I resist, pull up and across, and let me bring you back."* Finally, the patient is asked to move independently: *"Now, pull up and across on your own and roll onto your side."*

Clinical Note: The suggested VCs provided in this and later chapters should be used to guide and organize your thoughts when instructing a patient. VCs should be *concise, straightforward,* and *direct.* In clinical practice, VCs often require carefully guided repetition, modification, and expansion to ensure patient understanding and achieve optimal outcomes.

Comments

- The patient is instructed to turn the head and follow the hand with the eyes. Having the patient watch the movement promotes the use of visual sensory cues to improve movement control and promotes involvement of the head and neck in the overall movement of rolling. Watching the movement also prevents the limb from covering the mouth and nose as it moves up and across the face.
- Rhythmic initiation is ideal for initial motor learning of PNF extremity patterns. As the patient achieves some control, a progression is made from active-assistive to resisted movement, with the end result being independent movement.

Clinical Note: Neck flexion and extension patterns with rotation can also be used to promote rolling. From a sidelying (or supine) position, neck flexion and rotation is used to facilitate rolling toward prone. From a sidelying (or prone) position, neck extension and rotation is used to roll toward supine.

Red Flag: For the application to neck flexion and extension patterns, manual contacts and application of resistance must be used carefully and accurately and avoided when the symmetrical tonic neck reflex (STNR) influences tonal changes.

Lower Extremity Flexion/Adduction/External Rotation Pattern; D1 Flexion (LE D1F), Rhythmic Initiation

Application of the LE D1F pattern to rolling assumes functional ROM of the LE. The patient's LE is positioned in hip extension and abduction with the knee extended. If difficulty is

experienced initiating movement from this position, the hip and knee may be flexed slightly with the knee supported by the therapist's distal thigh (Fig. 3.11A); the hip remains abducted. The patient's UEs may be placed in shoulder flexion with elbows extended and hands clasped together. The therapist's position transitions from initial heel-sitting to the side of the patient's moving LE to half-kneeling behind the patient's moving pelvis/thigh during movement into sidelying (Fig. 3.11B). Movements are first passive, then active-assistive, and finally resisted. The therapist provides the return motion. For the resistive phase of rhythmic initiation, manual contacts are on the dorsal/medial foot and the anterior/medial thigh; resistance is applied to both the thigh and the foot as the LE moves up and across the body. During the other phases of rhythmic initiation, manual contacts provide passive and assistive movement.

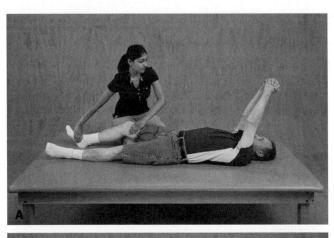

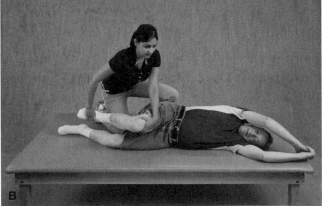

FIGURE 3.11 Application of lower extremity D1F pattern to rolling from supine to sidelying using rhythmic initiation (resistive phase). **(A)** Starting position; note modification of LE positioning using slight hip and knee flexion with the limb resting on the therapist's distal thigh to assist with the initiation of movement. **(B)** Approaching end range of pattern; note that manual contacts are positioned for the resistance phase of rhythmic initiation. During the other phases, manual contacts are positioned to provide passive and assisted movement.

Verbal Cues for LE D1F Pattern Rolling From Supine to Sidelying, Rhythmic Initiation Passive phase: *"Relax; let me move your leg up and across."* Active-assistive phase: *"Now move with me; lift your leg up and across. Let me bring you back."* Resistive phase: *"Continue to move as I resist; pull your leg up and across. Let me bring you back."* Finally, the patient is asked to move independently: *"Now, pull your leg up and across on your own and roll onto your side."*

Comments

• Quick (phasic) stretch can be applied to facilitate movement.
• Joint receptors are activated through the application of traction (in combination with resistance) during initial movement within the pattern.

Note: Rolling can also be promoted with simultaneous use of UE and LE D1F patterns. This combination assumes functional ROM and strength of the extremities on one side. In the simultaneous application of UE and LE D1F patterns, both the UE and the LE move together up and across the body. The therapist can assist or resist one extremity while the other extremity moves actively. Alternatively, the patient can be taught to move both limbs actively up and across the body. Note that the therapist's position transitions from heel-sitting to the side of the patient's pelvis/thigh to half-kneeling behind the patient's pelvis/thigh with movement into sidelying. Alternatively, the therapist can maintain the half-kneeling position throughout.

Reverse Chop (Chopping), Rhythmic Initiation

The reverse chop is a bilateral asymmetrical UE pattern that can also be used to promote rolling. It combines neck and upper trunk extension with rotation. Use of this pattern assumes functional strength of one UE (lead limb). Movement progresses from passive, to active-assistive, to resisted, and finally to independent. The patient is positioned in supine. The therapist's position transitions from initial heel-sitting (or squatting) to half-kneeling next to the patient's trunk on the side opposite the roll (alternatively, half-kneeling may be maintained throughout). Application of reverse chop for rolling from supine toward the left into sidelying involves the lead (right) UE moving in D1F; the patient's left hand grasps the top of the wrist of the lead limb. Initially, manual contacts are only on the forearm of the lead UE (Fig. 3.12A). As movement progresses, hand placement on the lead forearm remains and the opposite hand is placed on the posterior upper trunk (scapular region) (Fig. 3.12B). The therapist holds the right forearm (an open-handed, not tight, grasp should be used to allow rotation through the pattern) as it moves up and across the body in D1F; the therapist's other hand helps the patient roll to the left by assisting the trunk in the scapular region. The patient rolls to the sidelying position (see Fig. 3.12B).

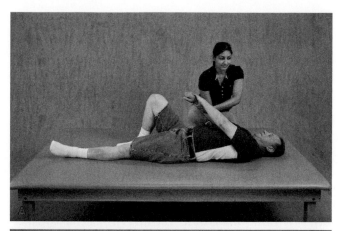

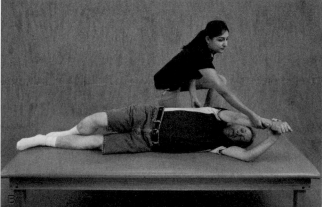

FIGURE 3.12 Reverse chop to facilitate rolling to the left from supine to sidelying. **(A)** Start position; note that the right LE is initially positioned in approximately 60 degrees of hip and knee flexion (modified hooklying) with foot flat on the mat to assist the roll. Although obscured in the photograph, the therapist's initial hand placements are on the patient's right forearm. **(B)** End position; note that the therapist's position has transitioned to half-kneeling. An alternative therapist positioning is to maintain half-kneeling throughout.

Verbal Cues for Reverse Chop Pattern Rolling From Supine to Sidelying, Rhythmic Initiation Passive phase: *"Relax; let me move your arms up and across your face."* Active-assistive phase: *"Now begin to move with me, pull up and across. I will bring you back."* Resistive phase: *"Continue to move as I resist; pull up and across. Let me move you back."* The patient is then asked to move independently: *"Now, turn your head. Pull up and across on your own and roll onto your side."*

Note: If the modified hooklying position is used to facilitate early rolling (with foot flat on mat to push into the roll), a verbal cue should be added—for example, *"Now turn your head, pull your arms up and across your face,* **push down with your foot,** *and roll onto your side."*

Comments

• To further promote rolling, the LE (on the side of the lead limb) can be flexed at the hip and knee with the foot flat on the mat (modified hooklying position [see Fig. 3.12A]), or it can actively move in a D1F pattern.

- Timing for emphasis may be used to facilitate movement by using stronger components of a pattern to facilitate weaker ones. A maximal contraction is elicited from stronger components of a movement to allow irradiation from stronger components to facilitate weaker components.
- Active-assistive and resistive movements occur in only one direction; movements in the opposite direction are passive.
- The reverse chop pattern increases the amount of upper trunk rotation that occurs with rolling as compared to unilateral limb patterns; this results from closing of the kinematic chain.

Lift, Rhythmic Initiation The lift is a bilateral asymmetrical UE pattern that combines UE flexion and neck and upper trunk extension with rotation. Movement progresses from passive, to active-assistive, to resisted, and finally to independent. The patient is supine. To begin, the therapist is heel-sitting next to the patient's trunk on the side of the roll (Fig. 3.13A); toward the end of the roll, the therapist may transition to a half-kneeling position to allow the UE to move through full range (Fig. 3.13B). Alternatively, the

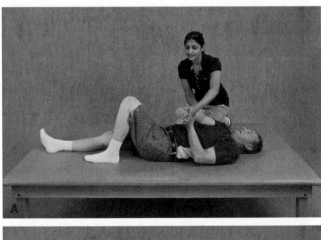

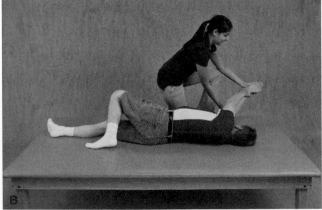

FIGURE 3.13 Lift pattern to facilitate rolling to the right from supine to sidelying using rhythmic initiation. **(A)** Beginning range of pattern; a modified hooklying position is used to assist the roll. **(B)** Ending range of pattern; the shoulders are flexed, and the neck and upper trunk are extending and rotating. Movement progresses from passive, to active-assistive, to resisted, and finally to independent.

therapist may assume half-kneeling throughout. Application of the lift for rolling from supine toward the right into sidelying involves the lead (right) UE moving in D2F; the patient's left hand grasps underneath the wrist of the lead limb. The therapist's manual contacts are on the right (lead) UE; one hand grasps the patient's hand (dorsal surface) while the other is positioned on the forearm. An open-handed (not a tight grasp) manual contact on the lead UE should be used to allow rotation through the pattern. Using rhythmic initiation, movements are first passive, then active-assistive, and lastly resisted.

Verbal Cues for Lift Pattern Rolling From Supine to Sidelying, Rhythmic Initiation Passive phase: *"Relax; let me move your arms up and toward me."* Active-assistive phase: *"Now begin to move with me, up and toward me. Let me move you back."* Resistive phase: *"Start to move against my resistance, lift up and toward me. Let me move you back."* Lastly, the patient is asked to move independently: *"Now, by yourself, turn your head, lift your arms up and toward me, and roll onto your left (or right) side."*

Comments
- To further promote rolling, the LE (opposite the lead limb) can be flexed at the hip and knee with the foot flat on the mat (modified hooklying position), or it can actively move in a D1F pattern.
- Active-assistive and resistive movements occur in only one direction; movements in the opposite direction are passive.
- The pattern represents a closed kinematic chain.

Clinical Note: Stronger extremity movements are used to assist rolling in the presence of weak trunk muscles. Irradiation from stronger limb movements facilitates weaker trunk muscle components.

Outcomes
Motor control goal: Mobility progressing to controlled mobility.
Functional skill achieved: The patient is able to roll independently from supine to prone position.

Indications Rolling is of functional significance for improved bed mobility, preparation for independent positional changes in bed (e.g., pressure relief), and as a lead-up (component skill) for LE dressing and independent transfers from supine to sitting. Rolling promotes the development of functional movement patterns (e.g., coordination of extremity and trunk movement) and is a frequent starting point of mat activities for patients with significant neurological (e.g., the patient with stroke or high-level spinal cord lesion) or musculoskeletal (e.g., motor vehicle accident or trauma) involvement. Although activities are typically initiated on a platform mat, rolling must also be mastered on the surface of a bed similar to the one the patient will use at home. See Box 3.4 Section Summary Student Practice Activity addressing treatment interventions to improve rolling.

BOX 3.4 SECTION SUMMARY STUDENT PRACTICE ACTIVITY: ROLLING

Preface to Student Practice Activity

When first learning the strategies to promote function included in this text, one's initial reaction might be that these approaches are too time consuming to use in a clinical setting. This notion should be cautiously considered. It speaks directly to the importance of careful understanding and mastery of the content. Once skill in the application and knowledge of these interventions is achieved, their use is generally no more time consuming than many other types of therapeutic interventions. An important consideration is that these interventions provide a rich source of treatment ideas. For example, after the first section of this chapter has been read, multiple treatment ideas should be available for addressing the needs of patients whose ability to roll is impaired. Sound clinical decision-making will guide identification of the most appropriate activities and techniques for an individual patient.

Another consideration is the foundation that these interventions provide for developing home management strategies to improve function. Although portions of the interventions described clearly require the skilled intervention of a physical therapist, many others can be modified or adapted for inclusion in a home exercise program (HEP) for use by the patient (self-management strategies), family members, or other individuals participating in the patient's care.

Description of Student Practice Activity

Each section of this chapter ends with a similarly challenging student practice activity titled *Section Summary Student Practice Activity (followed by the section title)*. A section outline for rolling to guide the activity is provided that highlights the key treatment strategies, techniques, and activities addressed in the preceding section. This activity is an opportunity to share knowledge and skills as well as to confirm or clarify understanding of the treatment interventions. Each student in a group will contribute his or her understanding of, or questions about, the strategy, technique, or activity being discussed and demonstrated. Dialogue should continue until a consensus of understanding is reached. (***Note:*** **These directions will be repeated for each subsequent section summary student practice activity, in the event that content is considered in a sequence different from that presented here.)**

Section Outline: Rolling

ACTIVITIES AND TECHNIQUES
- Sidelying, logrolling, using rhythmic initiation
- Sidelying, rolling using dynamic reversals
- Sidelying, rolling using replication
- Supine to sidelying rolling using UE D1F pattern and rhythmic initiation
- Supine to sidelying rolling using LE D1F pattern and rhythmic initiation
- Supine to sidelying rolling using reverse chop and rhythmic initiation
- Supine to sidelying rolling using lift pattern and rhythmic initiation

OBJECTIVE: Sharing skill in application and knowledge of strategies to promote improved rolling.

EQUIPMENT NEEDED: Platform mat.

DIRECTIONS: Working in groups of four to six students, consider each entry in the section outline. Members of the group will assume different roles (described below) and will rotate roles each time the group progresses to a new item on the outline.
- One person assumes the role of therapist (for demonstrations) and participates in discussion.
- One person serves as the subject/patient (for demonstrations) and participates in discussion.
- The remaining members participate in discussion and provide supportive feedback during demonstrations. One member of this group should be designated as a "fact checker" to return to the text content to confirm elements of the discussion (if needed) or if agreement cannot be reached.

Thinking aloud, brainstorming, and sharing thoughts should be continuous throughout this activity! As each item in the section outline is considered, the following should ensue:

1. An initial discussion of the *activity,* including patient and therapist positioning. Also considered here should be positional changes to enhance the activity (e.g., prepositioning a limb, hand placements to alter the BOS, and so forth).
2. An initial discussion of the *technique,* including its description, indication(s) for use, therapist hand placements (manual contacts), and VCs.
3. A *demonstration* of the activity and application of the technique by the designated therapist and subject/patient. Discussion during the demonstration should be continuous (the demonstration should not be the sole responsibility of the designated therapist and subject/patient). All group members should provide recommendations, suggestions, and supportive feedback throughout the demonstration. Particularly important during the demonstrations is discussion of strategies to make the activity either *more* or *less* challenging.
4. If any member of the group feels he or she requires practice with the activity and technique, time should be allocated to accommodate the request. All group members providing input (recommendations, suggestions, and supportive feedback) should also accompany this practice.

Sidelying

General Characteristics

The BOS in sidelying is large and the COM is low, making it a very stable posture; no upright postural control is required. The BOS may be increased by flexing either the lowermost or uppermost extremities (Fig. 3.14); in contrast, keeping the extremities extended reduces the BOS. Tonic reflex (symmetrical tonic labyrinthine reflex [STLR] and asymmetrical tonic neck reflex [ATNR]) activity and related muscle tone are reduced in sidelying. The posture may be used to promote the initiation of movement, increase ROM, promote trunk flexion or extension (stability), and encourage trunk rotation patterns in patients who lack upright (antigravity) control (e.g., weakness or disordered motor control).

Treatment Strategies and Considerations to Improve Trunk Control in Sidelying

- To promote stability (holding), treatment is initiated with the patient in sidelying with the trunk in midrange.
- The limbs should be prepositioned prior to beginning sidelying activities.
  - The lowermost extremities are flexed to increase the BOS (see Fig. 3.14).
  - The uppermost LE is in extension; the uppermost UE is flexed overhead (Fig 3.15). For patients without sufficient shoulder ROM to position the UE overhead, the UE can be held at the side of the trunk, with one hand on the pelvis.

Clinical Note: Good body mechanics for the therapist are important throughout all activities and application of techniques. In general, a wide BOS with dynamic positioning is recommended. This allows the therapist to weight shift during these activities when necessary. The back should be kept straight, with the elbows relatively extended. Bending forward over the patient and hyperextending the wrists should be avoided.

Sidelying: Interventions, Outcomes, and Management Strategies

Position and Activity: Sidelying, Holding

TECHNIQUES AND VERBAL CUES (TO IMPROVE SIDELYING CONTROL)

Stabilizing Reversals Stabilizing reversals involve alternating small-range isotonic contractions progressing to stabilizing (holding) in the posture. Resistance is applied in opposing directions within a relatively static sidelying posture; only minimal movement occurs.[2] The technique utilizes maintained isotonic contractions to promote stability, increase strength, and improve coordination between opposing muscle groups (trunk flexors and extensors). Resistance is first applied in the stronger direction (to promote irradiation to weaker muscles) and then in the opposite direction. For the application of stabilizing reversals in sidelying, the therapist is heel-sitting either behind (see Fig. 3.15) or in front of the patient. Manual contacts are on the upper trunk and on the pelvis. As resistance is applied in opposing directions, the therapist's hands alternate between the anterior and posterior surfaces of the upper trunk and pelvis; flat open hands (a lumbrical grip, using metacarpophalangeal flexion with interphalangeal extension) are used to apply resistance, not tightly grasped fingers. Using bilateral manual contacts, the therapist applies resistance first to trunk flexors until the patient's maximum is reached. (The patient is asked to maintain the sidelying position.) Once the patient is fully resisting flexion, one hand continues to resist while the opposite hand is positioned to resist trunk extensors. When trunk extensors begin to engage, the hand resisting flexion is also moved to resist extensors. The goal is to achieve small-range isotonic contractions progressing to stabilizing (holding). *Note:* Stabilizing reversals are a precursor to *rhythmic stabilization.*

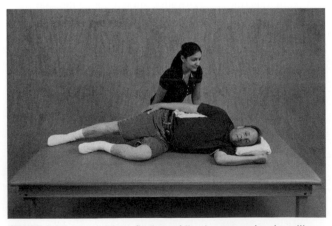

FIGURE 3.14 In sidelying, flexion of the lowermost extremities may be used to increase the BOS.

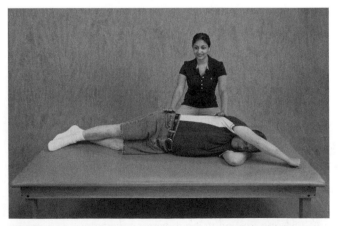

FIGURE 3.15 Application of stabilizing reversals in sidelying. In this example, the therapist's manual contacts for application of resistance are on the posterior upper trunk and the posterior pelvis. Note that the therapist is applying resistance with flat open hands; manual contacts alternate between the anterior and posterior surfaces of the upper trunk and pelvis.

Verbal Cues for Stabilizing Reversals in Sidelying

Resistance to trunk extensors: *"Don't let me push you forward."* Resistance to trunk flexors: *"Don't let me pull you backward."*

Comments

- The goal is maintained isotonic contractions and holding of the sidelying position.
- Therapist hand placements should provide smooth transitions between applications of resistance in opposite directions (this will prevent undesirable erratic or jerky movements).
- The patient is not allowed to relax between contractions.
- If the patient experiences difficulty holding the posture, dynamic reversals can be used initially (prior to stabilizing reversals) working toward decrements of ROM until improved holding is achieved.

Rhythmic Stabilization Rhythmic stabilization utilizes isometric contractions of antagonist patterns against resistance with emphasis on cocontraction; the patient does not attempt movement. Resistance is built up gradually as the patient responds to the applied force. The technique can be used to increase stability, strength, and ROM. Resistance is applied simultaneously to opposing directions (e.g., anterior rotation of shoulder and posterior rotation of pelvis *or* posterior rotation of shoulder and anterior rotation of pelvis). Although no movement occurs, resistance is applied as if twisting or rotating the upper and lower trunk in opposite directions.

For the application of rhythmic stabilization in sidelying, the therapist is positioned in heel-sitting behind the patient (Fig. 3.16); the patient is asked to hold the position while the therapist applies resistance. Resistance to isometric contraction is gradually increased until the patient's maximum is reached. Resistance is then reversed. For example, using the left hand, the therapist applies resistance to anterior rotation of the shoulder (pulling backward); with the right hand, resistance is simultaneously applied to posterior rotation of the

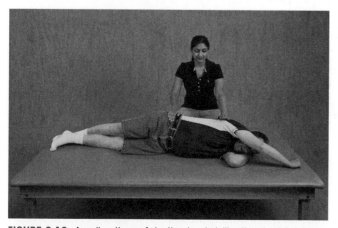

FIGURE 3.16 Application of rhythmic stabilization in sidelying. In this example, the therapist's left hand is positioned to resist posterior rotation of shoulder; the right hand is positioned to resist anterior rotation of the pelvis.

pelvis (pushing forward). Once the patient's maximum isometric response is achieved, the therapist moves the left hand to begin resisting posterior rotation of shoulder. As the patient responds to the new resistance, the right hand is moved to resist anterior rotation of the pelvis (see Fig. 3.16).

Verbal Cues for Rhythmic Stabilization in Sidelying

"Hold, don't let me move you. Hold, hold. Now don't let me move you the other way. Hold, hold."

Comments

- Resistance may first be applied to stronger muscles to facilitate those that are weaker.
- Resistance is built up gradually as the patient increases the force of isometric contraction.
- During any isometric contractions, the patient should be encouraged to breathe regularly. Breath holding increases intrathoracic pressures and can produce a Valsalva effect.

Outcomes

Motor control goals: Stability (static control).
Functional skill achieved: The patient is able to stabilize the trunk.

Indications Indications include weakness of trunk muscles and inability to stabilize the trunk. Both stabilizing reversals and rhythmic stabilization can be used in sidelying to promote stability and increase strength. Used in this context, stabilizing reversals place emphasis on the stabilizing action of the trunk flexors and extensors; rhythmic stabilization focuses on the stabilizing action of the trunk rotators.

Position/Activity: Sidelying, Upper or Lower Trunk Rotation (Segmental Rolling)

Isolated upper or lower trunk rotation can effectively be promoted with the patient in sidelying position. In upper trunk rotation, the patient moves the upper trunk/shoulder forward and backward while keeping the lower trunk/pelvis stationary. The sequence is reversed for lower trunk rotation: The pelvis/lower trunk moves forward and back while the upper trunk/shoulder remains stationary. This segmental rolling pattern is characterized by the shoulder/upper trunk segment leading the activity while the pelvis/lower trunk segment follows, or vice versa. During initial sidelying with upper or lower trunk rotation, the nonmoving segment is stabilized by the therapist. The therapist heel-sits behind or in front of the patient. Manual contacts are on the upper trunk and pelvis.

TECHNIQUES AND VERBAL CUES TO IMPROVE UPPER AND LOWER TRUNK ROTATION

Dynamic Reversals (Slow Reversals) Dynamic reversals use isotonic contractions to promote active concentric movement in one direction (*forward* or *backward* rotation) followed by active concentric movement in the reverse direction without relaxation. The technique involves continuous resisted movement in opposing directions, with VCs used to mark the initiation of movement in the opposite direction (continuous movement ↔ resistance ↔ VCs). To promote segmental rolling, the technique is applied separately to both the upper and lower trunk.

The therapist is in heel-sitting either behind (Fig. 3.17) or in front of the patient. Manual contacts for the application of resistance should promote smooth transitions between opposing directions of movement. For the application of dynamic reversals in sidelying with *upper trunk* rotation (see Fig. 3.17), the therapist's manual contacts include one hand placed on the stationary segment being stabilized (in this example, the lower trunk). The opposite hand resists movement, first on the anterior upper trunk (below the axilla) and then on the posterior upper trunk to resist the opposite movement. For the application to *lower trunk* rotation, one hand is placed on the stationary segment (upper trunk) and the opposite hand resists movement, first on the anterior lower trunk and then on the posterior lower trunk to resist the opposite movement. A smooth reversal of motion is the goal.

Verbal Cues for Dynamic Reversals in Sidelying, Trunk Rotation

Using the example of upper trunk rotation, the patient is directed to *"Keep your pelvis still; move your shoulder forward."* Prior to moving in the new direction (i.e., backward), a preparatory cue *"Now, reverse"* is used to direct the patient's attention to the new direction of movement. As the VC to change direction is given, the therapist repositions the hand to resist the new direction of motion and guides the patient: *"Now, push back."* If a hold (isometric contraction) is added to dynamic reversals, the VC is *"Pull forward (or backward), hold; now, push back."*

Outcomes

Motor control goal: Controlled mobility function.
Functional skill achieved: The patient is able to perform segmental trunk patterns (isolated upper trunk and lower trunk rotation).

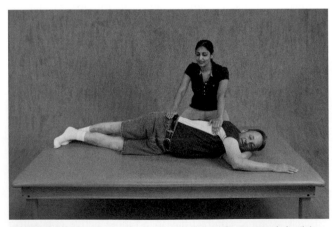

FIGURE 3.17 For the application of dynamic reversals in sidelying for upper trunk rotation, one of the therapist's hands is placed on the stationary segment (lower trunk). The opposite hand is on the anterior upper trunk (below the axilla) to resist forward movement. *Not shown:* The therapist's hand is then moved to the posterior upper trunk to resist the opposite movement.

Comments

- Resistance is applied first in the stronger direction (*forward* or *backward*) of movement.
- Movements begin with small-range control and progress to larger ranges and then to full-range control.
- Initially, movements are slow and controlled using graded resistance; progression is to variations in speed in one or both directions.
- An isometric hold may be added in the shortened range or at any point of weakness within the range. The hold is a momentary pause (the patient is instructed to *"Hold"*); the antagonist movement pattern is then facilitated. The hold can be added in one direction only or in both directions.
- Careful attention must be directed to the timing of the preparatory VC (such as *"Now, reverse"*). This will indicate to the patient that a change in movement direction is about to take place.
- A facilitatory quick stretch can be used, if needed to initiate the movement, and it should be timed to match with VCs.

Indications Indications include impaired segmental trunk patterns, impaired ability to make transitions between opposing muscle groups, weakness, and limitations in active ROM. Acquisition of segmental trunk patterns is an important lead-up skill for independent rolling, assumption of supine to sit, reaching across the body, and trunk counterrotation (reciprocal UE and trunk movements) during gait.

Clinical Note: Dissociation of the upper and lower trunk has several important clinical implications. It is often a useful strategy for patients with stroke, who typically move the trunk as a unit without separation of upper and lower segments. Patients with a retracted pelvic position (commonly seen in stroke) will benefit from lower trunk rotation with an emphasis on forward rotation; the reverse motion may be passive or assisted, but not resisted. It is also effective for patients with Parkinson's disease, whose overall trunk rotation is generally reduced, resulting in movement confined to a single plane of motion. Segmental rotation of the upper and lower trunk is effective in normalizing tone, allowing more normal patterns of movement to occur.

Position/Activity: Sidelying, Trunk Counterrotation

Prerequisite Requirements

Acquisition of segmental trunk patterns is a required lead-up skill for trunk counterrotation. Sidelying with trunk counterrotation involves simultaneous movement of both the upper and lower trunk in opposite directions. For example, the upper trunk moves *forward* at the same time the lower trunk is moving *backward*. The movements are then reversed (i.e., upper trunk moves *backward* as lower trunk moves *forward*). The therapist heel-sits behind or in front of the patient. Manual contacts are on the upper trunk (under the axilla) and the lower trunk/pelvis.

TECHNIQUES AND VERBAL CUES TO IMPROVE TRUNK COUNTERROTATION

Rhythmic Initiation Recall that rhythmic initiation is a technique that involves movements that are first passive, then active-assistive, and then appropriately resisted (passive → active-assistive → resisted); the patient is then asked to move independently. For the application of rhythmic initiation in sidelying for trunk counterrotation, the therapist's manual contacts are on the upper trunk (below the axilla) and on the lower trunk/pelvis (Fig. 3.18). The patient is instructed to relax while the therapist passively moves each trunk segment in opposite directions (e.g., the lower trunk/pelvis is moved forward while the upper trunk/shoulder is moved backward [see Fig. 3.18A]). This movement continues until passive movements are reasonably smooth and fluid. The patient is then instructed to begin active-assistive participation in the movement. The therapist provides the return

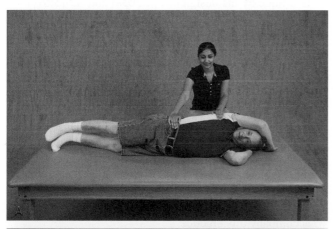

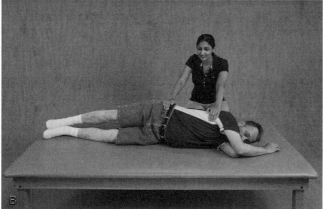

FIGURE 3.18 Sidelying, trunk counterrotation using rhythmic initiation. **(A)** The upper trunk moves *backward* at the same time the lower trunk moves *forward*. **(B)** For movement in the opposite direction, the upper trunk moves *forward* at the same time the lower trunk is moving *backward*. With rhythmic initiation, movements are first passive, then active-assistive, and then appropriately resisted (the return movement is provided by the therapist).

movements. Next is a gradual introduction of appropriate levels of resistance, typically beginning with light resistance. The final component of rhythmic initiation is progression to independent movement.

Verbal Cues for Rhythmic Initiation, Sidelying, Trunk Counterrotation VCs are timed with passive movements: *"Relax; let me move your shoulder forward (or backward) and your pelvis backward (or forward)."* VCs are timed with active-assistive movements: *"Now, move with me; shoulder forward (or backward) and pelvis backward (or forward)."* VCs are timed with resisted movements: *"Now, against resistance, push (or pull); shoulder forward (or backward) and pelvis backward (or forward)."* Alternative VCs: *"Twist your shoulder/pelvis in opposite directions; now reverse and twist again."*

Comments

- Resistance is used to facilitate muscle contraction.
- VCs should be soothing, slow, rhythmic, and carefully timed with all phases of movement (passive, active-assistive, and resisted) and facilitation (e.g., quick stretches).
- Trunk counterrotation can be a challenging movement to accomplish. Rhythmic initiation can be used to teach the motion (an effective technique for facilitating motor learning of difficult tasks). If resisted movement proves too difficult initially, the technique can be modified by using only passive to active-assisted movement, with later progression to resisted movements.
- If necessary, quick stretches can be used to facilitate movement in the desired direction.
- In combination with rhythmic initiation for sidelying trunk rotation, active reciprocal extremity movements simulating arm swing and stepping movements can be performed.
- Smooth reversal of direction of movement is the goal; movements should be coordinated and the movement sequence continuous.

Outcomes

Motor control goal: Skill-level control for the trunk.
Functional skill achieved: The patient is able to perform reciprocal trunk patterns required for gait.

Indications Indications are impaired reciprocal counterrotation trunk movements.

Clinical Note: From a hooklying position, an alternative activity to promote trunk counterrotation is to have the patient hold a small ball with the shoulders flexed to approximately 90 degrees and elbows extended. The patient is instructed to actively rotate ("twist") the ball and knees in opposite directions.

See Box 3.5 Section Summry Student Practice Activity on addressing treatment interventions to improve sidelying control.

BOX 3.5 SECTION SUMMARY STUDENT PRACTICE ACTIVITY: SIDELYING

Description of Student Practice Activity

Each section of this chapter ends with a similarly challenging student practice activity titled *Section Summary Student Practice Activity (followed by the section title)*. A section outline for sidelying to guide the activity is provided that highlights the key treatment strategies, techniques, and activities addressed in the preceding section. This activity is an opportunity to share knowledge and skills as well as to confirm or clarify understanding of the treatment interventions. Each student in a group will contribute his or her understanding of, or questions about, the strategy, technique, or activity being discussed and demonstrated. Dialogue should continue until a consensus of understanding is reached. (*Note:* **These directions will be repeated for each subsequent section summary student practice activity, in the event that content is considered in a sequence different from that presented here.**)

Section Outline: Sidelying

ACTIVITIES AND TECHNIQUES
- Sidelying, holding, using stabilizing reversals
- Sidelying, holding, using rhythmic stabilization
- Sidelying, upper trunk rotation using dynamic reversals
- Sidelying, lower trunk rotation using dynamic reversals
- Sidelying, trunk counterrotation using rhythmic initiation

OBJECTIVE: Sharing skill in the application and knowledge of treatment interventions used in sidelying.

EQUIPMENT NEEDED: Platform mat.

DIRECTIONS: Working in groups of four to six students, consider each entry in the section outline. Members of the group will assume different roles (described below) and will rotate roles each time the group progresses to a new item on the outline.

- One person assumes the role of therapist (for demonstrations) and participates in discussion.

- One person serves as the subject/patient (for demonstrations) and participates in discussion.
- The remaining members participate in discussion and provide supportive feedback during demonstrations. One member of this group should be designated as a "fact checker" to return to the text content to confirm elements of the discussion (if needed) or if agreement cannot be reached.

Thinking aloud, brainstorming, and sharing thoughts should be continuous throughout this activity! As each item in the section outline is considered, the following should ensue:

1. An initial discussion of the *activity,* including patient and therapist positioning. Also considered here should be positional changes to enhance the activity (e.g., prepositioning a limb, hand placements to alter the BOS, and so forth).
2. An initial discussion of the *technique,* including its description, indication(s) for use, therapist hand placements (manual contacts), and VCs.
3. A *demonstration* of the activity and application of the technique by the designated therapist and subject/patient. Discussion during the demonstration should be continuous (the demonstration should not be the sole responsibility of the designated therapist and subject/patient). All group members should provide recommendations, suggestions, and supportive feedback throughout the demonstration. Particularly important during the demonstrations is discussion of strategies to make the activity either *more* or *less* challenging.
4. If any member of the group feels he or she requires practice with the activity and technique, time should be allocated to accommodate the request. All group members providing input (recommendations, suggestions, and supportive feedback) should also accompany this practice.

Prone Extension (Pivot Prone)

General Characteristics

The prone position is very stable with a large BOS and low COM. Isometric contractions in the shortened range against gravity are required as the patient lies prone and lifts the head, UEs, upper trunk, and LEs off the mat in a total extension pattern (pivot prone position). No weightbearing occurs through the joints. The BOS of this posture will change relative to the number of body segments raised from the supporting surface; the COM of individual limb segments can also change based on positioning and the resultant change in lever arm (e.g., elbows flexed versus extended). Two UE positions can be used: (1) the shoulders may be extended,

externally rotated, and partially abducted, the scapulae adducted, and the elbows flexed to 90 degrees (Fig. 3.19A); or (2) the shoulders can be flexed overhead, the scapulae upwardly rotated, and the elbows extended (Fig. 3.19B). In both UE positions, the LEs are extended through the hips and knees. Stability control of postural extensors is the goal.

Position and Activity: Pivot Prone, Extremity Lifts
TREATMENT STRATEGIES AND CONSIDERATIONS
- The pattern of extremity lifts or combination of lifts can be varied to alter the challenge imposed or to meet specific treatment goals (e.g., activation of specific trunk musculature). For example, (1) both upper and LEs can

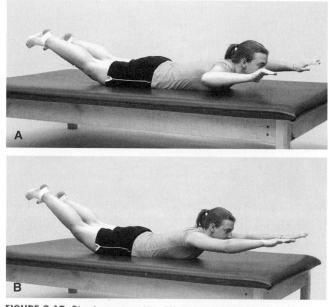

FIGURE 3.19 Pivot prone with different bilateral symmetrical UE positions. **(A)** Shoulders extended and elbows flexed; and **(B)** shoulders flexed with elbows extended.

be lifted off the support surface in a bilateral symmetrical pattern (see Fig. 3.19); (2) one UE or one LE can be lifted in a unilateral asymmetrical pattern; and (3) the opposite UE and LE can be lifted in a contralateral asymmetrical pattern.

Comments
- Prone activities are generally performed as active movements. The resistance of body weight and gravity provides sufficient challenge for most adults; at least fair (grade 3) muscle strength is required.
- Hip flexor or lumbar spine tightness may limit assumption and maintenance of the pivot prone position; some patients with ROM limitations may benefit from a firm pillow support placed under the abdomen/lower trunk.
- Owing to respiratory muscle weakness and/or compression of the chest wall, prone positions may be contraindicated in patients with cardiopulmonary involvement (e.g., cardiovascular disease, respiratory insufficiency) or respiratory muscle weakness (e.g., spinal cord injury [SCI]).
- Influence of the STLR will result in increased flexor tone in prone and impair active lifting.

PREREQUISITE REQUIREMENTS
Head and neck control and functional UE and LE ROM are necessary.

Prone on Elbows

General Characteristics
The prone on elbows posture is very stable with a large BOS and low COM. The head and upper trunk are elevated off the supporting surface, with weight distributed to the elbows and forearms. However, weight is not actually borne through the forearm or elbow joint in this flexed position, but through the shoulder and scapulothoracic joints. The UEs are in a bilateral symmetrical position with the elbows flexed to 90 degrees and positioned directly under the shoulders; the forearms are pronated. The lower body remains in contact with the supporting surface.

Prone on Elbows: Treatment Strategies and Considerations
- Scapular and/or shoulder weakness (e.g., diminished strength of the serratus anterior, trapezius, and rhomboids or shoulder stabilizers) may limit the patient's ability to assume or hold in this posture. A hallmark of serratus anterior weakness is scapular "winging" off the thorax.
- Shoulder pain or ROM limitations may also limit tolerance of the position and the amount of weight borne.
- A support (e.g., wedge cushion) can be positioned under the upper trunk to reduce loading of the UEs or to allow for progressive UE loading as tolerated.
- UE spasticity (typically flexion/adduction/internal rotation) may interfere with assuming the prone on elbows position by pulling the UE into an abnormal position of adduction and internal rotation of the shoulder with the hand closed. In such situations, appropriate inhibitory handling strategies such as rhythmic rocking movements may be indicated prior to assuming the position to diminish tone and promote relaxation. For example, the fisted (clenched) hand may be opened by gently grasping the thumb and gradually supinating the forearm; the hand may then be positioned open and flat on the supporting surface with the shoulder in neutral rotation; gentle stroking on top of the fingers can assist in relaxation.
- Rounding the thoracic spine in prone on elbows can help relax tone through active protraction movements. This is accomplished by having the patient push the elbows down into the mat and tuck the chin while lifting and rounding out the shoulders and upper thorax. The patient lowers the chin and upper chest to the mat again by allowing the scapulae to adduct.
- Abnormal reflex activity may interfere with the patient's ability to assume or hold the prone on elbows posture. Rotation of the head may activate the ATNR response, causing UE extension on the chin side and flexion, or collapse, on the skull side. Abnormal influence of the STLR may cause an increase in flexor tone in the prone position that can diminish head and trunk extension.
- Prone on elbows may be contraindicated in the presence of elbow pathology, recent chest surgery or trauma, and cardiopulmonary impairments.
- In the presence of initial low back discomfort, gradual increments of active holding in the posture may be indicated to improve prone extension in the lumbar spine.
- Tightness in the hip flexors may limit extension into this posture. This may be improved by stretching interventions

(e.g., prolonged stretch, contract-relax, hold-relax) and/ or using a pillow under the abdomen to assist initial positioning.

- Tightness in thoracic and cervical mobility may also limit attainment and maintenance of the posture. This may be improved through regular positioning using a series of graduated-height cushion wedges in combination with thoracic and cervical mobility exercises.

Clinical Note: Patients with activity limitations imposed by cardiopulmonary involvement or those with high levels of abnormal UE tone will not tolerate the prone on elbows position well. However, some benefits of the posture can be achieved using a modification of the position (termed *modified prone on elbows*). The modification is to position the patient in sitting with the elbows bearing weight on a tabletop. An alternative while sitting on a platform mat is to position the flexed elbow on a step stool (covered with a soft towel) or other firm surface placed next to, or on both sides of, the patient for either unilateral or bilateral weightbearing at the elbow. Modified prone on elbows can also be achieved in standing, using the plantigrade position.

Position and Activity: Prone on Elbows, Assist-to-Position
Assist-to-position transitions into prone on elbows can be accomplished from either *prone* or *sidelying on elbow*.

ACTIVITIES, STRATEGIES, AND VERBAL CUES: PRONE ON ELBOWS, ASSIST-TO-POSITION FROM PRONE LYING

Activities and Strategies For initial assisted movement transitions to the prone on elbows position (prone lying to prone on elbows position), the patient is in the prone position with the shoulders prepositioned at approximately 120 degrees of abduction with the elbows flexed to 90 degrees, forearms pronated, palms flat on supporting surface, and the head in a neutral position (or turned to one side for comfort) (Fig. 3.20A). The therapist is half-kneeling in straddle position over the patient or half-kneeling to the side of the patient. Both hands are on the patient's anterior trunk with fingers pointing toward the sternum; the hands are cupped over the clavicles to relieve any bony pressure. The therapist then assists the patient to assume the position by lifting and supporting the upper trunk. The patient actively assists with lifting the head and upper trunk and adducting the shoulders to pull both elbows under the shoulders to allow weightbearing (Fig. 3.20B).

Verbal Cues for Assist-to-Position From Prone Lying to Prone on Elbows The therapist lifts the patient on a count of three and assists the patient gently onto the elbows. VCs are *"On the count of three, I want you to lift your head up. I will help you lift up your upper trunk to come onto your elbows. One, two, three, now lift."*

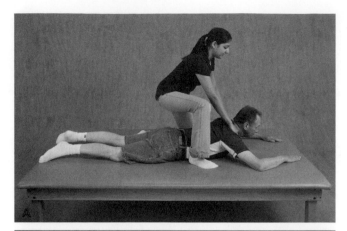

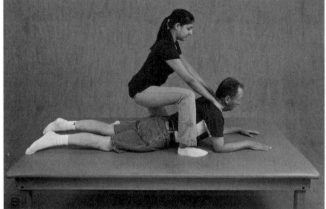

FIGURE 3.20 Active-assistive movement from prone to prone on elbows position. **(A)** Start position; the UEs are prepositioned in shoulder abduction with the elbows flexed, forearms pronated, palms flat, and the head in a neutral position. **(B)** End position; the patient lifts head and upper trunk and adducts the shoulders to move elbows into a weightbearing position.

Clinical Note: In this assist-to-position example, the patient is not yet able to independently assume the prone on elbows position. It should be noted that considerable functional gains may be made working within a posture well before the patient is actually able to assume the position independently.

Comments

- The assisted lift should be high enough (approximately 1 inch [2.5 cm] off the mat) so that as shoulders are adducted, gravity assists pulling the elbows into position for weightbearing.
- Once the patient is prone on elbows, manual approximation can be applied directly over the shoulders to facilitate stabilizing muscles (prior to use of approximation, the therapist must ensure that the glenohumeral joints are properly aligned).
- Following the lift, if one or both elbows are not accurately positioned to assume weightbearing (e.g., shoulders too abducted), the patient may be assisted to shift laterally to one side to unweight the opposite side. Gravity will then assist in pulling the opposite elbow under

the shoulder; this can be repeated to align the other side (e.g., if the right elbow were not positioned correctly, the patient would be laterally shifted toward the left).

• As control increases, the patient learns to lift the trunk actively and weight shift from elbow to elbow to pull both elbows under the shoulders.

ACTIVITIES, STRATEGIES, AND VERBAL CUES: PRONE ON ELBOWS, ASSIST-TO-POSITION FROM SIDELYING ON ELBOWS
Activities and Strategies The patient may also be assisted to prone on elbows from sidelying on one elbow. This movement transition begins with the patient in a sidelying on elbow position. The patient is supported and assisted with upper trunk rotation (lower trunk follows rotating toward prone) and movement into the prone on elbows position (Fig. 3.21A). The therapist is half-kneeling in a straddle position over the patient or half-kneeling to the side of the patient. Bilateral manual contacts are on the lateral aspect of the patient's upper trunk, under the axillae. The patient is assisted into the position by rotating the trunk until both elbows are resting on the mat (Fig. 3.21B). If required, the position of the elbows is then adjusted for bearing weight.

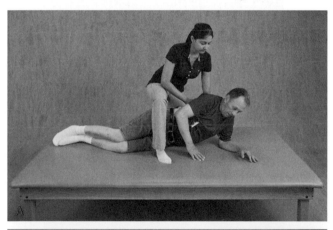

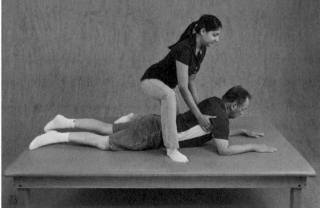

FIGURE 3.21 Assist-to-position from sidelying on elbow to prone on elbows position. **(A)** Start position; the patient is in a sidelying on elbow position as the therapist provides support and assistance with upper trunk rotation. **(B)** End position; the lower trunk rotates toward prone and both elbows are resting on the mat. The position of the elbows is then adjusted.

Verbal Cues for Assist-to-Position From Sidelying on Elbows to Prone on Elbows Position *"On the count of three, I want you to turn (rotate) your upper body and come down on your elbow so you're then supported by both elbows. One, two, three."*

Comments
• Influence of the STLR may cause an increase in flexor tone in prone position.
• Rotation of the head may activate an ATNR response, causing extension of the UE on the chin side and flexion or yielding on the skull side.
• For the patient with UE spasticity (e.g., the patient with stroke), the limb is positioned with the hand open and flat on the mat with neutral rotation of the shoulder.

Outcomes
Motor control goal: Mobility (active-assistive movements) progressing to controlled mobility (active movements).
Functional skill achieved: Lead-up skill to assumption of the prone on elbows position independently.

Indications Indications include weakness, lack of motor control, and poor proximal stability of shoulders. These *assist-to-position* activities are important lead-up skills for independent assumption of the prone on elbows position with carryover to bed mobility.

PREREQUISITE REQUIREMENTS
The prone on elbows position involves head and neck, upper trunk, and shoulder control. Active holding of the posture also requires scapular and shoulder stability (the serratus anterior stabilizes the scapula on the thorax; the rotator cuff muscles and pectoralis major stabilize the humerus under the body). Active holding of prone on elbows also requires midrange control of neck extensors.

Prone on Elbows: Interventions, Outcomes, and Management Strategies
Position/Activity: Prone on Elbows, Holding
Initial activities focus on holding (stability) the posture. The patient is in the prone on elbows position, with the head in midposition. Both scapulae are in midposition between protraction and retraction and should be flat on the thorax.

Clinical Note: Scapular winging (when the vertebral border of the scapula is lifted more than 1 inch [2.5 cm] off the thorax) indicates weakness of the serratus anterior muscle and is generally considered a contraindication for use of the prone on elbows posture. A modified prone on elbow posture that limits weightbearing may be considered. With slight winging, the therapist can place a hand in the midscapular region and ask the patient to flatten the upper back into the hand. The patient is then instructed to hold the position for several counts.

TECHNIQUES AND VERBAL CUES TO PROMOTE STABILITY
IN PRONE ON ELBOWS

Stabilizing Reversals Stabilizing reversals involve small-range alternating isotonic contractions progressing to stabilizing (holding) in the posture. Resistance is applied in opposing directions within a relatively static prone on elbows posture; only minimal movement occurs. For the application of this technique to prone on elbows, resistance is applied in both a *medial/lateral* and an *anterior/posterior direction* (both are described below).

Stabilizing Reversals, Medial/Lateral Resistance

For the application of stabilizing reversals with medial/lateral resistance in prone on elbows, the therapist is positioned in heel-sitting at the side of the patient's upper trunk or on a stool next to the mat. Using either an open or cupped hand (based on direction of movement), manual contacts are on either the vertebral or axillary borders of scapulae to apply resistance in opposing directions as the patient attempts movement both *toward* (open hand) and *away* (cupped hand) from the therapist. The patient is asked to maintain the prone on elbows position. As the patient pushes toward the therapist (Fig. 3.22A), one hand is positioned on the vertebral border of the contralateral scapula and one on the axillary border of the ipsilateral scapular. Once the patient is fully resisting (with progression to stabilizing holding), resistance is applied in the opposing direction (patient pulls away from therapist). One hand is moved to resist on the axillary border of the contralateral scapula. When the patient engages in movement in the opposite direction, the other manual contact is placed on the vertebral border of the ipsilateral scapula to resist movement away from the therapist (Fig. 3.22B). The therapist's hands alternate between the two positions. Resistance is applied until the patient's maximum is reached and then reversed.

Verbal Cues for Stabilizing Reversals, Medial/Lateral Resistance in Prone on Elbows

Pushing toward therapist: *"Don't let me push you away."* Pulling away from therapist: *"Don't let me pull you toward me."*

Stabilizing Reversals, Anterior/Posterior Resistance

For the application of stabilizing reversals with anterior/posterior resistance in prone on elbows, the therapist is positioned in a half-kneeling straddle position over the patient. Bilateral manual contacts move smoothly between resistance applied in *anterior* and *posterior* directions. As the patient attempts to move forward (as if *flexing* the upper trunk), the therapist's hands are positioned over the top of the shoulders on the anterior trunk (hands cupped over the clavicle), pulling backward. As the patient attempts to move backward (as if *extending* the upper trunk), the therapist's hands are on the inferior borders of the scapulae, pushing forward and downward.

Verbal Cues for Stabilizing Reversals, Anterior/Posterior Resistance in Prone on Elbows

As the patient attempts to shift forward: *"Don't let me pull you back."*

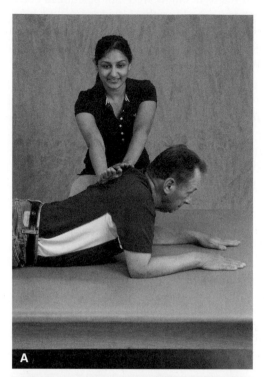

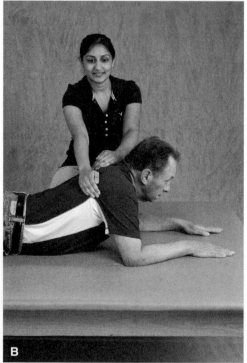

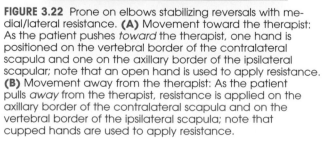

FIGURE 3.22 Prone on elbows stabilizing reversals with medial/lateral resistance. **(A)** Movement toward the therapist: As the patient pushes *toward* the therapist, one hand is positioned on the vertebral border of the contralateral scapula and one on the axillary border of the ipsilateral scapular; note that an open hand is used to apply resistance. **(B)** Movement away from the therapist: As the patient pulls *away* from the therapist, resistance is applied on the axillary border of the contralateral scapula and on the vertebral border of the ipsilateral scapula; note that cupped hands are used to apply resistance.

As the patient attempts to shift backward: *"Don't let me push you forward."*

Rhythmic Stabilization Recall that rhythmic stabilization utilizes isometric contractions against resistance; no movement occurs. Resistance is applied simultaneously in opposing directions (e.g., first to the *anterior* upper trunk and contralateral *posterior* upper trunk; hand placements are then reversed to the *posterior* upper trunk and contralateral *anterior* upper trunk). Although no movement occurs, resistance is applied as if twisting or rotating the upper trunk in opposite directions.

For the application of rhythmic stabilization in prone on elbows, the therapist is positioned in a half-kneeling straddle position over the patient. Alternatively, with the patient's upper body near the edge of the platform mat, the therapist may sit on a stool facing the patient. Manual contacts are positioned on the upper trunk. One hand is placed on the anterior (or *posterior*) upper trunk and the other on the contralateral posterior (or *anterior*) upper trunk; hand placements are then reversed. For example, once the patient is engaged in isometric contractions with the therapist's left hand resisting on the anterior upper trunk and the right on the posterior upper trunk, the hand placements are changed. The left hand is moved to resist at the posterior upper trunk. As the patient responds to the new resistance, the right hand is then also moved to resist on the anterior upper trunk. Resistance is applied in a twisting motion, as if attempting to rotate the upper trunk; the patient resists the movement (Fig. 3.23). No relaxation occurs as the direction of resistance is changed.

Verbal Cues for Rhythmic Stabilization in Prone on Elbows *"Hold, don't let me move (twist) you. Hold, hold. Now don't let me move you the other way. Hold, hold."*

Comments
- Isometric control (holding) is the goal. Resistance is built up gradually and smoothly as the patient increases the force of contraction; the hold should be steady, with no visible movement of the trunk.
- Rhythmic breathing should be encouraged during any isometric contractions; breath holding should be avoided.
- Good body mechanics for the therapist are important. The back should be kept straight, and wrist hyperextension should be avoided.
- Elastic resistive bands can be positioned around the patient's forearms; the patient is instructed to hold against the tubing, keeping the forearms apart. This will increase the proprioceptive loading and stabilizing actions of the shoulder muscles especially the rotator cuff muscles.

Outcomes
Motor control goals: Stability (static control) of the upper trunk.

Functional skill achieved: The patient is able to stabilize (actively hold) in prone on elbows.

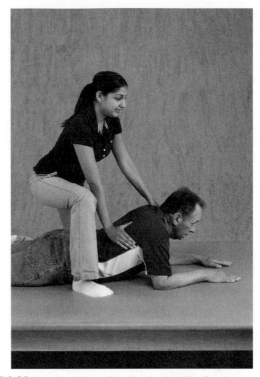

FIGURE 3.23 Application of rhythmic stabilization in prone on elbows. The patient is asked to hold the prone on elbows position as resistance is applied simultaneously to opposing muscle groups. In this example, resistance is applied in a "twisting motion" to the anterior upper trunk (left hand) and opposite posterior upper trunk (right hand) as if "pulling" upward with the anterior hand placement and pushing downward with the posterior hand placement.

Indications Indications include the inability to stabilize the glenohumeral and scapular musculature, an important prerequisite for using the UEs in weightbearing positions. These activities are effective for further improving head and upper trunk control in preparation for upright antigravity postures (sitting and standing).

Position/Activity: Prone on Elbows, Weight Shifting
For this activity, the patient is positioned in prone on elbows with the head in midposition. Weight shifts are accomplished in *medial/lateral* and *anterior/posterior* directions. Weight shifting is usually easiest in a medial/lateral direction with progression to anterior/posterior shifts. This activity improves dynamic stability, as the posture must be stabilized while moving.

TECHNIQUES AND VERBAL CUES
Dynamic Reversals: Medial/Lateral Shifts Dynamic reversals promote active concentric movement in one direction followed by active concentric movement in the reverse direction without relaxation. Smooth reversals of motion (normal transitions between opposing muscle groups) are the goal. Movements are continuously resisted in opposing directions, with VCs used to mark the initiation of movement in the opposite direction (continuous movement ↔ resistance ↔ VCs).

For the application of dynamic reversals with medial/lateral shifts in prone on elbows, the therapist heel-sits to the side of the patient's shoulders/upper trunk. As the patient shifts weight *toward* the therapist, one hand is positioned laterally on the upper trunk over the axillary border of the scapula to resist the motion; the opposite hand is positioned on the contralateral upper trunk over the vertebral border of the scapula (Fig. 3.24A). As the patient moves *away* from the therapist, the hands stay on the same side of the trunk but reverse their positions on the scapular borders to resist the opposite direction. As the patient moves away, one hand is positioned over the vertebral border of the scapula; the other hand is positioned laterally on the contralateral upper trunk over the axillary border of the scapula (Fig. 3.24B).

Verbal Cues for Dynamic Reversals, Medial/Lateral Shifts in Prone on Elbows Shifting toward therapist: *"Push toward me, push, push, push."* Transitional cue: *"Now, reverse."* Shifting away from therapist: *"Pull away from me, pull, pull, pull."* When the patient is ready to move in the new direction, a preparatory cue *("Now, reverse")* is used to direct the patient's attention to the new movement. At the same time as the VC to change direction, the therapist repositions the hands to resist the new direction of motion. If a hold (isometric contraction) is added to dynamic reversals, the VC is *"Pull, pull, pull, (or push, push, push) hold, hold, hold."*

Dynamic Reversals: Anterior/Posterior Shifts For the application of dynamic reversals with anterior/posterior shifts in prone on elbows, the position of the UEs is modified by placing the elbows slightly posterior and lateral to the shoulders (instead of directly under the shoulders). This positioning allows weight shifts in an anterior direction (further elbow flexion with head moving toward the mat) and posterior direction (decreasing elbow flexion with head moving back up and slightly beyond the starting prone on elbows position). The therapist is in a half-kneeling straddle position and applies resistance to the movement. For anterior shifts, manual contacts are on the anterior upper trunk (with hands cupped over the clavicles) to resist the downward anterior movement. To resist posterior shifts (return or slightly posterior to start position), manual contacts are on the posterior trunk (over inferior border of scapulae) to resist the reverse movement.

Verbal Cues for Dynamic Reversals, Anterior/Posterior Shifts in Prone on Elbows Shifting anteriorly from prone on elbows (head and shoulders move toward mat): *"Pull forward, move your head toward mat, pull, pull, pull."* Transitional cue: *"Now, reverse."* Shifting posteriorly back into or slightly beyond start position: *"Push up, push, push, push."*

Comments

• Initially, movements are slow and controlled with emphasis on careful grading of resistance; progression is to increasing range in one or both directions.

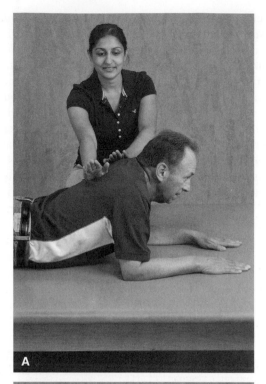

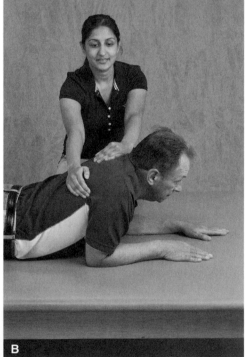

FIGURE 3.24 Dynamic reversals: medial/lateral shifts in prone on elbows. **(A)** Moving *toward* the therapist, manual contacts are on the axillary border of the ipsilateral scapula and the vertebral border of the contralateral scapula. **(B)** Moving *away* from the therapist, manual contacts are on the vertebral border of the ipsilateral scapula and on the axillary border of the contralateral scapula.

- Movements begin with small-range control and progress through increasing ROM (increments of ROM) to full-range control.
- Emphasis is on efficient reversal of opposing muscle groups; movement is continuous.
- Changing manual contacts should be carefully timed with transitional cues (*"Now, reverse"*) to ensure smooth reversal of movement.
- A facilitatory stretch can be used to initiate movement and should be well timed to coincide with the VCs.
- An isometric hold may be added in the shortened range to improve stability. The hold is a momentary pause (the patient is instructed to *"Hold for one count"*); the antagonist movement pattern is then facilitated. The hold can be added in one direction only or in both directions. An isometric hold can also be used at any point of weakness within the range.

Combination of Isotonics: Anterior/Posterior Shifts

Combination of isotonics is a technique that utilizes concentric, eccentric, and stabilizing (holding) contractions without relaxation.[2] Against continual resistance, the patient first moves to the end range of a desired motion (concentric) and then holds (stabilizing) in this end position. When stability is achieved, the patient is instructed to allow the body segment to be slowly moved back to the start position (eccentric). It should be noted that the direction and type of desired movement would determine whether the technique is begun with *concentric* or *eccentric* contractions.

For the application of combination of isotonics to anterior/posterior shifts in prone on elbows, the patient begins in the prone position with upper trunk resting on the mat surface (Fig. 3.25A). The patient shifts posteriorly and moves up toward prone on elbows against continual resistance to concentric contractions. When the end of motion is reached (Fig. 3.25B), the patient holds the position (stabilizing). In the prone on elbows position, the same positioning modifications are used as for dynamic reversals with anterior/posterior shifts (elbows slightly posterior and lateral to the shoulders). Once stability is achieved in prone on elbows, the patient begins to shift forward against (eccentric) resistance and returns to the original start position (see Fig. 3.25A). The therapist is in a half-kneeling straddle position over the patient. Manual contacts are on the posterior trunk (over the inferior border of the scapula); hand placements *do not change* during application of the technique.

It should be noted that the start position for this activity was selected arbitrarily. It can begin from either the prone or prone-on-elbows position.

Verbal Cues for Combination of Isotonics: Anterior/Posterior Shifts in Prone on Elbows

During concentric movement from prone (posterior shift): *"Push back, push, don't let me stop you."* During the middle stabilizing phase: *"Hold, hold, don't let me move you, hold."* During return to start position, using eccentric controlled lowering (anterior shift): *"Go down slowly, very slowly. Make me work at pushing you down."*

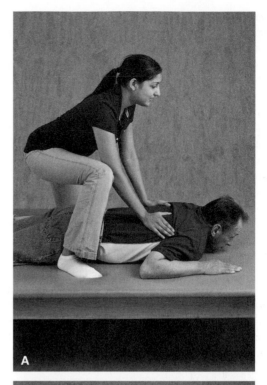

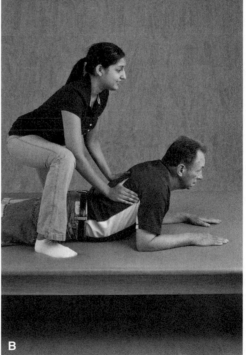

FIGURE 3.25 Combination of isotonics: anterior/posterior shifts in prone on elbows. **(A)** The activity begins with the patient in prone position. **(B)** Against continual resistance, the patient shifts weight posteriorly (concentric) and moves up into prone on elbows. When the end range of motion is reached, the patient holds (stabilizes) in the position. **(A)** Once stability is achieved, the patient returns (eccentric) to the original start position. The therapist's hand placements do not change during application of the technique. **(B)** In the prone on elbows position, note that the patient's elbows are positioned slightly posterior and lateral to the shoulders.

Outcomes

Motor control goal: Controlled mobility function of the upper trunk and shoulders.

Functional skill achieved: The patient has improved bed mobility (proximal stability of the glenohumeral and scapular musculature).

Indications Dependent function due to weakness is an indication, as well as disordered control of upper trunk and shoulder muscles. These activities are important lead-up skills for dynamic balance control in prone on elbows and for assuming the quadruped position.

Position/Activity: Prone on Elbows, Limb Movements

Extremity combinations can be used in prone on elbows to promote greater challenges by altering the pattern of muscle activation and imposing increased demands for trunk stability to support the weight of the dynamic limb; unilateral weightbearing also promotes further demands for stability on the static, supporting limb. For all static-dynamic activities, the COM must shift toward the weightbearing limb in order to free the dynamic limb for movement.

TECHNIQUES AND VERBAL CUES

Upper Extremity D1 Thrust and Reverse Thrust (Withdrawal) Pattern, Dynamic Reversals

The therapist is positioned in heel-sitting or half-kneeling in front and to the side of the patient, diagonally opposite the dynamic (unweighted) UE. The patient is positioned in prone on elbows, with the head in midposition. The patient is instructed to shift weight onto the static (weightbearing) UE. The dynamic UE is unweighted and passively moved through the motion several times before resistance is applied. The limb begins in a position of shoulder extension and scapular retraction, forearm supination, with elbow, wrist, and finger flexion (D1 reverse thrust) (Fig. 3.26A). The UE then moves forward and upward, crossing the midline of the patient's face, moving into scapular protraction, shoulder flexion and adduction, elbow extension, and forearm pronation, with wrist and finger extension (D1 thrust) (Fig. 3.26B). The patient then reverses direction and brings the UE back down to the start position (D1 reverse thrust). The dynamic UE is non-weightbearing at all times.

Dynamic reversals promote active concentric movement in one direction followed by active concentric movement in the reverse direction without relaxation; resistance is continual, with VCs used to mark the initiation of movement in the opposite direction. The therapist resists the motion of the dynamic UE with one hand grasping the patient's wrist or distal forearm. As the patient moves into the thrust pattern, the therapist's forearm must also move from supination to pronation. The therapist's other hand is positioned on or near the shoulder of the static limb; this hand can be used to apply approximation to increase stabilizing responses as needed. The amount of resistance applied to the dynamic limb is determined by the patient's ability to hold the static limb and trunk steady. A hold (isometric contraction) may

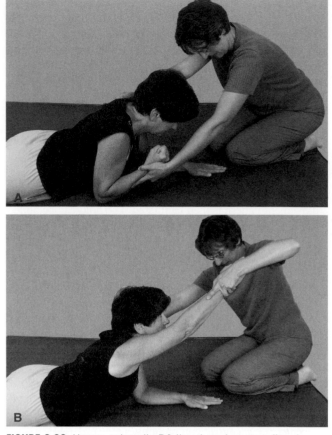

FIGURE 3.26 Upper extremity D1 thrust and reverse thrust (withdrawal) pattern using dynamic reversals in prone on elbows. **(A)** The dynamic UE begins in shoulder extension and scapular retraction, forearm supination, with elbow, wrist, and finger flexion (D1 reverse thrust). **(B)** The dynamic UE then moves forward and upward, crossing the midline of the patient's face, moving into scapular protraction, shoulder flexion and adduction, elbow extension, and forearm pronation, with wrist and finger extension (D1 thrust).

be added to dynamic reversals in either direction; the hold is most commonly applied to the D1 thrust pattern.

Verbal Cues for Upper Extremity D1 Thrust and Reverse Thrust (Withdrawal) Pattern, Dynamic Reversals in Prone on Elbows

"Shift your weight over onto your right (or left) elbow." For the thrust pattern: *"Now, lift your left (or right) arm up and across your face while I resist the movement, push, push, push."* Transitional cue: *"Now, reverse."* For the withdrawal pattern: *"Now, pull the arm back down and to your side, pull, pull, pull."*

Comments

- The therapist should be positioned to the side of midline to ensure that the thrust pattern is not blocked or inhibited.
- Activities that require resisted hand grasp of the static UE, such as squeezing a ball, will further support stability (cocontraction) of the static shoulder.

Clinical Note: An alternative activity involves active reaching alone (dynamic limb), or in combination with a cone-stacking task. This activity requires a series of 5- to 7-inch (12- to 17-cm) rigid plastic stacking cones; the cones typically have a nonslip textured surface. The therapist holds the target cone and asks the patient to place another cone on top of it. Initially, the therapist holds the target cone in front and diagonally to the patient's side to facilitate weight transfer onto the static limb. As control increases, the target cone can be shifted to other locations to challenge control. This task promotes dynamic stability as well as eye-hand coordination.

Outcomes

Motor control goals: Controlled mobility function and static-dynamic control of the upper trunk and UE. This activity is an important lead-up skill for bed mobility, as it promotes UE function in prone on elbows position.

Functional skills achieved: The patient is independent in maintaining the prone on elbows position with simultaneous performance of UE reach and grasp activities.

Indications An indication is impaired controlled mobility function (static-dynamic control) in prone on elbows.

Position/Activity: Prone on Elbows, Balance Activities
In prone on elbows, balance activities focus on improved static postural control (biomechanical alignment and symmetrical weight distribution) and dynamic postural control (musculoskeletal responses to support movement). Balance activities begin with static holding (static postural control) and progress to weight shifts in all directions (dynamic postural control). The patient's limits of stability (maximum distance the patient is able to lean in prone on elbows without loss of balance) must be reestablished, which is among the first activities in a balance sequence. The patient learns how far to shift in any one direction before losing balance and falling out of the position. Additional activities that challenge balance control in prone on elbows include UE reaching and placing activities (cone stacking) and turnarounds (head and upper trunk rotation to allow looking from side to side).

To challenge reactive balance control, the patient's forearms and elbows can be supported on a small inflatable dome or equilibrium board. After initial balance control is achieved on the dome or board, side to side weight shifts can be introduced; lateral curvature of head and upper trunk is a normal response to tilting (the head and upper trunk rotate toward the elevated side).

Outcomes

Motor control goals: Static and dynamic balance control in prone on elbows.

Functional skill achieved: The patient demonstrates functional balance skill in the prone on elbows posture.

Indications Indications include severely disordered balance control (e.g., the patient with TBI) and diminished proximal stability of shoulders and upper trunk. Balance activities in prone on elbows promote balance control in a stable posture with a large BOS. The patient is prepared for bed mobility on soft uneven surfaces (e.g., mattress).

See Box 3.6 Section Summary Student Practice Activity on treatment interventions used in prone on elbows.

BOX 3.6 SECTION SUMMARY STUDENT PRACTICE ACTIVITY: PRONE ON ELBOWS

Description of Student Practice Activity

Each section of this chapter ends with a similarly challenging student practice activity titled *Section Summary Student Practice Activity (followed by the section title)*. A section outline for prone on elbows to guide the activity is provided that highlights the key treatment strategies, techniques, and activities addressed in the preceding section. This activity is an opportunity to share knowledge and skills as well as to confirm or clarify understanding of the treatment interventions. Each student in a group will contribute his or her understanding of, or questions about, the strategy, technique, or activity being discussed and demonstrated. Dialogue should continue until a consensus of understanding is reached. (**Note: These directions will be repeated for each subsequent section summary student practice activity, in the event that content is considered in a sequence different from that presented here.**)

Section Outline: Prone on Elbows

MOVEMENT TRANSITIONS: ACTIVITIES AND STRATEGIES
▲ Prone to prone on elbows transitions using assist-to-position
▲ Sidelying on elbow to prone on elbows transitions using assist-to-position

ACTIVITIES AND TECHNIQUES
▲ Prone on elbows, holding using stabilizing reversals with medial/lateral resistance
▲ Prone on elbows, holding using rhythmic stabilization
▲ Prone on elbows, medial-lateral shifts using dynamic reversals
▲ Prone on elbows, anterior-posterior shifts using combination of isotonics
▲ Prone on elbows, upper extremity D1 thrust and withdrawal pattern using dynamic reversals

OBJECTIVE: Sharing skill in the application and knowledge of treatment interventions used in prone on elbows.

(box continues on page 70)

BOX 3.6 SECTION SUMMARY STUDENT PRACTICE ACTIVITY: PRONE ON ELBOWS (continued)

EQUIPMENT NEEDED: Platform mat.

DIRECTIONS: Working in groups of four to six students, consider each entry in the section outline. Members of the group will assume different roles (described below) and will rotate roles each time the group progresses to a new item on the outline.

▲ One person assumes the role of therapist (for demonstrations) and participates in discussion.

▲ One person serves as the subject/patient (for demonstrations) and participates in discussion.

▲ The remaining members participate in discussion and provide supportive feedback during demonstrations. One member of this group should be designated as a "fact checker" to return to the text content to confirm elements of the discussion (if needed) or if agreement cannot be reached.

Thinking aloud, brainstorming, and sharing thoughts should be continuous throughout this activity! As each item in the section outline is considered, the following should ensue:

1. An initial discussion of the *activity,* including patient and therapist positioning. Also considered here should

be positional changes to enhance the activity (e.g., prepositioning a limb, hand placements to alter the BOS, and so forth).

2. An initial discussion of the *technique,* including its description, indication(s) for use, therapist hand placements (manual contacts), and verbal cues.

3. A *demonstration* of the activity and application of the technique by the designated therapist and subject/patient. Discussion during the demonstration should be continuous (the demonstration should not be the sole responsibility of the designated therapist and subject/patient). All group members should provide recommendations, suggestions, and supportive feedback throughout the demonstration. Particularly important during the demonstrations is discussion of strategies to make the activity either *more* or *less* challenging.

4. If any member of the group feels he or she requires practice with the activity and technique, time should be allocated to accommodate the request. All group members providing input (recommendations, suggestions, and supportive feedback) should also accompany this practice.

Interventions to Improve Control in Quadruped, Hooklying, and Bridging

Quadruped

General Characteristics

Quadruped (kneeling on all fours, or prone kneeling) is a stable, four-limb posture with a large BOS; the COM is higher than in prone on elbows, but still low. The shoulders are flexed to 90 degrees, with the elbows extended and the hands positioned directly under the shoulders. The hips are flexed to 90 degrees, with the knees positioned directly under the hips; the back is straight (flat).

The quadruped posture involves increased demands for balance, especially with dynamic shifting activities. The influence of abnormal reflexes may interfere with the patient's ability to assume and maintain this position. The ATNR may cause one UE to flex if the head turns to the opposite side; the STNR may cause the UEs to flex with head/neck flexion or the hips to flex with head/neck extension.

Treatment Strategies and Considerations

Position and Activity: Quadruped, Assist-to-Position
Assist-to-position movement transitions into quadruped can be accomplished from either *prone on elbows* or *side-sitting.*

PREREQUISITE REQUIREMENTS
Assumption and maintenance of the quadruped posture requires head/neck, upper trunk, UE (shoulder/elbow), and lower trunk/hip control.

ACTIVITIES, STRATEGIES, AND VERBAL CUES: QUADRUPED, ASSIST-TO-POSITION FROM PRONE ON ELBOWS
Activities and Strategies For movement transitions from prone on elbows into quadruped, the patient starts in prone on elbows. The knees remain in position as the patient "walks" backward on the elbows until the knees are under the hips. The patient then extends both elbows one at a time, lifting the upper trunk into a hands-and-knees position.

To assist the patient to position, the therapist initially is in a squatting straddle position behind the patient with both hands on the patient's hips. The therapist lifts backward and upward, first on one hip then on the other, and the patient "walks" backward on elbows into quadruped (Fig. 3.27A). The therapist's lifts are coordinated with the patient's same-side backward movement of the elbow. Movement of the pelvis facilitates shoulder extension by stretching the latissimus dorsi on the same side. The therapist moves to a partially upright straddle position to assist with positioning the patient's knees under the hips (Fig. 3.27B). The therapist keeps both of his or her knees in contact with the patient's hips to stabilize the hip position. The therapist's hands then shift to the upper trunk to assist upper trunk/UE movement into quadruped. If the patient's knees are too far apart in quadruped, weight can be shifted onto one knee; the opposite unweighted knee will adduct into its proper alignment.

Verbal Cues for Assist-to-Position Movement Transitions Into Quadruped From Prone on Elbows
"On the count of three, I want you to take 'steps' backward on your elbows until your hips are over your knees.

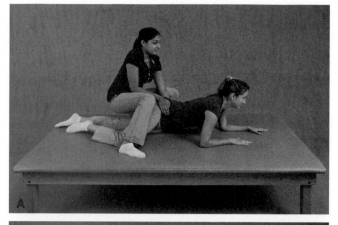

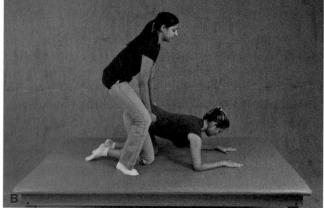

FIGURE 3.27 Assist-to-position movement transition from prone on elbows into quadruped. *Not shown:* Start position is prone on elbows. **(A)** The therapist alternating lifts each hip backward and upward, as the patient "walks" backward on elbows. **(B)** The patient continues to "walk" backward on elbows until the knees are approximately under the hips (some final positioning adjustments may be required). Note that both of the therapist's knees are used to stabilize the hip position. *Not shown:* Lastly, the patient extends elbows one at a time, lifting the upper trunk into quadruped.

At the same time, I will assist by lifting your hips one at a time up and back, starting on the right. Okay, one, two, three; step back with your right elbow. Now, the left side, step back with your left elbow." This sequence is repeated until the knees are under the hips. *"Now, push up with your hands and arms, and come up into the hands-and-knees position."*

ACTIVITIES, STRATEGIES, AND VERBAL CUES: QUADRUPED, ASSIST-TO-POSITION FROM SIDE-SITTING

Activities and Strategies Assist-to-position movement transitions into quadruped can also be accomplished from side-sitting. The patient is positioned in side-sitting with the upper trunk rotated to one side and the elbows extended; both hands are weightbearing on the support surface (the hands should be shoulder-width apart). The hips and knees are prepositioned to approximately 90 degrees of flexion (Fig. 3.28A). The patient begins to move the head and upper trunk from side to side to generate momentum and then, on the

count of three, twists and rotates the lower trunk from side-sitting into quadruped. The therapist is in the half-kneeling straddle position over the patient's legs. Manual contacts are on both hips. The therapist assists the movement of the hips (lower trunk rotation) into quadruped (Fig. 3.28B).

Verbal Cues for Assist-to-Position Movement Transitions Into Quadruped From Side-Sitting *"Begin to shift your head and upper trunk from side to side and then, on the count of three, move your hips up and over your knees. Begin to shift, one, two, three; swing your hips up and over your knees."*

Comments
- During assist to quadruped position, maximum assistance is required in the beginning of the movement; as the hips move closer to the final position, less assistance is given.
- Prepositioning of the limbs is a key element in achieving the desired final position.

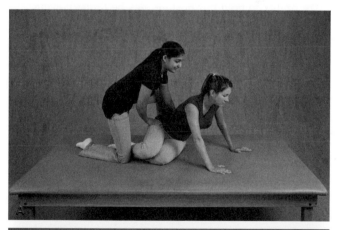

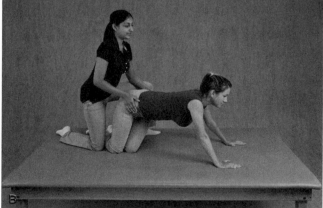

FIGURE 3.28 Assist-to-position movement transitions into quadruped from side-sitting. **(A)** The patient is side-sitting with hips and knees flexed, upper trunk rotated to one side with elbows extended and hands weightbearing; the therapist's manual contacts are on hips/pelvis. *Not shown:* The patient then rocks the head and upper trunk from side to side to generate momentum. **(B)** The patient then twists and rotates the lower trunk from side-sitting toward quadruped; the therapist's manual contacts remain on the hips/pelvis.

- A ball can be used to assist the movement of the hips while providing support for the trunk during early quadruped activities. *The ball size is important.* It should be large enough to support the trunk in quadruped, but not so large as to interfere with assumption of the posture or postural alignment in the position.
- The therapist must be in a dynamic position to allow for the required weight shifting while supporting and assisting the patient without losing balance.

Outcomes

Motor control goal: Mobility (active-assistive movements) progressing to controlled mobility (active movements).

Functional skill achieved: The patient is able to independently assume the quadruped position.

Indications
Weakness or diminished/disordered motor control is an indication. These activities are important lead-up skills for creeping and floor-to-standing transfers.

Comments

- The ability to hold this posture may be limited owing to weakness and/or instability. Modified holding in quadruped with limited weightbearing can be achieved by positioning the patient over an appropriately sized ball to support body weight.
- The ability to hold in this posture may also be limited due to inhibitory pressure on the quadriceps and wrist and finger flexor tendons (firm maintained pressure across tendons from prolonged positioning causes a dampening [inhibition] of muscle tone). An alternative is to position the hand over a sandbag, folded cuff weight, or the end of a platform mat (allowing fingers to flex), or weightbearing can occur on the base of a fisted hand to reduce inhibitory effects. Reducing the impact of inhibitory pressure on the quadriceps is more challenging. Some patients benefit from kneeling on a more resilient surface such as a small soft cushion under each knee. An alternative is to include several shorter time intervals in quadruped over the course of a treatment session (to reduce the effect of prolonged positioning).
- Patients with LE extensor or UE finger flexor hypertonicity may benefit from the effects of inhibitory pressure inherent in this posture. Quadruped can be a useful lead-up activity to relax tone before standing and walking or before UE hand and finger activities.
- Prior to work on the assist-to-position movement transition, patients with UE spasticity accompanied by a retracted scapula with shoulder internal rotation and adduction and elbow flexion (e.g., the patient with stroke) may benefit from initial practice rounding the back and then hollowing; this requires active scapular protraction movements. The UE should be positioned in elbow extension, forearm supination, and shoulder flexion and external rotation.

- Patients with knee pain (e.g., osteoarthritis) may find quadruped as well as kneeling activities uncomfortable. A folded towel or small pillow or cushion placed under the knees may be used to increase comfort level.
- Patients with shoulder pain and limited ROM (e.g., a painful, subluxed shoulder) may not tolerate the quadruped posture. In these situations, sitting with weightbearing on elbows using a stool placed next to the patient or on UEs with elbows extended on a low table in front of the patient may be used to achieve the benefits of early weightbearing.
- Quadruped posture may be contraindicated for patients with LE flexor spasticity.

Quadruped: Interventions, Outcomes, and Management Strategies

Position and Activity: Quadruped, Holding

The patient is in quadruped, actively holding the posture. Initially, attention is directed toward postural alignment. The hands are positioned directly under the shoulders, and weightbearing occurs at the shoulders and through the elbows and wrists, and on the hands. The head and spine are in midposition, and the back is flat. The knees are positioned under the hips; weightbearing occurs at the hips and on the knees.

If scapular instability is present, some winging may be evident. Placing a hand (manual contact) over the midscapular region and asking the patient to flatten the upper back into the hand and then hold the position will activate the scapular stabilizers. Lumbar lordosis may also be present initially, especially if the trunk is heavy. Improved alignment can be achieved by placing a hand over the lumbar region and asking the patient to flatten the back into the hand and then hold the back level (flat). This will activate the abdominal muscles to diminish the lordosis; the back extensors contribute to holding the flat-back position.

TECHNIQUES AND VERBAL CUES

Stabilizing Reversals Stabilizing reversals involve the application of resistance in opposing directions on the trunk in a relatively static quadruped posture; resistance is sufficient to prevent movement. The patient is asked to maintain the quadruped position. Using bilateral manual contacts, the therapist applies resistance first in the stronger direction of movement (agonists) until the patient's maximum is reached. Once the patient is fully resisting with agonists, one hand continues to resist while the opposite hand is positioned to resist the antagonists. When the antagonists begin to engage, the other hand is also moved to resist antagonists. The goal is small-range isotonic contractions progressing to stabilizing (holding).

For the application of stabilizing reversals to the quadruped position, resistance is applied at the scapula (upper trunk) and pelvis (lower trunk) in a *medial/lateral, anterior/posterior,* and *diagonal* direction (each is described below). Recall that stabilizing reversals use isotonic contractions to promote stability, increase strength, and improve coordination between opposing muscle groups. This is a precursor to rhythmic stabilization utilizing isometric contractions.

Stabilizing Reversals, Medial/Lateral Resistance

For the application of stabilizing reversals with medial/lateral resistance in quadruped, the therapist is positioned in half-kneeling at the patient's side (Fig. 3.29). Resistance is given in medial/lateral directions. One of the therapist's manual contacts is on the contralateral upper trunk (depending on the direction, over either the *axillary* or *vertebral* border of scapula); the other hand is positioned on the ipsilateral lower trunk (either on the *lateral aspect of the pelvis* or at the *midpelvic region*). The hand positions are then reversed. For example, if the patient is shifting *toward* the therapist, hand placements are on the vertebral border of the contralateral scapula and the lateral aspect of the ipsilateral pelvis (see Fig. 3.29). If the patient is shifting *away* from the therapist, one hand is on the axillary border of the contralateral scapula and the opposite hand is cupped and "pulls" on the ipsilateral midpelvic region. Alternatively, both hands can resist on the upper and lower sides of the trunk, switching from ipsilateral to contralateral.

Verbal Cues for Stabilizing Reversals, Medial/Lateral Resistance in Quadruped

As the patient attempts to shift toward the therapist: *"Don't let me push you away."* As the patient attempts to shift away from the therapist: *"Don't let me pull you toward me."*

Stabilizing Reversals, Anterior/Posterior Resistance

For the application of stabilizing reversals with anterior/posterior resistance in quadruped, the therapist is positioned in a half-kneeling position behind the patient (one knee may straddle the patient's feet). Bilateral manual contacts are on the pelvis (over either the iliac crests or the lower *pelvis/ischium/buttocks*) and move between resistance applied in *anterior* and *posterior* directions. As the patient attempts to

move forward, the therapist's hands are positioned over the top of the iliac crest (Fig. 3.30). As the patient attempts to move backward, the therapist's hands are positioned over the lower pelvis/ischium/buttocks. Alternatively, one hand can be on the upper trunk and one hand on the lower pelvis/ischium/buttock.

Verbal Cues for Stabilizing Reversals, Anterior/Posterior Resistance in Quadruped

As the patient attempts to shift forward: *"Don't let me pull you back."* As the patient attempts to shift backward: *"Don't let me push you forward."*

Stabilizing Reversals: Diagonal Resistance

For the application of stabilizing reversals with diagonal resistance in quadruped, the therapist is in a half-kneeling position diagonally behind the patient. The patient attempts to shift forward over one UE and then diagonally backward over the contralateral LE. Movement is then reversed to the opposite UE and contralateral LE. Bilateral manual contacts are on the pelvis (either over the *iliac crest* or over the *lower pelvis/ischium/buttocks*) and on the contralateral upper trunk (either over the *top of the shoulder* or at the *vertebral border of the scapula*). Manual contacts change between resistance applied in *anterior diagonal* and *posterior diagonal* directions. As the patient attempts to move diagonally forward, the therapist's hands are positioned over the top of the shoulder and over the iliac crest. As the patient attempts to move diagonally backward, the therapist's hands are positioned over the vertebral border of the scapula and the lower pelvis/ischium.

Verbal Cues for Stabilizing Reversals, Diagonal Resistance in Quadruped

As the patient attempts to shift diagonally forward over UE: *"Don't let me pull you back toward me."* As the patient attempts to shift diagonally backward over LE: *"Don't let me push you forward and away from me."*

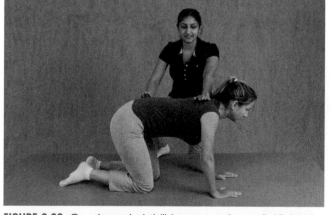

FIGURE 3.29 Quadruped, stabilizing reversals: medial/lateral resistance. In this example, the patient is attempting to shift *toward* the therapist. Manual contacts are on the vertebral border of the contralateral scapula and the lateral aspect of the ipsilateral pelvis.

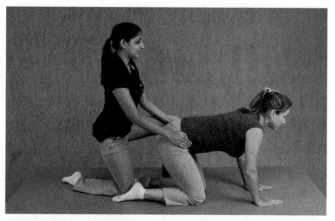

FIGURE 3.30 Stabilizing reversals, anterior/posterior resistance. In this example, the patient is attempting to move forward. Resistance is applied bilaterally with manual contacts over the top of the iliac crests.

Rhythmic Stabilization Rhythmic stabilization involves alternating isometric contractions of agonist/antagonist patterns against resistance. The patient is asked to hold the quadruped position without moving; no movement occurs. The therapist is positioned in half-kneeling behind and to the patient's side. Resistance is built up gradually and applied simultaneously in opposing directions as if twisting the upper and lower trunk in different directions. Resistance is continual; no relaxation occurs. Manual contacts are on the upper and lower trunk. One hand is positioned on the upper trunk, either over the axillary border of the scapula or over the shoulder using a cupped hand. The other hand is positioned on either the contralateral anterior/lateral or posterior/lateral pelvis. The therapist applies resistance by pushing forward and downward on the upper trunk while pulling upward and backward on the pelvis (as if "twisting" the upper and lower trunk in opposite directions). The patient resists the force, holding steady (Fig. 3.31). When the patient is responding with maximal isometric contractions of the agonist pattern, one of the therapist's hands is moved to resist the antagonist pattern. When the antagonists begin to engage, the therapist's other hand is also moved to resist the antagonist pattern. As manual contacts are reversed, their respective positions on the pelvis and upper trunk are maintained.

Verbal Cues for Rhythmic Stabilization in Quadruped
"Hold, don't try to move. Hold, hold. Now don't try to move the other way. Hold, hold." Alternative VCs: *"Hold, don't let me twist you. Hold, hold. Now don't let me twist you the other way. Hold, hold."*

Comments
• Isometric (holding) control is the goal. Resistance is built up gradually. The hold should be smooth and steady, with no visible movement of the trunk.

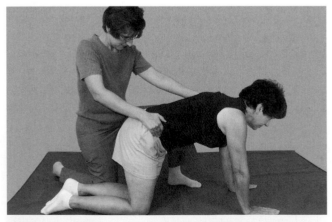

FIGURE 3.31 Rhythmic stabilization in quadruped. In this example, resistance is applied simultaneously in opposing directions as if attempting to twist the upper and lower trunk in opposite directions; hand placements are on the axillary border of the left scapula and on the right anterior/lateral pelvis. *Not shown:* Hand placements are then reversed and positioned over the shoulder (cupped hand) and on the contralateral posterior/lateral pelvis.

• The therapist's hands are moved smoothly during transitions; the patient should not be allowed to relax at any time.
• Rhythmic breathing should be encouraged. Breath holding should be avoided by the patient during all isometric work.
• Good body mechanics for the therapist are important: The back should be straight (not stooped or flexed), and wrist hyperextension should be avoided.
• Elastic resistive bands can be placed around the patient's arms (to increase lateral stabilization of the shoulders) or around the patient's thighs (to increase lateral stabilization of the hips). The patient is instructed to keep the limbs apart, holding against the resistive band.

Outcomes
Motor control goals: Stability and static control of the head, upper and lower trunk, shoulders, and hips.
Functional skill achieved: The patient is able to stabilize independently in the quadruped posture.

Indications Dependent function due to weakness and disordered motor control are indications. Kneeling on all fours is an intermediate posture and lead-up skill for independent assumption of floor-to-standing transfers.

Position and Activity: Quadruped, Weight Shifting
The patient is in quadruped position, with the head in midposition and the back flat. Weight is shifted in *medial/lateral, anterior/posterior*, and *diagonal* directions. This activity promotes dynamic stability, as it requires the patient to maintain the posture while moving. Movement begins with small-range control and progresses to full-range control (through increments of ROM).

TECHNIQUES AND VERBAL CUES
Dynamic Reversals: Medial/Lateral Shifts Dynamic reversals promote active concentric movement in the quadruped position, first in one direction followed by active concentric movement in the reverse direction without relaxation. Smooth reversals of motion (normal transitions between opposing muscle groups) are the goal. Movements are continuously resisted in opposing directions, with VCs used to mark the initiation of movement at the same time direction. The therapist's hands move at the same time the VC is given to ensure smooth reversals of movement.

For the application of dynamic reversals with medial/lateral shifts in quadruped, the therapist is half-kneeling at the patient's side. The patient shifts weight first onto the ipsilateral UE and LE and then shifts weight onto the contralateral limbs. As the patient shifts weight toward the therapist, manual contacts are at the side of the ipsilateral trunk. One hand is on the upper trunk; the other hand is on the pelvis. As the patient moves away from the therapist, hand placements on the upper trunk and pelvis are moved to the side of the contralateral trunk to resist movement. Using an alternative hand position, the therapist maintains one hand positioned on the side of the contralateral upper trunk, resisting first the vertebral border of the scapula and then the axillary border (changed as the patient moves *toward* and *away* from therapist); the other hand is positioned on the ipsilateral pelvis, resisting first on the lateral pelvis (movement *toward* therapist) and then on the midpelvis (movement *away* from therapist).

Verbal Cues for Dynamic Reversals, Medial/Lateral Shifts in Quadruped

Shifting toward therapist: *"Push toward me, push, push, push."* Transitional cue: *"Now, reverse."* Shifting away from therapist: *"Pull away from me, pull, pull, pull."* When the patient is ready to move in the new direction, a preparatory cue (*"Now, reverse"*) is used to direct the patient's attention to the new movement. At the same time as the VC to change directions, the therapist repositions the hands to resist the new direction of motion. If a hold (isometric contraction) is added to dynamic reversals, the VC is *"Pull away, pull, pull, and hold, now push back, push, push."*

Dynamic Reversals: Anterior/Posterior Shifts

For the application of dynamic reversals with anterior/posterior shifts in quadruped, the patient moves weight forward (anterior shift) onto both UEs (Fig. 3.32A) and then backward (posterior shift) onto both LEs (Fig. 3.32B). To resist the movement, the therapist is in a half-kneeling position behind the patient (one knee may straddle the patient's feet). Bilateral manual contacts are on the pelvis (either over the *iliac crest* or over the *lower pelvis/ischium/buttocks*) and change between resistance applied in *anterior* and *posterior* directions. As the patient moves forward, the therapist's hands are positioned over the top of the iliac crest (see Fig. 3.32A). As the patient moves backward, the therapist's hands are positioned over the lower pelvis/ischium/buttock (see Fig. 3.32B).

Verbal Cues for Dynamic Reversals, Anterior/Posterior Shifts in Quadruped

Shifting anteriorly from quadruped: *"Pull forward, pull, pull, pull."* Transitional cue: *"Now, reverse."* Shifting posteriorly: *"Push back, push, push, push."*

Dynamic Reversals: Diagonal Shifts

For the application of dynamic reversals with diagonal shifts in quadruped, the therapist is in a half-kneeling position diagonally behind the patient. The patient shifts diagonally forward over one UE and then diagonally backward over the contralateral LE; movement is then reversed to the opposite UE and contralateral LE. Bilateral manual contacts are on the ipsilateral pelvis (either over the *iliac crest* or over the *lower pelvis/ischium/buttocks*) and on the contralateral upper trunk (either over the *top of the shoulder* or at the *vertebral border of the scapula*). Manual contacts change between resistance applied in *anterior diagonal* and *posterior diagonal* directions. As the patient attempts to move diagonally forward, the therapist's hands are positioned over the top of the ipsilateral shoulder and over the contralateral iliac crest. As the patient attempts to move diagonally backward, the therapist's hands are

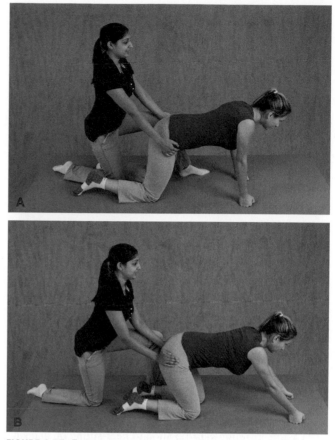

FIGURE 3.32 Dynamic reversals: anterior/posterior shifts in quadruped. **(A)** The patient is shifting forward; resistance is provided using bilateral manual contacts over the iliac crest. **(B)** The patient is shifting backward with manual contacts over the lower pelvis/ischium/buttocks. Note that the patient is using a fisted hand placement on the mat. This alternative hand position may be used if the patient experiences discomfort in weight shifting using an open, flat hand placement on the mat.

positioned over the ipsilateral vertebral border of the scapula and the contralateral lower pelvis/ischium/buttocks.

Verbal Cues for Dynamic Reversals, Diagonal Shifts in Quadruped

Shifting diagonally forward: *"Pull forward, pull, pull, pull."* Transitional cue: *"Now reverse."* Shifting posteriorly: *"Push back, push, push, push."*

Position and Activity: Quadruped, Movement Transitions Into Bilateral Heel-Sitting, Unilateral Heel-Sitting on One Side, and Side-Sitting

TECHNIQUES AND VERBAL CUES

Dynamic Reversals, Movement Transitions From Quadruped to Bilateral Heel-Sitting Position

Movement transitions can be made from the quadruped position down into heel-sitting (buttocks make contact with the heels). During this activity, the patient's hips, knees, and shoulders further flex until the buttocks make contact with the heels; the hands remain in contact with the mat as flexion is increased at the shoulder (Fig. 3.33). The patient then returns back up

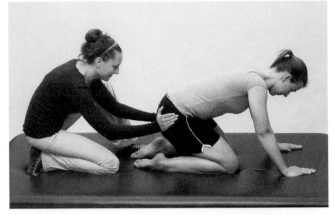

FIGURE 3.33 Dynamic reversals, movement transitions from quadruped to bilateral heel-sitting position. *Not shown:* Start position is quadruped. The patient's hips, knees, and shoulders further flex until the buttocks make contact with the heels; the patient's hands remain in contact with the mat. Manual contacts are on the lower pelvis/ischium/buttocks to resist active concentric movement into heel-sitting. *Not shown:* Manual contacts are then changed and placed over the *iliac crests* to resist movement back up into the starting quadruped position.

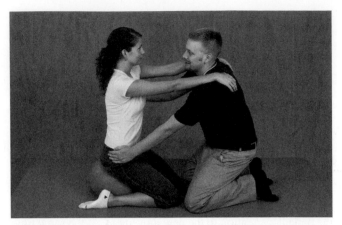

FIGURE 3.34 Heel-sitting on ball. A small ball placed between the patient's feet may be used to provide a more gradual assumption of the heel-sitting position. The therapist is guiding movement with manual contacts at the pelvis and contralateral upper trunk under the axilla. Placement of the patient's UEs on the therapist's shoulders assists with initial stabilization of the upper trunk.

into the starting quadruped position. To resist the concentric movement, dynamic reversals are used first in one direction followed by active concentric movement in the reverse direction without relaxation. The therapist's position transitions from a half-kneeling start position to heel-sitting on one side directly behind the patient. Bilateral manual contacts change between resistance applied over the *lower pelvis/ischium/ buttocks* (to resist movement into heel-sitting) (see Fig. 3.33) and over the *iliac crest* (to resist movement back up into the starting quadruped position).

Verbal Cues for Dynamic Reversals, Movement Transitions From Quadruped to Bilateral Heel-Sitting Position

Moving from quadruped into heel-sitting: *"Push back, all the way onto your heels, push, push, push."* Transitional cue: *"Now, reverse."* Moving from heel-sitting to quadruped: *"Pull back up to all fours, pull, pull, pull."*

Clinical Note: Movements from quadruped into heel-sitting can be used to improve shoulder ROM; this may be useful with unsuspecting patients who may be otherwise anxious about shoulder passive range of motion (PROM).

For patients with LE ROM limitations, those who require a more gradual assumption of the heel-sitting position, or those who find it difficult to get up from the full heel-sitting position, a small ball may be placed between the feet to sit on (Fig. 3.34). This will decrease the range of movement required (compared to full heel-sitting). Caution should be used in selecting the correct size ball. If the ball is too large, it will impose excessive internal rotation at the hips. Alternatively, a sufficiently large stool may be placed over the patient's heels to sit on.

Dynamic Reversals, Movement Transitions From Quadruped to Heel-Sitting on One Side

Dynamic reversals promote active concentric movement in one direction (agonist) followed by active concentric movement in the reverse (antagonist) direction without relaxation. The technique involves continuous resisted movement in opposing directions, with VCs used to mark the initiation of movement in the opposite direction. For the application of dynamic reversals to movement transitions from quadruped to heel-sitting on one side, the therapist transitions from a half-kneeling start position to heel-sitting on one side behind the patient (on the heel-sit side). The patient begins in quadruped and diagonally moves down into heel-sitting on one side and then returns to the start position. Bilateral manual contacts change between resistance applied over the *lower pelvis/ischium/buttocks* (to resist movement into heel-sitting on one side) and over the *iliac crest* (Fig. 3.35) (to resist movement back up into the starting quadruped position); no relaxation occurs. A foam cushion, firm bolster, or wedge may be placed next to the patient's hip on the heel-sit side to decrease the range of movement required (compared to full heel-sitting on one side). A footstool with appropriate padding (towel or cushion) may also be used. If needed, the footstool may be positioned closer to the patient by allowing it to straddle the patient's foot on the heel-sit side. Use of an elevated support surface is helpful for patients who find it difficult to get up from the full heel-sitting position.

Verbal Cues for Dynamic Reversals, Movement Transitions From Quadruped to Heel-Sitting on One Side

Moving backward toward heel-sitting on one side: *"Push back over your (right or left) foot, push, push, push."* Transitional cue: *"Now reverse."* Moving from heel-sitting on one side to quadruped: *"Pull back up to all fours,*

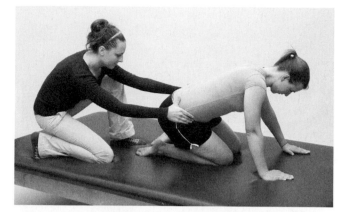

FIGURE 3.35 Dynamic reversals, movement transitions from quadruped to heel-sitting on one side. In this example, the patient has completed the movement down into heel-sitting on one side (right) and is beginning the return to the starting quadruped position. Therapist hand placement is over the *iliac crest* to resist movement back up into quadruped. As the patient progresses into quadruped, the therapist's position transitions from heel-sitting on one side back to the half-kneeling position.

*pull, pull, pull." **Note:*** An alternative verbal cue for moving backward toward heel-sitting on one side is *"Push back toward your (right or left) hip, push, push, push."*

Clinical Note: Movement transitions from quadruped to heel-sitting on one side are a useful activity to elongate the trunk (on the side opposite the heel-sit) and reduce spasticity (e.g., the patient with hemiplegia who demonstrates spasticity in the lateral trunk flexors).

Dynamic Reversals, Movement Transitions From Quadruped to Side-Sitting

This transition involves movement from quadruped to the side-sitting position using lower trunk rotation; the hands remain in contact with the mat. The therapist is in a half-kneeling position diagonally behind the patient (toward the side of the side-sit). The patient begins in quadruped and rotates the lower trunk to move down into side-sitting on one side and then returns to the start position. Bilateral manual contacts change between resistance applied over the *lower pelvis/ischium/buttocks* (to resist movement into side-sitting) and over the *iliac crest* (to resist movement back up into the starting quadruped position); no relaxation occurs. Patients with limited ROM can be instructed to move through the available ranges only or to sit on a foam cushion or firm bolster placed to the side. It should be noted that movement transitions from quadruped to side-sitting require considerable flexibility through the lower trunk and pelvis. Increasing flexibility and learning the movement requirements for transitions to side-sitting may be enhanced by initially supporting the patient's trunk on a ball (Fig. 3.36).

Verbal Cues for Dynamic Reversals, Movement Transitions From Quadruped to Side-Sitting

Moving back toward side-sitting: *"Swing your hips to the right (left)*

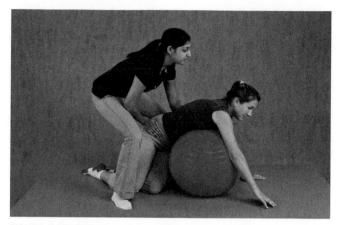

FIGURE 3.36 Movement transitions from quadruped to side-sitting using a ball to support the trunk. This activity may be used to enhance learning as well as to increase flexibility of the lower trunk and pelvis. In this example, the patient is moving toward side-sitting on the left.

and sit down. Push to that side, push, push, push." Transitional cue: *"Now, reverse."* Moving from side-sitting to quadruped: *"Pull your hips back up to all fours, pull, pull, pull."*

Outcomes

Motor control goals: Controlled mobility function of the upper trunk/shoulders and lower trunk/hips.

Functional skills achieved: The patient is able to assume and weight shift in the quadruped posture.

Indications Dependent function due to weakness and disordered motor control are indications. These activities are important lead-up skills for dynamic balance control in the quadruped position and in creeping (progression on hands and knees).

Position and Activity: Quadruped, Static-Dynamic Control, Upper and Lower Extremity Active Limb Lifts

For all static-dynamic activities (lifting one limb from support surface), the BOS decreases and the COM shifts toward the static weightbearing limb(s) to free the dynamic limb for movement. Static-dynamic activities further challenge postural stability; additional challenges can be imposed by movement (e.g., UE reaching, LE lifts) or application of resistance to the dynamic limb. In quadruped, static-dynamic activities are progressed from lifting a single upper or lower limb to simultaneously lifting contralateral upper and lower limbs.

QUADRUPED, UPPER EXTREMITY LIFTS

The patient is in quadruped position, with the head in midposition and the trunk in neutral alignment. The therapist is heel-sitting in front and to the side of the patient (Fig. 3.37). While maintaining the posture, the patient weight shifts onto one UE and lifts the opposite UE off the mat. For active reaching, the therapist can provide a target by holding an open hand in space (within the patient's reach) and asking the patient to touch it; this is repeated, changing the target

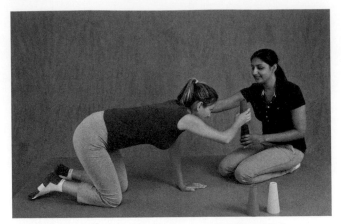

FIGURE 3.37 Quadruped, upper extremity lifting (static-dynamic control). The therapist moves the target cone into position and then actively reaches to place another cone on top. The activity is repeated changing target cone position.

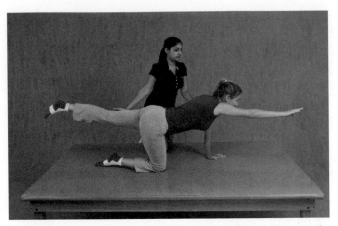

FIGURE 3.38 Quadruped, static-dynamic control, upper and lower extremity limb lifts. This example illustrates simultaneous lifting of contralateral upper and lower limbs to promote static-dynamic control.

hand position. Active reaching can also be combined with a cone-stacking task (see Fig. 3.37). The therapist holds the target cone and asks the patient to place another cone on top of it; the position can be varied with each trial. The initial location of the target (e.g., open hand or cone) should facilitate weight transfer onto the static limb. As control increases, the target can be shifted to other locations to challenge control.

QUADRUPED, LOWER EXTREMITY LIFTS

The patient is in quadruped position, with the head in midposition and the trunk in neutral alignment. The therapist is to the side of the patient in a guard position. While maintaining the posture, the patient is asked to weight shift onto one side and extend the LE backward and up behind the body. Further challenges can be imposed by movement of the dynamic limb (e.g., alternating from full hip and knee flexion with ankle dorsiflexion to full hip and knee extension with ankle plantarflexion or by the application of manual or mechanical resistance (e.g., ankle cuff weights). The amount of resistance applied to the dynamic limb is determined by the patient's ability to hold the static limb and trunk steady. Various combinations of static-dynamic activities can be used: alternating lifts of one UE, then the other; alternating lifts of one LE, then the other; or lifting the contralateral UE and LE (Fig. 3.38).

Position and Activity: Quadruped, Static-Dynamic Control, Application of PNF Extremity Patterns
TECHNIQUES AND VERBAL CUES (TO IMPROVE STATIC-DYNAMIC CONTROL)
Dynamic Reversals, Upper Extremity Extension/Adduction/Internal Rotation, D2 Extension (UE D2E) and Upper Extremity Flexion/Abduction/External Rotation, D2 Flexion (UE D2F) For the application of dynamic reversals using UE D2E and UE D2F to improve static-dynamic control, the patient is in quadruped

position, with the trunk in neutral alignment. The patient's head follows the extremity pattern. The therapist is halfkneeling on the dynamic limb side (Fig. 3.39A). To resist motion of the dynamic UE, one of the therapist's manual contacts is over the dorsal surface of the patient's hand with fingers on the radial side. The opposite hand is positioned over the shoulder to emphasize proximal movement; however, if needed, this hand may be used to apply approximation force over the shoulder of the static limb to increase stabilizing responses. Dynamic reversals involve continuously resisted concentric movement in opposing directions, with VCs used to mark the initiation of movement in the opposite direction. While maintaining the posture, the patient weightshifts onto the static UE and the dynamic UE is unweighted (to instruct the patient in the desired movement, the therapist may passively move the limb through the range once or twice before resistance is applied). The dynamic UE begins in shoulder extension, adduction, and internal rotation with elbow flexion, forearm pronation, and wrist and finger flexion (UE D2E); the fisted hand is placed near the opposite pelvis, at the level of the anterior superior iliac spine (ASIS) (see Fig. 3.39A). The hand opens, turns, and lifts up and out, moving the arm into shoulder flexion, abduction, and external rotation with elbow extension, forearm supination, and wrist and finger extension (UE D2F) (Fig. 3.39B). The patient then reverses direction and brings the UE back down to the start position. The dynamic UE is non-weightbearing at all times.

Verbal Cues for the Application of Dynamic Reversals Using UE D2E and UE D2F *"Shift weight over your right (or left, static limb) arm."* For UE D2F: *"Against my resistance, open your hand, turn, and lift your left (or right, dynamic limb) hand up and out toward me and straighten your elbow."* Transitional cue: *"Now, reverse."* For UE D2E: *"Close your hand, turn, and pull your hand down and across to your opposite hip. Bend your elbow."*

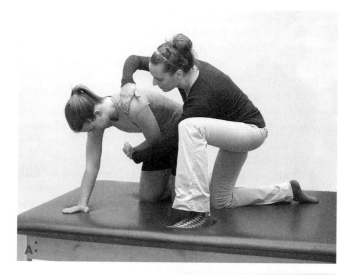

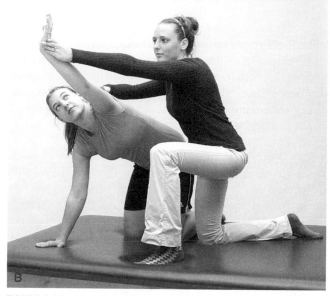

FIGURE 3.39 Application of dynamic reversals using UE flexion and extension patterns in quadruped. **(A)** Start position for the UE D2F pattern; **(B)** end position for the UE D2F pattern. Note that the therapist's right hand is positioned to emphasize shoulder movement.

Comments
- Dynamic reversals are used to increase strength and active ROM as well as promote normal transitions between opposing muscle groups; smooth reversals of motion are the goal.
- Initially, movements are slow and controlled with emphasis on careful grading of resistance; progression is to variations in speed in one or both directions.
- If an imbalance in strength is evident, resistance is typically applied first in the stronger direction of movement (irradiation from stronger components to facilitate weaker components).

Clinical Note: During the application of extremity patterns, hand placements are influenced by the specific goals of treatment. For example, hand placements would change if treatment goals called for emphasis on the scapula (e.g., vertebral border), the shoulder (e.g., proximal humerus), or the forearm (e.g., ulnar surface to control pronation).

Dynamic Reversals, Lower Extremity Flexion/ Adduction/External Rotation, D1 Flexion (LE D1F) With Knee Flexed and Extension/Abduction/ Internal Rotation, D1 Extension, (LE D1E) With Knee Extended For the application of dynamic reversals using LE D1F and LE D1E, the patient is in quadruped with the trunk in neutral alignment. The therapist is behind the patient in a half-kneeling position straddling the static leg (Fig. 3.40A). To resist motion of the dynamic limb, manual contacts are placed on the anterior distal (LE D1F) leg (see Fig. 3.40A) or the posterior distal (LE D1E) leg (Fig. 3.40B). The therapist's other hand is positioned over the top of the pelvis of the static limb. Approximation may be applied to the static lower limb to increase stabilizing responses as needed. While maintaining the posture, the patient weight shifts onto the static LE, and the dynamic LE is unweighted (to instruct

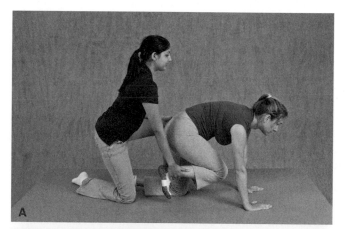

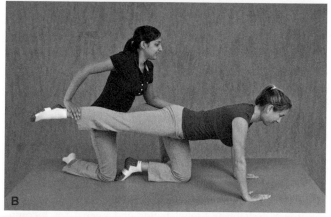

FIGURE 3.40 Application of dynamic reversals using LE flexion and extension patterns in quadruped. **(A)** Start position is the LE D1F pattern; **(B)** end position is the LE D1E pattern.

the patient in the desired movement, the therapist may passively take the limb through the range once or twice before resistance is applied). The dynamic LE begins in hip flexion, adduction, and external rotation with the knee flexed in a diagonal toward the opposite hand (LE D1F) (Fig. 3.40A). In the reverse diagonal direction, the knee then moves back and up into extension, moving the hip into extension, abduction, and internal rotation (see Fig. 3.40B). The patient then reverses direction and brings the dynamic limb back down to the start position. The dynamic LE is non-weightbearing at all times. An isometric hold may be added in the shortened range (either LE D1F or LE D1E) to increase the challenge to the postural trunk and static limb musculature.

Verbal Cues for the Application of Dynamic Reversals Using LE D1F and LE D1E
"Shift your weight over your right (or left, static limb) leg." For LE D1F: *"Against my resistance, pull your foot up and across your body to your opposite hand."* Transitional cue: *"Now, reverse."* For LE D1E: *"Push your leg back and up; straighten your knee."*

Outcomes
Motor control goals: Controlled mobility function and static-dynamic control of the trunk and extremities.

Functional skills achieved: The patient gains postural control and dynamic stability of the trunk in quadruped position and is able to perform UE reaching and LE movements.

Indications Impairments in static-dynamic control in quadruped are indications. These activities are important lead-up skills for function within the posture (i.e., creeping).

Position and Activity: Quadruped, Creeping
ACTIVITIES AND STRATEGIES TO PROMOTE MOVEMENT WITHIN QUADRUPED POSTURE

Movement Within Posture Movement within the quadruped position (creeping) has several important functional implications. It requires trunk counterrotation and contralateral limb movements, important prerequisites for locomotion. Creeping can also be used to improve strength (resisted progression), promote dynamic balance reactions, and improve coordination and timing. Movement within the quadruped posture is also an important precursor to assuming a standing position from the floor (e.g., following a fall, the patient can creep to a chair or other solid support prior to again assuming an upright posture).

To initiate creeping, the patient is in quadruped position, with the head in midposition and the trunk in neutral alignment. The patient moves forward or backward using the upper and lower limbs (hands and knees) for locomotion. Either a four- or two-point sequence is used. A four-point creeping pattern is often used initially, as it provides

maximum stability. The patient advances only one limb at a time (e.g., left hand, right knee; then right hand, left knee). This requires the patient to shift weight to the static limb as the dynamic limb is advanced. The sequence is repeated as the progression continues.

In a two-point creeping pattern, the patient advances one hand and the opposite knee simultaneously (e.g., left hand and right knee are moved together; then right hand and left knee are moved together). The sequence is repeated for continued progression. A two-point pattern allows for a more continuous movement sequence. Some patients may adopt an ipsilateral pattern in which the hand and the knee on the same side move together. This pattern should be discouraged in favor of a contralateral pattern, with the opposite hand and knee moving together.

Position and Activity: Quadruped, Creeping, Resisted Progression
TECHNIQUES AND VERBAL CUES

Resisted Progression This technique involves the application of manual resistance to the pelvis in quadruped (creeping) to resist both forward progression and the pelvic rotation that accompanies the advancement of the LEs (improved timing and control of pelvic rotation are the goals). A stretch can be used to facilitate the initiation of pelvic and LE movements. During the application of resisted progression, the patient is in quadruped position, with the head in midposition and the trunk in neutral alignment. The therapist moves with the patient and is positioned standing, with knees slightly flexed (partial squat position), behind the patient. Alternatively, the therapist may be positioned in half-kneeling behind the patient and slide forward as the patient progresses. Bilateral manual contacts are over the iliac crests (Fig. 3.41). A modification of this activity is for the therapist to assume a squatting position behind the patient, moving forward each time the patient moves; manual contacts are

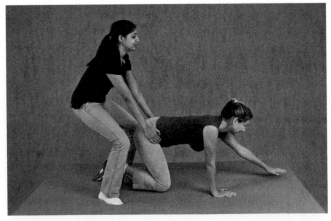

FIGURE 3.41 Quadruped, creeping, resisted progression. Bilateral manual contacts are over the iliac crests to provide resistance during forward movement. Maintaining manual contacts, the therapist moves forward with the patient.

then placed on the patient's ankles to resist forward progression. The level of resistance is graded so as not to disrupt the patient's momentum, coordination, and velocity.

 Clinical Note: An alternative resisted progression activity is the application of resistance using elastic resistance bands wrapped around the patient's hips/pelvis and held from behind by the therapist (Fig. 3.42). Resistance can also be provided using wrist and ankle cuff weights.

Verbal Cues for Quadruped, Creeping, Resisted Progression
"On three, 'step' forward, moving your opposite arm and leg together. One, two, three, and step, step." Movements should be well timed with VCs.

 Clinical Note: Some patients may be resistant to creeping as a treatment activity, feeling it is too childish. These feelings must be respected and explored; such feelings may indicate the patient is not fully aware of the rationale for the activity. The therapist should stress the clinical relevance of creeping to other functional activities. For example, the counterrotation pattern is important for gait; patients may need this skill following a fall to get to the nearest chair or support to pull themselves up.

Outcomes
Motor control goals: Development of skilled locomotion pattern and trunk counterrotation with contralateral UE and LE movements.

Functional skill achieved: The patient is able to move independently in quadruped using a reciprocal trunk and limb pattern.

Indications
Indications are impaired timing and control of limb and trunk/pelvic movements.

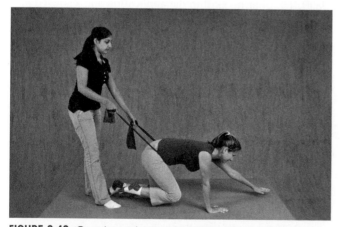

FIGURE 3.42 Quadruped, creeping, resisted progression using elastic resistance bands. For this activity, the therapist is standing holding the ends of the resistance bands and moves forward with the patient. Greater resistance is applied during forward movement of the dynamic limb.

Position and Activity: Quadruped, Balance Control
Many of the activities already presented address various aspects of balance control. However, patients who demonstrate significant impairments in dynamic postural control may be unable to control their postural stability and orientation while moving segments of the body. A number of impairments, either alone or in combination, may be contributing factors, including imbalances in tone (e.g., spasticity and rigidity), limitations in ROM, impaired voluntary control (e.g., ataxia and athetosis), inability to make smooth transitions between opposing muscle groups (e.g., cerebellar dysfunction), and inability to stabilize proximally. Functionally, these patients may have difficulty with movements that increase the demand for dynamic stabilization control owing to changes in the BOS or COM such as weight shifting in any direction and static-dynamic control in quadruped. For these patients, greater emphasis will be placed on balance strategies to improve static and dynamic postural control.

ACTIVITIES AND STRATEGIES TO IMPROVE BALANCE
Balance Strategies Balance activities in quadruped can begin with static holding (static postural control) and progresses to weight shifts in all directions (dynamic postural control). An important early element of a balance sequence is for the patient to learn his or her limits of stability (LOS). This requires the patient to learn how far he or she can shift in any one direction before losing balance and falling out of the quadruped posture. Balance practice begins with movements emphasizing smooth directional changes that engage antagonist actions (e.g., weight shifts). As control improves, the movements are gradually expanded through an increasing range (increments of range).

Although active movement is the goal, assistance may be required during initial movement attempts for both the dynamic movements and for stabilizing body segments. Dynamic movements can be facilitated using quick stretches, manual contacts, and graded resistance. Task-oriented dynamic movements (e.g., reaching) often hold more interest, especially if the task is important to the patient. The patient's attention should focus on performing the activity or task and not on the stabilizing postural components. This redirecting of cognitive attention is an important measure of developing postural control, as intact postural control functions largely on an automatic and unconscious level.

Additional activities that challenge *anticipatory balance control* in quadruped posture include arm lifts, leg lifts, and combined arm and leg lifts as well as "look-arounds" (the head and upper trunk rotate first to one side, then to the other) and transitions from quadruped to side-sitting and back to quadruped using pelvic/lower trunk rotation. PNF extremity patterns can be used to increase the level of difficulty.

Activities that can be used to challenge *reactive balance control* include side-to-side tilts on a large equilibrium board (self- or therapist-initiated). Lateral curvature of the head and upper trunk is a normal response; the head and trunk rotate toward the raised or elevated side. Progression is from four-limb support to three-limb to two-limb support while balancing on the equilibrium board. Self-initiated tilts challenge both anticipatory and reactive balance control.

Outcomes

Motor control goals: Static and dynamic balance control.

Functional skill achieved: The patient demonstrates appropriate functional balance in the quadruped position.

Indications Significant impairments in postural stability and dynamic postural control as well as inability to control postural stability and orientation while segments of body are moving.

See Box 3.7 Section Summary Student Practice Activity on treatment interventions used in quadruped.

Hooklying

General Characteristics

In *hooklying,* the patient is supine with both hips and knees flexed to approximately 60 degrees and feet flat on the supporting surface. With its large BOS, the posture is very stable. The COM is low. In hooklying, lower trunk rotation occurs as the knees move from side to side away from midline. The posture primarily involves lower trunk, hip, and knee control. For example, activation of the lower trunk rotators and hip abductors and adductors allows the patient to actively move the knees from side to side away from

---

BOX 3.7 SECTION SUMMARY STUDENT PRACTICE ACTIVITY: QUADRUPED

Description of Student Practice Activity

Each section of this chapter ends with a similarly challenging student practice activity titled *Section Summary Student Practice Activity (followed by the section title).* A section outline for quadruped to guide the activity is provided that highlights the key treatment strategies, techniques, and activities addressed in the preceding section. This activity is an opportunity to share knowledge and skills as well as to confirm or clarify understanding of the treatment interventions. Each student in a group will contribute his or her understanding of, or questions about, the strategy, technique, or activity being discussed and demonstrated. Dialogue should continue until a consensus of understanding is reached. (*Note:* **These directions will be repeated for each subsequent section summary student practice activity, in the event that content is considered in a sequence different from that presented here.**)

Section Outline: Quadruped

MOVEMENT TRANSITIONS: ACTIVITIES, STRATEGIES, AND TECHNIQUES
▲ Prone on elbows to quadruped transition using assist-to-position
▲ Quadruped from side-sitting transition using assist-to-position
▲ Quadruped to bilateral heel-sitting transitions using dynamic reversals
▲ Quadruped to heel-sitting on one side transitions using dynamic reversals
▲ Quadruped to side-sitting transitions using a ball to support trunk

ACTIVITIES AND TECHNIQUES
▲ Quadruped, holding using stabilizing reversals, medial/lateral resistance
▲ Quadruped, holding using stabilizing reversals, anterior/posterior resistance

▲ Quadruped, holding using rhythmic stabilization
▲ Quadruped, holding using dynamic reversals, anterior/posterior shifts

STATIC-DYNAMIC ACTIVITIES
▲ Quadruped, holding, UE lifts using active movements and cone stacking
▲ Quadruped, upper and lower extremity contralateral limb lifts using active movements

EXTREMITY PATTERNS AND TECHNIQUES
▲ Quadruped, holding, UE D2F and UE D2E patterns using dynamic reversals
▲ Quadruped, holding, LE D1F and LE D1E patterns using dynamic reversals

RESISTED PROGRESSION
▲ Quadruped, creeping, resisted progression (manual)
▲ Quadruped, creeping, resisted progression using elastic resistance bands

---

OBJECTIVE: Sharing skill in the application and knowledge of treatment interventions used in quadruped.

EQUIPMENT NEEDED: Platform mat, large ball, and elastic resistance bands.

DIRECTIONS: Working in groups of four to six students, consider each entry in the section outline. Members of the group will assume different roles (described below) and will rotate roles each time the group progresses to a new item on the outline.

▲ One person assumes the role of therapist (for demonstrations) and participates in discussion.
▲ One person serves as the subject/patient (for demonstrations) and participates in discussion.
▲ The remaining members participate in discussion and provide supportive feedback during demonstrations. One member of this group should be designated as a "fact checker" to return to the text content to confirm elements of the discussion (if needed) or if agreement cannot be reached.

BOX 3.7 SECTION SUMMARY STUDENT PRACTICE ACTIVITY: QUADRUPED (continued)

Thinking aloud, brainstorming, and sharing thoughts should be continuous throughout this activity! As each item in the section outline is considered, the following should ensue:

1. An initial discussion of the *activity,* including patient and therapist positioning. Also considered here should be positional changes to enhance the activity (e.g., prepositioning a limb, hand placements to alter the BOS, and so forth).
2. An initial discussion of the *technique,* including its description, indication(s) for use, therapist hand placements (manual contacts), and verbal cues.
3. A *demonstration* of the activity and application of the technique by the designated therapist and

subject/patient. Discussion during the demonstration should be continuous (the demonstration should not be the sole responsibility of the designated therapist and subject/patient). All group members should provide recommendations, suggestions, and supportive feedback throughout the demonstration. Particularly important during the demonstrations is discussion of strategies to make the activity either *more* or *less* challenging.

4. If any member of the group feels he or she requires practice with the activity and technique, time should be allocated to accommodate the request. All group members providing input (recommendations, suggestions, and supportive feedback) should also accompany this practice.

---

midline (knee rocks); activation of the hamstrings allows the patient to keep the knees flexed in the hooklying position.

Treatment Strategies and Considerations

Hooklying is an important lead-up activity for controlled bridging (hip extension from hooklying), kneeling, and bipedal gait. Abnormal reflex activity may interfere with assumption or maintenance of the posture. In supine, the STLR may cause the LEs to extend. A positive support reaction (applying pressure to the ball of the foot) may also cause the LE to extend; a heel-down position minimizing contact of the ball of the foot may need to be adopted. Active movements of the knees from side to side (lower trunk rotation) involve crossing the midline and can be an important treatment activity for patients with unilateral neglect (e.g., the patient with left hemiplegia). Patients with gluteus medius weakness (e.g., a Trendelenburg gait pattern) may benefit from hooklying activities to activate the abductors in a less stressful, non-weightbearing or modified weightbearing position. Lower trunk rotation should occur without accompanying upper trunk rotation or log rolling, which can be minimized by positioning the shoulders in abduction on the mat. UE positions can also be changed to alter the BOS in hooklying (e.g., difficulty is increased by folding the arms across the chest or holding the hands clasped together above the chest). For the patient recovering from stroke who demonstrates excess flexor tone in the UE, the hands-clasped position with both elbows extended and shoulders flexed to approximately 90 degrees should be used.

Clinical Note: In hooklying, some patients may initially experience difficulty maintaining foot position (i.e., heels slide away from the buttocks). In these situations, the feet should be blocked in position (e.g., manual contacts from the therapist or use of a weighted sandbag). In the presence of a positive support reaction, care should be taken not to block the feet such that pressure is applied to the ball of the foot, as this may cause the LE

to extend. As mentioned, a heel-down position minimizing contact of the ball of the foot may need to be adopted.

Hooklying: Interventions, Outcomes, and Management Strategies

Position/Activity: Hooklying, Lower Trunk Rotation

TECHNIQUES AND VERBAL CUES

Rhythmic Initiation Rhythmic initiation is a technique used to instruct the patient in the desired movement, to facilitate the initiation of movement, and to promote relaxation. Movements are first passive, then active-assistive, and then resisted (passive → active-assistive → resisted). The patient then moves independently. If needed, quick stretch can be used to facilitate the initiation of movement in the desired direction. Progression to each phase of movement is dependent on the patient's ability to relax and participate in the movements.

For the application of rhythmic initiation in hooklying to promote lower trunk rotation, the patient is in the hooklying position with both feet placed flat on the mat. The therapist is in the half-kneeling or heel-sitting position at the base of the patient's feet. To assist with movement, manual contacts for the passive and active-assistive components are on top of the patient's knees (Fig. 3.43). The therapist moves the patient passively through the desired movement (knees are moved laterally to and from midline in each direction). The patient is instructed to relax as the therapist slowly rocks the knees from side to side and the lower trunk is rotated. As relaxation is achieved, the range is gradually increased until the knees move laterally down close to the mat on each side. The movements to and from midline are first passive, next active-assistive, and then resisted.

During the resistive phase of rhythmic initiation, manual contacts change. The therapist remains in the half-kneeling position. Hand placements are now on the medial side of one knee (closest to therapist) and the lateral side of the opposite knee (farthest from therapist) to resist both knees as they pull away (Fig. 3.44). The therapist's hands need to

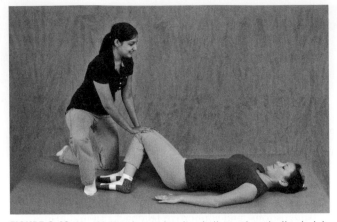

FIGURE 3.43 Hooklying, lower trunk rotation using rhythmic initiation (passive and active-assistive components). Therapist hand placements are on the tops of the knees. The knees are moved from side to side and the lower trunk is rotated.

"pivot" in order to resist the complete movement of the knees down to the mat. This sequence is repeated with the gradual introduction of appropriate levels of resistance typically beginning with light resistance. Manual contacts then move to the opposite sides of the knees to resist movement toward the therapist.

Verbal Cues for Rhythmic Initiation in Hooklying, Lower Trunk Rotation
Passive phase: *"Relax, let me move your knees out to the side and back up to the other side."* Active-assistive phase: *"Move with me, out to the side; now back up to the other side."* Resistive phase, knees moving away from midline and therapist: *"Move against my resistance. Pull your knees down toward the mat, pull, pull. Now, pull back up and to the other side "* If optional quick stretches are used, they should be well timed with VCs. VCs should be soothing, slow, rhythmic, and well timed with movements.

Clinical Note: An alternative application of the passive movement in hooklying for lower trunk rotation involves positioning the patient's legs on a ball (Fig. 3.45) with the hips and knees flexed to approximately 70 degrees. The therapist is half-kneeling on a diagonal to one side, with manual contacts on the anterior aspects of the patient's legs. The therapist slowly rocks the ball from side to side. This positioning eliminates tactile input to the bottom of the feet, thereby reducing the possible negative effects of a hyperactive positive support reflex. The ball also allows the patient to move from side to side easily and is an effective intervention to promote LE relaxation (e.g., for patients with multiple sclerosis or stroke and high levels of extensor spasticity). This positioning is also a good way to protect the lower back, if that is a concern.

Outcomes
Motor control goals: Initiation of movement (mobility) and relaxation.
Functional skills achieved: The patient learns the movement requirements of lower trunk rotation and strategies for initiating movement and relaxation.

Indications Indications include impaired function due to hypertonia (spasticity, rigidity) and inability to initiate or control lower trunk rotation.

Replication Recall that replication is a unidirectional technique, emphasizing movement in one direction. The patient is passively moved to the end of the desired motion (or available range) and asked to hold against resistance (isometric contraction). The patient then relaxes and is moved passively through a small range in the opposite direction; the patient then actively returns (concentric contraction) to the initial end range position. Movement is through increments of range until full range is achieved (passive movement to end range → hold against

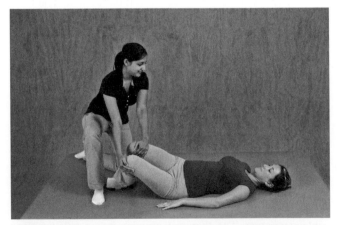

FIGURE 3.44 Hooklying, lower trunk rotation using rhythmic initiation (resistive component). For application of resistance, manual contacts are on the medial side of one knee and the lateral side of the opposite knee; the therapist provides the return motion. *Not shown:* Hand placements are then reversed for movement in the opposite direction.

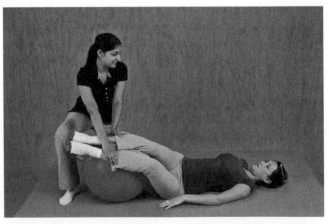

FIGURE 3.45 Hooklying, lower trunk rotation using a ball (passive phase of rhythmic initiation). The patient's hips and knees are flexed to approximately 90 degrees and supported on the ball. Manual contacts are on the anterior aspects of the legs.

resistance → relaxation → passive movement in opposite direction → active return to initial end range).

For the application of replication to promote lower trunk rotation in hooklying, the therapist is positioned in half-kneeling to the side. Manual contacts for passive movements are on the tops of the patient's knees; for resistive hold components, manual contacts are on the medial side of one knee and the lateral side of the opposite knee (Fig. 3.46). The patient's knees are passively moved toward one side (e.g., away from the therapist) one-quarter range. This is the initial start position. The patient then holds this position against resistance, and an isometric contraction is slowly built up. The patient then actively relaxes. Next, the therapist passively moves the knees past midline through a small range (e.g., one-quarter range) in the opposite direction (e.g., toward the therapist). The patient then actively contracts (concentric contraction) and moves through the range back to the initial start position. Movement is through increments of range; midrange control is achieved first. With successive replication of movement, the range is gradually increased until full range is accomplished.

Verbal Cues for Replication in Hooklying
"Let me move your knees to one side. Now hold this position against my resistance. Don't let me move you, hold, hold, hold. Now relax completely, and let me move your knees back toward me. Now pull all the way back to the starting position."

Comments
• Resistance to the isometric contraction (hold) is used to recruit gamma motor neurons and enhance contraction; resistance is built up gradually.

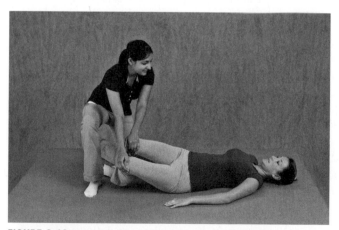

FIGURE 3.46 Application of replication to promote lower trunk rotation in hooklying. The example illustrates the *resistive (isometric) component.* Following passive movement of the patient's knees through partial range to one side (here knees have been moved toward the patient's left, away from the therapist), the patient holds this position against resistance and an isometric contraction is slowly built up. Manual contacts for the application of resistance are on the medial side of one knee and the lateral side of the opposite knee. Movement is through increments of range.

• Active relaxation is important; the patient should not be passively moved in the opposite direction until the contraction is completely released (relaxation is achieved).
• If needed, a quick stretch can be applied in the lengthened range to facilitate the return movement.
• Replication is a unidirectional technique, emphasizing holding and movement in one direction. The hold is built up slowly. The patient is moved back through the range once relaxation is achieved.
• Resistance (irradiation) can be used to facilitate weaker muscles (e.g., weak hip abductors on one side).

Outcomes
Motor control goal: Initiation of movement (mobility).
Functional skill achieved: The patient performs independent initiation of lower trunk rotation.

Indications Indications are to promote the initiation of lower trunk rotation in the presence of muscle weakness (e.g., lower trunk rotators, hip abductors) and hypotonia. The patient should be instructed in the end result (outcome) of the movement.

Position/Activity: Hooklying, Active Holding
ACTIVITY AND VERBAL CUES

Holding Static postural stability (holding) in hooklying is the focus of this activity. For the application of holding in hooklying, the therapist guards from a heel-sitting or half-kneeling position to one side of the patient's LEs. Manual contacts are used to assist if initial holding of the posture is difficult. The patient actively holds the hooklying position. Both of the patient's knees are stable (knees are not touching), feet are in contact with the mat surface, and biomechanical alignment and symmetrical midline weight distribution are maintained. As control increases, the position of the feet can be moved more distally, decreasing the amount of hip and knee flexion. Holding is imposed at each successive repositioning of the feet as hip and knee flexion is gradually decreased. This promotes development of selective knee control at different points in the range.

Verbal Cues for Active Holding in Hooklying
"Hold the position, keep your knees stable and apart, feet flat on the mat, and your weight evenly distributed. Hold, hold, keep holding the position."

Comments
• Progression can be achieved by altering the activity from bilateral to unilateral holding (modified hooklying) and by holding for gradually longer periods with varying amounts of hip and knee flexion.
• Elastic resistive bands can be placed around the patient's thighs to enhance proprioceptive loading and contraction of the stabilizing hip abductors.
• A small ball may be placed between the knees to promote contraction of hip adductors.

Outcomes
Motor control goal: Stability.
Functional skill achieved: The patient has improved static postural control in hooklying.

Indications Decreased strength, diminished lower trunk stability, and inability to stabilize hips and knees in flexion with feet supported are indications.

📄 **Clinical Note:** Trunk (core) and hip stability control (holding) is among the most critical elements for successful functional task execution. Initiated in dependent postures, trunk and hip stability is eventually progressed to upright positions and skill level activities. Trunk stability provides the foundation and support for extremity function as well as the individual's ability to interact with the environment.

Position/Activity: Hooklying, Resisted Holding
TECHNIQUES AND VERBAL CUES
Stabilizing Reversals This technique utilizes small-range isotonic contractions progressing to stabilizing (holding) in the posture to promote stability, increase strength, and improve coordination between opposing muscle groups. There is no relaxation with directional changes. For the application of stabilizing reversals in hooklying, the therapist is positioned in half-kneeling to one side of the patient's LEs. The patient is asked to hold the hooklying position while the therapist applies resistance to the knees (Fig. 3.47). Resistance is applied in a side-to-side direction; the therapist's manual contacts alternate between the *medial side* of one knee and the *lateral side* of the opposite knee. The hand placements are then reversed to resist holding in the other direction. Resistance is applied until the patient's maximum is reached and then reversed. This sequence is repeated with gradual introduction of appropriate levels of resistance, typically beginning with light resistance.

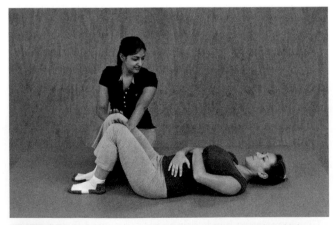

FIGURE 3.47 Application of stabilizing reversals in hooklying. The patient is asked to hold the hooklying position while the therapist applies resistance to the knees. Resistance is applied in a side-to-side direction, with the therapist's manual contacts alternating between the *medial side* of one knee and the *lateral side* of the opposite knee.

Verbal Cues for Stabilizing Reversals in Hooklying
"Don't let me move your knees to the side. Hold, hold. Now, don't let me move your knees to the other side. Hold, hold."

Outcomes
Motor control goal: Stability.
Functional skills achieved: The patient gains independent static postural control in hooklying.

Indications Indications include weakness and instability of the lower trunk (e.g., the patient with low back dysfunction or the patient with asymmetrical trunk control) and weakness and instability of the hip muscles (e.g., the patient with abductor weakness and a Trendelenburg gait). Independent static postural control in hooklying is an important lead-up skill for lower trunk/pelvic stabilization during locomotion.

Comments
- Resistance is first applied in the stronger direction (to promote irradiation to weaker muscles) and then in the opposite direction.
- Greater challenges can be imposed by gradually decreasing the amount of hip and knee flexion (e.g., from 60 to 40 to 20 degrees).
- Stabilizing reversals may also be applied diagonally; the manual contacts and position of therapist vary based on the desired direction of diagonal force. For example, diagonal resistance at the knees can be applied with manual contacts alternating between the *distal anterior medial* side of one knee and the *distal anterior lateral* side of the opposite knee. The hand placements are then reversed to the *proximal superior medial* side of one knee and the *proximal superior lateral* side of the other knee to resist holding in the opposite direction.
- Resistance can be applied to the ankles. Distal resistance can be used to further promote trunk stability. In addition, this variation shifts the focus more distally and can be used to recruit more activity of the knee muscles, especially the hamstrings.
- Therapist hand placements should provide smooth transitions between applications of resistance in opposite directions.
- Steady holding of the hooklying posture is the goal.

Position/Activity: Hooklying, Lower Trunk Rotation, Active Movement
TECHNIQUES AND VERBAL CUES
Dynamic Reversals Dynamic reversals promote active concentric movement in one direction followed by active concentric movement in the reverse direction without relaxation. The technique involves continuous resisted movement in opposing directions, with a transitional VC used to mark the initiation of movement in the opposite direction.

For the application of dynamic reversals in hooklying, the patient moves both knees together in side-to-side movements (i.e., toward the *right* and *left* away from midline).

Depending on the ROM available, the knees may move all the way down to the mat on one side and then the other. The therapist is positioned in half-kneeling slightly to one side of the patient's LEs. Resistance is applied as the knees move in a side-to-side direction, with the therapist's manual contacts alternating between the *medial side* of one knee and the *lateral side* of the opposite knee. The hand placements are then reversed to resist movement in the other direction. For example, as the knees move toward the therapist, hand placements are on the lateral side of the knee closest to the therapist and the medial side of the knee farthest from the therapist (Fig. 3.48). The hands then move to the opposite sides of the knees to resist movement away from the therapist. Manual contacts should allow smooth transitions between opposing directions of movement. An isometric hold may be added in the shortened range or at any point of weakness within the range. The hold is a momentary pause (the patient is instructed to *"Hold"*); the antagonist movement pattern is then facilitated. The hold can be added in one direction only or in both directions.

Dynamic reversals may be combined with repeated stretch if weakness exists. The purpose of repeated stretch (manual stretch or tapping over muscle) is to elicit the stretch reflex to support active movement. The repeated stretch is performed in the lengthened range and carefully timed to coincide with the patient's voluntary effort. For example, if the hip abductors were weak on the right side, the knees would be moved down to the mat on the left (placing right hip abductors in lengthened range). From this lengthened position, the patient's knees would be repeatedly pulled back down to the mat on the left (repeated stretches) while dynamic VCs *("Pull up, and pull up again, pull up, and pull up")* are given to facilitate the movement. Repeated stretch may also be superimposed on an existing contraction, applied at points of weakness within range, or applied through partial range with progression to full range (response will be influenced by the relative length of the muscle being stretched).

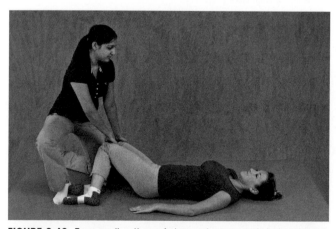

FIGURE 3.48 For application of dynamic reversals in hooklying, resistance is applied as the knees move in a side-to-side direction. In the example shown, manual contacts are on the *lateral* side of one knee and the *medial* side of the opposite knee as the knees move toward the therapist.

Verbal Cues for Dynamic Reversals in Hooklying

As knees move away from the therapist: *"Pull your knees away as I resist. Don't let me stop you, pull, pull, pull."* Transitional cue: *"Now, reverse."* As knees move toward the therapist: *"Now push back toward me. Don't let me stop you, push, push, push."* If a hold (isometric contraction) is added to dynamic reversals at the end range or point of weakness, the VC is *"Hold."*

Outcomes

Motor control goal: Controlled mobility function.

Functional skills achieved: The patient masters controlled lower trunk rotation. Control of lower trunk/pelvic movements is an important prerequisite requirement for standing and gait.

Indications Indications include weakness and instability of the lower trunk and hip muscles, impaired coordination and timing (e.g., patients with ataxia), and limitations in ROM. Lower trunk rotation in hooklying is an important lead-up skill for upright antigravity control in standing and gait.

Comments

- Resistance is typically applied first in the stronger direction of movement.
- Movements begin with small-range control (e.g., one-quarter range movement in each direction) and progress through increasing ROM (increments of ROM) to full-range control (the knees move all the way down to the mat on each side).
- Initially, movements are slow and controlled, with emphasis on careful grading of resistance.
- The successful application of dynamic reversals requires careful timing and coordination of the transitional VCs with changes in manual contacts between opposing directions of movement.
- Dynamic reversals are used to increase strength and active ROM as well as promote normal transitions between opposing muscle groups.
- A smooth reversal of motion is the goal.

See Box 3.8 Section Summary Student Practice Activity on treatment interventions used in hooklying.

Bridging

General Characteristics

From a hooklying position, *bridging* involves extending the hips and elevating the pelvis from the support surface with the lumbar spine in a neutral position (initial instruction in pelvic tilting may be required to identify the neutral position). Bridging is an important prerequisite requirement for moving in bed (positional changes) and for moving to the edge of the bed. It is also an important lead-up for later functional activities, such as developing sit-to-stand control and stance phase control of

BOX 3.8 SECTION SUMMARY STUDENT PRACTICE ACTIVITY: HOOKLYING

Description of Student Practice Activity

Each section of this chapter ends with a similarly challenging student practice activity titled *Section Summary Student Practice Activity (followed by the section title)*. A section outline for hooklying to guide the activity is provided that highlights the key treatment strategies, techniques, and activities addressed in the preceding section. This activity is an opportunity to share knowledge and skills as well as to confirm or clarify understanding of the treatment interventions. Each student in a group will contribute his or her understanding of, or questions about, the strategy, technique, or activity being discussed and demonstrated. Dialogue should continue until a consensus of understanding is reached. (*Note:* **These directions will be repeated for each subsequent section summary student practice activity, in the event that content is considered in a sequence different from that presented here.**)

Section Outline: Hooklying

ACTIVITIES AND TECHNIQUES
- Hooklying, lower trunk rotation using rhythmic initiation
- Hooklying, lower trunk rotation using a ball, passive movements
- Hooklying, lower trunk rotation using replication
- Hooklying, holding, using stabilizing reversals
- Hooklying, lower trunk rotation using dynamic reversals

OBJECTIVE: Sharing skill in the application and knowledge of treatment interventions used in hooklying.

EQUIPMENT NEEDED: Platform mat and large ball.

DIRECTIONS: Working in groups of four to six students, consider each entry in the section outline. Members of the group will assume different roles (described below) and will rotate roles each time the group progresses to a new item on the outline.

- One person assumes the role of therapist (for demonstrations) and participates in discussion.
- One person serves as the subject/patient (for demonstrations) and participates in discussion.
- The remaining members participate in discussion and provide supportive feedback during demonstrations. One member of this group should be designated as a "fact checker" to return to the text content to confirm elements of the discussion (if needed) or if agreement cannot be reached.

Thinking aloud, brainstorming, and sharing thoughts should be continuous throughout this activity! As each item in the section outline is considered, the following should ensue:

1. An initial discussion of the **activity,** including patient and therapist positioning. Also considered here should be positional changes to enhance the activity (e.g., prepositioning a limb, hand placements to alter the BOS, and so forth).
2. An initial discussion of the **technique,** including its description, indication(s) for use, therapist hand placements (manual contacts), and verbal cues.
3. A **demonstration** of the activity and application of the technique by the designated therapist and subject/patient. Discussion during the demonstration should be continuous (the demonstration should not be the sole responsibility of the designated therapist and subject/patient). All group members should provide recommendations, suggestions, and supportive feedback throughout the demonstration. Particularly important during the demonstrations is discussion of strategies to make the activity either *more* or *less* challenging.
4. If any member of the group feels he or she requires practice with the activity and technique, time should be allocated to accommodate the request. All group members providing input (recommendations, suggestions, and supportive feedback) should also accompany this practice.

---

gait as well as for stair climbing. The posture is very stable, with a large BOS and low COM (although compared to hooklying, the BOS is smaller and the COM is higher). Bridging is similar to hooklying in that it primarily involves the lower trunk, hip, and knee muscles. The lower trunk muscles and hip abductors and adductors stabilize the hip and lower trunk. The low back and hip extensors elevate the pelvis. The hamstrings keep the knees flexed and the feet positioned for weightbearing. During bridging, the gluteus maximus is primarily responsible for hip extension because knee flexion places the hamstrings in a position of active insufficiency.

To begin bridging activities, the patient is positioned in hooklying with the hips and knees flexed to approximately 60 degrees and the feet flat on the mat. The patient is instructed to raise the hips/pelvis from the mat (concentric contraction) until the hips are fully extended (0 degrees), the pelvis is elevated and level, and the lumbar spine is in neutral position (isometric contraction). For the return motion, the patient slowly controls lowering (eccentric contraction) of the hips/pelvis back down to the mat; collapsing back to the mat using body weight and gravity should be avoided.

Red Flag: During hip/pelvis elevation, the pelvis should not rotate. Patients with unilateral weakness of the gluteus maximus (for example, the patient recovering from a hip fracture) may be unable to hold the pelvis level and the pelvis will drop on the weaker side. The therapist can hold a wand or yardstick across the pelvis to demonstrate this rotation visually to the patient. Additional strengthening of the gluteus maximus or increasing the BOS through positioning (see the following paragraph) may be indicated until pelvic control improves.

The BOS in bridging may be altered to *increase* or *decrease* the challenge imposed. Initially, the activity may be made easier through positioning to increase the stability (BOS) of the posture. This is accomplished by extending the elbows, abducting the shoulders with forearms pronated and hands flat on the mat, and/or moving the feet apart. Reducing this stabilization can increase the difficulty. This is achieved by gradually adducting the shoulders (bringing the UEs closer to the trunk) with progression to the UEs folded across the chest, or the hands clasped together with shoulders flexed to approximately 90 degrees and elbows extended. The LEs can be brought closer together, the feet may be moved farther from the buttocks (decreasing knee flexion), or static dynamic activities may be introduced.

The therapist can also facilitate pelvic elevation by placing manual contacts on the patient's lower thighs and pushing down on the knees, pulling the distal thighs toward the feet (this may also be performed unilaterally). Tapping (quick stretch) over the gluteus maximus can be used to stimulate muscle contraction.

Treatment Strategies and Considerations

- Bridging allows early weightbearing at the foot and ankle without the body weight constraints of a fully upright posture. It is an appropriate early posture for patients recovering from ankle injury.
- Breath holding is common during bridging activities. This may present problems for the patient with hypertension and cardiac disability; breathing should be closely monitored. Patients should be encouraged to breathe rhythmically during all bridging activities.
- Elevating the hips higher than the head may be contraindicated for patients with uncontrolled hypertension or elevated intracranial pressures (e.g., the patient with acute TBI).
- As with hooklying, abnormal reflex activity may interfere with assumption or maintenance of the bridging posture. Influence of the STLR may cause the LEs to extend. Pressure to the ball of the foot may elicit a positive support reaction (a heel-down weightbearing position can be adopted).
- Bridging promotes selective control (out-of-synergy combination of hip extension with knee flexion) and may be indicated for patients recovering from stroke who demonstrate the influence of the mass movement synergies (when hip and knee extension may be firmly linked together with hip adduction and ankle plantarflexion).

Bridging: Interventions, Outcomes, and Management Strategies
Position/Activity: Bridging, Resisted Movement, Resisted Holding

PREREQUISITE REQUIREMENTS

Static postural control and controlled lower trunk rotation in hooklying as well as dynamic stability of the upper trunk and neck are necessary.

TECHNIQUES AND VERBAL CUES

Combination of Isotonics Recall that combination of isotonics is a technique that utilizes concentric, eccentric, and stabilizing (holding) contractions without relaxation. Against continual resistance, the patient first moves to the end range of a desired motion (concentric) and then holds and stabilizes (isometric) in this end position. When stability is achieved, the patient is instructed to allow the body segment to be slowly moved back to the start position (eccentric). Combination of isotonics allows the application of resistance to the hip extensors using several types of contractions. This is an important lead-up activity for the patient with poor eccentric control during stand-to-sit transitions.

For the application of combination of isotonics to bridging, concentric contractions are used first (the direction and type of desired movement determine whether the technique is begun with *concentric* or *eccentric* contractions). The patient is in the hooklying position. The therapist is in a half-kneeling position to one side (Fig. 3.49). Bilateral manual contacts are on the anterior pelvis (over anterior superior iliac spines); hand placements *do not change* during application of the technique. The hip extensors are resisted throughout. Resistance to concentric contractions is applied as the patient raises the pelvis from the mat until the hips are fully extended. When end range is reached, resistance continues to isometric contractions as the patient holds the

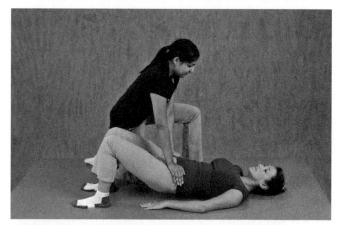

FIGURE 3.49 Combination of isotonics, bridging, resisted movement, holding. Bilateral manual contacts are on the anterior pelvis and *do not change* during the application of the technique. In this illustration, resistance to concentric contractions is applied as the patient raises the pelvis (and then holds the position (isometric contraction)). *Not shown:* The patient then moves slowly back to the original start position using eccentric contractions against resistance.

position. Once stability is achieved, the patient moves slowly back to the original start position using eccentric contractions against resistance.

Clinical Note: In combination of isotonics, resistance for the eccentric component of bridging should be carefully measured when applied, since gravity is already challenging the patient's control.

Verbal Cues for Combination of Isotonics: Bridging, Resisted Movement, Holding During concentric elevation of pelvis: *"Push your pelvis all the way up against my resistance, push, push, push."* During the middle holding, stabilizing phase: *"Now, hold, hold, don't let me push you down, hold."* During return to the start position using eccentric contractions: *"Now, go down slowly, very slowly. Make me work at pushing you down."*

Outcomes
Motor control goal: Controlled mobility.
Functional skills achieved: The patient acquires eccentric control of hip extensors.

Indications Weakness of hip extensors is an indication. Bridging is an important lead-up skill for sit-to-stand and stand-to-sit transfers and for ambulation up and down stairs.

Stabilizing Reversals, Anterior/Posterior Resistance

Stabilizing reversals involve the application of resistance in opposing directions without relaxation within a relatively static bridging posture; resistance is sufficient to prevent movement. The technique utilizes small-range isotonic contractions progressing to stabilizing (holding) in the posture to promote stability, increase strength, and improve coordination between opposing muscle groups.

For the application of stabilizing reversals in bridging, a prerequisite requirement is the ability to hold (maintain) the posture. Either *anterior/posterior* (Fig. 3.50) or *medial/lateral* (described below) resistance may be applied with manual contacts on the pelvis. In the following example, resistance is applied in an anterior/posterior direction. The therapist is positioned in half-kneeling to the side of the patient's hips/pelvis. The patient is asked to hold the bridge position while anterior/posterior resistance is applied to the pelvis. Steady holding is the goal. As resistance is applied in opposing directions, the therapist's hands alternate between the anterior (Fig. 3.50A) and posterior (Fig. 3.50B) surfaces of the pelvis. Resistance is first applied in the stronger direction (to promote irradiation to weaker muscles) and then in the opposite direction. Only minimal motion occurs. Resistance is applied until the patient's maximum is reached and then reversed. The technique is a precursor to rhythmic stabilization.

Verbal Cues for Stabilizing Reversals in Bridging, Anterior/Posterior Resistance
Anterior resistance at pelvis: *"Don't let me push your pelvis downward."* Posterior resistance at pelvis: *"Don't let me pull your pelvis up."*

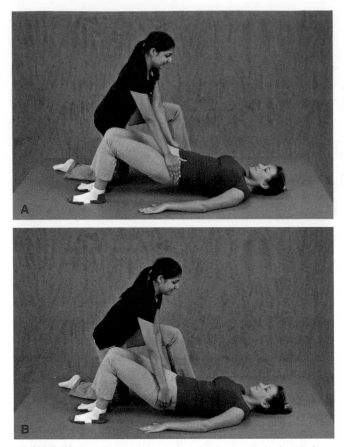

FIGURE 3.50 Stabilizing reversals in bridging, anterior/posterior resisted holding. Resistance (sufficient to prevent movement) is applied to the pelvis using both **(A)** anterior and **(B)** posterior manual contacts. The therapist's hands alternate between the two surfaces of the pelvis. Steady holding is the goal.

Stabilizing Reversals, Medial/Lateral Resistance
Stabilizing reversals in bridging can also be applied using *medial/lateral* resistance (Fig. 3.51). The therapist is positioned in half-kneeling to the side of the patient's hips/pelvis. The patient is asked to hold the bridge position while medial/lateral resistance is applied to the pelvis. Steady holding is the goal. For the application of medial/lateral resistance, manual contacts are over the medial aspect of one ASIS and the lateral aspect of the opposite ASIS. The therapist's hands alternate between the two surfaces. For example, if resisted movement is toward the therapist, hand placements are on the lateral aspect of the ipsilateral ASIS and on the medial aspect of the contralateral ASIS (see Fig. 3.51).

Verbal Cues for Stabilizing Reversals in Bridging, Medial/Lateral Resistance
Resisted movement toward the therapist: *"Don't let me push you away from me."* Resisted movement away from the therapist: *"Don't let me pull you toward me."*

Outcomes
Motor control goal: Stability of lower trunk and pelvis.
Functional skills achieved: The patient is able to stabilize the lower trunk and pelvis in the anterior/posterior and medial/lateral directions.

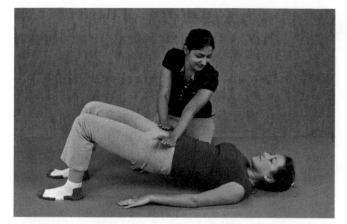

FIGURE 3.51 Stabilizing reversals in bridging, medial/lateral resisted holding. In this example, the resisted movement is *toward* the therapist with hand placements on the lateral aspect of the ipsilateral ASIS and on the medial aspect of the contralateral ASIS. Hand placements change to the opposite sides of the ASIS to resist movement away from the therapist.

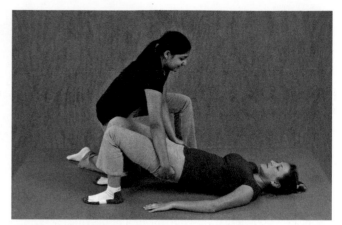

FIGURE 3.52 Application of rhythmic stabilization in bridging. The patient is asked to hold the bridge position while rotational resistance is applied to the pelvis. Manual contacts are on opposite sides and opposite surfaces of the pelvis. In this example, the therapist's left hand is on the anterior pelvis *pushing downward*, and the right hand is on the opposite posterior pelvis *pulling upward.*

Indications Indications include poor lower trunk and pelvis stability, weakness of the lower trunk and hip muscles, and impaired coordination between opposing lower trunk muscle groups.

Comments

- Medial/lateral resistance applied with bilateral manual contacts on the lateral pelvis is effective for facilitating hip abductors and adductors.
- Therapist hand placements should provide smooth transitions between applications of resistance in opposite directions.
- The patient is not allowed to relax between contractions.
- Elastic resistive bands can be placed around the distal thighs to facilitate contraction of the lateral hip muscles (gluteus medius).

Rhythmic Stabilization Rhythmic stabilization utilizes isometric contractions against resistance; no movement occurs. It can be used to increase lower trunk stability and strength. Resistance is applied simultaneously to opposing muscle groups. Although no movement occurs, resistance is applied as if twisting or rotating the lower trunk in opposite directions.

Similar to stabilizing reversals, a prerequisite requirement for the application of rhythmic stabilization to bridging is the ability to hold (maintain) the posture. The therapist is positioned in half-kneeling to the side of the patient. The patient is asked to hold the bridge position while rotational resistance is applied to the pelvis. Manual contacts for the application of rotational resistance are one hand on the *anterior pelvis pushing downward* and one hand on the *opposite posterior pelvis pulling upward*. As resistance is reversed, manual contacts remain on the same side of the pelvis but shift to the opposite surface (Fig. 3.52).

Verbal Cues for Rhythmic Stabilization in Bridging
"Hold, don't let me twist you. Hold, hold, hold. Now, don't let me twist you the other way. Hold, hold, hold."

Outcomes
Motor control goal: Stability of lower trunk and pelvis.
Functional skills achieved: The patient is able to stabilize the lower trunk and pelvis in all directions. These are important lead-up skills for stabilization needed during upright antigravity activities (e.g., standing and locomotion).

Indications Indications include lower trunk and pelvis instability, weakness of the lower trunk and hip and ankle muscles, and impaired coordination between opposing lower trunk muscle groups.

Comments

- Resistance is built up gradually as the patient increases the force of contraction.
- During any isometric contractions, the patient should be encouraged to breathe regularly.

See Box 3.9 Section Summary Student Practice Activity on task analysis and the selection and application of techniques and activities in bridging.

Position/Activity: Bridging, Weight Shifting and Advanced Stabilization Activities, Active Movement
ACTIVITIES AND STRATEGIES
Active Pelvic Shifts This controlled mobility activity involves movement in which the distal part is fixed (feet on mat) while the proximal segment (pelvis) is moving. Weight shifts are important because they promote the simultaneous action of synergistic muscles at more than one joint. From a bridged position, the patient actively shifts the pelvis from side to side (medial/lateral shifts). The focus of this activity

BOX 3.9 SECTION SUMMARY STUDENT PRACTICE ACTIVITY: BRIDGING

OBJECTIVE: Task analysis and selection and application of techniques and activities in bridging.

EQUIPMENT NEEDED: Platform mat.

DIRECTIONS: Working in groups of four to six students, complete the following *task analysis activity* and answer the *guiding questions*.

I. TASK ANALYSIS

Divide into two groups (subjects and therapists), complete the task analysis activity, and then reverse roles.

SUBJECT GROUP: Position yourself in a hooklying position on a mat.

▲ One at a time, each person performs four repetitions of bridging at a **comfortable pace**.
▲ Taking turns, each person performs four repetitions of bridging **slowly**.
▲ Finally, one at a time, each person performs four repetitions of bridging **quickly**.

The subject group should remain positioned on the mat to repeat any of the above movements as requested by members of the therapist group.

THERAPIST GROUP: From your observations of the subject group performing bridging, answer the following task analysis questions. If required to answer the questions, you may request that bridging movements be repeated. Once you have completed the questions, you should assume the role of subject (reverse roles). After both groups have completed the task analysis questions, reconvene into one group to discuss your answers and observations.

TASK ANALYSIS QUESTIONS

Compare and contrast the movement strategies used for bridging:

1. What differences were observed among the subject group during *initiation* (e.g., start position, alignment, use of UEs), *execution* (e.g., timing, force, direction of movement), and *termination* of the bridging activity?
2. What performance differences were observed among the different speeds of movement: *comfortable pace,*

slow, and *quick* (e.g., movement strategies used, postural control, musculoskeletal alignment)?

II. GUIDING QUESTIONS

Working with the whole group of four to six students, one person should serve as a subject (for purposes of demonstration). For each question, rotate the position of the subject. Discuss your ideas with group members as you formulate answers. (*Note:* Not all questions require demonstration.)

1. What individual component skills are needed to accomplish bridging (i.e., what prerequisite skills does a patient need prior to the application of activities and techniques in bridging)?
2. Demonstrate on the subject how you could use extremity positioning both to *reduce* and to *increase* the challenges imposed by the activity (i.e., easier or more difficult).
3. Identify the functional implications of bridging; that is, for what activities of daily living is bridging a prerequisite requirement?
4. Assume you are working with a patient who presents with poor eccentric control of low back and hip extensors. Demonstrate on the subject how you would address this clinical problem. Your demonstration should include position/activity, technique(s), therapist positioning, manual contacts, and verbal cues. Provide a rationale for the position/activity and technique(s) selected.
5. For each of the techniques listed below, demonstrate on the subject their application in bridging. Your demonstration should include position/activity, technique, therapist positioning, manual contacts, and verbal cues. Identify a motor control goal for each technique.
   • Stabilizing reversals (demonstration should include application of both anterior/posterior *and* medial/lateral resistance)
   • Rhythmic stabilization

---

is on control of small-range weight shifts. Weight shifting in bridging is an important lead-up activity for the pelvic lateral control required for gait.

Bridge and Place This is also a controlled mobility activity that involves movement in which the distal part is fixed (feet on mat) while the proximal segment (pelvis) is moving. From a bridged position, the patient actively shifts the pelvis laterally to one side and then lowers the pelvis down to the new side position (Fig. 3.53). A prerequisite requirement for this activity is the ability to actively shift the pelvis medially and laterally from a bridged position.

Clinical Note: Bridge and place is a valuable activity for the patient in the early stages of recovery from stroke. Movement of the pelvis toward the more affected side stretches and elongates the trunk muscles on that side. This counteracts the common problem of shortening of the lateral trunk flexors on the stroke side. The patient's hands may be clasped together with the shoulders flexed and the elbows extended. This positioning effectively counteracts the common flexor and adductor posturing of the UE following stroke. The functional carryover of bridge and place activities is to bed skills such as scooting side to side and scooting to the edge of the bed prior to sitting up.

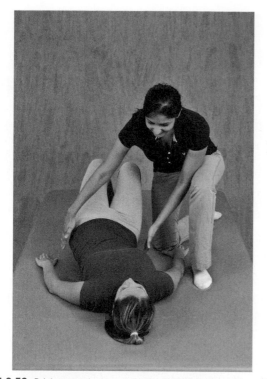

FIGURE 3.53 Bridge and place. From a bridged position, the patient actively shifts the pelvis laterally to one side. In this example, the patient is shifting toward the left. The therapist is in guard position. *Not shown:* The patient would then lower the pelvis down to the new side position.

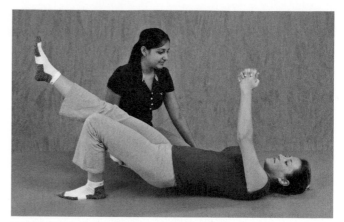

FIGURE 3.54 Bridging, static-dynamic single-leg lifts. Positional challenges are increased by flexing the shoulders and extending the elbows with the hands clasped together.

Position/Activity: Bridging, Advanced Stabilization Activities

ACTIVITIES AND STRATEGIES

Bridging, Single-Leg Lifts Static-dynamic activities involve unilateral LE weightbearing in bridging. The patient raises one LE (dynamic limb) from the mat while maintaining the bridge position using the opposite LE (static limb) for support. The dynamic limb may be held steady with the hip partially flexed and the knee extended (Fig. 3.54), or further challenges may be imposed by adding movement (e.g., alternating between partial hip flexion with knee extension to close to full hip and knee flexion). Further challenges may be imposed by removing UE support from the mat and moving the shoulders into flexion, with elbows extended and the hands clasped together (see Fig. 3.54).

Bridging, Alternating Leg Lifts, Marching in Place This activity alternates static and dynamic elements between the two lower limbs. From a bridge position, marching in place (hip and knee flexion) requires lifting one LE (dynamic) off the mat using hip and knee flexion, returning it to the start position (static), and then immediately lifting the opposite LE (dynamic) in the same pattern with return to the start position (static). Patients with instability will demonstrate a pelvic drop on the side of the dynamic, non-weightbearing limb. A wand or yardstick can be placed across the pelvis to provide visual feedback to assist keeping the pelvis level.

Static-dynamic movements in bridging can be facilitated with tactile (e.g., tapping) or verbal cueing. Initially,

increased stability of the posture may be required to free one lower limb. This may be accomplished by abducting the shoulders on the mat with elbows extended and forearms pronated with hands on the mat. As control progresses, difficulty can be increased by reducing the UE support (e.g., by increasing shoulder adduction or crossing the UEs over the chest or by flexing the shoulders with elbows extended and the hands clasped together). The speed and range of movements may be varied to increase the difficulty of the activities. Patients can work up to marching and then "running" in place or "running" from side to side. The latter activities impose considerable challenge to the bridging position.

Bridging, Mobile Base of Support Using a Ball, Knees Extended With the patient in a hooklying position, a medium-sized ball is placed under the patient's legs. Maintaining leg position on the ball, the patient then elevates the pelvis, extending the hips and knees (Fig. 3.55). This activity significantly increases the postural challenge of pelvic elevation because the BOS is not fixed. The patient must stabilize the legs on the ball and maintain the ball position in addition to elevating the pelvis. The more distally the ball is placed under the legs (toward the feet), the more difficult the activity. The hamstrings participate more fully in stabilization with the knees extended. Use of the UEs on the mat to increase the stability of the posture should be encouraged initially and reduced as control increases. A progression from this activity is bridging with a mobile base of support using a small ball to support the feet with the knees flexed (Fig. 3.56).

Sit to Modified Bridge Position, Movement Transitions Using a Ball This advanced stabilization activity presents considerable challenge to postural control. It involves movement transition from sitting on a ball to a modified bridge position (upper trunk supported by ball). The patient begins by sitting on an appropriately sized ball. The hips and knees should be flexed to 90 degrees. The patient "walks" both feet away from the ball maintaining knee flexion while the hips move toward extension. The ball will roll upward along the

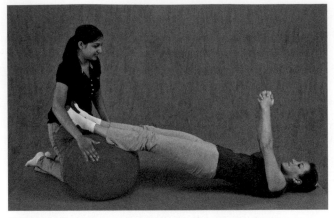

FIGURE 3.55 Bridging, mobile base of support using a medium-size ball to support the legs with the knees extended.

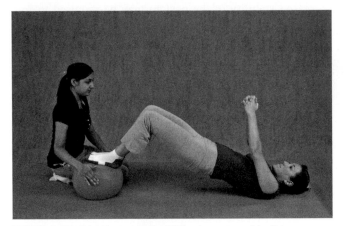

FIGURE 3.56 Bridging, mobile BOS using a small ball to support the feet with the knees flexed.

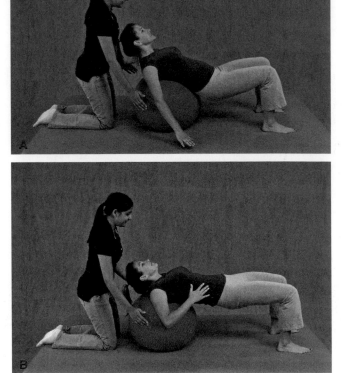

FIGURE 3.57 Sit to modified bridge position, movement transitions using ball. From a sitting position on a ball (not shown), the patient "walks" both feet away from the ball until the head and shoulders are resting on the ball. UE support may be required during early movement transitions. This may be accomplished by **(A)** positioning the patient's hands and fingertips for touch-down support, if needed; and **(B)** "locking" the elbows against the ball to increase stability.

center of the trunk until the head and shoulders are resting on the ball (Fig. 3.57). The patient maintains the hips in the extended position with the pelvis level. Initially, fingertip or hand touch-down support may be necessary; as control develops, hand contact is removed. Alternatively, additional stability can be accomplished by "locking" the elbows against the ball (with elbows flexed and shoulders extended and adducted against the ball). The progression would be to the UEs folded across the chest to the more difficult position of shoulder flexion to approximately 90 degrees and elbows extended with hands clasped together.

Modified Bridge Position, Static-Dynamic Activities Using a Ball Static-dynamic activities in a modified bridge position provide high-level challenges to postural control and should be reserved for late-stage rehabilitation (Fig. 3.58). These challenges can include lifting one LE (the dynamic limb can move in hip flexion or knee extension) while the static limb stabilizes the body and maintains the bridge position. Alternating LE lifts (marching in place) can then be performed. An additional activity while maintaining a

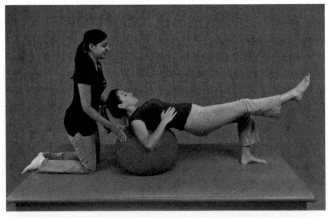

FIGURE 3.58 Static-dynamic activities in a modified bridge position.

single-limb bridge position on the ball is writing alphabet letters with the foot (or great toe) of the dynamic limb.

Outcomes

Motor control goals: Controlled mobility function and static-dynamic control.

Functional skills achieved: The patient is able to stabilize the hip/pelvis/ankle during upright antigravity activities.

Indications Advanced stabilization activities in bridging further promote dynamic stability required for upright antigravity activities such as standing and locomotion.

See Box 3.10 Section Summary Student Practice Activity on treatment interventions used in bridging.

BOX 3.10 SECTION SUMMARY STUDENT PRACTICE ACTIVITY: BRIDGING

Description of Student Practice Activity

Each section of this chapter ends with a similarly challenging student practice activity titled *Section Summary Student Practice Activity (followed by the section title).* A section outline for bridging to guide the activity is provided that highlights the key treatment strategies, techniques, and activities addressed in the preceding section. This activity is an opportunity to share knowledge and skills as well as to confirm or clarify understanding of the treatment interventions. Each student in a group will contribute his or her understanding of, or questions about, the strategy, technique, or activity being discussed and demonstrated. Dialogue should continue until a consensus of understanding is reached. (*Note:* **These directions will be repeated for each subsequent section summary student practice activity, in the event that content is considered in a sequence different from that presented here.**)

Section Outline: Bridging

ACTIVITIES AND TECHNIQUES

▲ Bridging, assumption of posture using combination of isotonics
▲ Bridging, holding, using stabilizing reversals, anterior/ posterior resistance
▲ Bridging, holding, using stabilizing reversal, medial/ lateral resistance
▲ Bridging, holding, using rhythmic stabilization
▲ Bridge and place using active-assistive movements
▲ Bridging, holding, single-leg lifts using active movements

BRIDGING, ADVANCED STABILIZATION ACTIVITIES

▲ Bridging, mobile BOS using a medium-sized ball to support legs with knees extended
▲ Bridging, mobile BOS using a small ball to support feet with knees flexed
▲ Sit to modified bridge position on therapy ball, movement transitions using ball
▲ Modified bridge position on therapy ball, leg lifts, active movements

OBJECTIVE: Sharing skill in the application and knowledge of treatment interventions used in bridging.

EQUIPMENT NEEDED: Platform mat and small and medium-sized balls.

DIRECTIONS: Working in groups of four to six students, consider each entry in the section outline. Members of the group will assume different roles (described below) and will rotate roles each time the group progresses to a new item on the outline.

▲ One person assumes the role of therapist (for demonstrations) and participates in discussion.
▲ One person serves as the subject/patient (for demonstrations) and participates in discussion.
▲ The remaining members participate in discussion and provide supportive feedback during demonstrations. One member of this group should be designated as a "fact checker" to return to the text content to confirm elements of the discussion (if needed) or if agreement cannot be reached.

Thinking aloud, brainstorming, and sharing thoughts should be continuous throughout this activity! As each item in the section outline is considered, the following should ensue:

1. An initial discussion of the *activity,* including patient and therapist positioning. Also considered here should be positional changes to enhance the activity (e.g., prepositioning a limb, hand placements to alter the BOS, and so forth).
2. An initial discussion of the *technique,* including its description, indication(s) for use, therapist hand placements (manual contacts), and verbal cues.
3. A *demonstration* of the activity and application of the technique by the designated therapist and subject/ patient. Discussion during the demonstration should be continuous (the demonstration should not be the sole responsibility of the designated therapist and subject/patient). All group members should provide recommendations, suggestions, and supportive feedback throughout the demonstration. Particularly important during the demonstrations is discussion of strategies to make the activity either *more* or *less* challenging.
4. If any member of the group feels he or she requires practice with the activity and technique, time should be allocated to accommodate the request. All group members providing input (recommendations, suggestions, and supportive feedback) should also accompany this practice.

SUMMARY

This chapter explored strategies, activities, and techniques to enhance bed mobility and control in prone on elbows, quadruped, hooklying, and bridging. Where appropriate, movement transitions between and within postures are addressed. The collective treatment value of these activities is their importance as *critical lead-up skills* for independent positional changes in bed (e.g., pressure relief), LE dressing, independent supine-to-sit transfers, reciprocal UE and trunk movements required for gait, and independent creeping and floor-to-standing transfers. Enhancing the importance of the strategies, activities, and techniques presented is their unique ability to promote functional movement patterns through the coordination of extremity and trunk movements while limiting the degrees of freedom as well as their application to a broad range of both *basic* and *instrumental* activities of daily living.

REFERENCES

1. American Physical Therapy Association. Guide to Physical Therapist Practice, ed 2. Phys Ther 81:9–744, 2001 (revised June 2003).
2. Adler, SS, Beckers, D, and Buck, M. PNF in Practice: An Illustrated Guide, ed 3. Springer, New York, 2008.

Interventions to Improve Sitting and Sitting Balance Skills

SUSAN B. O'SULLIVAN, PT, EdD

This chapter focuses on sitting control and interventions that can be used to improve sitting and sitting balance skills. Careful examination of the patient's overall status in terms of impairments and activity limitations that limit sitting control is necessary. This includes examination of musculoskeletal alignment, range of motion (ROM), and muscle performance (strength, power, and endurance). Examination of motor function (motor control and motor learning) focuses on a determination of weightbearing status, postural control, and neuromuscular synergies required for static and dynamic control. Utilization of sensory (somatosensory, visual, and vestibular) cues for sitting balance control and central nervous system (CNS) sensory integration mechanisms is also necessary. Finally, the patient must be able to safely perform functional movements (activities of daily living [ADL]) in sitting and in varying environments (clinic, home, work [job/school/play], and community).

Sitting Alignment

It is important to understand the foundational requirements of sitting. Sitting is a relatively stable posture with a moderately high center of mass (COM) and a moderate base of support (BOS) that includes contact of the buttocks, thighs, and feet with the support surface. During normal sitting, weight is equally distributed over both buttocks with the pelvis in neutral position or tilted slightly anteriorly. The head and trunk are vertical, maintained in midline orientation. The line of gravity (LoG) passes close to the joint axes of the spine (Fig. 4.1). Muscles of the cervical, thoracic, and lumbar spine are active in maintaining upright postural control and core stability. The BOS can be increased by using one or both hands for additional support.

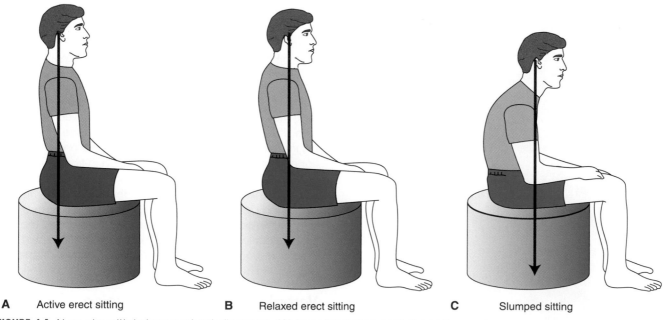

| A | Active erect sitting | B | Relaxed erect sitting | C | Slumped sitting |

FIGURE 4.1 Normal sagittal plane postural alignment. **(A)** In optimal alignment, the LoG passes close to the axes of rotation of the head, neck, and trunk. **(B)** During relaxed sitting, the LoG changes very little, remaining close to those axes. **(C)** During slumped sitting, the LoG is well forward of the spine and hips.

Common Impairments in Sitting Alignment

Although not all-inclusive, deficits in sitting can be broadly grouped into those involving alignment, weightbearing, and extensor muscle weakness. Changes in normal alignment result in corresponding changes in other body segments. For example, malalignment (e.g., slumped sitting posture or sacral sitting) results in increased passive tension on ligaments and joints (Fig. 4.2). Box 4.1 presents common impairments in sitting alignment and seated weightbearing.

Treatment Strategies for Improving Sitting Control

Patients with impairments in static postural control benefit from activities that challenge sitting control. Progression is obtained by varying the level of difficulty. For example, greater challenges can be incorporated into sitting activities by modifying the BOS, the support surface, the use of upper extremities (UEs) or lower extremities (LEs), and sensory inputs. See Box 4.2 for a description of varying postural stabilization requirements and level of difficulty.

Red Flag: The use of mirrors to improve postural alignment is contraindicated for patients with visual-perceptual spatial deficits (e.g., vertical disorientation or position-in-space deficits seen in some patients with stroke or traumatic brain injury [TBI]).

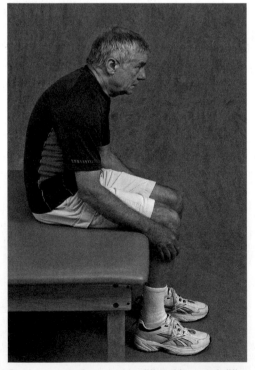

FIGURE 4.2 Abnormal alignment in sitting (slumped sitting posture). The patient exhibits a forward head position, dorsal kyphosis, flattening of the lumbar spine, and a posterior pelvic tilt resulting in sacral sitting.

BOX 4.1 Common Impairments in Sitting Alignment and Seated Weightbearing

- **Deficits in head/upper trunk alignment:** Patients with extensor weakness typically demonstrate a *forward head position,* rounded thoracic spine *(kyphosis),* with a flattened lumbar curve (Fig. 4.2).
- **Deficits in pelvic position:** Excessive posterior tilt of the pelvis results in flattening or reversal of the lumbar curve and *sacral sitting.* The typical cause of sacral sitting is tight or spastic hamstring muscles. Excessive anterior tilt of the pelvis results in increased lordosis and increased lateral rotation and abduction of the hips.
- **Deficits in seated weightbearing:** Patients may demonstrate asymmetrical alignment with increased weightbearing on one side (e.g., the patient with stroke).

Initial practice requires the patient to focus full attention on the task and its key elements. With repeated practice, the level of cognitive monitoring decreases as motor learning progresses. With an autonomous level of learning, postural responses are largely automatic, with little conscious thought for routine postural control. This level of control can be tested by introducing *dual-tasking* (e.g., the patient is required to sit without UE support and carry on a conversation, read aloud, or pour water from a pitcher into a glass). Progression to the next level of difficulty should not be attempted until the patient can safely perform the prerequisite task. For example, patients should demonstrate sitting stability on a stationary surface (e.g., a platform mat) before attempting sitting on a ball.

Clinical Note: Patients who are unstable in sitting are likely to demonstrate increased anxiety and fear of falling when first positioned in sitting. It is important for the therapist to demonstrate the ability to control for instability in order to instill patient confidence. Two therapists may be needed to assist severely involved patients (e.g., the patient with TBI). In this situation, one therapist sits immediately in front of the patient, and one is positioned behind the patient. If positioned in front, the therapist can lock his or her knees around the outside of the patient's knees and firmly stabilize them (Fig. 4.3). This assists the patient by extending the BOS. If positioned behind the patient, the therapist can sit on a ball. The ball is used to support the lumbar spine and maintain the upright posture. The patient's arms can rest on the therapist's knees for support (Fig. 4.4).

Verbal Instructions and Cueing

The therapist should instruct the patient in the correct sitting posture and demonstrate the position in order to provide an accurate *reference of correctness.* It is important to focus the patient's attention on key task elements and improve overall sensory awareness of the correct sitting posture and

BOX 4.2 Varying Postural Stabilization Requirements and Level of Difficulty

Base of Support (BOS)

A wide-based sitting posture (LEs abducted and externally rotated, UEs used for support) is a common compensatory change in patients with decreased sitting control. Postural control can be challenged through altering the BOS by moving from:

- Long-sitting to short-sitting
- Bilateral UE support to unilateral UE support to no UE support
- Hands positioned on the thighs to arms folded across the chest
- Both feet flat on the floor to no foot contact with the floor (e.g., sitting on a high seat)

Support Surface

The type of support surface can influence postural alignment and control:

- A firm surface (e.g., a platform mat) provides a stable base and promotes upright alignment.
- A soft, compliant surface (e.g., a bed or upholstered chair), a low seat, or a wheelchair with excessive seat depth encourages a flexed posture (kyphosis and forward head position) with sacral sitting.
- A chair with a firm surface and back support or sitting with the back against a wall maximizes somatosensory cues and support to the trunk, while sitting on a stool or mat with no back is more difficult.

- Moving from sitting on a stationary, fixed support surface to sitting on a mobile surface (e.g., an inflated disc, wobble board, or therapy ball) increases the difficulty.
- Moving from feet flat on a stationary surface to feet on a mobile surface (e.g., a small ball or roller) increases the difficulty.

Sensory Influence

Sensory support and modification can influence postural alignment and control.

- Eyes open (EO) provides maximum orientation to the environment; eyes fixed on a target directly in front of the patient helps to stabilize posture. Progression is to eyes closed (EC).
- Visual support can be increased by using a mirror to assist the patient in perceptual awareness of vertical and postural symmetry. Vertical lines improve awareness (e.g., the patient wears a vertical line drawn or taped on the front of a shirt and matches it to a vertical line taped on a mirror).
- Sitting against a wall can be used to provide feedback about alignment.
- Somatosensory inputs from the feet can be maximized by having the patient wear flexible-soled shoes and maintain foot contact with a fixed support surface. Progression is to sitting with feet placed on a foam cushion, an inflated dome, or a roller.

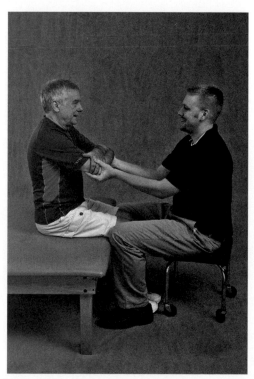

FIGURE 4.3 In sitting, the therapist stabilizes the patient from the front by locking both knees around the patient's knees. The patient's arms are cradled and held by the therapist. Note the improvement in erect posture compared to Figure 4.2.

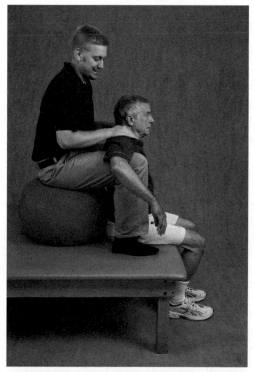

FIGURE 4.4 In sitting, the therapist stabilizes the patient from behind, sitting on a therapy ball. The ball is used to provide support to the lumbar spine. The patient's arms are resting on the therapist's knees (as shown) or can be folded across the lap.

BOX 4.3 Suggested Verbal Instructions and Cueing

- *"Sit tall, hold your head erect, and keep your chin tucked with your shoulders over your hips."*
- *" Look up and focus on the target directly in front of you."*
- *"Tuck your stomach muscles in and flatten your stomach."*
- *"Keep your weight equally distributed over both buttocks and feet."*
- *"Keep your feet flat and in contact with the floor."*
- *"Breathe normally and hold this posture as steady as as you can."*
- *"Imagine you are a puppet with a line from the top of your head pulling you straight up."*

position in space. Suggested verbal instructions and cueing are presented in Box 4.3.

Augmented feedback (e.g., tapping, light resistance, and verbal cueing) should focus attention on *key errors,* which are defined as those errors that when corrected result in considerable improvement of performance, with other elements of the task falling into place. Tactile cues can be used to call attention to missing elements. For example, tapping on the posterior head, neck, and/or trunk can be used to facilitate and engage the extensor muscles. Augmented feedback should also emphasize positive aspects of performance, providing reinforcement and enhancing motivation.

Sitting: Interventions, Outcomes, and Self-Management Strategies

Improving Stability Control

Stability (static postural control) is necessary for prolonged maintenance of upright sitting. Important factors when examining stability control include the ability to maintain correct sitting alignment and the ability to maintain the posture for prolonged times. The patient who can sit for only 30 seconds without losing control demonstrates poor sitting stability, while the patient who can sit for 5 minutes or longer demonstrates good sitting stability. Other control factors frequently examined in stability control include minimal postural sway (maintained center of alignment), the ability to sit without UE support, and the ability to sit without grasping the edge of the mat or hooking LEs onto the mat.

Position and Activity: Sitting, Active Holding

The patient sits with the head and trunk vertical, both hips and knees flexed to 90 degrees, and feet flat on the floor. Posture is symmetrical with equal weightbearing over both buttocks and feet.

One or both of the patient's UEs can be used for support as needed. The shoulder is abducted and extended and the elbow and wrist are extended with the hand open and

positioned at the side (Fig. 4.5A). This is a useful position to counteract UE flexor-adductor spasticity common in the patient recovering from stroke or TBI. Initially, the technique of *rhythmic rotation (RRo)* can be used to move the UE into position. Additional stimulation (tapping or stroking) over the triceps can be used to assist the patient in maintaining elbow extension. The fingers are extended with the thumb abducted (Fig. 4.5B). The dorsum of the hand can also be stroked to keep the hand open.

 Clinical Note: The patient with shoulder instability (e.g., the patient recovering from stroke who has a flaccid, subluxed shoulder) also benefits from

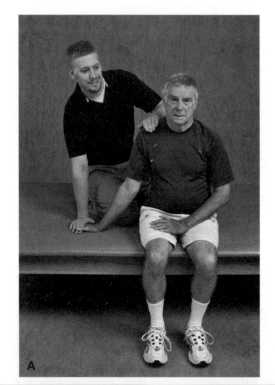

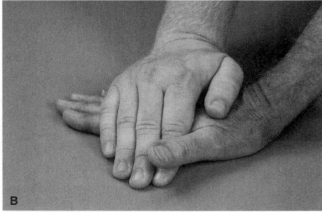

FIGURE 4.5 The patient sits with unilateral UE support. **(A)** The patient's right shoulder is abducted and externally rotated, the elbow is extended, and the wrist and fingers are extended. The therapist assists in shoulder and hand position. This is a useful position for the patient who exhibits UE flexor-adductor spasticity. **(B)** Close-up of the hand position. The fingers are extended with the thumb abducted.

weightbearing and compression through an extended UE. The proprioceptive loading that occurs increases the action of stabilizing muscles around the shoulder. The therapist can add additional stimulation by lightly compressing (approximation) the top of the shoulder downward while stabilizing the elbow as needed.

Clinical Note: The patient with elbow instability due to paralysis (e.g., the patient with a complete C6 tetraplegia who has no triceps function) can be assisted to maintain an extended UE position using shoulder girdle musculature. The patient first "tosses" the UE behind with the shoulder in external rotation and extension with the forearm supinated. Once the base of the hand makes contact with the mat, the humerus is flexed forward by contracting the anterior deltoid, causing the elbow to extend (closed kinetic chain). This is followed by rapid shoulder depression to maintain elbow extension. This technique will stabilize the UE in extension and external rotation. It is important to remember that this patient will need to keep the fingers flexed (interphalangeal flexion) during weightbearing for protection of tenodesis grasp.

Sitting, Active Holding in Long-Sitting Position

Long-sitting is an important posture for developing initial sitting control in patients with spinal cord lesions. Initially, the hands are positioned behind the patient to maximize the BOS (shoulders, elbows, and wrists are extended with base of hand bearing weight). As control develops, the position of the hands can be varied by placing them in front and finally at the sides of the hips. Sitting then progresses to short-sitting activities, with the knees flexed over the side of a mat. Adequate range of the hamstrings (90 to 110 degrees) is required in order for the patient to sit with a neutral or slightly anteriorly tilted pelvis. Decreased range results in a posterior pelvic tilt with sacral sitting and overstretching of low back muscles (Fig. 4.6).

Side-Sitting, Active Holding

In the side-sitting position, the patient sits on one hip with the LEs flexed and tucked to the opposite side. Since this

posture elongates the trunk on the weightbearing side, this is a useful activity for the patient recovering from stroke. The position provides stretch and inhibition to spastic lateral trunk muscles. The more affected UE can be extended and weightbearing (Fig. 4.7), or both UEs can be held in front in a hands-clasped position (hands clasped together with both elbows extended and shoulders flexed), which imposes greater challenge.

Sitting, Resisted Holding

Generally extensor muscles demonstrate greater weakness and the patient may benefit initially from assistance to assume and maintain the correct upright position.

Light resistance to the head and upper trunk can be used to facilitate and engage the extensor muscles to hold. As extensor control increases, resistance/assistance is gradually removed and the patient actively holds.

Clinical Note: Light approximation (joint compression) through the spine can be used to stimulate postural stabilizers; the therapist places both hands on the shoulders and gently compresses downward. Approximation is contraindicated in patients with spinal deformity or an inability to assume an upright position (e.g., the patient with osteoporosis and kyphosis) and in patients with acute pain (e.g., disc pathology or arthritis). The therapist may have the patient sit on a ball and

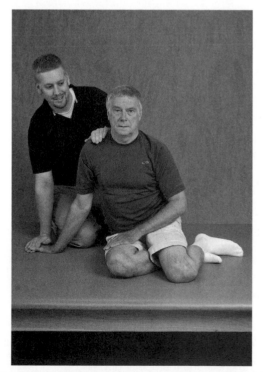

FIGURE 4.7 Side-sitting. The patient is positioned in side-sitting, with knees flexed and tucked to one side. Weight is borne more on the right hip and UE, which is extended and weightbearing. Sitting in this position places a stretch on the trunk lateral flexors, which can demonstrate spasticity and shortening (e.g., the patient with stroke).

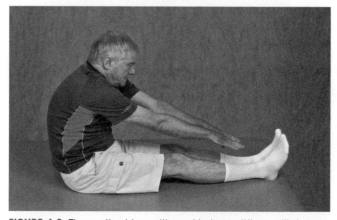

FIGURE 4.6 The patient is positioned in long-sitting, with knees extended. This patient exhibits tight hamstrings with resultant dorsal kyphosis, posterior pelvic tilt, and sacral sitting.

gently bounce up and down to activate extensor muscles and promote upright sitting via activation of joint propriocepters in the spine.

Sitting, Holding, Stabilizing Reversals

In *stabilizing reversals,* the patient is asked to hold the sitting position while the therapist applies resistance first in one direction and then in the opposite direction. During medial/lateral (M/L) resistance, the therapist applies resistance as if pushing the upper trunk sideward away from the therapist (Fig. 4.8), then pulling the upper trunk toward the therapist. During anterior/posterior (A/P) resistance, the therapist applies resistance as if pushing the upper trunk backward and then pulling the upper trunk forward toward the therapist. Manual contacts are varied, first on one side of the upper trunk and then on the other. The resistance is built up gradually, starting from very light resistance and progressing to more moderate resistance. Initially, only a small amount of motion is allowed, progressing to holding steady. Verbal cues (VCs) include *"Push against my hands"* and *"Don't let me push you."* The therapist provides a transitional command (*"Now don't let me pull you the other way"*) before sliding the hands to resist the opposite muscles. This allows the patient the opportunity to make appropriate anticipatory postural adjustments. The position of the therapist will vary according to the line of force that needs to be applied.

Sitting, Holding, Rhythmic Stabilization

In *rhythmic stabilization (RS),* the patient is asked to hold the sitting position while the therapist applies rotational resistance to the upper trunk. One hand is placed on the posterior trunk of one side (the lower axillary border of the scapula) pushing forward, while the other hand is on the opposite side, anterior upper trunk, pulling back (Fig. 4.9). The therapist's hands are then reversed for the opposite movement (each hand remains positioned on the same side of the trunk). No motion is allowed. VCs for RS include *"Don't let me move you. Now don't let me move you the other way."*

📄 **Clinical Note:** Interventions to promote stability are an important lead-up for many ADL (e.g., dressing, grooming, toileting, and feeding) as well as for later transfer training.

Outcomes

Motor control goals: Improved stability (static control) and postural alignment in sitting.

Functional skill achieved: The patient is able to maintain the sitting position independently with minimal sway and no loss of balance for extended times.

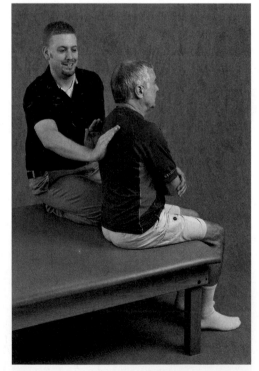

FIGURE 4.8 Sitting, holding using stabilizing reversals. The patient is sitting with feet flat on the floor and the UEs folded across the chest. The therapist is applying lateral resistance while the patient allows only small-range movement and progresses to holding steady. The left hand is placed on the axillary border of scapula, while the right hand is positioned on the vertebral border of the scapula on the other side of the trunk. Hand placements are then reversed to apply resistance in the opposite direction.

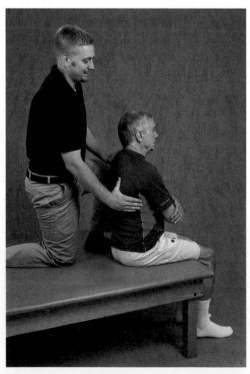

FIGURE 4.9 Sitting, holding using rhythmic stabilization. The patient is sitting with feet flat on the floor and the UEs folded across the chest. The therapist is applying resistance with the left hand on the anterior upper trunk pulling backward, while the right hand is on the lower scapula pushing forward. The patient resists all attempts for movement, holding steady.

Improving Controlled Mobility

In sitting, controlled mobility (dynamic postural control) is necessary for moving in the posture (e.g., weight shifting, turning) or moving the limbs (e.g., reaching, lifting) while maintaining postural stability. These movements produce disturbances of the COM and require ongoing anticipatory postural adjustments in balance in order to maintain upright sitting. Initially the patient's attention is directed to the key task elements required for successful postural adjustments and movement. With increased practice, the postural adjustments become more automatic.

Sitting, Active Weight Shifts

The patient is encouraged to shift weight from side to side, forward-backward, and diagonally with trunk rotation. Re-education of the *limits of stability (LOS)* is one of the first goals. The patient is encouraged to shift as far as possible in any one direction without losing balance and then to return to the midline position. Initially, weight shifts are small range, but gradually the range is increased (i.e., moving through *increments of range*). The patient may begin with bilateral or unilateral UE support and progress to no UE support (e.g., UEs are folded on the chest). The LEs may begin with both feet in contact with the support surface, progressing to one foot in contact (e.g., crossing one leg over the other) and then to no foot contact (e.g., sitting on a treatment table).

Clinical Note: Patients with ataxia (e.g., cerebellar pathology) exhibit too much movement and have difficulty holding steady (maintaining stability). Weight shifts are large to begin with and are progressed during treatment to smaller and smaller ranges (moving through *decrements of range*). Holding steady is the final goal of this progression.

Sitting, Active Weight Shifts With Extended Arm Support

Patients with excess UE flexor tone (e.g., the patient with stroke or TBI) may benefit from weight shifting forward and backward with the elbow extended and the hand weightbearing. The rocking promotes relaxation to the spastic muscles, most likely through mechanisms of slow vestibular stimulation (Fig. 4.10).

Sitting, Active Weight Shifts With Hands on a Large Ball

The patient sits with both shoulders flexed, elbows extended, and hands resting on a large ball placed in front. The patient is instructed to move the ball slowly forward and backward and side to side. Initially, the therapist stands on the opposite side of the ball to assist in controlling the range and speed of movements. This activity has a number of benefits. The ball can provide UE support and inhibitory positioning for the patient with a spastic UE (e.g., the patient recovering from stroke). It also reduces anxiety that may occur with weight

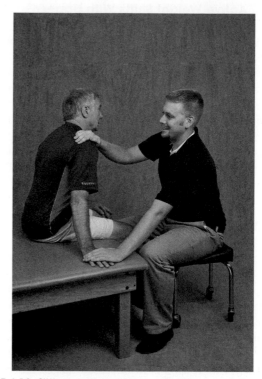

FIGURE 4.10 Sitting, weight shifting with UE support. The patient is sitting with both feet flat on the floor and the right UE extended and weightbearing. The therapist is holding on top of the patient's hand to prevent finger flexion, while the right hand is on top of the shoulder applying approximation. The weight shifting enhances relaxation of the patient's right UE.

shifting forward, since the patient does not feel threatened with falling forward to the floor. Movements can be easily assisted using the ball. The movements forward and backward can be used to promote shoulder ROM in unsuspecting patients who may be otherwise anxious about passive range of motion (PROM) of a tight, restricted shoulder (Fig. 4.11).

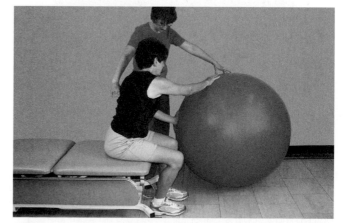

FIGURE 4.11 Sitting, weight shifting with hands on a ball. The patient is sitting with both feet flat on the floor and both hands on top of a large therapy ball. The therapist instructs the patient to roll the ball over to the left. The upper trunk rotates as the patient moves the ball to that side. The activity is then repeated to the opposite side.

Sitting, Active Weight Shifts With Upper Trunk Rotation

Upper trunk rotation (UTR) is a difficult movement for many patients (e.g., the patient with Parkinson's disease who has difficulty with all rotation activities). The patient holds the UEs folded across the chest in a cradle position and is instructed to *"Turn slowly first to one side and then the other."* The head also begins to turn with this activity. The patient is then instructed to *"Turn your head and look over your shoulder."* The therapist monitors the position and directs the patient to keep both hips down in contact with the support surface allowing only small-range trunk flexion (Fig. 4.12).

Sitting, Active Weight Shifts With Voluntary Limb Movements (Static-Dynamic Control)

Active movements of the UE or LE can be used to promote controlled mobility function. Postural adjustments are required during each and every limb movement. Movements can be performed individually or in combination (bilateral symmetrical or alternating from one limb to the other). The therapist can provide a target *("Reach out and touch my hand"),* or a functional task like cone stacking can be used (Fig. 4.13). Progression is to increased range and speed of movements and increased time on task. The patient holds the

elevated limb position for three counts and performs an increasing number of repetitions. If the patient starts to lose control, he or she is directed to reduce the speed or range of movements and regain control before continuing on with the activities.

Additional examples of voluntary limb movments in sitting include the following:

- Raising one or both UEs to the forward or side horizontal
- Raising one or both UEs overhead
- Stacking cones
- Reaching down to touch the floor or pick up objects from the floor
- Raising both UEs diagonally from the floor from one side to overhead on the opposite side or lifting a ball diagonally up and across the body
- Extending one knee out to horizonal and returning
- Marching in place, alternating lifing one foot up, then the other
- Performing toe-offs and heel-offs in sitting
- Holding one foot off the floor and performing toe circles or "writing" the letters of the alphabet with the great toe
- Crossing one limb over the other, then repeating with the other side (Fig. 4.14)

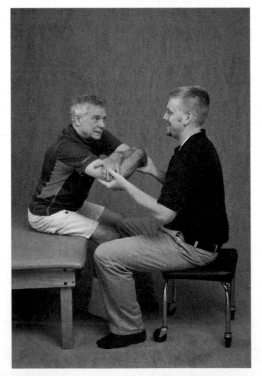

FIGURE 4.12 Sitting, active weight shifting. The patient is sitting with both feet flat on the floor and both UEs flexed across the chest, in an arms cradled position. The therapist sits in front on a rolling stool. The patient lifts both UEs up while leaning forward (as shown). The arms are moved to one side or the other, combining movements of upper trunk rotation with flexion. This is a good early sitting activity because the therapist provides support for the patient and the position of the therapist reduces fear of falling. Light stretch and resistance can be added to enhance movement.

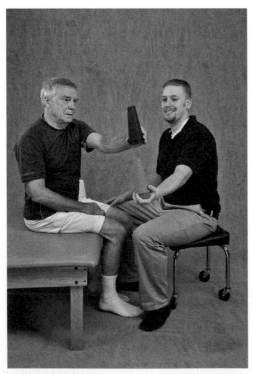

FIGURE 4.13 Sitting, reaching using cone stacking. The patient practices upper trunk rotation with UE reach, grasp, and release. The therapist varies the position of the target stacking cone to vary the amount of movement and weight shifting. The patient with an asymmetrical sitting position (e.g., the patient with stroke) can be encouraged to lean to the more affected side.

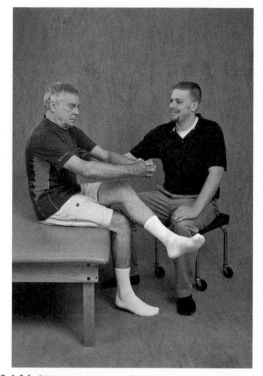

FIGURE 4.14 Sitting, dynamic LE movements. The patient practices crossing and uncrossing the left leg over the right. This activity requires a weight shift toward the static side and away from the side of the dynamic limb. The UEs are held steady in front, shoulders flexed, elbows extended, and hands clasped together in a hands-clasped position. This forces the dynamic adjustments to occur in the lower trunk and pelvis and does not permit the patient to use an upper trunk lateral tilt.

Sitting, Weight Shifts, Dynamic Reversals

The patient moves from side to side (medial-lateral shifts) or forward and backward against graded resistance. The therapist alternates hand placement, first on one side of the upper trunk to resist the upper body pulling away and then on the other side to resist the return movement. Manual contacts alternate between the anterior and posterior surfaces of the upper trunk to resist forward-backward movement. To resist medial-lateral shifts, manual contacts are on the lateral aspect of the upper trunk under the axilla. The therapist can also provide resistance with one hand on the lateral trunk and the other hand on the scapula on the opposite side of the trunk (Fig. 4.15). It is important to keep from resisting directly on the lateral shoulders (humerus). Smooth reversals of antagonists are facilitated by well-timed VCs *("Pull away"* or *"Push back")* and a transitional cue *("Now")* to indicate the change in direction. A quick stretch is used to initiate the reverse movement. Progression is from partial-range to full-range control. Shifts may also be resisted in diagonal and in diagonal with rotation directions.

A hold may be added in one or both directions if the patient demonstrates difficulty moving to one side (e.g., the patient with stroke). The hold is a momentary pause (held for one count); the antagonist contraction is then facilitated.

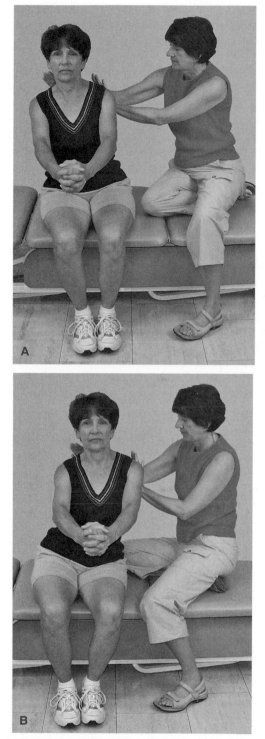

FIGURE 4.15 Sitting, weight shifting, dynamic reversals. The patient practices weight shifting side to side. The UEs are held steady in front, shoulders flexed, elbows extended, and hands clasped together in a hands-clasped position. The therapist provides light stretch and resistance to enhance movement. The patient has moved away from the therapist (not shown) and then **(A)** pushes back toward the therapist. The end position **(B)** shows the patient with weight shifted onto the left side.

Clinical Note: Interventions to promote weightshifting are important lead-up activities for more advanced sitting balance activities, pressure relief, and transfers.

Sitting, Resisted UE Movements

The addition of graded resistance to limb movements strengthens and enhances control of the limbs (e.g., the patient with weakness following brain injury). It also serves the valuable function of directing the patient's attention to the control of limb movements and away from actions of the trunk. This helps to promote automatic control of postural mechanisms required for sitting. Resistance can be in the form of lightweight cuffs, elastic resistive bands, pulleys, or manual resistance.

Proprioceptive Neuromuscular Facilitation (PNF) patterns can be used effectively to provide a dynamic challenge to postural control and stabilization. The patient can be instructed to actively move in the pattern(s), or the pattern(s) can be resisted. The benefits of using PNF patterns are many. They promote muscle activity in naturally occurring synergistic combinations. Diagonal and rotational movements are combined with elements of flexion/extension and abduction/adduction, representing advanced control work for many patients. The patterns can be more easily translated into ADL skills as compared to straight plane motions. The therapist starts with unilateral patterns and progresses to combination or trunk patterns (e.g., chop or lift patterns).

With resisted patterns, the level of resistance is determined by the ability of the trunk to stabilize and maintain upright sitting, not by the strength of the UEs. If stabilization is lacking, resistance may be contraindicated and active movements should be promoted.

The therapist chooses which pattern(s) to use based on the patient's level of control. Unilateral patterns are often used initially, when patients are unfamiliar with PNF patterns or when one extremity is needed for weightbearing and support. As control develops, the therapist progresses to more difficult bilateral or upper trunk patterns (e.g., chop or lift patterns).

Sitting, PNF Unilateral UE D1 Patterns

D1F, FLEXION-ADDUCTION-EXTERNAL ROTATION, DYNAMIC REVERSALS

The hand of the dynamic limb is positioned near the side of the ipsilateral hip (Fig. 4.16A), with hand open and thumb facing down. The patient is instructed to close the hand, turn, and pull the hand up and across the face while following the movement with the eyes (Fig. 4.16B).

D1E, EXTENSION-ABDUCTION-INTERNAL ROTATION, DYNAMIC REVERSALS

In the return pattern, the patient opens the hand, turns, and pushes the hand down and out to the side. In dynamic reversals, movements are assisted for a few repetitions to ensure that the patient knows the movements expected. The movements are then lightly resisted using graded resistance. The therapist alternates hand placement, first in one direction

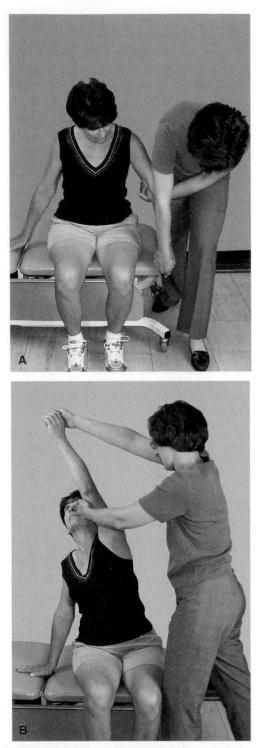

FIGURE 4.16 Sitting, resisted PNF UE D1 flexion pattern. **(A)** The patient begins with the left UE held abducted and extended out to the side, hand open. **(B)** The patient is instructed to close the hand, turn, and pull the UE up and across the face. The patient's right UE is used for support. The therapist provides light stretch and resistance to the movement. As trunk control improves, the activity can be performed with no right UE support.

and then the other. Smooth reversal of antagonists is facilitated by well-timed VCs.

Sitting, PNF Unilateral UE D2 Patterns

D2F, FLEXION-ABDUCTION-EXTERNAL ROTATION, DYNAMIC REVERSALS

The hand of the dynamic limb is positioned across the body with the UE extended, adducted, and internally rotated on the opposite hip, with hand closed and thumb facing down (Fig. 4.17A). The patient is instructed to open the hand, turn, and lift the hand up and out while following the movement with the eyes (Fig. 4.17B).

D2E, EXTENSION-ADDUCTION-INTERNAL ROTATION, DYNAMIC REVERSALS

In the return pattern, the patient closes the hand, turns, and pulls the hand down and across the body toward the opposite hip.

Red Flag: UE PNF D2 patterns are contraindicated for patients recovering from stroke who are in early to mid recovery and firmly locked into abnormal synergy patterns.

Sitting, PNF Chop/Reverse Chop, Dynamic Reversals

This is an upper trunk flexion and rotation pattern that involves both UEs moving together. The lead limb moves in D1E; the hand of the assist limb holds on from on top of the wrist/distal forearm (Fig. 4.18A). The limbs move down and across the body with head and trunk rotation and flexion (Fig. 4.18B). In the reverse chop pattern, the lead limb is positioned in D1F (Fig. 4.19A) and the limbs move up and across the face (Fig. 4.19B). In order to resist this pattern, the therapist is positioned slightly in front and to the side of the patient (wide, dynamic BOS) in the direction of the chop.

Sitting, With PNF Lift/Reverse Lift, Dynamic Reversals

This is an upper trunk extension and rotation pattern that involves both UEs moving together. The lead limb moves in D2F; the hand of the assist limb holds on from underneath the wrist/distal forearm (Fig. 4.20A). The limbs move up and out with head and trunk rotation and extension (Fig. 4.20B). In the reverse lift pattern, the lead limb begins in D2E (Fig. 4.21A); the limbs move down and across the body (Fig. 4.21B). To resist this pattern, the therapist is positioned slightly behind and to the side of the patient in the direction of the lift.

Clinical Note: The therapist selects either a chop or lift pattern. One is not a progression from the other, and there is no need to use both in order to improve sitting control. PNF patterns, especially chop/reverse chop and lift/reverse lift, promote crossing the midline, an important activity for patients with unilateral neglect of one side (e.g., the patient with stroke).

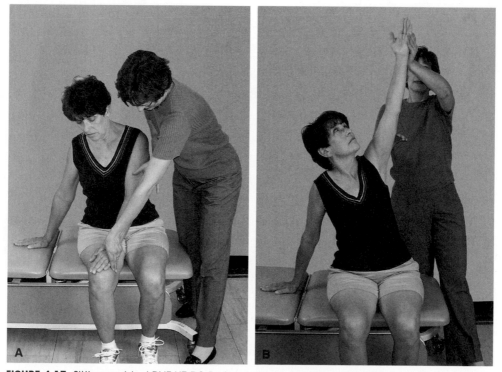

FIGURE 4.17 Sitting, resisted PNF UE D2 flexion pattern. **(A)** The patient begins with the left UE extended, adducted, and internally rotated across the body. **(B)** The patient is instructed to open the hand, turn, and lift the left UE up and out. The patient's right UE is used for support. The therapist provides light stretch and resistance to the movement while weight shifting backward to allow for full limb excursion.

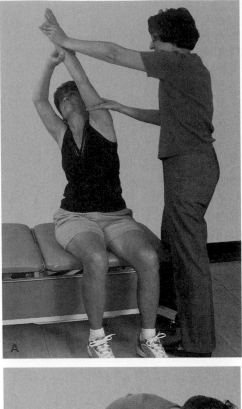

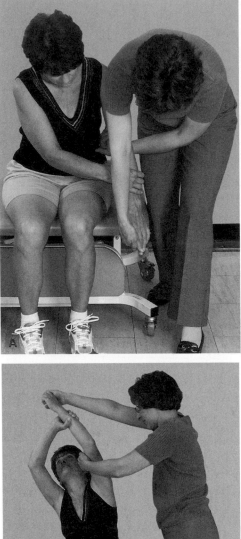

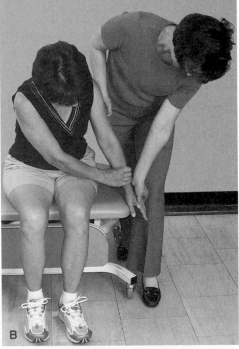

FIGURE 4.18 Sitting, resisted PNF chop pattern. **(A)** The patient's lead left UE moves in the D1 extension pattern; the assist arm holds onto the top of the wrist/distal forearm. **(B)** The patient is then instructed to open the hand, turn, and push both UEs down and out to the side. The therapist resists the movement, ensuring that trunk flexion with rotation and weight shift to the left side occurs.

FIGURE 4.19 Sitting, resisted PNF reverse chop pattern. **(A)** The patient's lead left UE moves in the D1 flexion pattern; the assist arm holds onto the top of the wrist/distal forearm. **(B)** The patient is instructed to close the hand, turn, and pull both UEs up and across the face. The therapist resists the movement, ensuring that trunk extension and rotation with weight shift to the right side occurs.

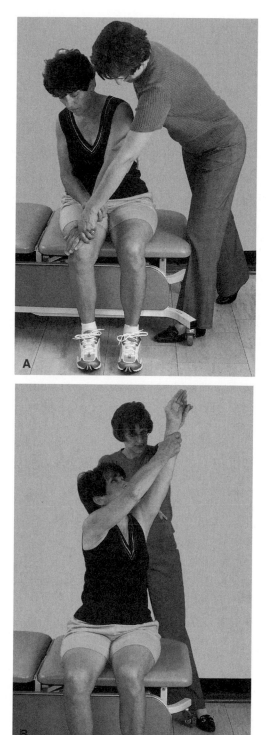

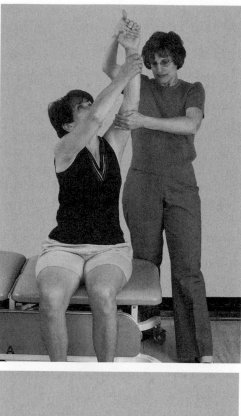

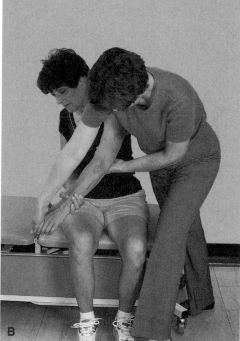

FIGURE 4.20 Sitting, resisted PNF lift pattern. **(A)** The patient's lead left UE moves in the D2 flexion pattern; the assist arm holds onto the bottom of the wrist/distal forearm. **(B)** The patient is instructed to open the hand, turn, and lift both UEs up and out to the side. The therapist resists the movement, ensuring that trunk extension and rotation with weight shift to the left occurs.

FIGURE 4.21 Sitting, resisted PNF reverse lift pattern. **(A)** The patient's lead left UE moves in the D2 extension pattern; the assist arm holds onto the bottom of the wrist/distal forearm. **(B)** The patient is instructed to close the hand, turn, and pull both UEs down and across the body. The therapist resists the movement, ensuring that trunk flexion and rotation with weight shift to the right occurs. Note that the therapist uses a wide, dynamic BOS that allows weight shifting for continuous application of resistance throughout the pattern.

Sitting, Bilateral Symmetrical (BS) PNF D1 Thrust and Withdrawal, Dynamic Reversals

In the thrust pattern, the hands are closed, the elbows flexed and forearms supinated, and the shoulders extended (Fig. 4.22A). The UEs move together up and across the face, with hands opening, forearms pronating, elbows extending, and shoulders flexing above 90 degrees (Fig. 4.22B). This is a protective pattern for the face and promotes actions of shoulder flexion and elbow extension with scapular protraction. In withdrawal or reverse thrust, the hands close, the forearms supinate with elbow flexion, and the shoulders extend, pulling the arms back and to the sides. Holding in the withdrawal pattern is a useful activity to promote symmetrical scapular adduction, trunk extension, and upright sitting posture.

Sitting, Bilateral Symmetrical (BS) PNF D2F, Dynamic Reversals

The patient moves both UEs together in a BS D2F pattern. The pattern begins with the UEs in extension, adduction, and internal rotation (Fig. 4.23A). The hands open and the

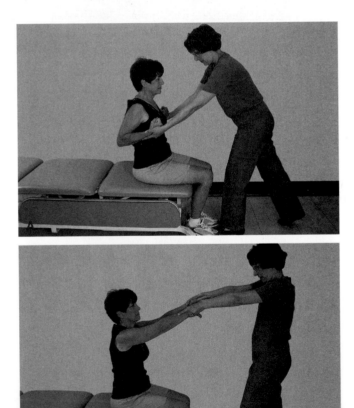

FIGURE 4.22 Sitting, resisted PNF D1 thrust pattern. **(A)** The patient begins with both UEs flexed and adducted, forearms supinated, hands flexed, and arms tucked close to the side. **(B)** The patient is instructed to open both hands, turn, and push up and across, extending both elbows and crossing both hands (thrust position). The therapist resists the movement and must weight shift backward to ensure that both elbows extend fully. During reverse thrust, the therapist resists the UEs as they flex and move back to the sides.

limbs turn and lift up and out. As the UEs move up and out, trunk extension is promoted (Fig. 4.23B). The therapist is positioned behind the patient to resist the UEs as they move. The therapist can position manual contacts on the proximal forearm or just above the elbow on the arm, depending on the length of the arm. A hold may be performed in the D2F position to further emphasize trunk extension.

Clinical Note: This is a useful activity for the patient with kyphosis and rounded, forward shoulders (e.g., the patient with Parkinson's disease). The patient is instructed to "*Slowly breathe in*" during BS D2F and to "*Slowly breathe out*" during BS D2E. This helps to enhance respiration so often limited with restrictive lung conditions.

Note: The technique of rhythmic initiation (RI) can also be used with any of the above UE patterns. The patient is passively moved through the patterns for several repetitions. The patient is then asked to actively move with the therapist through the range (active-assistive movements). Movements are then lightly resisted. Progression to the next phase is dependent on the patient's ability to relax and participate in the active and resistive phases. This is an ideal technique to use with the patient who has difficulty with initiation of movement (e.g., the patient with Parkinson's disease or with dyspraxia).

Outcomes

Motor control goal: Improved controlled mobility (dynamic control).

Functional skills achieved: The patient demonstrates appropriate functional balance in sitting, allowing independence in reaching and ADL (e.g., bathing, grooming, and dressing).

Activities and Strategies to Improve Adaptive Balance Control

Balance is defined as the ability to maintain the COM within the BOS while controlling the alignment of body segments and orientation of the body to the environment. Balance control is achieved through the actions of a number of different body systems working together. These include the sensory systems (visual, somatosensory, and vestibular inputs as well as sensory strategies), musculoskeletal system (muscle synergies), neuromuscular system (postural tone, automatic postural synergies; anticipatory, reactive, and adaptive mechanisms), and cognitive/perceptual systems (internal representations, interpretation of sensory information, motor planning). Reactive balance control refers to the ability to maintain or recover balance when subjected to an unexpected challenge and is based on feedback-driven adjustments. These include manual perturbations (disturbances in the COM) and changes in the support surface (disturbances in the BOS), such as force platform perturbations. Anticipatory balance control allows the CNS to modify (preset) the nervous system in advance of voluntary movements. The central set or overall state of readiness of the

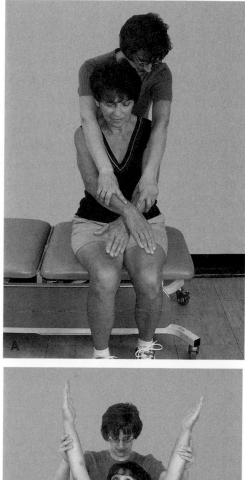

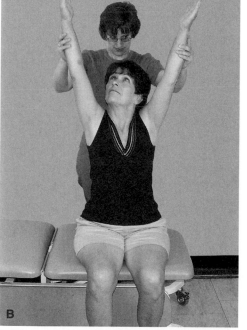

FIGURE 4.23 Sitting, resisted PNF bilateral symmetrical D2 flexion pattern. **(A)** The patient begins with both UEs extended and adducted across the body. **(B)** The patient is instructed to open the hands, turn, and lift both UEs up and out. The therapist resists the movement, ensuring that the patient lifts both UEs up and extends the upper trunk. The therapist needs to be positioned behind the patient with both hands holding over the upper forearm or lower arm. For improved respiratory control, the patient can be instructed to breathe in deeply during D2 flexion, and breathe out during the reverse movement (D2 extension).

CNS is influenced by feedforward adjustments based on prior instructions, prior experience, and the context of the balance experience. For example, the responses of a patient to catch a ball would produce far different results if instructions included that the ball was inflated versus weighted (e.g., 3 lb [1.36 kg]). Optimal function is achieved when all aspects of balance control are working.

Interventions selected are based on a careful examination of the systems contributing to balance control and the functional outcomes of impairments (e.g., functional performance and fall history). For most patients, balance training is a multifaceted program. It frequently begins in the sitting posture and is progressed through other upright postures that serve to increase the challenge by raising the COM and decreasing the BOS (e.g., kneeling and standing). More severely involved patients (e.g., the patient with TBI or spinal cord injury [SCI]) may spend considerable time in rehabilitation working on sitting balance responses. For other patients who are less involved, it may represent only a brief part of the balance training program, with greater emphasis placed on standing balance training. The following section offers suggested training activities.

Sitting, Manual Perturbations

The patient sits on a stationary surface (platform mat) with feet flat on the floor. The therapist provides quick, small-range manual perturbations (nudges/pulls) in various directions, forward-backward, side to side, and diagonal. Manual contacts should be on the trunk, not on the shoulders. It is important to ensure appropriate postural responses. For example, with backward displacements, trunk and neck flexors are active. With forward displacements, trunk and neck extensors are active. UE protective extension reactions can be initiated if the displacements move the COM near or past the LOS, and are more easily activated with sideward displacements. If patient responses are inappropriate or lack countermovements, the therapist may need to guide the initial attempts either verbally or manually. The patient can then progress to active movements. Perturbations should be appropriate for the patient's level of control. It is important to use gentle perturbations; violent shoves are not necessary to stimulate balance responses. The therapist can vary the BOS to increase or decrease difficulty during the perturbations. Progression is from predictable perturbations (*"Don't let me push you backward"* and *"Now don't let me pull you forward"*) to unpredictable perturbations applied with no preliminary instructions. In the former situation, both anticipatory and reactive control mechanisms are activated, whereas in the latter, primarily reactive control mechanisms are used.

Clinical Note: It is important to know the patient's capabilities and to anticipate the patient's ability to respond. Exceeding the patient's capabilities may induce anxiety and fear of falling. *Postural fixation* is the likely response to this situation and is often seen in the patient with cerebellar ataxia. It is equally important to adjust responses, increasing the level of difficulty appropriate to the patient's improving capabilities.

Sitting on a Moveable Surface

Activities on a moveable surface (wobble or rocker board, inflated disc, or ball) can be used to disturb the patient's BOS and engage postural mechanisms. Wobble boards are constructed to allow varying motion. The type and amount of motion are determined by the design of the board. A curved-bottom (bidirectional) board allows motion in two directions; a dome-bottom board allows motion in all directions. The degree of curve or size of the dome determines the amount of motion in any direction; motion is increased in boards with large curves or high domes. The type of board used is dependent on the patient's capabilities and the type and range of movements permitted.

An inflated disc is a dome-shaped cushion that is positioned under the patient while sitting. It allows limited motion in all directions (Fig. 4.24A). Challenge can be varied by the level of inflation (a firm disc provides a greater challenge than a soft disc) or by varying the BOS (Fig. 4.24B).

During sitting on the wobble board or disc, the patient's feet should be flat on the floor. A step or stool may be needed for some patients. Initial activities include having the patient maintain a balanced, centered, or aligned sitting position. The patient can then progress to active weight shifts, tilting the board or moving on the disc in varying directions. These patient-initiated challenges stimulate balance using both anticipatory and reactive balance mechanisms. The therapist can also manually tilt a wobble board to stimulate reactive balance responses.

Various names have been used to describe the balls used for therapeutic interventions, including therapy ball, balance ball, stability ball, and Swiss ball. Sitting on the ball facilitates postural mechanisms through intrinsic feedback mechanisms (visual, proprioceptive, and vestibular inputs) and challenges CNS adaptive postural control. The use of the ball also adds novelty to rehabilitation programs and can be easily adapted to group classes. Patients may feel initially insecure and should be carefully guarded. The therapist may sit directly behind the patient, shadowing the patient's body with his or her own (Fig. 4.25), or the therapist can stabilize from the front. If the patient is very insecure, the ball can initially be positioned on a floor ring that prevents the ball from moving in any direction. A ball that is slightly underinflated and positioned on a soft floor mat will roll less easily than a hard (fully inflated) ball positioned on a tile floor. Initially the therapist can provide manual and VCs or manual assistance to guide the patient in the correct movements. As control develops, active movement control is expected (a hands-off approach).

Choosing the right size ball is important to ensure proper sitting posture. When the patient sits on the ball, the hips and knees should be flexed to 90 degrees (*the 90-90 rule*) with knees aligned over the feet. Feet should be flat on the floor and positioned hip width apart. The patient's hands

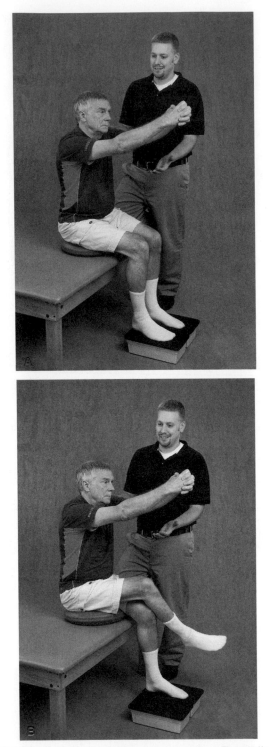

FIGURE 4.24 Sitting on an inflated disc, holding. The patient sits on an inflated disc with both feet flat on a small step. **(A)** The hands are clasped together in a forward position (elbows extended, shoulders flexed). The therapist instructs the patient to maintain a steady posture. **(B)** The patient then is instructed to maintain balance while crossing the right leg over the left, a movement that reduces the patient's BOS and increases the challenge to balance.

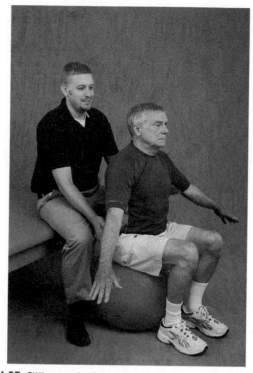

FIGURE 4.25 Sitting on ball, holding. Initially, as the patient sits on a therapy ball, the therapist can shadow and support the patient from behind by sitting on a mat (for maximum security) or on another ball. The therapist maintains both hands near the patient's hips but does not hold onto the patient. The patient is instructed to maintain a steady position on the ball. Both UEs are held out to the sides in a low guard position with hips and knees flexed to 90 degrees and feet apart.

can be used initially to stabilize by holding onto the thighs; progression is to hands off the thighs (e.g., out to the side or folded on the chest). Guidelines for choosing the correct ball size based on patient height are presented in Box 4.4.

Clinical Note: Patients with restricted hip flexion during sitting (e.g., the patient with a new total hip replacement) will benefit from using a ball that is a size larger to decrease the angle of the hip. Patients who are overweight or obese may require a larger ball with greater surface area.

Sitting on the Ball, Static Activities

Initially the patient is instructed to maintain a neutral position in sitting (toes and knees pointing forward, feet hip-width apart, knees aligned over the feet, pelvic neutral position) (Fig. 4.26A). The patient is instructed to *"Sit tall*

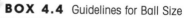

BOX 4.4 Guidelines for Ball Size

Patient Height	Size of Ball
Below 5 ft 0 in	45-cm ball
5 ft 0 in to 5 ft 7 in	55-cm ball
5 ft 8 in to 6 ft 3 in	65-cm ball
Above 6 ft 3 in	75-cm ball

and hold steady" and *"Don't let the ball roll in any direction."* Sitting off to one side will result in instability and movement off the ball. Approximation can be given during early sitting by having the patient gently bounce up and down. An improvement in posture (i.e., the patient sits up straight) is often seen with this stimulation. Initially the hands can rest on the knees (a position of maximum stability). As control develops, the patient is instructed to hold the UEs in a forward position with the elbows extended and the hands clasped together (hands-clasped position). Alternatively, the patient can hold the arms out to the sides, with shoulder abduction and elbow extension (Fig. 4.26B). The patient should also be instructed to focus on a visual target.

Sitting on the Ball, Dynamic Activities

Dynamic activities should be attempted only after static control is achieved. Examples include the following:

• *Anterior/posterior pelvic shifts.* The patient rolls the ball forward and backward using anterior/posterior pelvic tilts, holds for three counts, and then returns to neutral position (Fig. 4.27).

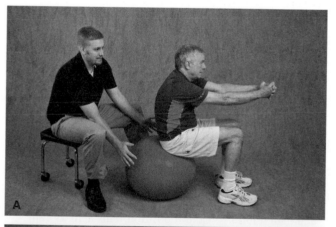

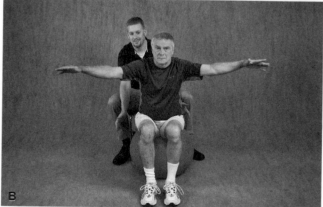

FIGURE 4.26 Sitting on ball, holding. **(A)** The patient maintains steady sitting on the ball while holding both hands clasped together in a forward position (elbows extended and shoulders flexed). **(B)** For added balance control, the UEs can be held with shoulders abducted out to the sides and elbows extended.

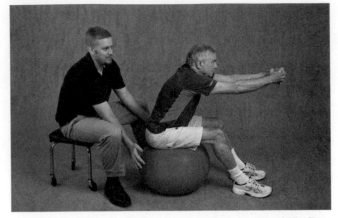

FIGURE 4.27 Sitting on ball, anterior-posterior pelvic shifts. The patient sits on a ball, holding both hands clasped together in a forward position (elbows extended and shoulders flexed). The head, upper trunk, and UEs are held steady. The therapist instructs the patient to roll the ball forward and backward, moving the ball by using pelvic movements (backward or posterior pelvic tilts and forward or anterior pelvic tilts).

Clinical Note: It is important for the patient to actively stabilize the upper body, preventing any attempts to move by tilting the upper trunk. This can be promoted by having the patient maintain the UEs steady (e.g., holding both hands clasped together or holding a second ball). The patient is instructed to *"Hold your upper trunk steady. Don't lean forward, backward, or side to side."*

- *Lateral weight shifts.* The patient rolls the ball from side to side (Fig. 4.28) with medial/lateral weight shifts, holds for three counts, and then returns to neutral position.
- *Pelvic clock.* The patient rotates the ball by using hip actions around in a full circle, first clockwise and then counterclockwise.
- *UE lifts.* The patient raises one UE to the forward horizontal position or overhead, holds for three counts, and then returns to neutral position. This activity can progress to the opposite UE or to bilateral movements (e.g., symmetrical lifts or reciprocal lifts).
- *UE circles.* The patient holds both UEs out to the sides and rotates first forward (clockwise) and then backward (counterclockwise).
- *Knee lifts.* The patient lifts one knee up into hip flexion, holds for three counts, and then returns to neutral position; this activity is repeated with the other limb.
- *Marching in place (alternate knee lifts).* The patient marches rhythmically in place, first slowly and then with increasing speed.
- *Marching in place (contralateral UE and LE lifts).* The patient raises the right UE and the left knee, lowers them, and then repeats with the left UE and right knee (Fig. 4.29).
- *Knee extension.* The patient straightens the knee and holds the foot out in front for three counts and then returns to neutral position (Fig. 4.30). This activity can progress to alternate knee extensions, including ankle

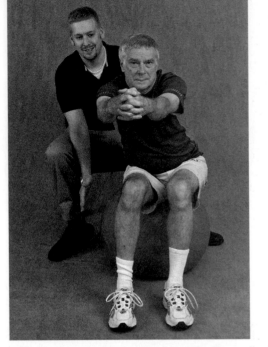

FIGURE 4.28 Sitting on ball, lateral pelvic shifts. The patient sits on a ball, holding both hands clasped together in a forward position (elbows extended and shoulders flexed). The head, upper trunk, and UEs are held steady. The therapist instructs the patient to roll the ball from side to side, moving the ball to the side using pelvis movements (lateral tilts).

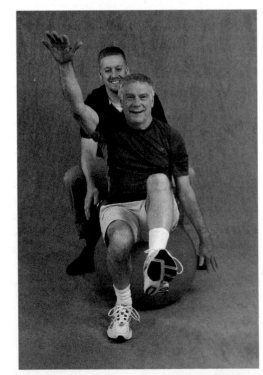

FIGURE 4.29 Sitting on ball, marching. The patient practices marching (alternate hip and knee flexion movements) while maintaining stable sitting on the ball. These movements are combined with reciprocal UE movements (shoulder flexion and extension). This is a four-limb movement pattern that requires considerable dynamic stability while sitting on the ball.

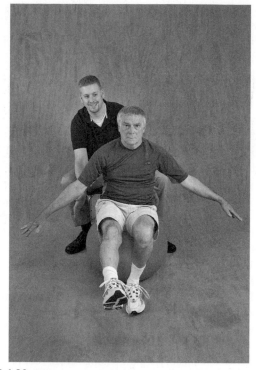

FIGURE 4.30 Sitting on ball, knee extension. The patient practices lifting one foot up and extending the knee while maintaining stable sitting on the ball. The UEs are held out to the sides in a guard position. The activity can be progressed by having the patient trace letters or numbers with the dynamic foot.

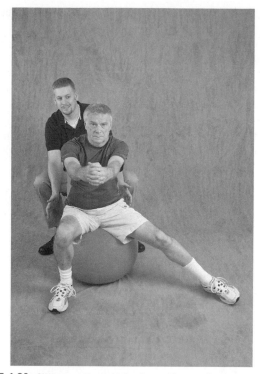

FIGURE 4.31 Sitting on ball, side steps. The patient practices stepping out to the side, moving one LE into hip abduction with knee extension while maintaining stable sitting on the ball. The UEs are held with both hands clasped together in a forward position (elbows extended and shoulders flexed).

circles, or writing letters of the alphabet in space with the great toe of the dynamic foot.

- *Side-steps*. The patient moves the LE out to the side into hip abduction and knee extension (Fig. 4.31), holds for three counts, and then returns to neutral position. This activity can progress to hip abduction with the knee flexed, moving down into unilateral kneeling while half-sitting on the ball (a modified half-kneeling position).
- *Heel-lifts*. The patient lifts both heels off the floor while keeping the toes in contact, holds for three counts, and then lowers slowly.
- *Toe-lifts*. The patient lifts both toes off the floor while keeping the heels in contact with the floor, holds for three counts, and then lowers slowly.
- *Lateral trunk rotation*. The patient extends both UEs out to the sides, rotates (twists) as far as possible to the left, returns to midline, and then twists to the right. This activity can be combined with head/neck rotations (look arounds). Trunk rotations can also be performed holding a small ball (Fig. 4.32); rotations can also be performed diagonally.
- *Jumping jacks*. The patient raises both UEs overhead, claps the hands, and returns hands to the start position (along sides of ball). This activity can be combined with bouncing on the ball and alternating reciprocal knee extension and flexion.
- *Passing, catching, and throwing a ball*. The patient practices passing, catching, and throwing a ball or batting a

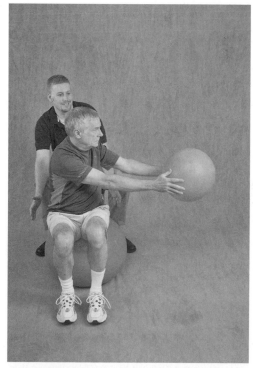

FIGURE 4.32 Sitting on ball, head and trunk rotation. The patient practices head and trunk rotation to the left while holding a small ball and maintaining sitting stability. The patient then twists to the other side, moving the ball as far as possible in the new direction.

balloon in a variety of directions. The ball can be inflated or weighted (Fig. 4.33).

- *Kicking a ball.* A small ball is rolled toward the patient, who then kicks it back to the therapist.

Red Flag: Patients with vestibular insufficiency may experience increased dizziness, nausea, or anxiety during activities on the therapy ball. This should be carefully monitored and the level of challenge decreased to tolerable levels. For some severely involved patients, ball activities may be contraindicated.

Clinical Note: During episodes of instability, ball activities should be modified to ensure patient safety (e.g., decrease range or speed of movements, increase BOS). The therapist should be attentive and utilize appropriate guarding techniques. For some patients (e.g., the patient with TBI and cerebellar ataxia), this may mean utilizing a safety belt.

Adaptive Sitting Balance Activities

Adaptive balance control can be enhanced by modifying or changing task or environmental demands. Examples include the following:

- Change the support surface. Change from an inflatable disc to a ball with a floor ring holder to a ball with no ring holder; change from a hard floor to dense foam.
- Modify the BOS. Change from feet wide apart to feet together to one leg crossed; change from hands on thighs to hands folded across the chest.

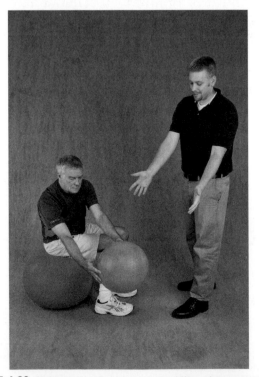

FIGURE 4.33 Sitting on ball, catching and throwing a small ball. The patient practices catching and throwing a small ball while maintaining sitting stability. The therapist varies the direction and speed of the throws to alter the challenge to balance.

- Progress from unilateral to bilateral limb movements.
- Utilize combinations of limb movements: UE, LE, two-limb or four-limb activities.
- Increase the number of repetitions.
- Increase the height of the extremity lifts.
- Increase the speed of the activity.
- Pace the activity using rhythmic timing devices (a metronome or music).
- Increase the time a position is held.
- Increase the weight or size of the ball during catching and throwing activities.
- Change the direction of the throw. The ball is thrown at or near the LOS or toward the side of an instability.
- Add resistance. Elastic resistive bands can be applied to the hips to provide resistance during pelvic shifts or to the knees to strengthen hip abductors. Resistance can be added to UE or LE movements using resistive bands or lightweight cuffs.
- Use dual-tasking. The patient performs two tasks simultaneously (e.g., hold a tray or count backward by 7s from 100 while performing leg lifts while sitting on the ball).
- Modify visual input: eyes open (EO) to eyes closed (EC).
- Modify somatosensory input. Change from feet on a sticky mat (yoga mat) to a tile floor to a soft mat to a foam cushion to an inflatable disc.
- Modify the environment. Progress from a closed environment (quiet room) to an open environment (busy treatment area).

Outcomes

Motor control goal: Improved sitting balance control.
Functional skills achieved: The patient demonstrates appropriate functional balance skills in sitting for independence in ADL.

Activities to Improve Mobility in Sitting

Scooting is the ability to move the hips forward or backward while sitting. It requires a weight shift onto one hip in order to partially unweight the other hip for movement. The patient advances forward or backward by walking on his or her bottom ("butt walking"). Clasping the hands together with arms extended and held in front helps isolate the motion to the lower trunk and pelvis while restricting upper trunk movements. The patient is instructed to: *"Hold your hands together directly in front; I want you to shift your weight to one side and move forward. Now shift to the other side and move the other limb forward."* Scooting is an important lead-up activity for independent bed mobility (moving in bed) and for sit-to-stand transfers (scooting forward to the edge of the seat before standing up). This activity is appropriate to both long- and short-sitting positions.

Scooting in the Long-Sitting Position

The patient sits in a long-sitting position. The therapist is positioned at the patient's feet and assists the motion by holding both feet off the mat, reducing friction effects. The patient is instructed to shift to one side and move the opposite limb forward. The process is then reversed as the patient moves forward. Adequate range of the hamstrings (90 to 110 degrees) is essential to prevent sacral sitting and overstretching of low back muscles.

Scooting, in the Short-Sitting Position

The patient sits at the edge of the mat, with both feet flat on the floor. The therapist initially assists the forward motion by lifting and supporting the thigh of the dynamic limb to reduce friction effects. Forward movement of the dynamic limb can be lightly resisted at the front of the knee (manual contacts on the upper tibia, avoiding the patella) to enhance muscular responses (Fig. 4.34). Scooting in the short-sitting position is an important lead-up activity for independent sit-to-stand transfers, which require that the patient initially come forward to the edge of the seat before standing up.

Scooting off a High Table Into Modified Standing

The patient sits on a high table with both feet off the floor. The patient is instructed to scoot forward to the edge of the table (Fig. 4.35A). The patient then rotates the pelvis forward on the dynamic side while extending the hip and knee on the same side. The patient places the foot on the floor, keeping the other hip resting on the table (half-sitting on the table) (Fig. 4.35B). This activity promotes unilateral weightbearing and is a useful

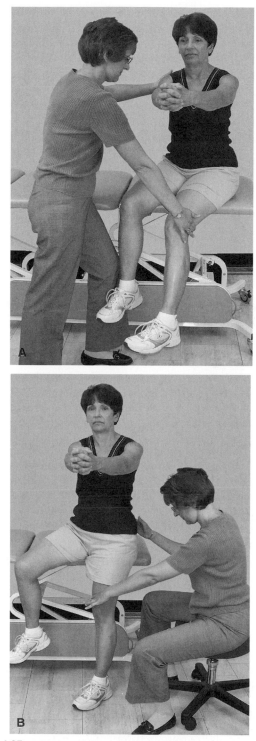

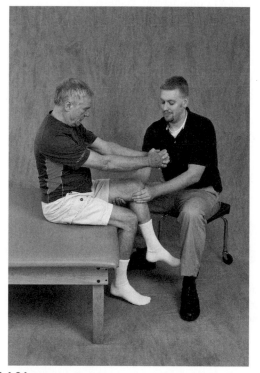

FIGURE 4.34 Sitting, scooting in short-sitting. The patient sits with both hands clasped together in a forward position (elbows extended and shoulders flexed). The patient practices weight shifting to one side while moving the opposite limb forward. The therapist instructs the patient in the movements and provides some unweighting of the dynamic limb and resistance to enhance the forward movement of the limb. The patient then shifts to the other side and moves the opposite limb forward, scooting forward to the edge of the mat.

FIGURE 4.35 Sitting, scooting off a high table into unilateral standing. **(A)** The patient sits with both hands clasped together in a forward position (elbows extended and shoulders flexed). The patient practices weight shifting to one side while moving one limb forward. The therapist instructs the patient in the movements and provides some unweighting of the dynamic limb and resistance to enhance the forward movement of the limb. The patient then shifts to the other side and moves the opposite limb forward, scooting forward to the edge of the table. **(B)** The patient then moves one LE into weightbearing (modified standing) while keeping the other hip on the table. The therapist provides light pressure to the quadriceps to enhance extension. An adjustable-height table is required to ensure proper standing height.

activity for patients who lack symmetrical weightbearing in standing (e.g., the patient recovering from stroke who demonstrates asymmetrical weightbearing; this requires the patient to stand on the more affected LE). Proper height of the treatment table is important to facilitate standing posture; thus an adjustable-height table is required for this activity.

Student Practice Activities in Sitting

Sound clinical decision-making will help identify the most appropriate activities and techniques to improve sitting and sitting balance skills for an individual patient. Many of these interventions presented will provide the foundation for developing home management strategies to improve function. Although some of the interventions described clearly require the skilled intervention of a physical therapist, many can be modified or adapted for inclusion in a home exercise program (HEP) for use by the patient (self-management strategies), family members, or other individuals participating in the patient's care.

Student practice activities provide an opportunity to share knowledge and skills as well as to confirm or clarify understanding of the treatment interventions. Each student in a group contributes his or her understanding of, or questions about, the strategy, technique, or activity, and participate in the activity being discussed. Dialogue should continue until a consensus of understanding is reached. Box 4.5 Student Practice Activity presents an activity that focuses on task analysis of sitting. Box 4.6 Student Practice Activity presents activities that focus on techniques and strategies to improve sitting and sitting balance control.

BOX 4.5 STUDENT PRACTICE ACTIVITY: TASK ANALYSIS OF SITTING

EQUIPMENT NEEDS: Adjustable-height platform mat or treatment table and a dome-shaped wobble board.

PROCEDURE: Work in groups of two or three. Begin by having each person in the group sit on the mat, first in short-sitting (knees flexed, feet flat on the floor) and then in long-sitting (knees extended). Then have each person practice weight shifts to the LOS in both postures. Finally, have each person sit on a dome-shaped wobble board placed on a hard sitting surface. Have each person practice sitting centered on the board (no tilts); then have each person sit on the wobble board with reduced BOS (one leg crossed over the other; sitting on a high seat without contact of the feet on the floor).

OBSERVE AND DOCUMENT: Using the following questions to guide your analysis, observe and record the variations and similarities observed among the different sitting patterns represented in your group.

▲ What is the person's normal sitting alignment?
▲ What changes are noted between short- and long-sitting postures?
▲ During weight shifts exploring LOS, are the shifts symmetrical in each direction?
▲ During sitting on a wobble board, how successful is the person at maintaining centered alignment on the board (no touch down support)? What is the position of the UEs? What changes are noted when one leg is crossed over the other? When both feet are off the ground using a high seat?
▲ What types of pathology/impairments might affect a patient's ability to sit?
▲ What compensatory strategies might be necessary?
▲ What environmental factors might constrain or impair sitting? What modifications are needed?

BOX 4.6 STUDENT PRACTICE ACTIVITY: TECHNIQUES AND STRATEGIES TO IMPROVE SITTING AND SITTING BALANCE CONTROL

OBJECTIVE: To provide practice oportunities for developing skill in interventions designed to improve sitting and sitting balance control.

EQUIPMENT NEEDS: Platform mat, treatment table, therapy balls (inflated, weighted), cones, balloons, water pitcher, and glass.

DIRECTIONS: Work in groups of three or four students. Practice and demonstrate the activities and techniques presented in the outline below (titled *Outline of Activities and Techniques for Demonstration and Practice*). Members of the group will assume different roles (described below) and will rotate roles each time the group progresses to a new item on the outline.

▲ One person assumes the role of therapist (for demonstrations) and participates in discussion.
▲ One person serves as the subject/patient (for demonstrations) and participates in discussion.
▲ The remaining members participate in task analysis of the activity and discussion. Following the demonstration, members provide supportive and corrective feedback. One member of this group should be designated as a "fact checker" to return to the text content to confirm elements of the discussion (if needed) or if agreement cannot be reached.

BOX 4.6 STUDENT PRACTICE ACTIVITY: TECHNIQUES AND STRATEGIES TO IMPROVE SITTING AND SITTING BALANCE CONTROL (continued)

Thinking aloud, brainstorming, and sharing thoughts should be continuous throughout this activity! As each item in the section outline is considered, the following should ensue:

1. An initial discussion of the *activity,* including patient and therapist positioning. Also considered here should be positional changes to enhance the activity (e.g., prepositioning a limb, hand placements to alter the BOS, and so forth).
2. An initial discussion of the *technique,* including its description, indication(s) for use, therapist hand placements (manual contacts), and VCs.
3. A *demonstration* of the activity and application of the technique by the designated therapist and subject/ patient. All group members should provide supportive and corrective feedback, highlighting what was correct and providing recommendations and suggestions for improvement. Particularly important is a discussion of strategies to make the activity either *more* or *less* challenging for the patient.
4. If any member of the group feels he or she requires additional practice with the activity and technique, time should be allocated to accommodate the request.

Outline of Activities and Techniques for Demonstration and Practice

▲ Sitting, holding
  • Stabilizing reversals
  • Rhythmic stabilization
▲ Sitting, weight shifts, cone stacking
▲ Sitting, weight shifts, dynamic reversals

▲ Sitting, application of PNF UE patterns, using dynamic reversals
  • UE D1 flexion and extension
  • UE D2 flexion and extension
  • Chop and reverse chop
  • Lift and reverse lift
  • Bilateral symmetrical D1 thrust and withdrawal
  • Bilateral symmetrical D2 flexion, rhythmic initiation
▲ Sitting, manual perturbations
▲ Sitting, ball activities
  • Pelvic shifts (anterior-posterior, side to side, pelvic clock)
  • UE lifts (unilateral, bilateral symmetrical, bilateral asymmetrical, reciprocal with marching)
  • LE lifts (hip flexion, knee extension, with ankle circles or writing letters, side-steps, heel-lifts, toe-offs)
  • Head and trunk rotation (lateral rotations, diagonal rotations)
  • Marching in place (contralateral UE and LE lifts)
  • Jumping jacks (bouncing with UE lifts overhead)
  • Catching and throwing a ball (inflated ball, weighted ball); batting a balloon
  • Kicking a rolling ball
▲ Dual-task activities: simultaneously sitting on the ball and pouring a glass of water; counting backward from 100 by 7s
▲ Scooting in short-sitting or in long-sitting, assisted
▲ Scooting off a high table into modified standing

SUMMARY

This chapter has presented the requirements for sitting and sitting balance control. Multidimensional exercises that promote static and dynamic control as well as reactive, anticipatory, and adaptive balance skills have been addressed. Ensuring patient safety while progressively challenging control using a variety of exercises and activities is key to improving functional performance.

Interventions to Improve Kneeling and Half-Kneeling Control

THOMAS J. SCHMITZ, PT, PhD

Kneeling Postures

Kneeling postures offer the benefit of achieving improved trunk and hip control without the demands required to control the knee and ankle. Inherent to these upright, antigravity postures are important prerequisite requirements for standing. For example, kneeling postures are particularly useful for developing initial upright postural control and for promoting hip extension and abduction stabilization control required for standing. By eliminating the demands of upright standing, patient anxiety and fear of falling are typically diminished. Kneeling activities also provide important lead-up skills for independent floor-to-standing transfers.

The postures addressed in this chapter are *kneeling* (Fig. 5.1A) and *half-kneeling* (Fig. 5.1B). In kneeling, both hips are extended, with bilateral weightbearing occurring primarily at the knees and upper tibia with the legs and feet resting on the support surface. This creates a relatively narrow base of support (BOS). In contrast, the BOS in half-kneeling is wider. One hip remains extended, with weightbearing at the knee and upper leg; the opposite hip and knee are flexed to approximately 90 degrees, with weightbearing occurring at the foot placed forward on the supporting surface. In kneeling postures, the center of mass (COM) is intermediate in height.

Kneeling

In kneeling, the BOS is decreased compared to quadruped. The COM is intermediate; it is higher than in supine or prone positions and lower than in standing. The BOS is influenced by the relative length of the leg and foot and is positioned largely posterior to the COM. Thus, this posture is more stable posteriorly than anteriorly. Owing to this relative anterior instability, any forward shift in the COM must be compensated for by trunk and hip extensors. This is an important safety issue. Without the ability to compensate (e.g., trunk and hip extensor weakness), anterior displacement may cause the patient to fall forward.

Kneeling involves head, trunk, and hip muscles for upright postural control. The head and trunk are maintained vertical in midline orientation, with normal spinal lumbar and thoracic curves.

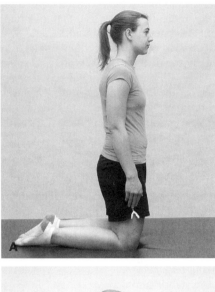

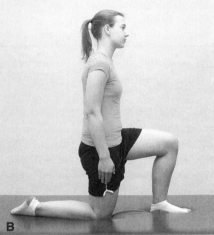

FIGURE 5.1 **(A)** Kneeling posture. Both hips are extended, with bilateral weightbearing occurring at the knees and legs; the BOS is narrow. **(B)** Half-kneeling posture. One hip is extended, with weightbearing at the knee and legs. The opposite hip and knee are flexed to approximately 90 degrees with slight abduction; the foot is forward and placed flat on the support surface. The BOS is wide and angled on a diagonal between the posterior and anterior limbs.

The pelvis is level in horizontal orientation. Weight-bearing in kneeling is through the hips and on the knees and legs. Both hips are extended with the knees flexed to approximately 90 degrees. This position represents an advanced lower extremity (LE) pattern (initiated during bridging) of hip extension with knee flexion required for gait (i.e., terminal phase of stance).

General Characteristics

- The relatively low COM (compared to standing) makes kneeling a safe posture for initially promoting upright trunk and hip control. If the patient inadvertently loses control, the distance to the mat is small; with contact guarding from the therapist, a fall would be unlikely to result in injury.
- Compared to standing, the degrees of freedom are reduced. In kneeling, control of the knee or foot and ankle is not required to maintain upright trunk and hip control.
- Prolonged positioning in kneeling provides strong inhibitory influences (inhibitory pressure on patellar tendon) acting bilaterally on the quadriceps. It is therefore a useful intervention to dampen hypertonicity for patients with LE extensor spasticity.
- Owing to the inherent inhibitory influences of the posture, kneeling may be an important intervention to immediately precede standing and gait activities for the patient with LE extensor spasticity and a scissoring gait pattern.

Clinical Notes:

- Patients with strong abnormal flexor synergy influence (e.g., the patient with stroke) will have difficulty maintaining the hip in extension; the tendency will be to recruit hip flexors with knee flexors. In this situation, the therapist may use manually guided (active assistive) movement to assist with hip extension (manual contacts on posterior hip/pelvis).
- For the patient whose foot pulls strongly into dorsiflexion when positioned in kneeling, a small pillow or towel roll may be placed under the dorsum of the foot to relieve pressure on the toes.
- For the patient with limitations in plantarflexion range of motion (ROM), the ankle/foot may be positioned over the edge of a platform mat.
- Patients who experience knee discomfort and knee pain from prolonged positioning may benefit from kneeling on a more resilient surface such as a small cushion placed under both knees. An alternative is to incorporate several shorter time intervals in kneeling over the course of a treatment session to reduce the discomfort.

Red Flag: Kneeling may be contraindicated in some patients, such as individuals with rheumatoid or osteoarthritis affecting the knee, patients with knee joint instability, or patients recovering from recent knee surgery.

Kneeling: Prerequisite Requirements

Prior to the use of kneeling as an activity, several important requirements for assuming the posture need consideration. Full hip flexor ROM is necessary; if limitations exist, the patient's ability to achieve the needed hip extension will be compromised. Sufficient strength of the trunk and hip extensor muscles is necessary to keep the head and trunk upright and the hips extended. This is particularly important given the relative anterior instability inherent in the posture. Although kneeling provides an important opportunity for improving posture and balance control, adequate static postural control (ability to keep the COM over the BOS) is needed for initial maintenance of the upright posture.

Position and Activity: Kneeling, Assist-to-Position

Assist-to-position movement transitions into kneeling can be effectively accomplished from a bilateral heel-sitting position. For some patients, heel-sitting is most easily assumed from quadruped (see Chapter 3, *Interventions to Improve Bed Mobility and Early Trunk Control*, for a description of movement transitions from *quadruped* into *heel-sitting*).

ACTIVITIES, STRATEGIES, AND VERBAL CUES FOR KNEELING, ASSIST-TO-POSITION FROM BILATERAL HEEL-SITTING

Activities and Strategies For assisted movement transitions into kneeling, both the patient and the therapist are initially positioned in heel-sitting facing each other (Fig. 5.2A). The therapist places one hand on the posterior upper trunk passing under the axilla; the opposite manual contact is on the contralateral posterior hip/pelvis. These hand placements allow the therapist to assist with lifting the trunk into the upright position as well as with moving the patient's hips toward extension. The patient's hands are supported on the therapist's shoulders, which assists in guiding the upper trunk in the desired direction of movement. The patient and therapist then move together into a kneeling position (Fig. 5.2B).

Verbal Cues for Assist-to-Position From Bilateral Heel-Sitting to Kneeling The therapist provides the patient with assistance to the kneeling position on a count of three, and both move together toward kneeling. *"On the count of three, lift your trunk and move your hips forward toward me. I will help with the movement. One, two, three, now lift your trunk up and bring your hips forward; come up into kneeling."*

Kneeling: Interventions, Outcomes, and Management Strategies

Position and Activity: Kneeling, Holding

ACTIVITIES AND STRATEGIES TO IMPROVE POSTURAL STABILITY IN KNEELING

Active Holding Static postural stability (holding) in a functional position (kneeling) is the focus of this activity. Recall that postural stability control is the ability to maintain

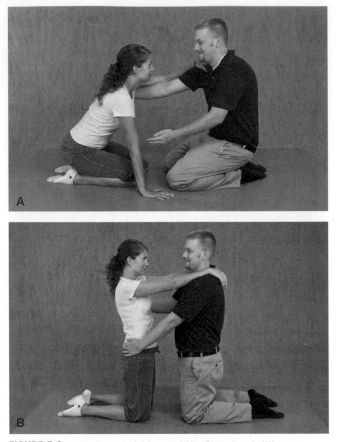

FIGURE 5.2 Kneeling, assist-to-position from heel-sitting.
(A) Initial preparation for movement transition; one of the therapist's hands is on the posterior upper trunk and the other is moving toward placement on the posterior hip/pelvis. Note that one of the patient's hands is on the therapist's shoulder and will progress to bilateral placement. The patient and therapist move together into kneeling. **(B)** The completed movement transition into kneeling.

a position (stability) with the COM over the BOS with the body at rest (no motion). The patient is in kneeling, actively holding the posture. Initially, attention is directed toward postural alignment. The head and trunk are upright (vertical) and symmetrical (midline orientation), with normal spinal lumbar and thoracic curves; the pelvis is level. Both hips are extended, with the knees flexed to approximately 90 degrees. Symmetrical weightbearing occurs at the knees positioned in a comfortable kneeling base width (i.e., distance between knees). The legs and feet are supported posteriorly on the mat surface; the ankles are plantarflexed.

For the application of holding in kneeling, the therapist guards from a kneeling or half-kneeling position facing the patient. Manual contacts are used only if contact guard is required or to assist if initial holding of the posture is difficult. As used for assist-to-position (heel-sitting to kneeling), therapist hand placements are on the posterior upper trunk passing under the axilla; the opposite

manual contact is on the contralateral posterior hip/pelvis (see Fig. 5.2B). Alternatively, each of the therapist's hands may be cupped around the lateral aspect of the hip/pelvis on both sides. The patient's hands are supported on the therapist's shoulders. As control increases, manual contacts are removed. The patient's bilateral hand placement on the therapist's shoulders is reduced from bilateral to unilateral and then to touch-down support as needed. For touch-down support, the therapist continues kneeling in front of the patient with elbows flexed, forearms supinated, and hands open to provide support as needed while postural stability is established.

Verbal Cues for Active Holding in Kneeling *"Hold the kneeling position. Keep your head and trunk upright and your weight evenly distributed on your knees. Hold, hold, keep holding the position."*

Clinical Note: During initial holding in kneeling, the patient with weakness and instability may benefit from upper extremity (UE) support. This can be accomplished by vertically positioning bolsters (or high stools) on each side or in front of the patient for weightbearing support on the elbows or on the hands (shoulders flexed and elbows extended). Alternatively, support can be provided by placing the patient's hands on a large ball positioned in front. A wall or wall ladder next to a mat can also be used effectively for this purpose.

Stabilizing Reversals: Anterior/Posterior Resistance Recall that stabilizing reversals involve small-range alternating isotonic contractions progressing to stabilizing (holding) in the posture. Resistance is applied to opposing muscle groups (agonist/antagonist) within a relatively static kneeling posture; resistance is sufficient to prevent movement. The patient is asked to maintain the kneeling position. Using bilateral manual contacts, the therapist typically applies resistance first in the stronger direction of movement (agonists) until the patient's maximum is reached. Once the patient is fully resisting with agonists, one hand continues to resist while the opposite hand is positioned to resist the antagonists. When the antagonists begin to engage, the other hand is also moved to resist antagonists. The goal is maintained holding.[1] Only minimal motion is permitted. The technique is a precursor to rhythmic stabilization utilizing isometric contractions.

For the application of stabilizing reversals with anterior/posterior resistance, the patient is asked to hold the kneeling position. The therapist is also kneeling, facing the patient. The therapist's manual contacts reverse position between the *anterior* (Fig. 5.3) and *posterior* aspects of the pelvis and contralateral shoulder/upper trunk as the patient attempts to shift toward and away from the therapist. Resistance is applied until the patient's maximum is reached and then gradually reversed. Owing to the relative

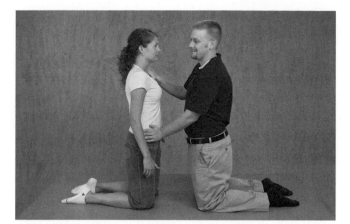

FIGURE 5.3 Stabilizing reversals: anterior/posterior resistance in kneeling. The therapist's hands are positioned to apply posteriorly directed resistance on the upper trunk and contralateral pelvis; note that the posterior BOS is comparatively large. *Not shown:* Hands are then reversed to the posterior aspects of the pelvis and contralateral shoulder/upper trunk to apply anteriorly directed resistance; because the anterior BOS is minimal, only slight resistance is applied.

anterior instability of the posture, the patient will be able to withstand relatively little resistance directed in an anterior direction and greater resistance directed posteriorly. As the patient holds the posture, posteriorly directed resistance is applied from the front, as if pushing the trunk and pelvis away from the therapist. Manual contacts then reverse and an anteriorly directed resistance is applied from behind, as if pulling the trunk and pelvis toward the therapist.

Verbal Cues for Stabilizing Reversals, Anterior/Posterior Resistance in Kneeling As the patient attempts to shift toward the therapist: *"Don't let me push you away."* As the patient attempts to shift away from the therapist: *"Now, don't let me pull you toward me."*

Directed by the goals of the intervention, several variations in manual contacts can be used for application of stabilizing reversals in kneeling. Some examples follow:

• Bilateral manual contacts alternating between the anterior and posterior surfaces of the pelvis can be used for application of anterior/posterior resistance.
• Bilateral manual contacts alternating between the anterior and posterior surfaces of the upper trunk/shoulder can be used for application of anterior/posterior resistance.
• Bilateral manual contacts on the lateral aspects of the pelvis allow application of medial/lateral resistance.

Outcomes
Motor control goals: Stability (static postural control).
Functional skill achieved: The patient is able to stabilize during upright kneeling.

Comments
• During initial activities in kneeling, the patient with instability may benefit from additional support provided by placing hands on the therapist's shoulders (see Fig. 5.2B).
• Elastic resistive bands can be placed around the distal thighs to increase proprioceptive input and contraction of the lateral hip muscles (gluteus medius).
• The patient may be positioned with the knees in the step position (with one knee slightly in front of the other) and resistance applied on the diagonal.

Indications Diminished postural stability of the lower trunk and pelvis is an indication.

Rhythmic Stabilization Rhythmic stabilization utilizes alternating isometric contractions of agonist/antagonist patterns against resistance. The patient is asked to hold the kneeling position without moving (no movement occurs) as resistance is applied simultaneously to opposing muscle groups (e.g., upper trunk flexors and lower trunk extensors *or* upper trunk extensors and lower trunk flexors; trunk rotators are also activated). With bilateral manual contacts, resistance is built up gradually as the patient responds to the applied force. When the patient is responding with maximal isometric contractions of the agonist pattern, one of the therapist's hands is moved to resist the antagonist pattern. When the antagonists begin to engage, the therapist's other hand is also moved to resist the antagonist pattern. The technique can be used to promote cocontraction and increase stability, strength, endurance, and ROM. Although no movement occurs, resistance is applied as if twisting or rotating the upper and lower trunk in opposite directions. No relaxation occurs as the direction of resistance is changed.

For the application of rhythmic stabilization in kneeling, the patient is asked to hold the position while the therapist applies rotational resistance to the trunk. One hand is on the anterior upper trunk/shoulder to resist the upper trunk flexors, while the other hand is on the contralateral posterior pelvis to resist the lower trunk extensors (Fig. 5.4). Resistance is then reversed so that one hand is on the posterior upper trunk/shoulder to resist upper trunk extensors, while the other hand is on the contralateral anterior pelvis to resist lower trunk flexors. Alternatively, rotational resistance may be applied with both hands on the pelvis or both hands on the upper trunk/shoulders.

Verbal Cues for Rhythmic Stabilization in Kneeling
"Hold, don't let me twist you. Hold, hold. Now, don't let me twist you the other way. Hold, hold."

Outcomes
Motor control goals: Stability (static postural control).
Functional skill achieved: The patient is able to independently stabilize during upright kneeling.

Indications Diminished postural stability of the lower trunk/pelvis and weakness of the trunk and hip muscles are

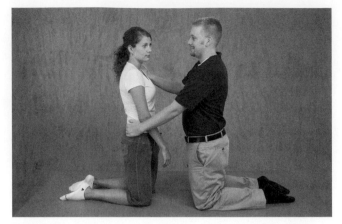

FIGURE 5.4 Application of rhythmic stabilization in kneeling. Manual contacts are on the anterior upper trunk/shoulder to resist the upper trunk flexors and rotators; the other hand is positioned on the posterior pelvis to resist the lower trunk extensors and rotators. *Not shown:* Manual contacts are then reversed so that one hand is on the posterior upper trunk/shoulder to resist upper trunk extensors, and the other hand is on the contralateral anterior pelvis to resist lower trunk flexors.

indications. Kneeling is an important lead-up activity to upright stance in plantigrade and standing.

Position/Activity: Kneeling, Weight Shifting

Weight shifting in kneeling is a closed-chain exercise that involves motions in which the distal part (knees) is fixed while the proximal segment (pelvis) is moving. Weight-shifting activities provide the important benefit of promoting the simultaneous action of synergistic muscles at more than one joint. In addition, the joint approximation and stimulation of proprioceptors further enhance joint stabilization (cocontraction). Since the kneeling posture must be stabilized while moving, weight shifting also improves dynamic stability.

ACTIVITIES, STRATEGIES, TECHNIQUES, AND VERBAL CUES TO
IMPROVE WEIGHT SHIFTING IN KNEELING

Active Weight Shifting For *medial/lateral* weight shifting in kneeling, the patient actively shifts the pelvis from side to side with the knees in a comfortable symmetrical stance position. For *anterior/posterior* diagonal weight shifting, the patient's knees are placed in a step position (with one knee slightly in front of the other). During weight-shifting activities, the therapist is positioned in front or to the side of the patient in a kneeling or half-kneeling guard position. Small-range shifts are stressed and are important lead-up skills for normal gait.

Active reaching activities can be used to promote weight shifting in all directions or in the direction of instability (e.g., the patient with hemiplegia). The therapist provides a target (*"Reach out and touch my hand"*) or uses a functional task such as cone stacking to promote reaching. With the hands on a large ball placed in front, the patient can also practice moving the ball from side to side or forward and backward.

Dynamic Reversals, Medial/Lateral Shifts Dynamic reversals utilize isotonic contractions of first agonists and then antagonists performed against resistance without relaxation. The technique involves continuously resisted concentric movement in opposing directions.[1] A transitional verbal cue (VC) is used to mark the initiation of movement in the opposite direction (*"Now, reverse"*) and alerts the patient to make the needed preparatory postural adjustments (continuous movement ↔ resistance ↔ VCs). Dynamic reversals are used to increase strength and active ROM as well as promote normal transitions between opposing muscle groups. A smooth reversal of motion is the goal.

For the application of dynamic reversals with medial/lateral shifts in kneeling, the therapist is positioned in kneeling or half-kneeling in front and to the side of the patient (diagonally in front). The therapist's manual contacts are on the lateral aspect of each side of the pelvis; application of resistance alternates between hand placements. Initially, side-to-side movement of the pelvis may be assisted (guided) for several repetitions to ensure that the patient knows the desired movements. As the patient shifts *toward* the therapist, resistance is applied to the side of the pelvis closest to the therapist. Without relaxation, movement is then reversed (transitional verbal cue required) and resistance is applied to the contralateral side of the pelvis as the patient shifts *away* from the therapist.

Verbal Cues for Dynamic Reversals, Medial/Lateral Shifts in Kneeling Shifting toward the therapist: *"Push toward me, push, push, push."* Transitional cue: *"Now, reverse."* Shifting away from the therapist: *"Pull away from me, pull, pull, pull."* When the patient is ready to move in the new direction, a preparatory cue (*"Now, reverse"*) is used to direct the patient's attention to the new movement. If a hold (isometric contraction) is added to dynamic reversals, the VC is *"Pull, pull, pull, (or push, push, push) and hold."*

Dynamic Reversals, Diagonal Shifts For the application of dynamic reversals with diagonal shifts, the patient is kneeling with the knees in step position (one knee is advanced in front of the other, simulating a step length). The therapist kneels or half-kneels diagonally in front of the patient. Resistance is applied to the pelvis as the patient shifts diagonally forward over the knee in front and then diagonally backward over the opposite knee (Fig. 5.5).

Verbal Cues for Dynamic Reversals With Diagonal Shifts Shifting toward the therapist over the knee placed in front: *"Shift forward and toward me, push, push, push."* Transitional cue: *"Now, reverse."* Shifting away from the therapist over the posterior knee: *"Shift back and away from me, pull, pull, pull."*

Dynamic Reversals, Diagonal Shifts With Rotation Once control is achieved in diagonal shifts, the diagonal shifts are combined with rotation. The patient is kneeling

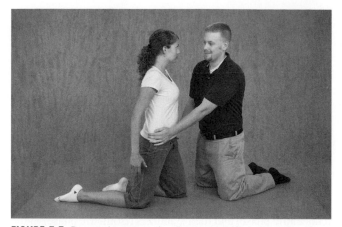

FIGURE 5.5 Dynamic reversals, diagonal shifts in kneeling. In step position, the patient alternates between shifting weight diagonally over the forward knee (shown here) and backward over the posterior knee. Resistance is applied to active concentric movement in each direction without relaxation.

with the knees in step position. The therapist is kneeling or half-kneeling diagonally in front of the patient with bilateral manual contacts at the pelvis. The patient is instructed to shift weight diagonally forward onto the knee in front while rotating the pelvis forward on the opposite side; then to shift diagonally back onto the posterior knee while rotating the pelvis backward.

With some patients, the upper trunk may move forward (or backward) as the pelvis rotates forward (or backward), producing an ipsilateral trunk pattern. In these situations, improved isolation of pelvic motion can be achieved by having the patient cross the arms before placing the hands forward on the therapist's shoulders (Fig. 5.6). The patient is instructed to keep both elbows straight and move only the pelvis forward and backward during the weight shifts. The

therapist's shoulder support for the crossed arms "locks" the upper trunk in place and promotes isolated pelvic motion. As an alternative, UE support may be provided by a wall adjacent to a platform mat.

Verbal Cues for Dynamic Reversals, Diagonal Shifts With Rotation Shifting over the knee in front with contralateral pelvic forward rotation: *"Shift forward and twist your pelvis forward, push, push, push."* Transitional cue: *"Now, reverse."* Shifting backward over the posterior knee with same-side pelvic posterior rotation: *"Shift backward and twist your pelvis back, pull, pull, pull."*

Outcomes
Motor control goal: Controlled mobility (dynamic postural control).
Functional skill achieved: The patient is able to weight shift independently in kneeling position.

Comments
• Weight shifting and pelvic rotation in kneeling are important lead-up skills for the weight transfers and pelvic motion needed for normal gait.
• Movements begin with small-range control and progress through increasing ROM (increments of ROM) to full-range control.
• If an imbalance of strength exists, resistance is applied first in the stronger direction of movement.
• Initially, movements are slow and controlled with emphasis on careful grading of resistance.
• An isometric hold may be added in the shortened range or at any point of weakness within the range. The hold is a momentary pause for one count (the patient is instructed to *"Hold"*); the antagonist movement pattern is then facilitated.
• Careful attention must be directed to providing the patient a preparatory VC (such as *"Now, reverse"*) to indicate that a change in movement direction is about to take place.

Indications Indications include weakness and incoordination of postural muscles (trunk and hip muscles) and an inability to accomplish smooth transitions between opposing postural muscle groups.

Position and Activity: Kneeling, Movement Transitions Into Bilateral Heel-Sitting and Side-Sitting
TECHNIQUES AND VERBAL CUES TO IMPROVE MOVEMENT TRANSITIONS TO AND FROM KNEELING
Combination of Isotonics, Movement Transitions Between Bilateral Heel-Sitting and Kneeling Position
Movement transitions are made from bilateral heel-sitting (buttocks make contact with the heels) up into the kneeling position and reverse. To begin, the patient is heel-sitting; the therapist is also heel-sitting diagonally in front of the patient, with bilateral manual contacts on the anterior pelvis

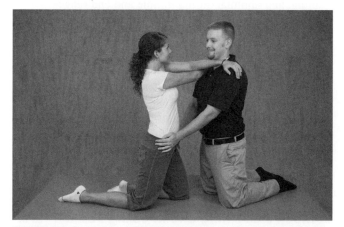

FIGURE 5.6 Dynamic reversals, diagonal shifts with pelvic rotation. The patient shifts weight diagonally forward onto the knee in front while rotating the pelvis forward on the opposite side and then diagonally backward onto the posterior knee while rotating the pelvis backward. In this example, the patient's upper limbs are crossed, with hands supported on the therapist's shoulders and elbows extended to prevent movement of the upper trunk (dissociated from pelvic movement).

(Fig. 5.7A). If needed, the therapist may assist or guide movement for one or two repetitions to ensure that the patient knows the desired movements. The patient initially flexes the trunk forward and concentrically moves up into the kneeling position by extending both hips to achieve full upright extension (Fig. 5.7B). The patient then holds the kneeling position against resistance (isometric phase). When stability is achieved, the movement transition is reversed. From the kneeling position with the knees in a comfortable stance position, the patient then flexes the trunk forward (shifting the COM anteriorly) and eccentrically controls lowering as the hips and knees flex until the buttocks make contact with the heels (see Fig. 5.7A). The UEs may be positioned with both shoulders flexed to approximately 90 degrees, elbows extended, and hands clasped together. This is an important lead-up activity for the patient with poor eccentric control who has difficulty sitting down slowly or going down stairs slowly.

As with transitions between sitting and standing, forward trunk flexion (i.e., instructing the patient to lean forward)

is important to ensure success in assuming the upright kneeling position and should be verbally cued. The therapist should encourage the patient to control lowering of the body slowly rather than "plopping" or collapsing down.

Recall that combination of isotonics is a technique that utilizes concentric, eccentric, and stabilizing (holding) contractions without relaxation.[1] For the application of this technique to movement transitions between bilateral heel-sitting and the kneeling position, the patient begins in the heel-sitting position (see Fig. 5.7A). The therapist's bilateral manual contacts are on the anterior pelvis; hand placements *do not change* during application of the technique. The therapist applies resistance as the patient first moves up into kneeling (concentric phase) and then stabilizes (isometric phase) in the kneeling position (see Fig. 5.7B). When stability is achieved, the patient is instructed to slowly move back to the heel-sitting position (eccentric phase).

Verbal Cues for Combination of Isotonics, Movement Transitions Between Bilateral Heel-Sitting and Kneeling Position

During concentric movement toward kneeling: *"Now, push up to kneeling, push, don't let me stop you."* During the middle holding phase: *"Now, don't let me move you, hold."* During eccentric controlled lowering: *"Now, go down slowly, very slowly. Make me work at pushing you down."*

Comments

- Resistance is variable in different parts of the range. As the patient moves from heel-sitting toward kneeling, resistance is minimal through the early and middle range where the effects of gravity are maximal. Resistance then builds up by the end of the transition to kneeling, as the patient moves into the shortened range to emphasize hip extensors. In the reverse movement, resistance is greatest initially, as the patient starts to move down into heel-sitting, and minimal during middle and end ranges, where the maximum effects of gravity take hold.
- If difficulty is experienced in achieving full hip extension in kneeling, the therapist may verbally cue the patient or tap over the gluteal muscles to facilitate muscle contraction.
- For patients who require a more gradual assumption of the heel-sitting position, or those who find it difficult to get up from the full heel-sitting position, a small ball may be placed between the feet to sit on (Fig. 5.8). This will decrease the range of movement required (compared to full range heel-sitting).

Combination of Isotonics, Movement Transitions Between Side-Sitting and Kneeling Position

To begin, the therapist assists or guides movement for several repetitions to ensure that the patient knows the desired movements. The patient begins in side-sitting with the UEs positioned in shoulder flexion, both elbows extended, and hands clasped together and supported on one of the therapist's shoulders (Fig. 5.9). The therapist is heel-sitting in front of the patient.

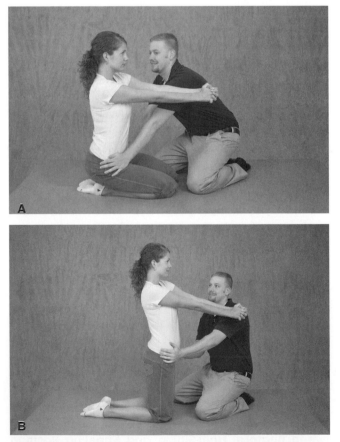

FIGURE 5.7 Combination of isotonics, movement transitions between bilateral heel-sitting and kneeling position. **(A)** From heel-sitting, concentric movement is resisted as the patient moves up toward kneeling. **(B)** Once in the kneeling position, the patient holds against continued resistance. *Not shown:* From kneeling, eccentric movement is resisted as the patient returns to heel-sitting.

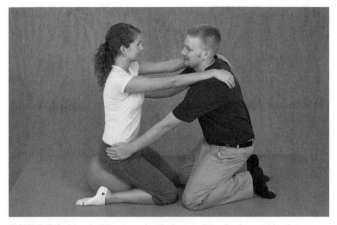

FIGURE 5.8 Heel-sitting on ball. A small ball placed between the patient's feet may be used to provide a more gradual assumption of the heel-sitting position.

From side-sitting, the patient initially flexes the trunk forward, extends both hips, and concentrically moves up into the upright kneeling position. The therapist may assist the movement by guiding upper trunk rotation and providing verbal and tactile cues. The patient then holds the kneeling position against resistance (isometric phase). From kneeling, the patient then flexes and rotates the lower trunk toward one side and controls lowering of both hips down into a side-sitting position. The trunk elongates on one side; the patient must rotate the head and upper trunk slightly to keep the UEs in position on the therapist's shoulder.

For the application of combination of isotonics to movement transitions between side-sitting and kneeling, the patient begins in the side-sitting position. Bilateral manual contacts are on the anterior pelvis; hand placements *do not change* during application of the technique. The therapist

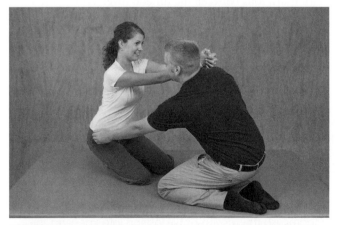

FIGURE 5.9 Combination of isotonics, movement transitions between side-sitting and kneeling position. The patient is in the starting side-sitting position. *Not shown:* Continual resistance is applied as the patient first moves up to into kneeling (concentric phase) and then stabilizes (holding phase) in the kneeling position. When stability is gained, against uninterrupted resistance, the patient slowly controls movement back to the side-sitting position (eccentric phase).

applies continual resistance as the patient first moves from side-sitting up to into kneeling (concentric phase) and then stabilizes (holding phase) in the kneeling position. When stability is achieved, the patient is instructed to slowly control movement back to the side-sitting position (eccentric phase). Resistance is variable in different parts of the range. As the patient moves from side-sitting up toward kneeling, resistance is minimal through the early and middle range where the effects of gravity are maximal. Resistance then builds up by the end of the transition to kneeling as the patient moves into the shortened range to emphasize hip extensors. The patient then stabilizes (isometric phase) in upright kneeling. As the patient starts to move back down into heel-sitting, resistance is greatest initially and then minimal during the middle and end ranges, where the maximum effects of gravity take hold.

Verbal Cues for Combination of Isotonics, Movement Transitions Between Side-Sitting and Kneeling Position During concentric movement toward kneeling: *"Now, push up to kneeling, push, don't let me stop you."* During the middle holding phase: *"Now, don't let me move you, hold."* During eccentric controlled lowering: *"Now, go down slowly, very slowly. Make me work at pushing you down."*

Red Flag: Patients with weak hip extensors or decreased lower trunk/hip flexibility may not be able move down into, or up from, the full side-sitting position. In these situations, the patient can be instructed to move through the available ranges only or to sit on a foam cushion or firm bolster placed to the side to decrease the range of excursion and provide a platform for sitting.

Clinical Note: Moving from kneeling to side-sitting is a useful treatment activity for the patient with decreased lower trunk/pelvic mobility (e.g., the post-acute patient with low back dysfunction or the patient recovering from stroke with spasticity or shortening of lateral trunk flexors). For patients with stroke, side-sitting on the more affected side lengthens the trunk side flexors and inhibits spasticity in the trunk (hands may be clasped together in front).

Dynamic Reversals, Movement Transitions Between Bilateral Heel-Sitting and Kneeling Using the PNF Bilateral Symmetrical UE Extension/Adduction/Internal Rotation, D2 Extension (UE D2E) Patterns, and UE Flexion/Abduction/External Rotation, D2 Flexion (UE D2F) Transitions from heel-sitting to kneeling can be performed with bilateral symmetrical UE Proprioceptive Neuromuscular Facilitation (PNF) patterns (D2E and D2F) using dynamic reversals (continuously resisted concentric movement in opposing directions with VCs used to mark the initiation of movement in the opposite direction). The patient is heel-sitting, with the head in midposition and the trunk in neutral alignment. The therapist is standing directly behind the patient with the LEs positioned to provide a dynamic BOS (Fig. 5.10A). To resist motion of the UEs, the therapist's bilateral manual contacts are typically positioned over the patient's forearms; however, positioning for this activity may require placement over the distal arms (see the Red Flag below). To begin, the patient's UEs are positioned in UE D2E with the shoulders toward extension, adduction, and internal rotation, the elbows are extended with forearms pronated, and the hands are closed and crossed (see Fig. 5.10A). Using dynamic reversals and UE D2F, continuous resistance is applied during transition into kneeling as the patient's hands open and the shoulders move toward flexion, abduction, and external rotation with forearm supination and wrist and finger extension (Fig. 5.10B). The patient then returns to heel-sitting with the arms moving back down into D2E. This activity recruits upper trunk extensors as the patient moves up into kneeling and upper trunk flexors as the patient moves down into heel-sitting.

⊘ **Red Flag:** This application of UE PNF patterns represents some modification in application. Typically, resistance is applied over the patient's forearm. However, the posterior positioning of the therapist and height variations of either the therapist or the patient may require that this positioning be altered (e.g., resistance applied

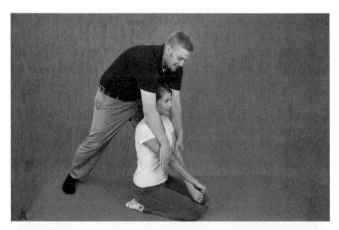

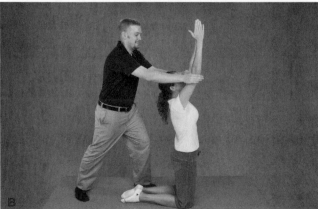

FIGURE 5.10 Dynamic reversals, movement transitions between bilateral heel-sitting and kneeling position. **(A)** Start position: heel-sitting UE D2E pattern; **(B)** end position: kneeling UE D2F pattern.

at the distal arms, just above the elbows). In addition, UE D2E normally includes movement of the patient's fisted hand toward the opposite pelvis. In the reverse movement transition going from kneeling to heel-sitting, the fisted hands actually move toward the opposite knees.

Verbal Cues for Application of Dynamic Reversals to Movement Transitions Between Bilateral Heel-Sitting and Kneeling Using PNF Bilateral Symmetrical UE D2E and UE D2F Patterns

Movement into kneeling (D2E): *"Push up against me, open your hands, lift your arms up and out, straighten your elbows, and slowly lift up into kneeling."* Transitional cue: *"Now, reverse."* Movement into heel-sitting (D2F): *"Close your hands; pull your arms down and across your body. Don't let me stop you; move slowly down into sitting on heels."*

Dynamic Reversals, Movement Transitions Between Bilateral Heel-Sitting and Kneeling Using PNF Lift and Reverse Lift Patterns

Heel-sitting to kneeling transitions can be performed with the lift (D2F) and reverse lift (D2E) PNF patterns. The patient is heel-sitting; the therapist is standing behind and to the side with the LEs positioned to provide a dynamic BOS. To begin, the patient's *lead* limb is positioned in the reverse lift (D2E) pattern across the body (toward shoulder extension, adduction, and internal rotation with forearm pronation and hand closed). The hand of the *assist* limb grasps underneath the wrist of the lead limb (Fig. 5.11A). The therapist's manual contact is on the lead UE using a loose-hand (not tight) grasp to allow rotation through the movement. Using the lift pattern, the patient then moves from heel-sitting up into kneeling, bringing the *lead* limb into D2F (shoulder flexion, abduction, and external rotation; elbow extension with forearm supination and hand open) (Fig. 5.11B). Resistance to the concentric movement in opposing patterns is continuous, with VCs used to mark transitions between the lift and reverse-lift. (The chop and reverse chop patterns may also be used.) The lead limb then moves back down into D2E as the patient returns to heel-sitting. The emphasis of this movement transition is on recruitment of the upper trunk rotators and extensors as the patient moves up into kneeling. It also involves crossing the midline, making it a useful activity for patients with unilateral neglect (e.g., the patient with stroke).

📥 **Clinical Note:** When movement transitions are combined with UE PNF bilateral symmetrical D2F or lift patterns, careful grading of resistance is required because muscle strength is not constant throughout the ROM. Resistance should not limit the patient's ability to accomplish the movement transition into kneeling. Initially, to instruct the patient in the desired movement, the UEs may be passively moved or guided (active-assistive) through the patterns before resistance is applied. At first, movements are slow and controlled with emphasis on the grading of resistance. For patients who demonstrate weakness, active movements against gravity (no manual

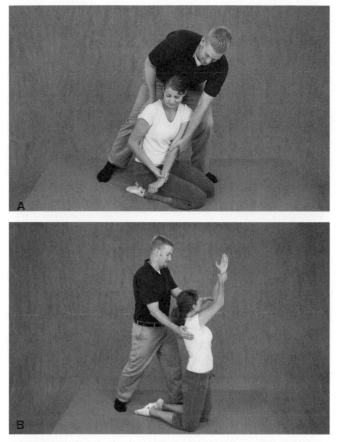

FIGURE 5.11 Dynamic reversals, movement transitions between bilateral heel-sitting and kneeling position using PNF reverse lift and lift patterns. **(A)** Reverse lift pattern: the lead limb is positioned in D2E with the patient in heel-sitting in preparation for transition into kneeling. **(B)** Lift pattern: the lead limb moves toward D2F as the patient moves up into kneeling.

resistance) may be the appropriate starting point. The therapist can subsequently initiate application of light resistance, with increased resistance as the patient approaches full kneeling. Weight cuffs can also be used to provide resistance.

Verbal Cues for Dynamic Reversals, Movement Transitions Between Bilateral Heel-Sitting and Kneeling Using PNF Lift and Reverse Lift Patterns
Movement into kneeling (lift [D2F]): *"Push up against me, open your hand, lift your arms up and out toward me, and slowly lift up into kneeling."* Transitional cue: *"Now, reverse."* Movement into heel-sitting (reverse lift [D2E]): *"Close your hand, pull your arms down and across your body. Don't let me stop you, move slowly down into sitting on heels."*

Outcomes
Motor control goals: Controlled mobility (static-dynamic control).
Functional skill achieved: The patient is able to assume the kneeling position independently.

Indications Indications include weakness and incoordination of postural muscles (trunk and hip muscles). These activities are important lead-up skills for the assumption of an upright stance position (floor-to-standing transfers).

Position and Activity: Kneeling, Forward and Backward Progression (Kneel-Walking)
TECHNIQUES AND VERBAL CUES FOR MOVEMENT PROGRESSION WITHIN KNEELING POSTURE
Resisted Progression In the kneeling position, the patient moves forward or backward using small "knee steps" with weightbearing on the knees (kneel-walking). This requires weight shifting onto one knee combined with contralateral hip hiking and forward pelvic rotation. The therapist can assist the timing and sequence of motion by providing verbal or tactile cues. Weight shifting with pelvic rotation is stressed. To begin, the therapist is kneeling directly in front of the patient (Fig. 5.12). If the patient is initially unstable, the hands may be placed on the therapist's shoulders (for light support) with a progression to no UE support. The therapist's manual contacts may be on the pelvis to provide tactile cues while the patient is instructed in weight shifting and pelvic rotation. Manual contacts then progress to the application of graded resistance and facilitation of movement using the technique of resisted progression. With this technique, resistance, stretch, and approximation are applied to facilitate weight acceptance, pelvic rotation, lower trunk motion, and forward (or backward) progression. The therapist provides steady resistance to the forward or backward progression by placing both hands on the pelvis. The therapist then takes reverse "knee steps" moving backward as the patient moves forward in time with the patient's movements. A backward knee-walking progression is also practiced; the therapist moves forward as the patient moves backward. A key element of application is careful grading of resistance. In general, resistance to kneel-walking is relatively light (facilitatory) to encourage proper timing of the pelvic movements but also not to disturb the momentum, coordination, and velocity of movement. Approximation can be applied down through the top of the pelvis to assist in stabilizing responses as weight is taken on the stance limb.

Red Flag: Safety is always a top priority when interacting with a patient or client. Although interventions confined to a padded mat surface with the therapist in a protective guard position provide considerable inherent safety, some situations require additional precautions. Use of a guarding (transfer) belt may be warranted during early movement transitions (e.g., quadruped to kneeling, heel-sitting to kneeling) and during forward or backward progressions such as kneel-walking. Reinforced fabric guarding belts with hook-and-loop fasteners are relatively inexpensive and easy to don. They not only provide improved overall safety but also enhance patient confidence when first progressing to activities that involve a higher COM and decreased BOS.

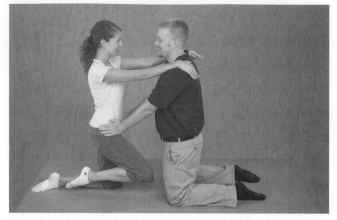

FIGURE 5.12 Resisted forward progression in kneeling (kneel-walking). Steady resistance is applied to forward (or backward) progression by placing both hands on the pelvis. Manual contacts are on the anterior (forward) or posterior (backward) pelvis. Resistance is relatively light so as not to disturb the patient's timing, momentum, and coordination.

Verbal Cues for Kneeling, Forward and Backward Progression (Kneel-Walking)

Overall timing of kneel-walking can be facilitated with appropriate verbal commands. Forward progression: *"On three I want you to step forward, beginning with your right knee. One, two, three and step, step, step."* Backward progression: *"On three I want you to step backward, beginning with your left knee. One, two, three and step, step, step."*

Clinical Notes: Kneel-walking is an activity that is generally limited to a small number of patients. Patients with bilateral LE extensor spasticity may benefit from practice in kneel-walking. Inhibition is provided to the knee extensors while the patient is free to practice the elements needed for trunk and hip control. Patients with incomplete paraplegia and intact hip control (e.g., cauda equina injury) may also benefit from initial gait activities in kneel-walking. Assistive devices (e.g., bilateral mat crutches) can be appropriately sized for this activity.

Kneel-walking is generally contraindicated for patients with significant arthritic changes of the knee or other knee pathologies.

Outcomes

Motor control goal: Skill.

Functional skill achieved: The patient is able to move independently in kneeling by using a reciprocal trunk and limb pattern.

Indications Impaired timing, coordination, or control of pelvis and lower trunk segments is an indication. Kneel-walking is a lead-up activity for bipedal (upright) walking.

ACTIVITIES AND STRATEGIES TO IMPROVE BALANCE IN KNEELING

Some of the activities already presented provide strategies for improving balance. However, patients who demonstrate significant impairments in *dynamic postural responses* may

be unable to control kneeling posture stability and orientation when movement of body segments is superimposed.

Kneeling, Active Holding, and Weight Shifting As presented earlier, activities to improve balance in kneeling begin with static holding (static postural control) (Fig. 5.13A) and progress to weight shifting (Fig. 5.13B) or reaching activities in all directions (dynamic postural control). Recall that *static postural control* is necessary for maintenance of the upright kneeling posture. *Dynamic postural control* is required for the control of movements performed in the kneeling posture (weight shifting and reaching). *Anticipatory balance control* is needed for preparatory postural adjustments that accompany voluntary movements. Examples of activities that challenge anticipatory balance include practicing postural sway in all directions with gradual trajectory increments, "look-arounds" (turning the head with trunk rotation), and UE reaching. *Reactive balance control* is needed for adjustments in response to changes in the COM or changes in the support surface. Activities that can be used to challenge reactive balance in kneeling include manual perturbations that disturb the patient's COM and balance activities on a tilting support surface (inflated disc) that disturb the patient's BOS. Reactive

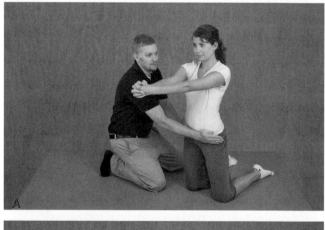

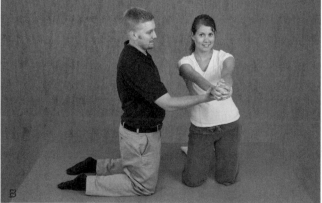

FIGURE 5.13 (A) Kneeling, active holding of posture. This activity promotes postural stability control (ability to maintain a position with the COM over the BOS with the body at rest). **(B)** Kneeling, medial/lateral weight shifts. This activity promotes dynamic stability as the kneeling posture must be stabilized during weight shifting.

balance control allows for rapid and efficient responses to environmental perturbations required during transitions from kneeling to standing, maintenance of standing posture, and walking.

Kneeling, Manual Perturbations Manual perturbations initiated by the therapist involve gentle displacement of the COM from over the BOS. Perturbations require that the patient provide a direction-specific movement response to return the COM over the BOS (state of equilibrium). To begin, the patient is kneeling on a stationary mat surface. The therapist is also in a kneeling position next to the patient (therapist positioning relative to patient will change based on the direction of perturbations). Manual contacts alternate between a guard position and application of displacing forces (manual contact perturbations) to the trunk. During initial use of perturbations, a guarding belt may be an important consideration. An additional early safety precaution is to have a second person present to assist with guarding.

During the application of perturbations, it is important to ensure that the patient is using appropriate compensatory responses relative to the direction of displacement. With posterior displacements in kneeling, hip and trunk flexor activity is required. With forward displacements, hip and trunk extensor activity is required. Lateral displacements require head and trunk inclination. Rotational displacements (twisting and displacing the trunk) require combinations of trunk movements. Protective extension of the UEs will be initiated if the displacements move the COM beyond the limits of stability (LOS) or outside of the BOS. If patient responses are lacking, the therapist may intervene with verbally and/or manually guided practice of initial attempts at direction-specific movement responses. The patient will then progress to active movements.

Clinical Note: Perturbations should be appropriate for the patient's available ROM and speed of control. It is important to use gentle disturbances with varied, asymmetrical manual contacts (tapping or nudging the patient out of position). Violent perturbations (pushes or shoves) are never appropriate. They place the patient "rigidly on-guard," defeating the purpose of the activity, and they are not necessary to stimulate balance responses. The therapist can vary the patient's BOS to increase or decrease the relative challenge of the activity (e.g., moving the knees apart or closer together).

Kneeling, Inflated Disc The patient is positioned in kneeling on an inflated disc with knees comfortably apart and ankles plantarflexed with feet supported on the mat. The UEs may be positioned with shoulders flexed to approximately 90 degrees with both elbows extended and hands clasped together (Fig. 5.14). The therapist is kneeling or half-kneeling to the side of the patient in a guard position. Initially, the patient holds the position by maintaining a balanced or centered kneeling position (holding the disc steady). A progression is then made to patient-initiated active weight shifts,

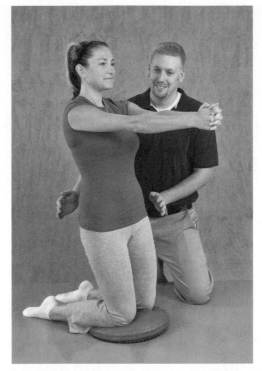

FIGURE 5.14 Kneeling on an inflated disc. Initially, the patient holds the position (holding the disc steady). *Not shown:* A progression is then made to patient-initiated active weight shifts in different directions (e.g., anterior/posterior and medial/lateral).

shifting in different directions to stimulate balance responses (e.g., anterior/posterior, medial/lateral). These patient-initiated challenges to balance stimulate both *feedforward* (anticipatory adjustments in postural activity) and *feedback-driven* (response produced information) adjustments to balance. Challenge can be increased by progressing to a higher inflated dome (e.g., a BOSU® dome). With a higher dome, the knees are the primary support; the feet are not in contact with the support surface (reducing the BOS).

Prone to Kneeling on Ball, Movement Transition This is a useful activity to improve balance (and stabilizing) responses of the trunk muscles as well as strengthen the core and UEs. The therapist is standing next to the patient in a guard position; if contact guard is required, manual contacts are on the pelvis. The patient begins in quadruped position over a ball that is large enough to support the patient's upper trunk. The patient then "walks" forward on the hands until the ball is positioned under the thighs (Fig. 5.15A). The patient then fully flexes both hips and knees, bringing the knees up toward the chest and the ball underneath the legs. The patient is now kneeling on the ball in a tucked position with the UEs extended and weightbearing on the mat (Fig. 5.15B). The movements are reversed to return to the start position. The therapist can initially assist the patient into the tucked position by manually stabilizing and/or lifting the pelvis. Progression is to active movement control. A variation of this activity is to have the patient bring both knees up into a tucked position to one side

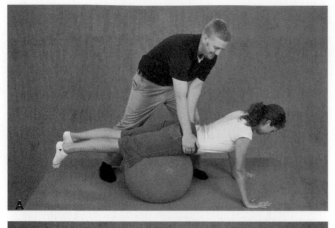

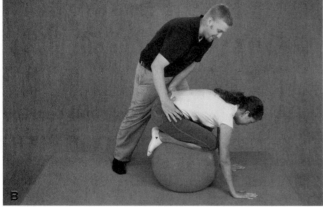

FIGURE 5.15 Prone to kneeling on a ball from a quadruped position (not shown). **(A)** The patient moves forward on the hands; as the patient rolls forward on the ball, the hips and knees extend. **(B)** Once the ball is under the thighs, the patient flexes both hips and knees to bring the ball under the legs.

(knees moving on a diagonal toward one shoulder as if moving toward a side-sitting position on the ball).

Outcomes
Motor control goals: Static and dynamic balance control.
Functional skill achieved: The patient demonstrates functional balance in the kneeling position.

Indications Indications include impaired lower trunk control and impaired balance in movement transitions from kneeling to standing.

Red Flag: Kneeling activities using a ball represent very challenging activities that require a great deal of lower trunk flexibility and postural control. It is important to observe the patient's responses carefully and use appropriate safety precautions, guarding the patient while on the ball.

Half-Kneeling

In half-kneeling, the COM is the same as in kneeling (intermediate); however, the BOS is wider and on a diagonal between the posterior and anterior limbs. One hip remains extended, with weightbearing on the stance limb; the opposite hip and knee are flexed to approximately 90 degrees with slight abduction and the foot is placed flat on the support surface (see Fig. 5.1B). Compared to kneeling, the position imposes greater weightbearing and stability demands on the hip of the stance limb. The posture can also be used to promote ankle stabilizing responses and movements of the forward limb as well as increase proprioceptive input through the foot.

General Characteristics
The posture is more stable than kneeling. Half-kneeling involves head, trunk, and hip muscles for upright postural control. The head and trunk are maintained on the vertical in midline orientation with normal spinal lumbar and thoracic curves. The pelvis is maintained in midline orientation with the hip fully extended on the posterior stance limb. As with kneeling, *static postural control* is necessary for the maintenance of upright posture. *Dynamic postural control* is necessary for control of movements performed in the posture (e.g., weight shifting or reaching). *Reactive balance control* is needed for adjustments in response to changes in the COM (perturbation) or changes in the support surface (tilting). *Anticipatory balance control* is needed for preparatory postural adjustments that accompany voluntary movements.

 Clinical Notes:

- Holding in the posture and weight-shifting activities in the half-kneeling position provide an early opportunity for partial weightbearing on the forward foot; the position can also be used to effectively mobilize the foot and ankle muscles (e.g., for the patient with ankle injury).
- As in kneeling, prolonged compression provides inhibitory influences on the stance-side quadriceps; there is no inhibitory pressure on the quadriceps of the forward limb.
- The asymmetrical limb positioning (one stance limb and one limb forward with foot flat) can be used to disassociate (break up) symmetrical limb patterns. Half-kneeling is a useful activity for the patient with spastic diplegia (cerebral palsy).
- As with kneeling, half-kneeling may be contraindicated in some patients, such as individuals with rheumatoid or osteoarthritis affecting the knee, patients with knee joint instability, or patients recovering from recent knee surgery.

Position and Activity: Half-Kneeling, Assist-to-Position
Assist-to-position movement transitions into half-kneeling can be effectively accomplished from a kneeling position. This movement transition is an important lead-up skill to independent floor-to-standing transfers.

ACTIVITIES, STRATEGIES, AND VERBAL CUES FOR HALF-KNEELING, ASSIST-TO-POSITION FROM KNEELING
Activities and Strategies From a kneeling position, the patient brings one limb up into the forward position with the hip and knee flexed and the foot placed flat on the mat. The opposite stance knee remains in a weightbearing position. The

therapist is in a half-kneeling position in front and slightly to the side of the patient. The therapist's manual contacts are on the pelvis (Fig. 5.16). The therapist may assist weight shifting toward the stance limb by gently rotating the pelvis backward on that side. This partially unloads and facilitates movement of the forward limb into position. To reduce the postural stability demands during initial practice, the patient's hands may be placed on the therapist's shoulders (for light support) with a progression to no UE support. During initial learning of the movement transitions, movement of the patient's forward limb can be assisted by the therapist sliding an assist hand under the upper thigh and moving the manual contact from upper to lower thigh as the patient lifts the LE. Practice in half-kneeling should include alternating the LEs between the stance and forward position.

Verbal Cues for Assist-to-Position From Kneeling to Half-Kneeling

The therapist provides the patient with assistance to the half-kneeling position on a count of three. *"On the count of three, shift your weight onto the left knee and bring the right knee up and place your foot flat on the mat. I will help. One, two, three, now shift and bring your right knee up and place your foot forward onto the mat."*

Half-Kneeling: Interventions, Outcomes, and Management Strategies

Position and Activity: Half-Kneeling, Holding
ACTIVITIES AND STRATEGIES TO IMPROVE POSTURAL STABILITY IN HALF-KNEELING

Active Holding This activity focuses on static postural stability (holding) in a functional position (half-kneeling). The patient is in half-kneeling, actively holding the posture with weight equally distributed between the posterior stance knee and the foot of the forward limb. Postural alignment is maintained with the head and trunk upright and the COM kept over the BOS with the body at rest (no motion).

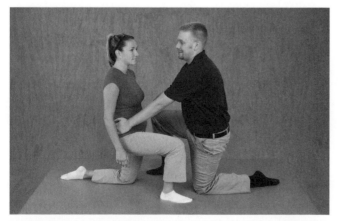

FIGURE 5.16 Half-kneeling, assist-to-position from kneeling. This figure illustrates the completed movement transition into half-kneeling; manual contacts are on the pelvis. Alternatively, manual contacts on the stance side are on the posterior upper trunk passing under the axilla and on the lateral hip/pelvis on the forward limb side.

For the application of holding in half-kneeling, the therapist is in half-kneeling in front of the patient in a *reverse mirror-image* position (patient and therapist use opposite limbs for the stance and forward positions) (see Fig. 5.16). Manual contacts are used only if contact guard is required or to assist if initial holding of the posture is difficult. Therapist hand placement on the stance side is on the posterior upper trunk passing under the axilla and on the lateral hip/pelvis on the forward limb side. Alternatively, each of the therapist's hands may be cupped around the lateral aspect of the hip/pelvis on both sides (see Fig. 5.16). To reduce the postural stability demands during initial practice, the patient's hands may be positioned on the elevated forward knee for support. Alternatively, both hands may be placed on the therapist's shoulders for light support. A progression is made to using only one hand, then to touch-down support as needed, and finally to no UE support. As with kneeling, to provide touch-down support, the therapist remains in front of the patient with elbows flexed, forearms supinated, and hands open to provide support as needed while postural stability is established.

Verbal Cues for Active Holding in Half-Kneeling

"Hold the position. Keep your head and trunk upright and your weight evenly distributed between your knee behind and the foot in front. Hold, hold, keep holding the position."

Stabilizing Reversals: Anterior/Posterior Resistance

Since the BOS in half-kneeling is on a diagonal, resistance is used only in the direction of the BOS. Resistance is applied on a diagonal in opposing (anterior/posterior) directions within a relatively static half-kneeling posture; the technique utilizes isotonic contractions progressing to stabilizing holds to promote stability.

For the application of stabilizing reversals with anterior/posterior resistance, the patient is asked to hold the half-kneeling position. The therapist is also half-kneeling, facing the patient. The therapist's manual contacts reverse position between the *anterior* and *posterior* aspects of the pelvis. Immediately before the hands slide to the opposite surfaces, a transitional cue is given such as *"Now, reverse."* Resistance is applied to the pelvis, first as if pushing the pelvis diagonally back toward the posterior stance knee (Fig. 5.17A) and then reversed as if pulling the pelvis frontward toward the forwardly placed limb. Resistance is applied until the patient's maximum is reached and then reversed. Resistance is applied only diagonally, in the direction of the BOS. The challenge of this activity may be progressed by placing the foot of the forward limb on an inflated disc (Fig. 5.17B). This increases the control demands imposed on the forward knee and ankle.

Verbal Cues for Stabilizing Reversals, Anterior/Posterior Resistance in Half-Kneeling.

As the patient attempts to shift forward toward the therapist: *"Don't let me push you away, and hold."* Transitional cue: *"Now reverse."* As the patient attempts to shift backward away from the therapist: *"Don't let me pull you toward me, and hold."*

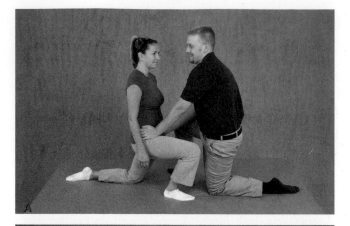

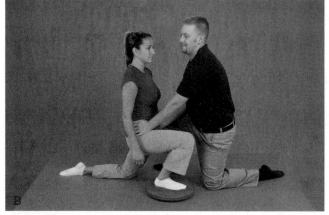

FIGURE 5.17 Stabilizing reversals: anterior/posterior resistance in half-kneeling. **(A)** The patient is asked to maintain the position. The therapist's hand placements are positioned to apply posteriorly directed resistance as if pushing the pelvis diagonally back toward the posterior stance knee (resistance is sufficient to prevent movement). *Not shown:* Hand placements are then reversed to the posterior aspects of the pelvis to apply anteriorly directed resistance as if pulling the pelvis frontward toward the forwardly placed limb. **(B)** A progression is made to placing the forward foot on an inflated disc.

Outcomes

Motor control goals: Stability (static postural control).
Functional skill achieved: The patient is able to stabilize independently in the half-kneeling position.

Indications
Indications include impaired postural control with altered BOS, diminished knee flexion control, and ankle instability.

Position/Activity: Half-Kneeling, Diagonal Weight Shifting

TECHNIQUES AND VERBAL CUES TO IMPROVE DIAGONAL WEIGHT SHIFTING IN HALF-KNEELING

The patient actively weight shifts diagonally over the forward limb and then diagonally backward over the stance limb.

Dynamic Reversals, Diagonal Weight Shifts Continuous resistance is applied to concentric movement as the patient weight shifts diagonally frontward over the forward limb and

foot and then diagonally backward over the stance limb without relaxation. For the application of dynamic reversals with diagonal shifts, the patient is positioned in half-kneeling. The therapist is also half-kneeling diagonally in front of the patient (reverse mirror image position). Manual contacts change position between the *anterior* and *posterior* pelvis to apply resistance to both forward and backward diagonal movement. The goal is to achieve a smooth transition between opposing muscle groups.

Verbal Cues for Dynamic Reversals With Diagonal Weight Shifts in Half-Kneeling Shifting toward the therapist over the foot placed in front: *"Shift forward and move toward me, push, push, push."* Transitional cue: *"Now, reverse."* Shifting away from the therapist over the posterior knee: *"Shift back and move away from me, pull, pull, pull."*

Position/Activity: Half-Kneeling, Advanced Stabilization Activities

ACTIVITIES AND STRATEGIES TO IMPROVE STATIC-DYNAMIC CONTROL DURING WEIGHT SHIFTING IN HALF-KNEELING POSITION

Half-Sitting/Half-Kneeling on a Ball This activity may be used to promote static-dynamic control. To begin, the patient is sitting on a medium-sized ball with the hips and knees flexed to 90 degrees and the feet flat on the floor. The therapist is in a kneeling or half-kneeling guard position to the side and slightly behind the patient. The patient shifts weight over toward one side, partially unweighting one limb for dynamic movement. The patient moves the unweighted limb down into the kneeling position and shifts weight over onto this knee. The ball is still underneath (partially supporting) the patient as the patient assumes the half-sitting/half-kneeling position (Fig. 5.18). The movements can then be reversed to return to a centered sitting position on the ball. The

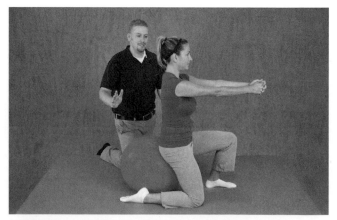

FIGURE 5.18 Half-sitting/half-kneeling position on a ball. The patient shifts weight to one side, moving down into kneeling on one knee. Shoulders are flexed with elbows extended and hands clasped together. Progression is made to alternating movements into half-kneeling on one side, then to sitting on the ball, and then to half-kneeling on the opposite side.

challenge to static-dynamic control may be increased by having the patient practice alternate movements, moving down into half-kneeling on one side, then to sitting, and then to half-kneeling on the other side. The positioning of the patient's UEs can also be used to alter the challenge imposed, beginning with hands placed on the elevated forward knee for support, then to arms folded across the chest, and finally positioned with both elbows extended, shoulders flexed to 90 degrees, and hands clasped together.

Outcomes

Motor control goals: Controlled mobility (static-dynamic control).

Functional skill achieved: Improved static-dynamic control during weight shifting in half-kneeling position.

Indications Diminished stability and controlled mobility function in half-kneeling are indications.

Position/Activity: Movement Transition to Standing
ACTIVITIES AND STRATEGIES TO IMPROVE MOVEMENT TRANSITIONS FROM HALF-KNEELING TO STANDING

Movement Transition, Half-Kneeling to Standing

For this activity, the therapist is standing in a guard position to the side and behind the patient. The patient is in a half-kneeling position with the hands supported on the elevated forward knee to assist with the rise to standing by pushing off. The patient then flexes and rotates the trunk, transferring weight diagonally forward over the foot of the forward limb (Fig. 5.19A). The patient then moves up toward the standing position by extending the hip and knee (Fig. 5.19B) and placing the other foot parallel to the weightbearing foot. The UEs can also be held with elbows extended, shoulders flexed to 90 degrees, and hands clasped together. This position assists with the forward transition of weight over the anterior limb. Initially, if physical assistance is required to assume standing, manual contacts may be placed on the upper trunk under the axillae. During initial practice, if the patient is unsteady or expresses anxiety, the activity can be first practiced with a chair or low table in front of the patient. With the hands supported on the chair or table in front, the patient then comes up into standing position using both UEs for weightbearing and push-off. Practice can then progress to unassisted movement transitions with no UE support.

Outcomes

Motor control goal: Controlled mobility (active-assistive movements progressing to active movements).

Functional skill achieved: The patient is able to independently accomplish movement transitions from floor to standing.

Indications Practicing movement transitions from half-kneeling to standing is generally a late-stage activity undertaken after the patient is walking. Functionally, this activity

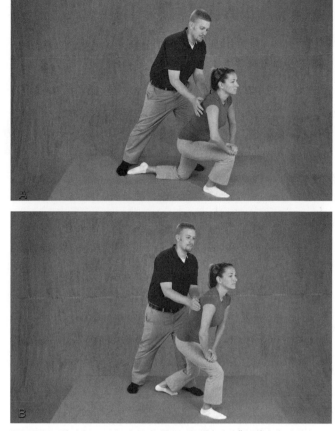

FIGURE 5.19 Movement transition, half-kneeling to standing. The therapist is standing in a guard position to the side of and behind the patient. **(A)** The patient flexes and rotates the trunk, shifting weight diagonally forward over the foot of the forward limb. **(B)** The patient then pushes off with the hands supported on the forward knee and moves up toward standing by extending the hip and knee. *Not shown:* The patient then places the feet together in upright standing.

is important to ensure that the patient who falls will be able to return to standing independently.

Clinical Note: Practice and feedback are critical to learning a new motor skill and to successful functional outcomes. The therapist's selection of practice strategies and feedback mechanisms will directly affect the achievement of optimal outcomes. Another important consideration is that integrating practice and feedback into functional interventions is highly *patient-specific.* For example, a patient with significant multisystem involvement, such as a traumatic brain injury (TBI), will require very different approaches to practice and feedback than will a patient who sustained a trimalleolar ankle fracture. The therapist must consider multiple factors when developing a feedback plan, such as the *mode* (type of feedback), *intensity* (how much should be used), and *scheduling* (when it will be given). Other important feedback elements include the patient's stage of motor learning (cognitive, associated, or autonomous) and whether feedback will be *intrinsic* (provided by the actual movement) or *extrinsic,* also called *augmented* (provided by external sources such as VCs or manual contacts). Essential elements of practice include *distribution* (intervals of practice and rest), *variability* (what tasks are included), *order* (sequencing of tasks), and *structuring of the environment* (closed versus open). For a discussion of the use of feedback and practice to enhance motor learning, refer to Chapter 2.

Student Practice Activity

Box 5.1 Student Practice Activity presents activities to promote the sharing of knowledge and skills about improving kneeling and half-kneeling control. The activity is divided into two parts. Part I addresses stability and balance control and Part II considers interventions in kneeling and half-kneeling.

BOX 5.1 STUDENT PRACTICE ACTIVITY: KNEELING AND HALF-KNEELING

OBJECTIVE: Sharing knowledge and skill in the application of treatment interventions used in kneeling and half-kneeling.

EQUIPMENT NEEDS: Platform mat, large ball, and inflatable disc.

STUDENT GROUP SIZE: Four to six students.

Part I: Postural Stability and Reactive Balance Control: Kneeling and Half-Kneeling

1. Using a platform or floor mat, each member of the group should alternate between the *kneeling* and *half-kneeling* positions; while in each position, practice holding for at least 45 seconds. Next, repeat the same activity, but this time superimpose a gentle postural sway in all directions (medial/lateral, anterior/posterior, and diagonally). During the postural sway, start with small-range movements and work toward increments of range. Be careful to maintain the trajectory of postural sway within your LOS. While transitioning between postures, focus your attention on the *postural stability demands* required of each position. When the activity is complete, convene the whole group to compare and contrast your individual perceptions of the relative stability of each posture.

Guiding Questions
▲ Which position was most stable?
▲ Within each position, which directions of postural sway did you feel were *most* and *least* stable?

2. Again alternate between the *kneeling* and *half-kneeling* positions and focus your attention on *postural stability demands*. Within each position, alter the UE positions as follows (hold each UE position for a minimum of 20 seconds): (1) resting at sides, (2) folded across chest, (3) shoulders abducted to 90 degrees with elbows extended, and (4) shoulders flexed to 90 degrees with elbows extended and hands clasped together. Alter the visual input from eyes open (EO) to eyes closed (EC). When the activity is complete, convene the whole group to compare and contrast your individual experiences with altering the UE position.

Guiding Questions
▲ What did you learn about changes in postural stability demands when altering the UE position?
▲ Within a given position, which UE positions provided the *greatest* and *least* challenges to stability?
▲ What did you learn about changes in postural stability demands when altering the visual input from EO to EC?

▲ What insights did this activity provide that can be applied clinically?

3. This activity involves the application of manual perturbations (gentle nudges) and observation of *reactive balance control*. Recall that manual perturbations initiated by the therapist involve gentle displacement of the COM from over the BOS. Reactive balance control allows for rapid and efficient responses to environmental perturbations required during standing and walking. One or more group members will assume the role of subject. One member will serve as the therapist for the application of perturbations. The subject will begin in kneeling with an inflated disc (or BOSU® dome) under the knees. The therapist will also assume a kneeling position. The therapist's manual contacts alternate between a guard position and application of displacing forces (manual contact perturbations) to the trunk. If more than one person is serving as a subject, the therapist should provide gentle anterior, posterior, and lateral perturbations to the trunk of each subject *individually* (*not* simultaneously) to allow careful observation of movement responses.

Guiding Questions
▲ What movement responses were used to return the COM over the BOS? Were the movements direction-specific?
▲ Were any UE protective extension responses noted? If they were, what does this indicate about the position of the COM with respect to the BOS?
▲ With posterior displacements, what muscle groups were activated (this question requires input from subjects)?
▲ With forward displacements, what muscle groups were activated?
▲ What compensatory responses were observed during lateral displacements?

Part II: Interventions in Kneeling and Half-Kneeling

DESCRIPTION OF STUDENT PRACTICE ACTIVITY
A chapter outline is provided below to guide the activity. The outline highlights the key treatment strategies, techniques, and activities addressed in the chapter. This activity is an opportunity to share knowledge and skills as well as to confirm or clarify understanding of the treatment interventions. Each student in a group will contribute his or her understanding of, or questions about, the strategy, technique, or activity being discussed and

BOX 5.1 STUDENT PRACTICE ACTIVITY: KNEELING AND HALF-KNEELING (continued)

demonstrated. Dialogue should continue until a consensus of understanding is reached.

Directions: Working in groups of three or four students, consider each entry in the outline below. Members of the group will assume different roles (described below) and will rotate roles each time the group progresses to a new item in the outline.

▲ One person assumes the role of therapist (for demonstrations) and participates in discussion.
▲ One person serves as the subject/patient (for demonstrations) and participates in discussion.
▲ One remaining member of the group should be designated as a "fact checker" to return to the chapter content to confirm elements of the discussion (if needed) or if agreement cannot be reached.
▲ All remaining group members participate in discussion and provide feedback after the demonstration.

Thinking aloud, brainstorming, and sharing thoughts should be continuous throughout this activity! As each item in the outline is considered, the following should ensue:

1. An initial discussion of the *activity,* including patient and therapist positioning.
2. An initial discussion of the *technique,* including its description, indication(s) for use, therapist hand placements (manual contacts), and verbal cues.
3. A *demonstration* of the activity and application of the technique by the designated therapist and subject/patient. Discussion follows the demonstration. All group members should provide recommendations, suggestions, and supportive feedback about the demonstration. Particularly important is discussion of strategies to make the activity either *more* or *less* challenging.
4. If any member of the group feels he or she requires additional practice with the activity and technique, time should be allocated to accommodate the request. All group members should provide input (recommendations, suggestions, and supportive feedback) during the practice.

Outline: Kneeling and Half-Kneeling

KNEELING
Assist-to-position and holding
▲ Kneeling, assist-to-position from heel-sitting
▲ Kneeling, holding, using stabilizing reversals

Weight shifting
▲ Kneeling, medial/lateral shifts, using dynamic reversals
▲ Kneeling, diagonal shifts (knees in *step position*), using dynamic reversals
▲ Kneeling, diagonal shifts with rotation (knees in *step position*), using dynamic reversals

Movement transitions
▲ Movement transitions between kneeling and bilateral heel-sitting positions using combination of isotonics
▲ Movement transitions between kneeling and side-sitting positions using combination of isotonics
▲ Movement transitions between kneeling and bilateral heel-sitting positions using PNF lift and reverse lift patterns and dynamic reversals
▲ Kneel-walking using resisted progression
  • Forward progression
  • Backward progression

Activities and strategies to improve balance
▲ Kneeling, manual perturbations (nudges)
▲ Kneeling on an inflated disc, active holding
▲ Sitting on ball to half-kneeling, active movements to each side

HALF-KNEELING
Assist-to-position and holding
▲ Half-kneeling, assist-to-position from kneeling
▲ Half-kneeling, holding using stabilizing reversals, anterior/posterior resistance

Weight shifting
▲ Half-kneeling, diagonal shifts using dynamic reversals

Advanced stabilization activities
▲ Sitting on ball to half-kneeling, active movements to each side

Movement transitions
▲ Half-kneeling to standing, assist-to-position
▲ Half-kneeling to standing, active movements

SUMMARY

This chapter explored strategies, activities, and techniques to enhance posture and balance control using the kneeling and half-kneeling postures. These postures provide a unique opportunity to enhance stability without the control requirements of standing. Kneeling and half-kneeling are ideal for developing critical lead-up skills required for standing and gait, including pelvic rotation, static and dynamic upright postural control, reactive and anticipatory balance control, and reciprocal trunk and limb patterns. The inherent patient safety provided by the relatively low COM and reduced degrees of freedom of these postures (compared to standing) enhances their importance as effective transitional postures between prone progressions and upright standing.

REFERENCE
1. Adler, SS, Beckers, D, and Buck, M. PNF in Practice: An Illustrated Guide, ed 3. Springer, New York, 2008.

Interventions to Improve Transfers and Wheelchair Skills

George D. Fulk, PT, PhD

The ability to transfer from a seated position to standing *(sit-to-stand transfers)* or to another surface is an essential skill that many people who receive rehabilitation services need to reacquire after an injury or illness. Being able to transition from sitting to standing or from a bed to a wheelchair allows the individual to be in a position to begin locomotion and to interact with the environment. Although there are various types of transfers, the ability to transfer from a seated surface to standing (and back again) (Fig. 6.1) is the most basic and the foundation for other types of transfers. An individual who cannot bear weight through his or her lower extremities (LEs) and stand (e.g., a person with a complete spinal cord injury [SCI]) may transfer from one surface to a wheelchair using a sit pivot technique (Fig. 6.2). This chapter examines various training strategies that can be used to enhance an individual's ability to perform these vital skills. The chapter also provides an introduction to basic wheelchair propulsion skills.

Task Analysis

Task analysis using critical observation skills serves as the foundation for examining how the patient performs the task[1]

and for developing task-oriented interventions to improve the patient's ability to transfer. Analyzing how the patient performs the movement in combination with an examination of any underlying body structure and function impairments allows the physical therapist to determine what factors may be causing the difficulties in performance. With this information, the physical therapist can then develop a plan of care (POC) designed to enhance motor learning that will result in improved performance.

Overview of Biomechanics

It is important to have a good understanding of the normal biomechanics of the sit-to/from-stand motion. The physical therapist uses this information as part of the task analysis to compare how the patient is performing the task and to identify possible impairments that may be causing the activity limitations observed. Sit-to-stand is commonly broken down into two phases: *pre-extension* and *extension*.[2] The pre-extension phase involves a forward or horizontal translation of body mass, and the extension phase involves a vertical translation of body mass. The point in time when the thighs come off the sitting surface (thigh off) is the transition between the two phases. It should be kept in mind that this

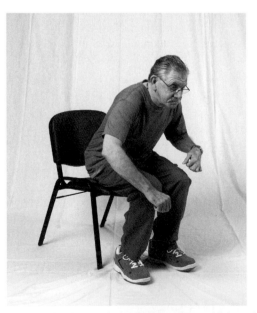

FIGURE 6.1 A patient with stroke (left hemiparesis) transfers from sitting to standing.

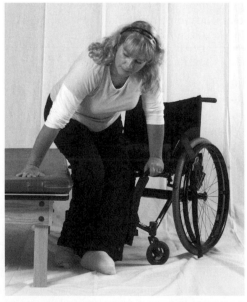

FIGURE 6.2 A patient with a T12 incomplete SCI transfers from a wheelchair to a mat.

breakdown into two distinct phases is done to organize the clinical analysis of the movement. Normally, the movement occurs in one smooth motion.

Initially, the majority of the body mass is resting on the thighs and buttocks in a stable sitting posture (Fig. 6.3A). During the pre-extension phase, the upper body (head and trunk) rotates forward at the hip joints and the lower legs rotate forward over the ankle joints (dorsiflexion) (Fig. 6.3B). Once the trunk and head rotate forward, causing the body mass to translate horizontally, the extension phase begins, with extension at the knees, closely followed by extension at

the hips and ankles.[2] The thighs come off the seat (Fig. 6.3C). During the extension phase, the greatest muscle force occurs to lift the body mass up off the sitting surface. During the rest of the extension phase (Fig. 6.3D), the hips and ankles continue to extend together with the knees to bring the body to an upright posture.

During the pre-extension phase, the iliopsoas and tibialis anterior are the primary muscles activated to propel the body mass forward. The trunk extensors and abdominal muscles contract isometrically to stabilize the trunk while it rotates forward at the hips. During the extension phase, the hip (gluteus

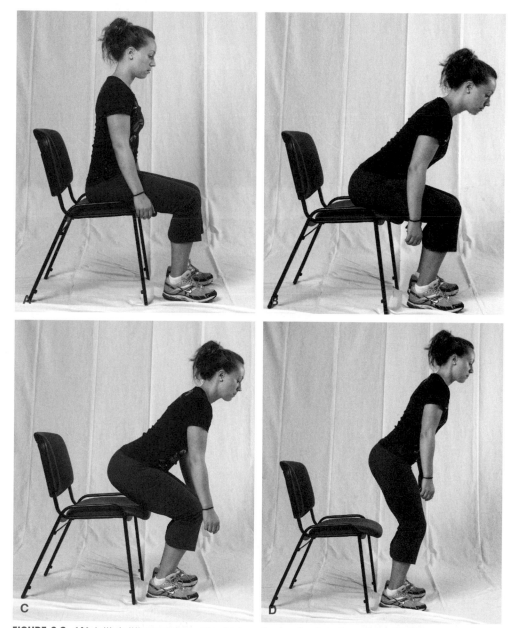

FIGURE 6.3 (A) Initial sitting posture prior to transferring to standing. Note that the upper trunk is erect and the pelvis is in a neutral position. **(B)** During the pre-extension phase, the body mass is shifted horizontally as the trunk rotates forward at the hips and the lower legs rotate forward at the ankles. Keeping the upper trunk extended and the pelvis in neutral is important for translating the body mass horizontally over the feet. **(C)** The extension phase begins as the thighs come off the seating surface. **(D)** During the extension phase, the hips and knees extend to bring the body to a standing position.

maximus), knee (rectus femoris, vastus lateralis, and vastus medialis), and ankle extensors (gastrocnemius and soleus) are activated to lift the body up to standing.

People generally utilize two basic strategies to transfer from sitting to standing: momentum-transfer strategy and zero-momentum strategy.[3] The *momentum-transfer strategy* involves generating forward momentum as the trunk and head translate in a horizontal direction (flexion at the hips) causing the center of mass (COM) to shift toward and over the feet. The trunk extensor muscles then contract eccentrically to brake the horizontal motion. This is followed by a strong concentric contraction of the extensor muscles of the LEs to lift the body vertically.

The *zero-momentum strategy* entails forward flexion of the trunk until the COM is within the base of support (BOS) of the feet. Then there is a vertical lift of the body mass into a standing position. The zero-momentum strategy is more stable than the momentum-transfer strategy but requires greater muscle force to perform. Individuals with LE weakness who utilize this strategy may also require armrests to push off of with their upper extremities (UEs). The

momentum-transfer strategy requires less force because the body is in motion as the legs begin the lift. However, there is a trade-off with stability. The person is less stable during the transition period.

The motion (angular displacement) of transitioning from standing to sitting is similar to the motions that occur during sit-to-stand, only in reverse.[4] However, the timing and type of muscle contraction are different. While transitioning from standing to sitting, the body mass is moving backward and downward. Flexion of the hips, knees, and ankles is controlled by eccentric contraction of the LE extensor muscles. Additionally, the patient cannot directly see the surface upon which he or she is about to sit.

Task Analysis of Sit to and From Stand Transfers

Movement tasks can generally be broken down into four stages: initial conditions, initiation, execution, and termination (Table 6.1).[1] Critically examining the *initial conditions* encompasses the patient's posture and the environment in

Table 6.1 Task Analysis for Sit-to-Stand Transfers

Sit-to-Stand Transfer	Initial Conditions	Initiation of Movement	Execution of Movement	Termination of Movement
Elements of Task Analysis	• Starting posture • Environment conditions	• Timing • Direction	• Direction • Speed • Smoothness • Weight shift • Vertical lift • Balance	• Timing • Stability • Accuracy
Common Difficulties Exhibited/ Encountered by Individuals With Neurological Disorders	• Initial foot placement too far forward (e.g., decreased ankle ROM) • Sitting in posterior pelvic tilt position • Increased thoracic kyphosis • Sitting too far back on the seating surface • Seat surface too low or too soft	• Delay in initiation • Multiple attempts to initiate movement • Movement initiated too quickly • Direction of movement not efficient	• Lack of strength/ power • Muscle activation not in optimal sequence (e.g., begin extending too early) • Forward weight shift not complete • Anterior weight shift by thoracic flexion instead of hip flexion • Too much weight shift onto less affected side • Speed too slow, does not build sufficient momentum to assist with extension phase • Fear of falling	• Over- or undershoot termination of movement • Unsteady on completion of movement transition

which the motor task is being performed. Common abnormalities in posture that may affect an individual's ability to transfer from sitting to standing include asymmetrical weightbearing (Fig. 6.4), sitting with a posterior pelvic tilt causing an increased thoracic kyphosis (Fig. 6.5), and incorrect placement of the feet (Fig. 6.6). The environmental context of the transfer should also be examined. This includes the seating surface (firm or cushioned), the height of the

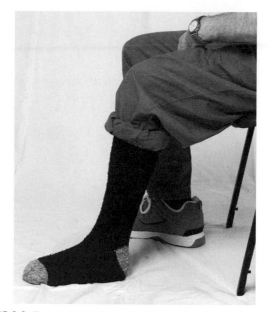

FIGURE 6.6 The patient does not place his left foot back far enough. This will make it difficult to translate the body mass horizontally during the pre-extension phase and to effectively utilize the left LE to push up during the extension phase. The inability to position the foot farther posterior could be due to a contracture of the gastrocnemius-soleus complex or to hamstring weakness.

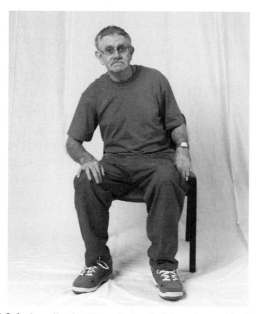

FIGURE 6.4 A patient with a stroke (left hemiparesis) sits with weightbearing primarily on his less affected (right) side.

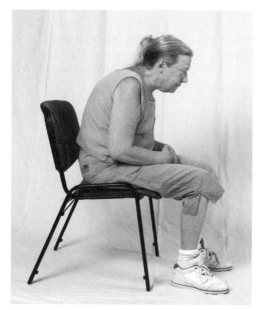

FIGURE 6.5 A patient with stroke (right hemiparesis) sits with an increased thoracic kyphosis and posterior pelvic tilt. This makes it difficult to translate the body mass horizontally during the pre-extension phase. When the patient extends to attempt to stand up, most of the body mass will be too far posterior. This will either cause the patient to lose her balance posteriorly and fall back as she attempts to stand or require increased effort and strength to come to standing.

seating surface, the floor surface (tiled or carpeted), lighting conditions, the presence or absence of armrests and backrest, and other environmental distractors such as noise.

After examining the initial conditions, the physical therapist should observe how the patient performs the movement task, including the initiation, execution, and termination of the transfer. During the ***initiation*** phase, the physical therapist should make note of the timing (e.g., Does the patient require multiple attempts to begin the movement?) and direction of the initial movement. Common issues during the initiation of the sit-to-stand transfer include delayed initiation and initiation of the movement in the wrong direction. Next, the ***execution*** of the movement is observed. The speed, direction, and coordination of movement between different body segments as well as balance and weight shifting ability are all elements that affect performance and should be critically analyzed during the execution phase. Common issues that occur during the execution of the movement that may cause difficulties or the inability to successfully transfer include weakness, inability to fully shift weight forward (Fig. 6.7), sequencing errors in the movement pattern, slowed pace, uneven weight distribution, and inability to maintain balance during the movement. Initial foot placement too far forward or decreased ROM at the ankle can also impair initial movement transfer during sit-to-stand transfers (Fig. 6.8). Finally, how the movement is terminated is observed and analyzed. Common issues that occur during the ***termination*** phase of the transfer are inability to stop the transfer at the appropriate place and time (overshooting or undershooting) and inability to maintain balance upon completion. In these cases, the patient may need to take a step (i.e., stepping

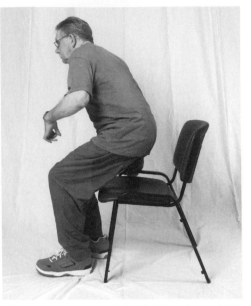

FIGURE 6.7 The patient with stroke (left hemiparesis) has not shifted his weight forward enough during the pre-extension phase. He compensates for this by using his right UE to push up from the chair.

strategy) upon reaching standing to reestablish the COM within the BOS.

Student Practice Activities: Task Analysis of Sit-to/From-Stand Transfers

Although it is not possible to exactly replicate the effects of different types of patient impairments on the sit-to/from-stand transition in healthy individuals, the activities presented in Box 6.1 Student Practice Activity may provide further insight into some of the difficulties that patients may encounter.

Sit to and From Standing: Intervention Strategies

Information gained from the task analysis and examination of body structure and function along with knowledge of the patient's goals will allow the physical therapist to design a comprehensive and effective intervention program. Intensive and task-oriented rehabilitation strategies are necessary to induce use-dependent neurological reorganization to enhance motor and functional recovery.[5,6] Incorporating strategies to enhance motor learning (see Chapter 2) in combination with intensive, task-oriented interventions provide the foundation for the POC.

Environment

During the initial stages of motor learning (cognitive stage), the physical therapist should set up the transfer practice environment to allow the patient to succeed, while minimizing compensatory movement strategies. This usually entails the use of a firm, raised surface. A high-low treatment table (Fig. 6.9) or mat is ideal for initial practice sessions. It allows the physical therapist to set the height at a point that is challenging for the patient, but not so challenging that the patient cannot successfully complete the transfer without excessive compensatory movements. Additionally, the intervention sessions should take place in a quiet, closed environment that is well lighted. Verbal cues can be used to provide *knowledge of results* and *knowledge of performance,* but they should be faded over time or summarized after a certain number of trials. Verbal cues can also be used to direct the patient's attention to the task.

During the later stages of motor learning (associative and autonomous), as the patient's ability to perform the movement improves, the environment should more realistically

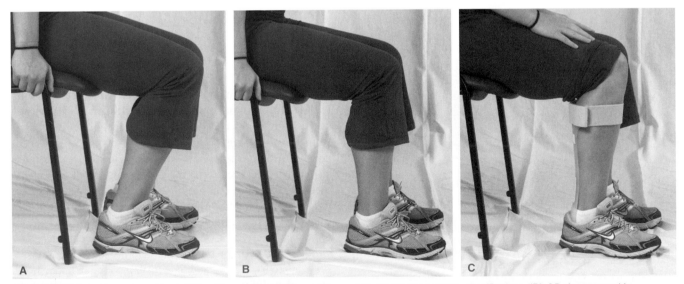

FIGURE 6.8 Sit-to/from-stand transfers with varying ankle positions: **(A)** 15-degree ankle dorsiflexion, **(B)** 15-degree ankle plantarflexion, and **(C)** with an off-the-shelf ankle foot orthotic (AFO).

BOX 6.1 STUDENT PRACTICE ACTIVITY: TASK ANALYSIS OF SIT-TO/FROM-STAND

OBJECTIVE: To analyze sit-to-stand transfers of healthy individuals.

EQUIPMENT NEEDS: Normal-height chair without armrests, a low seat surface, off-the-shelf ankle foot orthotic, and a small ball.

DIRECTIONS: Work in groups of two or three students. Members of the group will assume different roles and will rotate roles each time the group progresses to a new practice item.

▲ One person serves as the subject/patient and participates in discussion.

▲ The remaining members participate in task analysis of the activity and discussion and rotate turns as the subject/patient. One member of this group should be designated as a "fact checker" to return to the text content to confirm elements of the discussion (if needed) or if agreement cannot be reached.

Procedure/Guiding Questions

Have the subject/patient perform the following:

1. Sit-to/from-stand transfers from a normal-height chair (seat surface approximately 17.5 in. [44 cm] from the floor) without armrests three to five times
   a. What is the subject's initial sitting alignment?
   b. Which strategy was used? Timing, direction, smoothness? Postural stability and balance during and at end of movement?
2. Sit-to/from-stand transfers from a low seat surface (less than 16 in. [41 cm] from the floor) three to five times
   a. Did the strategy change compared to a normal-height chair?
   b. What was different about the movement pattern used?
   c. Did it require more or less effort?

3. Sit-to/from-stand transfers from a normal-height chair without armrests under three different starting conditions: 90 degree angle between thighs and trunk (sitting erect), trunk flexed forward 30 degrees, and trunk flexed forward 60 degrees
   a. What differences are there in the movement patterns used to transfer to standing in the three different starting positions?
   b. Which starting position required the least effort to transfer to standing?
   c. Which starting position was the most steady at the termination of the transfer?
4. Sit-to/from-stand transfers from a normal-height chair without armrests with a small ball (6 to 8 in. [15 to 20 cm] in diameter) that is partially inflated under one foot
   a. How was the movement pattern used in this transfer different from the one used without a ball under one foot?
   b. Was postural stability altered during or at the end of the transfer?
   c. Which LE provided more force during the transfer?
5. Sit-to/from-stand transfers from a normal-height chair without armrests with one foot behind the knee (in approximately 15 degrees of dorsiflexion) and the other foot in four different positions: 15 degrees of dorsiflexion (same as the other foot), neutral (ankle directly under the knee) (Fig. 6.8A), 15 degrees of plantarflexion (foot out in front of the knee) (Fig. 6.8B), and with an off-the-shelf ankle foot orthotic (AFO) (Fig. 6.8C)
   a. How was the movement pattern different among the four conditions?
   b. Which condition required the most effort?
   c. Which LE provided the most force in each of the conditions?

---

reflect conditions that are likely to be encountered in the home and community. Although the environment should be made more realistic, it should still be shaped to allow the patient to succeed and gradually be made more challenging. Specific intervention strategies can include the use of various seating surfaces (Fig. 6.10) and practice in an open environment where there are more external distractors. Verbal cues should be minimized at these later stages of learning. If difficulties are encountered, the patient should be encouraged to problem-solve in order to identify where or what the problem is.

 Clinical Note: Initially, a firm sitting surface at an appropriate height (usually higher than normal) should be used (see Fig. 6.9). Progression is to a lower (standard) seat height and then to various types of sitting surfaces (sofa, bed, toilet, stool, and so forth). The environment should be progressed from a closed to an open environment.

Posture

An erect sitting posture on the anterior portion of the seat surface, with weight evenly distributed, pelvis in a neutral position or tilted slightly anteriorly, and feet behind the knees (ankle in approximately 15 degrees of dorsiflexion) (Fig. 6.11), is the ideal starting posture. Limitations in ankle range of motion (ROM) may reduce the ability to position the foot. In such situations, stretching the gastrocnemius-soleus complex and/or performing joint mobilization to stretch the joint capsule may be indicated. Stretching can be done in both sitting and standing (Fig. 6.12). The stretch should be held for at least 30 seconds and repeated 5 to 10 times. Patients should be instructed to perform these stretches independently so they can practice multiple times a day. If the patient does not have sufficient hamstring strength to position the feet, a task-oriented strengthening program can be implemented. A towel under the foot can be used to reduce friction, or a

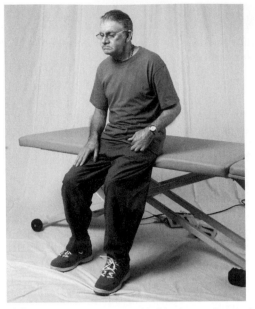

FIGURE 6.9 A high–low treatment table (or mat) may be used to vary the height of the seating surface. As the patient improves, the table can be lowered to make it more challenging.

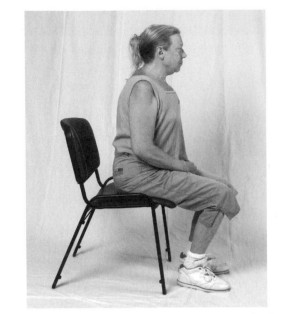

FIGURE 6.11 Positioning the ankles slightly posterior to the knee will allow the patient's weight to be translated horizontally during pre-extension.

small skateboard (Fig. 6.13) can be used as part of a task-specific strengthening program. Tape on the floor can be used to provide a target for the patient to position the foot.

Chapter 4 provides a variety of interventions designed to enhance sitting posture and balance that can be used to improve the initial sitting posture for transfers. As mentioned, the ideal sitting posture includes an erect, extended upper trunk, the pelvis in neutral alignment or slight anterior tilt, and the feet placed behind the knee (with the ankle in approximately 15 degrees of dorsiflexion).

Executing the Movement

The initial motion in transferring from sitting to standing is the forward translation of the upper body by flexing at the hips. Patients who sit with a posterior pelvic tilt (sacral sitting), have increased thoracic kyphosis, and have a fear of falling when leaning forward may try to bring their body weight forward by increasing thoracic kyphosis as they flex the hips. This brings the head forward but does not effectively translate the body mass horizontally (Fig. 6.14). From

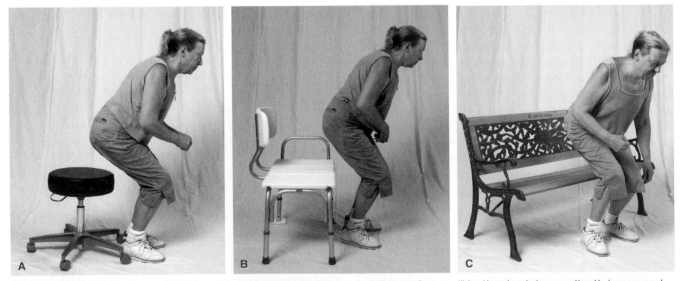

FIGURE 6.10 Practice of sit-to/from-stand transfers using a variety of seating surfaces will better simulate a patient's home and community environment.

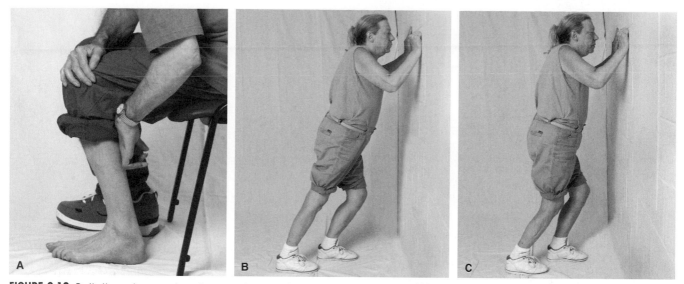

FIGURE 6.12 Both the soleus and gastrocnemius muscles should be stretched: **(A)** sitting soleus stretch; **(B)** standing gastrocnemius stretch with knee extended; **(C)** standing soleus stretch with knee flexed.

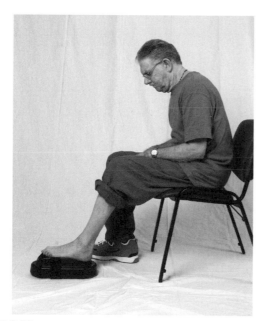

FIGURE 6.13 Using a skateboard under the foot will reduce friction between the foot and the floor, making it easier for the patient to initially practice placing the foot in the correct position. The patient could also practice this activity independently as a component of a home exercise program.

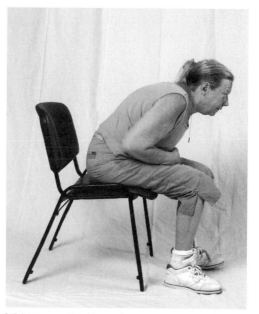

FIGURE 6.14 The patient has brought her head forward by increasing thoracic kyphosis and posterior pelvic tilt. The patient would likely lose her balance posteriorly and fall backward into the seat if she attempted to stand up from this position.

this position, it is difficult to transfer to standing because much of the body weight is too far posterior and restricts vision primarily to the floor.

An important element of practice is moving the upper body forward over the feet (i.e., hip flexion with upper trunk extension). Having the patient cross the arms in front while guided to flex forward at the hips assists in keeping the upper trunk extended and minimizes upper trunk flexion (Fig. 6.15). Alternatively, the patient's arms can be supported on a rolling tray table that can be guided

forward and backward (Fig. 6.16) or on a large therapy ball (Fig. 6.17). Care should be taken to protect the integrity of the shoulder joint when performing these interventions, particularly with patients who have experienced stroke and have a subluxed shoulder. This can be done by manually supporting the shoulder (Fig. 6.18).

The patient's feet may also need to be stabilized initially so that the lower leg rotates forward over the foot. As the patient progresses, assistance from the physical therapist is lessened and eventually removed.

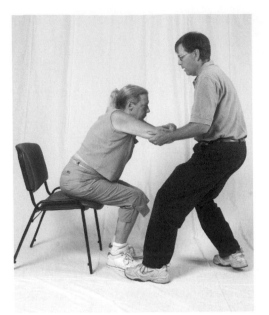

FIGURE 6.15 With the patient's UEs crossed in front, the therapist guides forward translation during pre-extension while the patient maintains upper trunk extension as the lower trunk rotates forward at the hips.

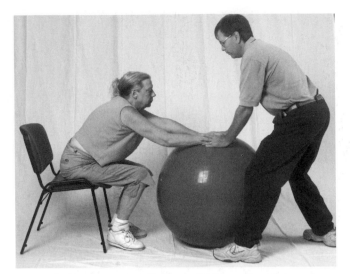

FIGURE 6.17 A therapy ball can assist the patient in learning how to effectively translate the body mass horizontally during the pre-extension phase by keeping the upper trunk extended while the trunk rotates forward at the hips.

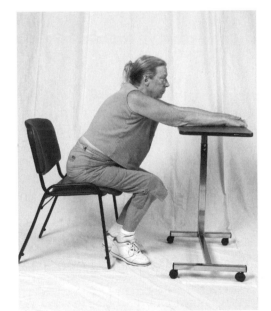

FIGURE 6.16 A tray table can assist with practicing maintaining upper trunk extension while the lower trunk rotates forward at the hips in preparation for effectively translating body mass horizontally during the pre-extension phase.

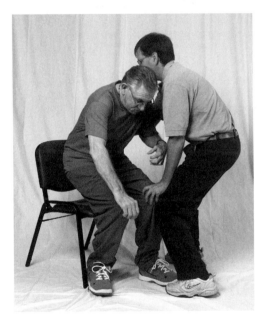

FIGURE 6.18 This patient with stroke (left hemiparesis) has a subluxed shoulder, which is manually supported by the therapist. The patient should never be assisted to standing by pulling on the shoulder joint.

Red Flag: Caution should be used when handling the shoulder to prevent trauma to the joint. All caregivers should be carefully instructed in how to effectively support the shoulder during movement transitions. The patient should never be assisted to standing by pulling (traction force) on the upper arm.

As mentioned earlier, during the initial stages of learning a higher seating surface can be used. This is particularly useful with patients who are weak. A higher surface encourages weightbearing on the more involved limb and minimizes compensatory overloading of the less involved limb. For patients who require physical assistance owing to weakness, the physical therapist can push downward and slightly posterior through the knee (Fig. 6.19). This will also help stabilize the foot. Forward translation of the trunk can be guided with the other hand placed at the pelvis or upper trunk.

Therapist positioning should not be so close to the patient that anterior rotation of the lower leg is blocked (Fig. 6.20).

A visual target on which to focus should be provided for the patient while moving to standing. The target should be in front and at eye level (when standing). Use of a target helps the patient keep the upper trunk extended when the weight is shifted forward as well as provides a sense of postural alignment and vertical orientation and discourages looking down at the feet.

Other strategies to increase loading on the more affected LE include the following:

- Placing the less affected LE slightly ahead of the more affected LE
- Placing the less affected LE on a slightly elevated surface such as a small block or step (Fig. 6.21)
- Using a force platform to provide visual feedback about the amount of weightbearing on both LEs

Comments

- A higher seating surface may be used initially for patients with weakness to promote symmetrical weightbearing.
- Manual assistance at the more affected knee will assist with extension.
- Therapist positioning should not block forward weight translation when assisting or guarding.
- A visual target can be used to promote upper trunk extension.

Repetitive Practice and Strengthening

Ample opportunity to practice a functional task is extremely important for enhancing motor learning and retention of the skill for use in the patient's environment. This is also true for transfers. Repetitive practice (11 to 14 times a day) of sit-to-stand transfers has been shown to improve the ability to transfer independently without UE assistance, improve quality of life, and increase physical mobility in people with stroke who are undergoing in-patient rehabilitation.[7] A key component of any intervention strategy designed to improve the ability to transition between sitting and standing is multiple practice repetitions.

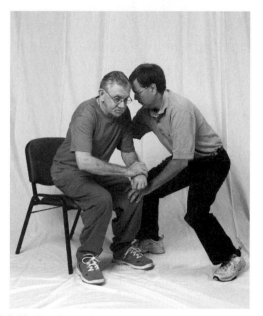

FIGURE 6.19 The therapist assists the patient by pushing down and slightly posteriorly through the knee. This will help stabilize the foot and provide assistance to extend the knee. The opposite hand is used to guide the trunk forward.

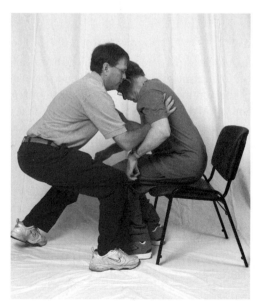

FIGURE 6.20 While providing physical assistance to stand up, the therapist should not stand so close to the patient as to block forward rotation of the trunk and lower leg. Such positioning will make it even more difficult for the patient to stand and will require more assistance from the therapist. Shown here is appropriate positioning for assisting sit-to-stand transition.

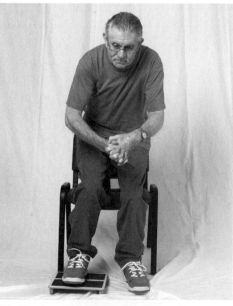

FIGURE 6.21 Placing a small raised surface (e.g., a block or step) under the less involved LE forces the patient to place more weight on the more involved LE. This helps strengthen the more involved LE and reduces reliance on the less involved LE to provide the necessary force to stand.

Strength training in people with stroke increases the strength of the more involved LE and improves self-reported function and decreased level of disability.[8] Lower extremity strength training can be achieved through task-oriented movements and progressive resistance using weights. Protocols should follow established guidelines such as those published by the American College of Sports Medicine (ACSM).[9] In general, strengthening exercises should be done two or three times a week. Patients should perform two or three sets of 8 to 12 repetitions at their 10-repetition maximum.

Red Flag: During any standing exercises, patients who may be at a risk of falling should be closely supervised and guarded. They may need to stand next to a wall, a rail, or another object to assist with balance. Light touch-down support (fingertip support) is preferred.

Task-oriented strengthening interventions in standing can include wall slides, step-ups (Fig. 6.22) and step-downs, and partial ("mini") lunges (Fig. 6.23) (see Chapter 7). Progressive resistance training can be accomplished with ankle weights, weights with pulleys, or isokinetic machines and can include leg presses (unilateral or bilateral), squats on a Total Gym®, knee extension and flexion, and standing hip extension and abduction with ankle weights.

Comments
• Repetitive practice is essential to motor learning.
• Strength training can be accomplished using task-oriented movements or progressive resistance training with weights.

Stand-to-Sit Transfers

During practice sessions, the stand-to-sit component of the transfer should also be emphasized. One way to do this

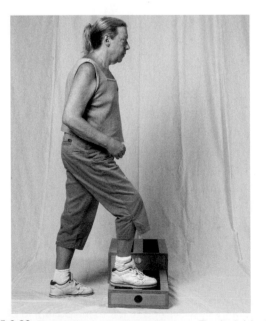

FIGURE 6.22 The patient practices step-ups. The height of the step can be increased as the patient's LE strength increases. Practice has direct functional carryover to improved stair and curb climbing.

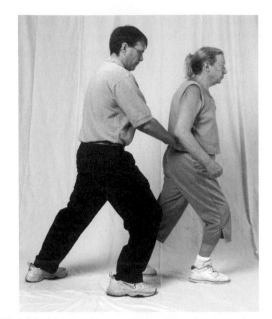

FIGURE 6.23 The patient practices partial lunges. The length of the forward step and the amount of knee and hip flexion during the lunge can be increased as the patient's strength increases. Practice has direct functional carryover to improved stair and curb climbing.

effectively is to have the patient control the descent from standing. This can be achieved by having the patient stop in mid-descent on cue and either hold the position for a short interval (1 to 3 seconds) or push back up to standing. The range and speed of descent can be varied according to the patient's ability. The patient can also be asked to sit slowly and come right back up to standing as soon as the sitting surface is felt. These intervention strategies will improve eccentric control while transitioning from standing to sitting.

Skill Practice

Once patients have mastered the basic skill of transferring and are in the associative or autonomous stage of motor learning, interventions should be designed to promote skill acquisition. A "transfer course" can be set up that requires the patient to transfer to and from many types of seating surfaces in a random order. The course can be set up such that the patient must walk a short distance to the different seating surfaces (Fig. 6.24).

To progress the complexity of the task to better reflect the patient's real-world environment, a dual- or multitask paradigm can also be introduced. In this scenario, the patient is required to hold an object while practicing transfers. Either unilateral or bilateral use of the UEs can be incorporated. For example, the patient may be asked to hold a cup (Fig. 6.25A) or hold a tray filled with objects (Fig. 6.25B) while transferring. The patient can also be asked to perform a cognitive task such as counting backward from 100 by 7s or provide the name of an animal that starts with a given letter. To make it more challenging, the patient can be asked to perform both the UE task and the cognitive task at the same time while practicing the movement pattern.

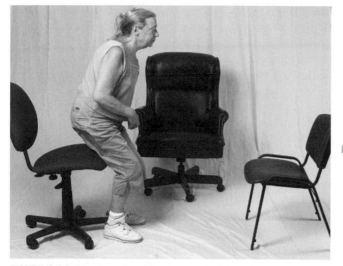

FIGURE 6.24 A "transfer course" can be set up in a circular, semicircular (shown here), or linear arrangement using a variety of seating surfaces. The transfer course should be arranged such that the patient must walk a short distance between the different seating surfaces. This activity will promote development of transfer skills necessary in the patient's home and community and enhance motor learning.

Other environmental conditions can be modified as well. The floor surface can be changed to a plush carpet or dense foam. The lighting can be changed so the patient is practicing transfers in a low or no light environment (similar to what would occur when a person gets up in the middle of the night to use the bathroom). Different noises can be introduced as distracters. As with intervention strategies utilized early on, repetitive practice is key to enhancing motor learning.

Comments
- Practice should include random transferring to and from a variety of seating surfaces.
- Other motor and cognitive tasks may be incorporated when practicing.
- Practice strategies should include modifications to the environment, including lighting and floor surface.

Transfers to and From a Wheelchair

During the initial stages of rehabilitation, particularly while in the acute care or rehabilitation hospital settings, patients often use a wheelchair for mobility purposes when they are not in therapy. Some patients, especially those with cognitive impairments or those who have never used a wheelchair before, may be unable to correctly sequence the steps needed to safely position the wheelchair for transfers. In these cases, it may be appropriate to write down the sequence of steps necessary to transfer safely and tape it to the armrest of the patient's wheelchair.

Stand Pivot Transfers

Although it may need to be adapted to the cognitive abilities and circumstances of the individual patient, the steps in a *stand pivot transfer* include the following:

- Position wheelchair.
- Manage wheel locks.
- Manage footrests.
- Scoot to edge of wheelchair.
- Move feet apart and behind knees.

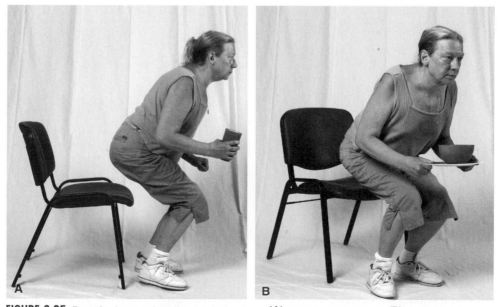

FIGURE 6.25 Transferring to standing while holding **(A)** a glass of water or **(B)** a plate with objects on it. Dual-task performance challenges the patient's control in order to prevent the contents from spilling from the glass or plate. This also serves to make the transfer more automatic as the patient's attention is on holding the glass or plate and not spilling the contents and not on the act of the transfer itself.

- Sit tall, keep back straight.
- Lean forward with nose over toes.
- Push to stand up.
- Turn 90 degrees toward other surface; feel surface on back of legs.
- Sit down slowly and safely.

A similar generic list can be developed for use with all sit-to-stand transfers, without the information about managing the wheelchair, as a way to remind the patient of the necessary steps.

Sit Pivot Transfers

Individuals who use a wheelchair as their primary method of mobility in their home and community, such as those with SCI, multiple sclerosis, or spina bifida, often must transfer into and out of their wheelchair using only their UEs *(sit pivot transfer)*. For a person with a complete SCI, the level of injury generally dictates the functional capacity for transfers. The lower the level of injury, the easier and more diverse the transfers will be. Factors other than level of preserved motor function will also influence the ability to independently perform sit pivot transfers, including body weight, spasticity, pain, ROM, and anthropometric characteristics.

Preservation of triceps function is a key element for independence with transfers. However, even individuals with a C6 level of injury can transfer to even (level) surfaces independently. Without triceps function the elbow can be locked in extension by positioning the shoulder in external rotation, the elbow and wrist in extension, and the forearm in supination. To accomplish this, the patient first tosses the shoulder into extension with the forearm supinated. Once the base of the hand is in contact with the mat, the humerus is flexed to cause the elbow to extend, since the arm is in a closed kinetic chain.

The elbow is maintained in extension by contracting the anterior deltoid, shoulder external rotators, and pectoralis major. To lift the trunk and hips from this position to transfer, the patient retracts and depresses the scapulae. The fingers should be flexed to preserve the tenodesis grip during all activities involving weightbearing on the hands with the wrists extended.

Unlike sit-to-stand transfers, there is very little research on how people with SCI (or other similar disorders) perform sit pivot transfers to and from their wheelchair. Perry and colleagues[10] identified three components to the sit pivot transfer: preparatory phase, lift phase, and descent phase. During the *preparatory phase,* the trunk flexes forward, leans laterally, and rotates toward the trailing arm (Fig. 6.26A). The *lift phase* starts when the buttocks lift off the sitting surface and continues while the trunk is lifted halfway between the two surfaces (Fig. 6.26B). The *descent phase* denotes the period when the trunk is lowered to the other seating surface, from the halfway point until the buttocks are on the other surface (Fig. 6.26C).

The preparatory phase includes shifting body weight from the buttocks onto the hands by flexing the trunk forward so that the shoulders are in front of the hands.[11] The ability to flex the trunk forward so that the shoulders are in front of the hands is a key component of the movement. The trailing hand is placed close to the upper thigh, anterior to the hip joint. The leading hand is placed farther away from the upper thigh to provide a space into which the buttocks and thighs can transfer. The upper trunk rotates toward the trailing hand, away from the target transfer surface. Initially, this may be difficult, as patients often want to see the surface they are transferring toward.

In the lift phase, the trunk and hips are lifted off the seating surface. The lower trunk is shifted toward the leading hand. The upper trunk rotates toward the trailing hand. During

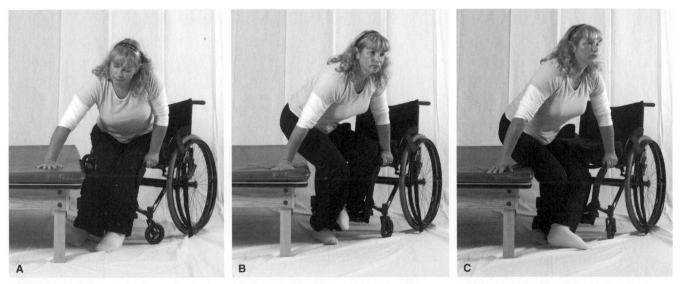

FIGURE 6.26 Sit pivot transfer from wheelchair to mat. **(A)** During the preparatory phase, the patient with incomplete SCI (T6) has the trailing hand on the wheelchair and the lead hand on the surface to which she is going to transfer. She flexes her trunk and begins to rotate her trunk toward the trailing hand. **(B)** During the lift phase, momentum from the forward trunk flexion and rotation with triceps extension and scapular depression serve to lift the trunk and pelvis off the wheelchair. **(C)** During the descent phase, eccentric muscle contraction serves to lower the body to the mat.

the descent phase, the trunk and hips continue to be lifted off the seating surface and the trunk rotates toward the trailing hand while the body is lowered onto the seating surface. Peak force generated at the trailing hand generally occurs right before the buttocks are lifted off the seating surface and while the buttocks are in the air for the lead hand.[11] Greater force is generated by the trailing than the lead UE, suggesting that the weaker UE or one that has a painful shoulder should be the lead.[10,11]

Comments

• Head and upper trunk should flex forward and rotate away from the lead hand.
• If one UE is painful or weak, it should be the lead UE.

Clinical Note: Many individuals who use a sit pivot transfer to and from their wheelchair are at risk of developing skin breakdown. During transfers, shearing forces on the skin should be avoided. Patients should be instructed to lift their body rather than sliding along the surface. Multiple small lifts and pivots are better than sliding along the surface. Early in a rehabilitation program, individuals with traumatic SCI may have orthopedic precautions that include avoiding excessive stress on healing, unstable fracture sites in the spine. These precautions need to be strictly adhered to. As described above, individuals with a C7 level injury and above should keep their fingers flexed when weightbearing on their hands with an extended wrist and elbow in order to preserve tightness in the longer finger flexors to maintain the ability to use a tenodesis grasp.

Red Flag: Shearing forces should be avoided during transfers to prevent skin breakdown. Orthopedic precautions should be carefully followed to avoid excessive force at healing, unstable spinal fracture sites.

Strategies and Activities

Very little, if any, research has been conducted that examines effective intervention strategies for developing skill in performing sit pivot transfers. The interventions presented here are based on task-oriented balance and strengthening strategies. It is important to keep in mind that multiple movement strategies should be practiced and that no one approach will work for every patient. Slight variations in hand placement, foot placement, or direction of trunk flexion/rotation may allow a patient to become independent or perform the transfer more efficiently. Patients should be encouraged to problem-solve and experiment in order to find an approach that is efficient and safe.

Long-sitting is an ideal initial position to practice beginning transfer skills. This position is more stable than short-sitting and patients feel more secure when flexing forward to initiate the transfer. However, an important precaution when using this position is to avoid overstretching low back muscles. Tightness in the low back muscles can provide lower trunk and pelvic stability in sitting. Patients should have approximately 100 degrees of passive straight leg raise ROM

before assuming long-sitting and performing these activities. Task-oriented activities that may be performed in long-sitting include:

• Push-ups with bars or blocks (weight cuffs instead of blocks can be used for individuals lacking full hand function) (Fig. 6.27)
• Push-up and scoot to the left and right
• Lower limb management: lifting and positioning LEs while in long-sitting
• Dips in parallel bars in a long-sitting position (Fig. 6.28)

Lead-Up Skills

Many lead-up skills are required in preparation for transferring into or out of a wheelchair. Table 6.2 provides information on these skills.

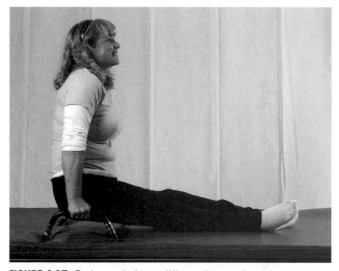

FIGURE 6.27 Push-ups in long-sitting using push-up bars (shown here) or blocks is a task-oriented method for strengthening triceps and scapular depressors necessary for transferring to and from a wheelchair.

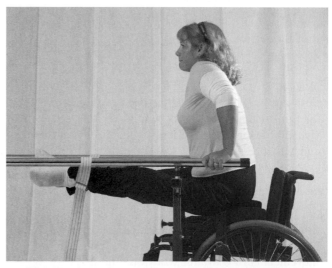

FIGURE 6.28 Dips in the parallel bars with the LEs supported by a gait belt. Initially, lowering the parallel bars closer to the wheelchair seat height makes it easier to perform the dip. As a progression, the bars can be gradually raised.

TABLE 6.2 Lead-Up Skills for Transferring to and From Wheelchair

Lead-Up Skill	Comments
Position wheelchair	Wheelchair should be positioned at a 20°–30° angle from the target transfer surface. Casters positioned backward provide more stability to the wheelchair.
Set wheel locks	Different wheel locks are available (e.g., push to lock, pull to lock, or scissor locks).
Remove and replace armrests	Armrest styles vary; some may swing away, while others may be removed completely.
Remove and replace legrests	Some individuals transfer by keeping the feet on the footplate; others remove the legrests and place their feet on the floor. To provide stability, the thighs should be parallel or angled slightly higher in relation to the surface the individual is transferring to.
Manage transfer board	Individuals with high-level SCI may require the use of a transfer board to transfer into and out of the wheelchair safely and independently.
Manage lower extremities	This includes moving LEs on and off footplates. Some patients may prefer to transfer with the LEs positioned on the surface he or she is transferring toward (i.e., in a long-sitting position).
Manage body position in wheelchair	Scooting to the edge of the seating surface and positioning the buttocks in front of the wheel are important lead-up skills.

Activities in prone and quadruped are beneficial to strengthen key muscles necessary for sit pivot transfers (see Chapter 3). Prone-on-elbows activities may be beneficial, especially for patients without active triceps, to strengthen scapular depressors required to lift the body during transfers. The prone-on-elbows position should be used with caution, as some patients with thoracic or lumbar involvement may be unable to tolerate the increased lordosis imposed by the position. Suggested activities in prone-on-elbows and quadruped include the following:

- Prone-on-elbows push-ups (Fig. 6.29)
- Prone-on-elbows scapular retraction (Fig. 6.30)
- Prone-on-elbows scapular retraction with downward rotation
- Push-ups in quadruped (the therapist may need to support the trunk, either manually or with a ball, to avoid excessive lumbar lordosis in patients with mid-thoracic level and higher SCI)

Interventions presented in Chapter 5 to improve sitting balance are useful, as well as the following additional activities in sitting:

- Sitting push-ups (with or without push-up bars or blocks): As described above, a key component of the movement is forward trunk flexion (Fig. 6.31).
- Sitting push-up and scoot to left and right: The head and trunk should flex forward and rotate away from the direction of the scoot.

Transfer Surfaces

Patients should also practice transferring to a variety of surfaces at varying heights as compared to their wheelchair height. These transfers should be specific to the patient's needs but typically include surfaces such as a sofa, toilet, bathtub, shower chair, or car. The technique used to transfer to these surfaces is the same as that described above. When

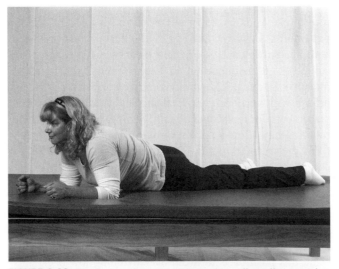

FIGURE 6.29 Prone-on-elbow push-ups strengthen the serratus anterior. As a progression, push-up height may be increased by instructing the patient to tuck the chin while lifting and rounding out the shoulders and upper thorax.

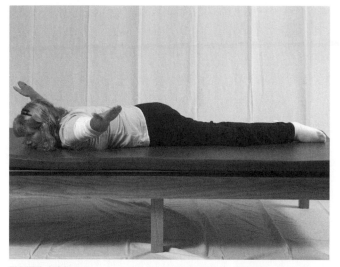

FIGURE 6.30 This prone scapular retraction exercise can be used to strengthen the middle and lower trapezius and rhomboid muscles.

there is a large difference between the heights of the wheelchair and the target transfer surface, the patient must generate more momentum and force with even greater forward flexion and rotation of the trunk and head in order to achieve enough lift to raise the buttocks up onto the higher surface (Fig. 6.32). When going to a lower surface, the patient must learn to control the descent.

Floor-to-Wheelchair Transfers: Intervention Strategies

The ability to transfer out of a wheelchair and onto the floor and back is an important skill. It allows the patient who is a

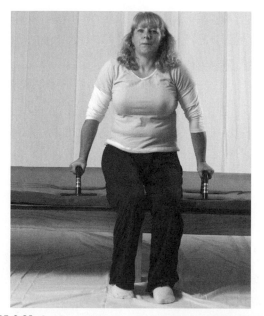

FIGURE 6.31 Seated push-ups using push-up bars are more challenging in short-sitting compared to long-sitting due to the smaller anterior BOS and lack of lengthened hamstrings providing pelvic stability.

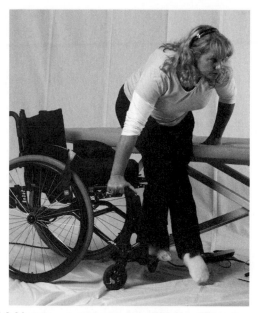

FIGURE 6.32 When transferring to a higher surface, the patient must flex forward and rotate even more than usual to generate sufficient momentum to lift the body up onto the higher surface.

wheelchair user to perform many important activities, such as getting into a pool and playing with children on the floor. Although the patient may not plan on it, it is likely that he or she may fall out of the wheelchair at some point in time. The ability to transfer back into the wheelchair is essential when this happens. There are three basic floor-to-wheelchair techniques: backward approach, forward approach, and sideways approach. If possible, the casters of the wheelchair should be positioned as if the wheelchair was moving backward to provide a longer wheelbase to the wheelchair, making it more stable.

Backward Approach
Using the *backward approach,* the individual sits slightly in front of and between the casters of the wheelchair, with hands on the edge of the seat facing away from the wheelchair (Fig. 6.33A). This hand position requires a great deal of shoulder ROM. Some individuals may not have sufficient flexibility in the shoulders to be able to use this technique. Once in this position, the patient lifts up his or her buttocks and trunk by pushing down forcefully using the UEs (Fig. 6.33B). When the buttocks are over the edge of the seat, the patient flexes the trunk forward, causing the buttocks to rise farther up and into the wheelchair (Fig. 6.33C).

Forward Approach
In the *forward approach,* the individual is initially side-sitting on one hip in front of the wheelchair. The knees are between and slightly in front of the casters; one hand is on the floor and one on the edge of the wheelchair (Fig. 6.34A). The individual lifts the buttocks off the floor by pushing down with both hands and comes up into a kneeling position facing

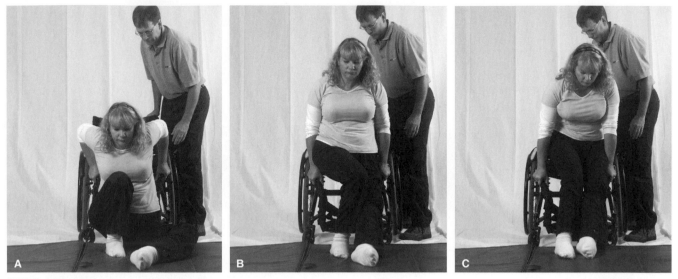

FIGURE 6.33 Floor-to-wheelchair transfer using a backward approach. **(A)** Starting position for backward approach with hands on the wheelchair and knees flexed. **(B)** The patient lifts herself off the floor using forceful extension of the elbows. **(C)** Once the buttocks clear the seat, the head and trunk are flexed slightly forward and the scapulae depressed to lift herself up and into the wheelchair.

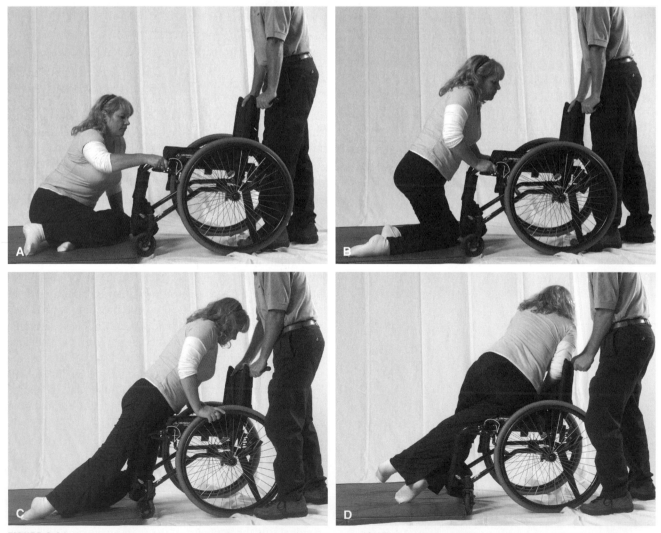

FIGURE 6.34 Floor-to-wheelchair transfer using a forward approach. **(A)** The starting position for the forward approach is side-sitting in front of wheelchair, with one hand on the floor and one on the wheelchair. **(B)** Next, the patient lifts herself into a kneeling position facing the wheelchair. **(C)** The patient lifts herself as high as possible, using the wheels or armrests on the wheelchair and then **(D)** rotates her body to turn into a sitting position in the wheelchair.

the wheelchair (Fig. 6.34B). From the kneeling position, the individual pushes down on the seat of the wheelchair with both hands to lift the body up as high as possible to raise the buttocks higher than the seat (Fig. 6.34C). If armrests are available, pushing down on them will provide greater leverage and lift the body up higher. Once the buttocks are as high as possible, the individual initiates trunk rotation while letting go with one hand and then continues to rotate the trunk and turns to land sitting in the wheelchair (Fig. 6.34D).

Sideways Approach

The *sideways approach* requires a great deal of skill and hamstring flexibility but does not require as much strength as the other two techniques. To start, the individual sits diagonally in front of the wheelchair, with one hand on the seat of the wheelchair and one on the floor (Fig. 6.35A). The individual next lifts the buttocks up onto the edge of the seat by rotating the head and upper trunk down and away from the wheelchair (toward the hand on the floor) (Fig. 6.35B). This motion must be done quickly and forcefully to lift the buttocks up onto the wheelchair. Next, the individual places the hand that is on the floor onto the leg (progressing to the thigh) and "walks" the hand up the lower limb until he or she is sitting upright in the wheelchair (Fig. 6.35C).

Strengthening to Improve Transfer Skills

Strengthening of key muscle groups using cuff weights, elastic resistive bands, free weights, pulleys, or other exercise equipment is another important component of a comprehensive POC. In general, strengthening exercises should be completed two or three times a week. Patients should perform two or three sets of 8 to 12 repetitions at their 10-repetition maximum. Key targeted muscle groups include elbow extensors, pectoralis major, deltoids, shoulder external rotators, scapular depressors, and serratus anterior.

Outcome Measures of Transfer Ability

It is important to use standardized outcome measures to document the patient's transfer ability. One of the most commonly used methods of measuring transfer ability is the transfer section of the Functional Independence Measure™ (FIM™).[12,13] The FIM™ measures the amount of physical assistance a person requires to transfer using a seven-point ordinal scale. Scores range from 1 (total assistance) to 7 (independent). Other standardized outcome measures that include examination of transfer skills include the Motor Assessment Scale,[14] the Berg Balance Scale,[15,16] the Wheelchair Skills Test,[17,18] and the Rivermead Motor Assessment.[19] All of these measures are to some degree based on the amount of assistance required and the quality of the movement. Another method of measuring transfer

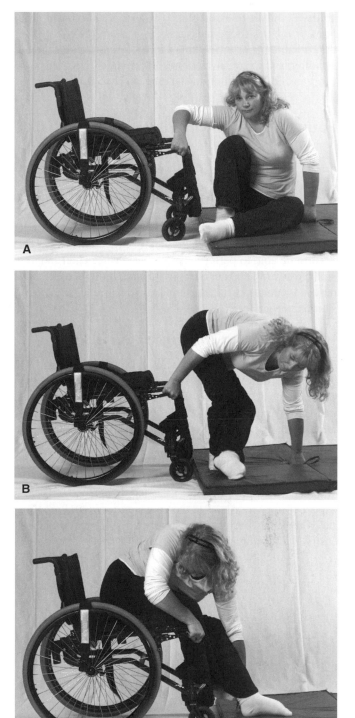

FIGURE 6.35 Floor-to-wheelchair transfer using a sideward approach. **(A)** The starting position for the sideward approach is sitting diagonally in front of the wheelchair with one hand on the floor and one on the wheelchair. **(B)** The patient lifts the buttocks up off the floor by flexing the head and trunk down toward the hand on the floor while pushing down with that hand. This motion assists in lifting the buttocks off the floor and into the wheelchair. **(C)** The hand that is on the floor is moved onto one leg (partially obscured) and "walks" the hand up the limb to bring the trunk up to a sitting position. Alternatively, the patient can use the hand on the floor together with the one on the wheelchair to quickly push up to bring the trunk to a sitting position.

ability is the sit-to-stand test.[20-23] There are two basic variations of this test: One measures the amount of time it takes the patient to transfer five times in succession from sitting to standing, and the other measures how many times the patient can transfer from sitting to standing in 30 seconds.

Foundational Manual Wheelchair Mobility Skills

For individuals who use a manual wheelchair, the ability to propel and maneuver over and around various obstacles and terrains in their home and community is essential for functional independence. To propel a manual wheelchair independently in the home and community environments, patients need to be able to perform certain basic wheelchair mobility skills: forward and backward propulsion, turning, ascend and descend inclines, assume and maintain a wheelie, and propulsion on uneven terrain.

Propulsion and Turning on Even Surfaces

To propel the wheelchair forward, the patient reaches back and grasps the wheelchair handrims (Fig. 6.36) and then pushes forward, releasing the handrim after the hands have passed in front of the hips. Patients should practice reaching as far back as possible on the handrims to initiate the stroke and pushing as far forward as possible before releasing the handrims. A longer pushing stroke is more efficient. Patients who do not have the ability to grasp the handrims propel the wheelchair by pushing with their palms against the lateral aspect of the handrims and then pushing forward. Propelling the wheelchair backward is performed in a similar manner. Instead of reaching back on the handrims to start, the patient

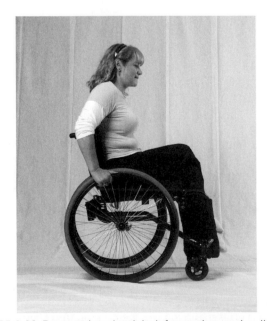

FIGURE 6.36 To propel a wheelchair forward, grasping the handrims behind the hips before beginning a push provides a longer arc through which to propel the wheels forward.

reaches forward on the handrims and pulls back. Patients who do not have the ability to grasp the handrim will place their palms on the wheel behind their hips and push backward by extending their triceps or depressing their scapulae. A wheelchair with a rigid frame is more energy efficient to propel than one with a folding frame.

The technique used to turn depends on how quickly the patient needs to turn as well as the size of the turning radius. To make a large radius or slow turn, the patient pushes harder on a single handrim using one arm (e.g., if turning to the right, the patient pushes harder with the left arm). To make a tight and/or quick turn, the patient pushes forward with one handrim while pulling back on the other (e.g., if turning to the right quickly, the patient pushes forward with the left handrim while pulling back with the right).

Propulsion on Inclines

There are a variety of surfaces with inclines that wheelchair users need to negotiate to be independent in their home and community. These include ramps, curb cutouts, slopes, and hills. The basic techniques used to ascend and descend these inclines are the same. To ascend an incline, the patient takes shorter and quicker strokes and pushes on the handrims more forcefully. If possible, the patient should lean forward with the head and trunk while pushing forward to prevent the chair from tipping backward. Patients with stronger UEs will be able to ascend inclines more easily and negotiate steeper inclines. However, even an individual with a C6 level SCI can ascend inclines with a modest grade.

When descending an incline, patients need to control the speed of descent. This is done by gripping the handrim and slowly releasing the grip in a controlled manner to slow the descent of the wheelchair. Patients without finger flexion function control the descent of the wheelchair by applying pressure to the handrims with the palms of the hands, slowly releasing the pressure to control the descent of the wheelchair. Cycling gloves are often used to protect the hands.

Wheelies

Although wheelchair accessibility has improved over recent years with the availability of curb cutouts and ramps, there are still many areas of the community that are not easily accessible with a wheelchair. The ability to perform a wheelie (Fig. 6.37) is an essential skill in order to negotiate curbs, steep declines, and uneven terrain. To attain a wheelie, the patient reaches back on the handrim and forcefully pushes forward to lift the front casters off the ground (as if attempting to tip the wheelchair over backward). When first learning any skill that involves a wheelie, there is a risk of the wheelchair tipping over. The patient should always be closely supervised and guarded. To ensure safety while practicing wheelies, a gait belt is looped through the frame of the wheelchair (Fig. 6.38). The therapist is positioned behind the wheelchair, holding the gait belt in one hand with the other hand placed on the patient's shoulder or the push handle of the wheelchair (Fig. 6.39). If the wheelchair starts to tip too far backward, the therapist pulls up on the gait belt, preventing the wheelchair from tipping backward. Alternatively, the therapist can use the push handles of the wheelchair alone. In either case, the therapist should refrain from pushing or pulling on the wheelchair unless required to prevent the chair from tipping over.

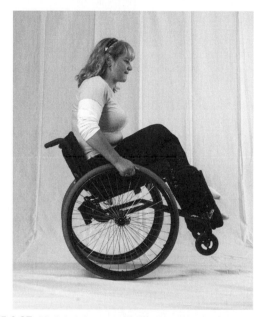

FIGURE 6.37 Maintaining a wheelie involves balancing with the front casters off the ground. Note the position of the patient's hands on the handrims near the hips. This position allows for greater control of the wheelie than with the hands either farther forward or backward on the handrims.

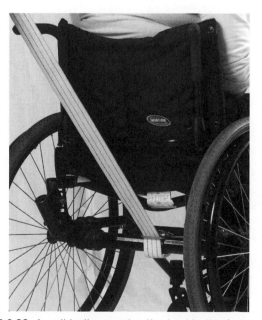

FIGURE 6.38 A gait belt securely attached to the frame of the wheelchair can be used to spot (guard) patients as they practice wheelies and other wheelchair skills.

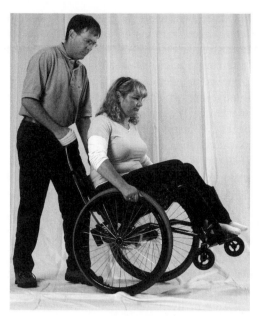

FIGURE 6.39 The therapist demonstrates how to safely spot a patient performing wheelies. Using a gait belt securely attached to the frame of the wheelchair, the therapist can pull up on the gait belt to prevent the patient from tipping over backward. The hand on the push handle of the wheelchair can be used to assist the patient in maintaining the wheelie.

The type of wheelchair and its configuration have an impact on how easy or difficult it is to perform a wheelie. Achieving a wheelie in a heavier wheelchair is more difficult. The position of the axle plate also affects the ease of attaining a wheelie. An axle that is more forward, so that the user's COM is behind the axle, causes the wheelchair to be less stable and more likely to tip backward. This makes it easier to perform a wheelie. A wheelchair is more stable with the axle plate positioned farther backward, but this configuration makes it more difficult to attain a wheelie.

The ability to maintain a wheelie should be learned in conjunction with attaining a wheelie. Both of these skills are important lead-up activities to more advanced wheelie skills, such as ascending and descending curbs and propulsion on uneven terrain. The therapist should assist the patient into the *balance point,* in which the front casters are off the ground with the wheelchair in equilibrium (i.e., the wheelchair is not going to tip over backward or forward [onto the casters]). To guide the patient in learning the location of this position, the therapist should gently tip the wheelchair forward and backward. This allows the patient to "feel" where his or her balance point is located. Next, the patient should learn how to tip the wheelchair forward and backward. The patient's hands should lightly grip the handrim in a position near the hips. To tip the wheelchair backward, the patient should push forward on the handrims; to tip the wheelchair forward onto the casters, the patient should pull the handrims backward. When doing this, and when practicing other wheelie skills, the patient should allow the handrim to slide backward or forward while gripping. The patient should not keep the hands tightly gripped on the handrim.

Now the patient requires practice maintaining the balance point by slightly pushing or pulling on the handrims. The patient can also assist by moving the head/upper trunk forward and back to maintain the wheelchair in equilibrium. Throughout this process, the therapist needs to closely supervise and guard the patient to provide a safe learning environment. Initially, patients may be fearful of falling and reluctant to practice wheelies. The therapist needs to reassure the patient that he or she will not allow the patient to fall.

When propelling a wheelchair on uneven surfaces (e.g., gravel or grass), there is a possibility of tipping the wheelchair over in a forward direction. On these types of surfaces, the casters can become "stuck" in a divot or stopped by a small object (e.g., a rock), causing the wheelchair to tip forward. Being able to propel the wheelchair forward while maintaining a wheelie can minimize this risk and allow the patient to propel the wheelchair independently over a variety of terrains.

To propel the wheelchair forward while maintaining the wheelchair in its balance point, the patient practices leaning forward while in a wheelie (this causes the wheelchair to tip forward) and then pushes the handrims forward to bring the wheelchair back to the balance point. When learning this maneuver, the patient should be instructed not to use a firm grip but to allow the handrims to "slide" within his or her grip ("sliding grip"). As the patient becomes more skilled, he or she can glide farther forward with each push of the handrims. Using similar techniques, the patient can learn to propel the wheelchair backward (the same technique but in reverse) and turn while maintaining a wheelie (similar to making a tight turn on all four wheels, by pulling backward on one handrim and pushing forward on the other).

On some uneven surfaces it may be easier to "pop" a wheelie for only a brief time (not maintain the wheelie) and push forward. The patient then crosses the surface in a series of short wheelies while pushing forward (Fig. 6.40). *Note:* The terms "pop" and "popped" are commonly used in reference to wheelies. They refer to generating a wheelie position (e.g., the patient *popped* a wheelie).

Ascending and Descending Curbs Using Wheelies

Performing wheelies is the easiest and most efficient method of ascending and descending a curb. When initially learning to ascend or descend curbs, the patient should practice on small curbs (2 in. [5 cm] high) and progress to larger curbs (6 in. [15 cm] high). There are two basic methods of ascending a curb: (1) powering up the curb from a stop and (2) popping up the curb on the go (while moving). The first method does not require as much skill with wheelies, but it requires much more strength. Some patients do not have the strength to perform this technique. To start this skill, the patient propels the wheelchair up to the front edge of the curb, pops a wheelie, and pushes slightly forward while in the wheelie so that the front casters rest on the top of the curb with the wheels on the surface below the curb (Fig. 6.41). Once in this position, the patient reaches far back on the handrims

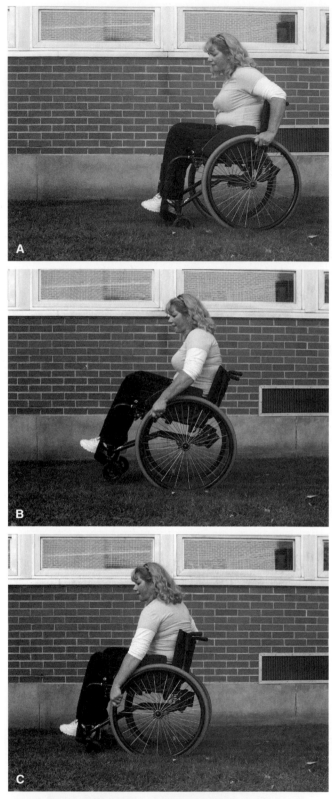

FIGURE 6.40 While propelling the wheelchair over uneven ground (A), the patient performs a continuous series of wheelies to prevent the front casters from catching and causing the wheelchair to tip over forward (B, C).

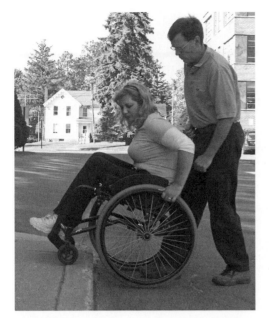

FIGURE 6.41 Ascending curbs: powering up the curb from a stopped position. The ability to ascend a curb from a stopped position without forward momentum requires a great deal of upper body strength. The casters are positioned on the curb (front edge), leaving some space between the wheels and the curb before forcefully pushing up and over the curb.

and pushes as hard as possible forward while throwing the head and trunk forward at the same time. The momentum from the push lifts the back wheels up onto the curb.

To ascend a curb on the go, the patient pops a wheelie while moving forward just before reaching the curb. This lifts the front casters so they are up on top of the curb. As the wheels make contact with the curb, the patient pushes forward on the handrims and leans the head and trunk forward. The forward momentum of the wheelchair (it is moving forward throughout this skill) lifts the back wheels up onto the curb (Fig. 6.42). Because the wheelchair is moving forward continuously, this technique does not require as much strength as the other method. However, more skill with popping a wheelie is required. The patient must be able to pop a wheelie while moving forward and must accurately time the wheelie. If the wheelie is popped too soon, the front casters will fall back down and won't clear the curb; if the wheelie is popped too late, the front end of the wheelchair will hit the curb. In both instances, the wheelchair is in danger of tipping over forward.

The backward and forward approaches are the two basic methods of descending a curb. Using the backward approach, the patient backs up to the edge of the curb so that the back wheels are on the edge of the curb. The patient then leans forward and places his or her hands far back on the handrims and controls the descent of the wheelchair as the back wheels roll off the curb. When the back wheels are off the curb, the patient pops a wheelie and turns 90 degrees to the right or left to prevent the footplate(s) from hitting the top of the curb (Fig. 6.43).

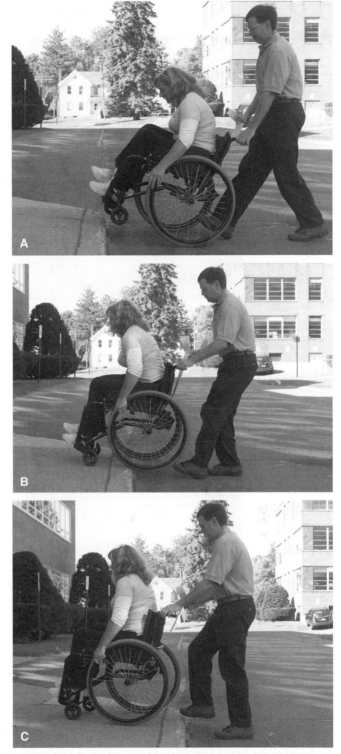

FIGURE 6.42 Ascending curbs: popping up the curb on the go (while moving). **(A)** The patient must carefully time popping the wheelie when ascending curbs with forward momentum. If the wheelie is popped too soon, it will be difficult to maintain the wheelie and the casters will drop down and hit the curb. If the wheelie is popped too late, the casters won't clear the curb. **(B)** The patient needs to give only a slight push forward after the casters clear the curb. **(C)** Momentum carries the back wheels up and over the curb.

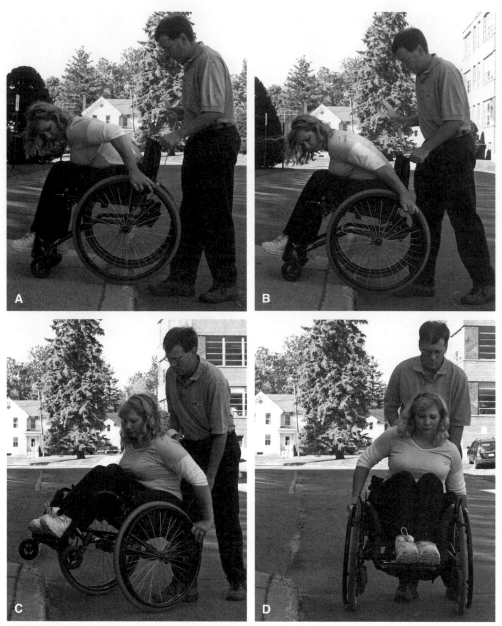

FIGURE 6.43 Backward approach to descending a curb. **(A)** The patient gradually approaches the edge of the curb and leans forward. **(B)** The back wheels are lowered slowly over the edge of the curb. Once the back wheels are safely on the ground, the patient **(C)** pops a wheelie and **(D)** rotates 90 degrees to prevent the footplate from getting stuck on or hitting the edge of the curb.

To descend a curb using the forward approach, the patient pushes the wheelchair forward and, just as the casters approach the edge of the curb, the patient pops a wheelie. The wheelie is maintained as momentum carries the back wheels off the curb. The patient maintains the wheelie so that the back wheels land first and then the casters land (Fig. 6.44). If the casters land first, the wheelchair will most likely tip over forward. This technique is analogous to an airplane landing, with the back wheels underneath the wings touching the ground before the front wheels underneath the cockpit.

As illustrated in the figures and mentioned earlier, the therapist should closely guard the patient until he or she becomes independent with these wheelchair skills.

There are a variety of other more advanced wheelchair skills that patients should learn, such as falling from a wheelchair and picking up objects off the floor. Two excellent resources for these and other more advanced wheelchair skills are a website developed by researchers at Dalhousie University called the Wheelchair Skills Program (http://www.wheelchairskillsprogram.ca) and a textbook by Martha

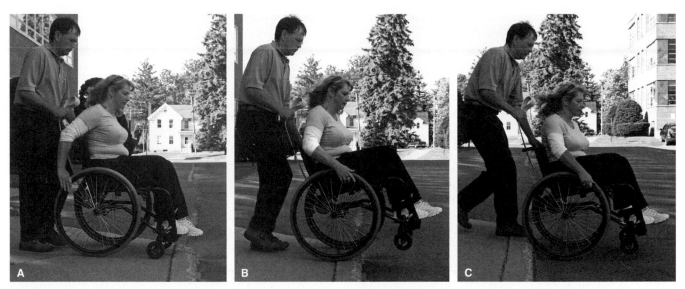

FIGURE 6.44 Forward approach to descending a curb. **(A)** The patient approaches the curb while moving forward. **(B)** A wheelie is popped as the front casters approach the edge of the curb. **(C)** The wheelie is maintained until the back wheels contact the ground. This prevents the wheelchair from tipping over forward.

Somers.[24] The Wheelchair Skills Program website includes short video clips of skills and includes the Wheelchair Skills Test,[17] which is an outcome measure designed to test a variety of basic wheelchair skills.

Student Practice Activities

Sound clinical decision-making will help identify the most appropriate activities and techniques to improve transfer skills for an individual patient. These activities provide the foundation for home and community independence. Student practice activities provide an opportunity to share knowledge and skills as well as to confirm or clarify understanding of the treatment interventions. Each student in a group contributes his or her understanding of, or questions about, the strategy, technique, or activity, and participates in the activity being discussed. Dialogue should continue until a consensus of understanding is reached. Box 6.1 Student Practice Activity, presented earlier in the chapter, focuses on task analysis of sit-to/from-stand transfers. Box 6.2 Student Practice Activity presents activities that focus on techniques and strategies to improve transfers to and from a wheelchair and wheelchair mobility skills.

BOX 6.2 STUDENT PRACTICE ACTIVITY: TECHNIQUES AND STRATEGIES TO IMPROVE TRANSFERS TO AND FROM A WHEELCHAIR AND WHEELCHAIR MOBILITY SKILLS

OBJECTIVE: To provide practice oportunities for developing skill in interventions designed to improve transfer and wheelchair skills.

EQUIPMENT NEEDS: Platform mat, adjustable treatment table, wheelchair, floor mat.

DIRECTIONS: Work in groups of three or four students. Practice and demonstrate the activities presented in the outline below ("Outline of Activities and Techniques for Demonstration and Practice"). Members of the group will assume different roles (described below) and will rotate roles each time the group progresses to a new item on the outline.

▲ One person assumes the role of therapist (for demonstrations) and participates in discussion.
▲ One person serves as the subject/patient (for demonstrations) and participates in discussion.

▲ The remaining members participate in task analysis of the activity and discussion. Following the demonstration, members provide supportive and corrective feedback. One member of this group should be designated as a "fact checker" to return to the text content to confirm elements of the discussion (if needed) or if agreement cannot be reached.

Thinking aloud, brainstorming, and sharing thoughts should be continuous throughout this activity! As each item in the section outline is considered, the following should ensue:

1. An initial discussion of the *activity,* including its description, indications for use, verbal cues, and patient and therapist positioning. Also considered here should be approaches to enhance the skill such as

(box continues on page 162)

BOX 6.2 STUDENT PRACTICE ACTIVITY: TECHNIQUES AND STRATEGIES TO IMPROVE TRANSFERS TO AND FROM A WHEELCHAIR AND WHEELCHAIR MOBILITY SKILLS (continued)

hand placement, use of body weight and momentum, and type of seating surface.

2. A ***demonstration*** of the activity and application of the technique by the designated therapist and subject/patient. All group members should provide supportive and corrective feedback, highlighting what was correct and providing recommendations and suggestions for improvement. Particularly important is a discussion of strategies to make the activity either *more* or *less* challenging for the patient.

3. If any member of the group feels he or she requires additional practice with the transfer or wheelchair skill, time should be allocated to accommodate the request.

Outline of Activities and Techniques for Demonstration and Practice

▲ Stand pivot transfers
▲ Sit pivot transfers: even surfaces
  • With transfer board (with and without triceps)
  • Without transfer board
▲ Sit pivot transfers: uneven surfaces
▲ Wheelchair-to/from-floor transfers
▲ Wheelchair mobility skills
  • Propulsion on even and uneven surfaces
  • Propulsion on inclines
  • Wheelies: attain and maintain wheelies
  • Ascending and descending curbs using wheelies

SUMMARY

This chapter has presented the skills necessary for developing and implementing a POC designed to improve transfer and basic wheelchair mobility skills. Task analysis serves as the foundation for analyzing functional movement patterns. The results of the task analysis are used to develop task-oriented interventions. The environment and task should be shaped to challenge the patient, enhance motor learning, and promote neuroplastic changes. Repetition is also an important component of the POC.

REFERENCES

1. Hedman, LD, Rogers, MW, and Hanke, TA. Neurologic professional education: Linking the foundation science of motor control with physical therapy interventions for movement dysfunction. Neurol Rep 20(1):9–13, 1996.
2. Shepherd, RB, and Gentile, AM. Sit-to-stand: Functional relationship between upper body and lower limb segments. Hum Movement Sci 13(6):817–840, 1994.
3. Schenkman, M, Berger, RA, Riley, PO, et al. Whole-body movements during rising to standing from sitting. Phys Ther 70(10):638–648; discussion 648–651, 1990.
4. Kralj, A, Jaeger, RJ, and Munih, M. Analysis of standing up and sitting down in humans: Definitions and normative data presentation. J Biomech 23(11):1123–1138, 1990.
5. Harvey, RL. Motor recovery after stroke: New directions in scientific inquiry. Phys Med Rehabil Clin N Am 14(1 Suppl):S1–S5, 2003.
6. Nudo, RJ. Functional and structural plasticity in motor cortex: Implications for stroke recovery. Phys Med Rehabil Clin N Am 14(1 Suppl):S57–S76, 2003.
7. Barreca, S, Sigouin, CS, Lambert, C, et al. Effects of extra training on the ability of stroke survivors to perform an independent sit-to-stand: A randomized controlled trial. J Geriatr Phys Ther 27(2):59–64, 2004.
8. Ouellette, MM, LeBrasseur, NK, Bean, JF, et al. High-intensity resistance training improves muscle strength, self-reported function, and disability in long-term stroke survivors. Stroke 35(6):1404–1409, 2004.
9. American College of Sports Medicine. ACSM's Exercise Management for Persons with Chronic Diseases and Disabilities, ed 2. Champaign, IL, Human Kinetics, 2003.
10. Perry, J, Gronley, JK, Newsam, CJ, et al. Electromyographic analysis of the shoulder muscles during depression transfers in subjects with low-level paraplegia. Arch Phys Med Rehabil 77(4):350–355, 1996.
11. Forslund, EB, Granstrom, A, Levi, R, et al. Transfer from table to wheelchair in men and women with spinal cord injury: Coordination of body movement and arm forces. Spinal Cord 45(1):41–48, 2007.
12. Stineman, MG, Shea, JA, Jette, A, et al. The Functional Independence Measure: Tests of scaling assumptions, structure, and reliability across 20 diverse impairment categories. Arch Phys Med Rehabil 77(11):1101–1108, 1996.
13. Ottenbacher, KJ, Hsu, Y, Granger, CV, et al. The reliability of the functional independence measure: A quantitative review. Arch Phys Med Rehabil 77(12):1226–1232, 1996.
14. Carr, JH, Shepherd, RB, Nordholm, L, et al. Investigation of a new motor assessment scale for stroke patients. Phys Ther 65(2):175–180, 1985.
15. Berg, KO, Wood-Dauphinee, SL, Williams, JI, et al. Measuring balance in the elderly: Validation of an instrument. Can J Public Health 83(Suppl 2):S7–S11, 1992.
16. Berg, K, Wood-Dauphinee, S, and Williams, JI. The Balance Scale: Reliability assessment with elderly residents and patients with an acute stroke. Scand J Rehabil Med 27(1):27–36, 1995.
17. Kirby, RL, Swuste, J, Dupuis, DJ, et al. The Wheelchair Skills Test: A pilot study of a new outcome measure. Arch Phys Med Rehabil 83(1):10–18, 2002.
18. Kirby, RL, Dupuis, DJ, Macphee, AH, et al. The Wheelchair Skills Test (version 2.4): Measurement properties. Arch Phys Med Rehabil 85(5):794–804, 2004.
19. Lincoln, N, and Leadbitter, D. Assessment of motor function in stroke patients. Physiother 65(2):48–51, 1979.
20. Bohannon, RW, Shove, ME, Barreca, SR, et al. Five-repetition sit-to-stand test performance by community-dwelling adults: A preliminary investigation of times, determinants, and relationship with self-reported physical performance. Isokinet Exerc Sci 15(2):77–81, 2007.
21. Bohannon, RW. Reference values for the five-repetition sit-to-stand test: A descriptive meta-analysis of data from elders. Percept Motor Skills 103(1):215–222, 2006.
22. Eriksrud, O, and Bohannon, RW. Relationship of knee extension force to independence in sit-to-stand performance in patients receiving acute rehabilitation. Phys Ther 83(6):544–551, 2003.
23. Bohannon, RW. Sit-to-stand test for measuring performance of lower extremity muscles. Percept Motor Skills 80(1):163–166, 1995.
24. Somers, M. Spinal Cord Injury: Functional Rehabilitation, ed 3. Prentice-Hall, Upper Saddle River, NJ, 2001.

CHAPTER 7

Interventions to Improve Standing Control and Standing Balance Skills

Susan B. O'Sullivan, PT, EdD

This chapter focuses on standing control and interventions that can be used to improve standing and standing balance skills. Careful examination of the patient's overall status in terms of impairments and activity limitations that affect standing control is necessary. This includes examination of musculoskeletal alignment, range of motion (ROM), and muscle performance (strength, power, endurance). Examination of motor function (motor control and motor learning) focuses on determining the patient's weightbearing status, postural control, and intactness of neuromuscular synergies required for static and dynamic control. Examination of sensory function includes utilization of sensory (somatosensory, visual, and vestibular) cues for standing balance control and central nervous system (CNS) sensory integration mechanisms. Finally, the patient must be able to safely perform functional movements (activities of daily living [ADL]) in standing and in varying environments (clinic, home, work [job/school/play], and community).

Standing

General Characteristics

It is important to understand the foundational requirements of standing. Standing is a relatively stable posture with a high center of mass (COM) and a small base of support (BOS) that includes contact of the feet with the support surface. During normal symmetrical standing, weight is equally distributed over both feet (Fig. 7.1). From a lateral view, the line of gravity (LoG) falls close to most joint axes: slightly anterior to the ankle and knee joints, slightly posterior to the hip joint, and posterior to the cervical and lumbar vertebrae and anterior to the thoracic vertebrae and atlanto-occipital joint (Fig. 7.2). Natural spinal curves (i.e., normal lumbar and cervical lordosis and normal thoracic kyphosis) are present but flattened in upright stance depending on the level of postural tone. The pelvis is in neutral position, with no anterior or posterior tilt. Normal alignment minimizes the need for muscle activity during erect stance.

Postural stability in standing is maintained by muscle activity that includes: (1) postural tone in the antigravity muscles throughout the trunk and lower extremities (LEs), and (2) contraction of antigravity muscles. The gluteus maximus and hamstrings contract to maintain pelvic alignment; the abdominals contract to flatten the lumbar curve; the

paravertebral muscles contract to extend the spine; the quadriceps muscles contract to maintain knee extension; and the hip abductors contract to maintain pelvic alignment during midstance and during lateral displacements.

Limits of stability (LOS) is the amount of maximum excursion possible in any one direction without losing balance. It is determined by the distance between the feet and the length of the feet as well as the height and weight of the individual. The normal anterior/posterior LOS is approximately 12 degrees; the normal medial/lateral LOS is approximately 16 degrees. Together they make up the *sway envelope,* the path of the body's movement during normal standing. In an intact person, sway cycles intermittently, with the midpoint of sway being *centered alignment.*

Stability (static postural control) is required for maintaining the standing position. *Controlled mobility* (dynamic postural control) is necessary for control of movements within the posture (e.g., weight shifting or upper extremity [UE] reaching or lower extremity [LE] stepping movements).

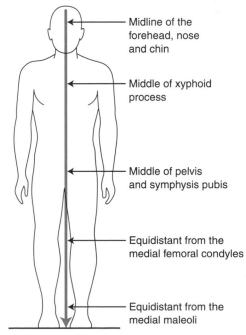

Midline of the forehead, nose and chin

Middle of xyphoid process

Middle of pelvis and symphysis pubis

Equidistant from the medial femoral condyles

Equidistant from the medial maleoli

FIGURE 7.1 Normal postural alignment—frontal plane. In optimal alignment, the LoG passes through the identified anatomical structures, dividing the body into two symmetrical parts.

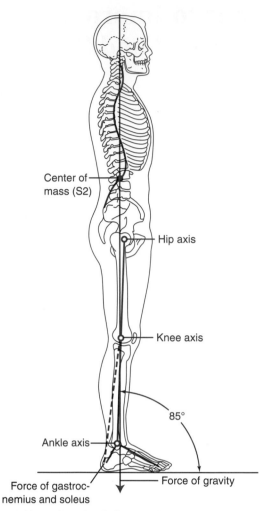

Center of mass (S2)

Hip axis

Knee axis

85°

Ankle axis

Force of gastroc-
nemius and soleus

Force of gravity

FIGURE 7.2 Normal postural alignment—saggital plane. In optimal alignment, the LoG passes through the identified anatomical structures.

Anticipatory postural control refers to adjustments that occur in advance of the execution of voluntary movements. The postural system is pretuned to stabilize the body; for example, an individual readies his or her posture before lifting a heavy weight or catching a weighted ball. *Reactive balance control* refers to adjustments that are not planned in advance but rather occur in response to unexpected changes in the COM (e.g., perturbations) or changes in the support surface. *Postural fixation reactions* stabilize the body against a thrust force (e.g., a perturbation or nudge). *Tilting reactions* reposition the COM within the BOS in response to changes in the support surface (e.g., standing on an equilibrium board). *Adaptive balance control* refers to the ability to adapt or modify postural responses relative to changing task and environmental demands. Prior experience influences the adaptability of an individual.

Sensory Components

Vertical postural orientation is maintained by multiple and overlapping sensory inputs; the CNS organizes and integrates sensory information and generates responses for controlling body position.

The *vestibular system* responds to gravity acting on the head. It stabilizes gaze during movements of the head using the vestibulo-ocular reflex (VOR). It provides input to labyrinthine righting reactions (LRR) of the head, trunk, and limbs and contributes to upright head position and normal alignment of the head and body. It helps to regulate postural tone through the action of vestibulospinal pathways.

The *somatosensory (tactile and proprioceptive) system* responds to support-surface inputs about the relative orientation of body position and movement. The somatosensory systems influence postural responses through the stretch reflexes, postural tone, and automatic postural reactions.

The *visual system* responds to visual cues about the environment and the relationship of the body to objects in the environment. It provides input for optical righting reactions of the head, trunk, and limbs and contributes to upright head position and normal alignment of the head and body. It assists in regulating postural tone and guides safe movement trajectories.

Normal Postural Synergies

Normal postural strategies for maintaining upright stability and balance include:

• *Ankle strategy* involves small shifts of the COM by rotating the body about the ankle joints; there is minimal movement of the hip and knee joints. Movements are well within the LOS (Fig. 7.3A).
• *Hip strategy* involves larger shifts of the COM by flexing or extending at the hips. Movements approach the LOS (Fig. 7.3B).
• *Change of support strategies* are activated when the COM exceeds the BOS and strategies must be initiated that reestablish the COM within the LOS. These include the *stepping strategy,* which involves realignment of the BOS under the COM achieved by stepping in the direction of the instability (Fig. 7.3C). They also include UE *grasp strategies,* which involve attempts to stabilize movement of the upper trunk, keeping the COM over the BOS.

Common Impairments in Standing

Although not all-inclusive, impairments in standing can be broadly grouped into those involving alignment, weight-bearing, and specific muscle weakness. Changes in normal alignment result in corresponding changes in other body segments; malalignment or poor posture results in increased muscle activity, energy expenditure, and postural stress. Box 7.1 presents common impairments in standing posture and weightbearing.

Clinical Note: The patient with bilateral LE paralysis (e.g., paraplegia) can obtain foot/ankle and knee stability through bilateral knee-ankle-foot orthoses (KAFOs); the hips can be stabilized by leaning forward on the iliofemoral (Y) ligament.

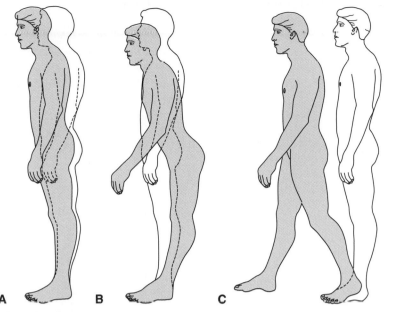

FIGURE 7.3 Normal postural strategies. Three automatic postural strategies used by adults to maintain balance (COM over BOS) are the (A) ankle strategy, (B) hip strategy, and (C) stepping strategy.

BOX 7.1 Common Impairments in Standing Postural Alignment and Weightbearing

- Asymmetrical standing with weight borne primarily on one LE with little weight on the other LE results in increased ligament and bone stress on the weight-bearing side; the knee is usually fully extended on the stance limb (e.g., the patient with stroke who stands with weight borne more on the less affected side).
- Extensor weakness is typically associated with a *forward head position*, rounded thoracic spine *(kyphosis)* with a flattened lumbar curve, creating a forward displacement of the COM near or at the anterior LOS. The hips and knees are typically flexed (Fig. 7.4). This flexed, stooped posture is seen in many elderly individuals (Fig. 7.5).
- A flexed-knee posture increases the need for quadriceps activity; it also requires increased hip extensor and soleus activity for accompanying increases in hip flexion and dorsiflexion.
- Excessive anterior tilt of the pelvis increases lumbar lordosis and produces a compensatory increase in thoracic kyphosis; lumbar interdiscal pressures are increased. The abdominals are stretched, and the iliopsoas becomes shortened. Excessive lumbar lordosis produces shortening of the lumbar extensors.
- Excessive dorsal kyphosis produces stretching of the thoracic trunk extensors and shortening of the anterior shoulder muscles.

- Excessive cervical lordosis produces shortening of the neck extensors.
- Genu valgum produces medial knee joint stresses and pronation of the foot with increased stress on the medial longitudinal arch of the foot.
- Pes planus (flat foot) results in depression of the navicular bone and compressive forces laterally; increased weight is borne on the metatarsal heads.
- Pes cavus (high-arched foot) results in increased height of the longitudinal arch with a depressed anterior arch and plantarflexion of the forefoot; toe deformity (claw toes) may also be present.
- Gastrocnemius-soleus weakness results in limited sway and a wide BOS.
- Quadriceps weakness results in unstable sway; the knees are hyperextended (genu recurvatum) and the trunk may be inclined forward to increase stability.
- The patient without active knee control compensates by keeping the hips slightly flexed, with increased lordosis.
- The patient with spasticity of the LEs demonstrates decreased mobility; the actions of the foot/ankle muscles and balance reactions are compromised. The LEs are typically adducted and internally rotated (scissoring) with feet plantarflexed and inverted.

(box continues on page 166)

BOX 7.1 Common Impairments in Standing Postural Alignment and Weightbearing (continued)

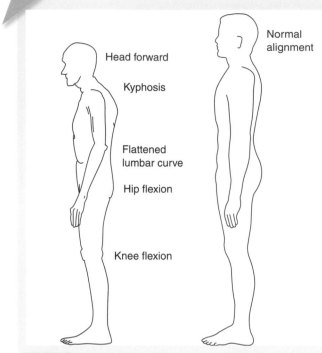

Head forward

Kyphosis

Flattened lumbar curve

Hip flexion

Knee flexion

Normal alignment

FIGURE 7.4 Postural changes seen in many older adults. Loss of spinal flexibility and strength can lead to a flexed, stooped posture with a forward head, dorsal kyphosis, and increased hip and knee flexion.

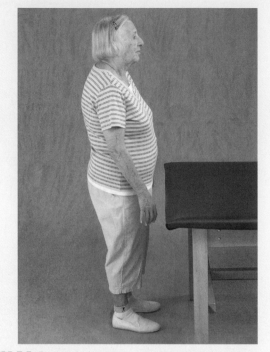

FIGURE 7.5 Postural changes associated with aging in this patient are slight forward head and dorsal kyphosis.

Strategies for Improving Standing Control

Flexibility and Strengthening Exercises

Adequate core (trunk) stability and extremity flexibility and strength are required for normal posture and balance. Table 7.1 presents standing activities that can be used to achieve these goals. The patient should be positioned next to a treatment table and instructed to use light touch-down, fingertip support as needed for balance during these activities. The patient is cautioned not to "hold on tight" and to use the minimal amount of touch-down support necessary, progressing from bilateral support to unilateral support as soon as possible. When these activites are part of a home exercise program (HEP), the patient can stand at the kitchen counter for support (sometimes called "kitchen sink exercises").

Before exercises are performed, it is important to ensure that there is an adequate warm-up to elevate muscle temperature and improve flexibility. Flexibility exercises (stretching) should be performed slowly, with gradual progression to the point of tightness (end range). Ballistic or dynamic stretching (repetitive bouncing) is contraindicated. Exercises to improve muscular strength and endurance can be performed as active exercises or against resistance (using weight cuffs or elastic resistive bands). Key muscles (major muscles of the trunk and extremities) important for posture and balance are targeted.

The patient performs a set of exercises (8 to 12 repetitions), working to the point of volitional fatigue while maintaining good form. The therapist should incorporate appropriate exercises for specific muscle groups as indicated. Holding (isometric exercise), lifting (concentric exercises), and lowering (eccentric exercises) should be incorporated as well as adequate rest to ensure good form. Patients should be cautioned to maintain a normal breathing pattern and to avoid breath-holding. Patients should also be cautioned to stop exercising if the exercise feels unsafe or if unusual pain develops.

Strategies to Vary Postural Stabilization Requirements and Level of Difficulty

Patients with impairments in static postural control benefit from activities that challenge standing control. Progression is obtained by varying the level of difficulty. For example, greater challenges can be incorporated into standing activities by modifying the BOS, the support surface, the use of UEs, and sensory inputs (Box 7.2). During initial practice, the patient should be encouraged to focus full attention on the standing task and its key elements. With repeated practice, the level of cognitive monitoring will decrease as motor learning progresses. Once an autonomous level of learning is achieved, postural responses are largely automatic, with little conscious thought for routine postural adjustments. This level of control can be tested by introducing *dual tasking,* in

(text continues on page 170)

TABLE 7.1 Standing Activities to Improve Flexibility and Strength

Activity	Purpose
Flexibilty Exercises	
Standing, full-body stretches, arms overhead: reaching toward ceiling	Improves ROM of trunk flexors and anterior shoulder muscles
Standing, anterior chest stretches: elbows flexed, shoulders pulling back into extension (Fig. 7.6)	Improves ROM of anterior chest and shoulder muscles
Standing, side stretches: leaning over to one side	Improves ROM of trunk lateral flexors
Standing, trunk twists (rotation), shoulders abducted: twisting around to one side, then the other; head turns, eyes follow the movement	Improves ROM of trunk and head rotators
Standing, arm circles (through increments of shoulder abduction)	Improves ROM in upper back, shoulders, and chest
Standing, hamstring stretch: limb extended in front on a small stool or step, hands pushing knee into full extension	Improves ROM of hamstrings
Standing, hip abductor stretch: standing sideways next to a wall, crossing the outside foot over the closer foot to the wall and leaning toward wall	Improves ROM of hip abductors
Standing, heel-cord stretches: leaning forward with both knees extended or leaning in a lunge position with one foot forward and knee flexed; hands may be placed against a wall in front for support	Improves ROM of Achilles tendon: leaning forward with both knees extended stretches gastrocnemius-soleus; lunge position with one knee flexed stretches soleus

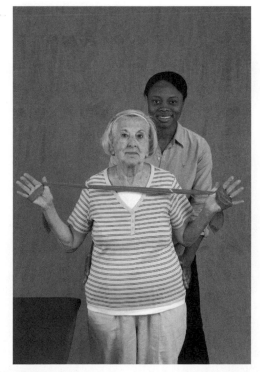

FIGURE 7.6 Standing, anterior chest stretch using an elastic resistance band.

(table continues on page 168)

TABLE 7.1 Standing Activities to Improve Flexibility and Strength *(continued)*

Activity	Purpose
Strengthening Exercises	
Standing, heel rises	Improves gastrocnemius-soleus muscle strength
Standing, toe-offs	Improves anterior tibial muscle strength
Standing, side kicks: lateral leg lifts (Fig. 7.7)	Improves gluteus medius strength
Standing, backward kicks: backward leg lifts (Fig. 7.8)	Improves gluteus maximus strength
Standing, knee curls: knee flexion with hip extension	Improves gluteus maximus and hamstring strength
Standing, hip and knee flexion (Fig. 7.9)	Improves hip flexor and hamstring strength
Standing, hip flexion with knee extension (Fig. 7.10)	Improves hip flexor and quadricep strength
Standing, marching in place	Improves hip flexor and hamstring strength
Standing, arms overhead	Improves shoulder and upper back strength
Standing, UE horizonal pull with resistive band held in each hand (shoulders in 90° of flexion, hands together; hands then pull apart as shoulders move toward abduction)	Improves chest and UE strength
Standing, elbow extensions, shoulder fully flexed using resistive band anchored with opposite hand behind back or hand weight	Improves triceps strength
Standing, elbow flexion with resistive band (distal end fixed) or using hand weight	Improves biceps strength
Standing, partial wall squats	Improves quadriceps and hip extensor strength

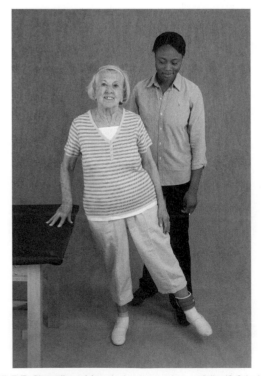

FIGURE 7.7 Standing, hip abduction using a 2-lb (0.9-kg) weight cuff and light fingertip support with one hand.

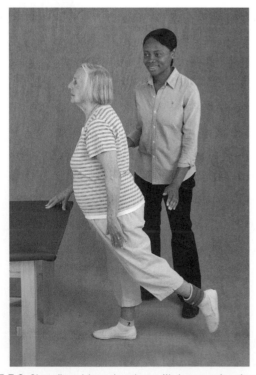

FIGURE 7.8 Standing, hip extension with knee extension using a 2-lb (0.9-kg) weight cuff and light fingertip support with one hand.

TABLE 7.1 Standing Activities to Improve Flexibility and Strength *(continued)*

Activity	Purpose
Chair rises (sit-to-standing)	Improves quadriceps and hip extensor and trunk strength
Standing, partial lunges (movement through partial ROM)	Improves quadriceps and hip extensor and trunk strength

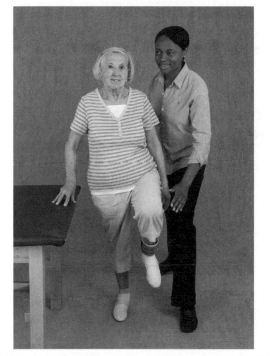

FIGURE 7.9 Standing, hip and knee flexion using a 2-lb (0.9-kg) weight cuff and light fingertip support with one hand.

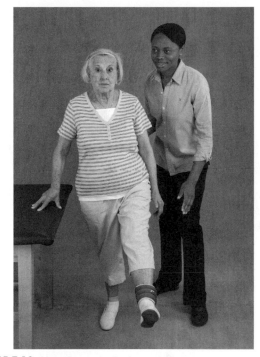

FIGURE 7.10 Standing, hip flexion with knee extension using a 2-lb (0.9-kg) weight cuff and light fingertip support with one hand.

BOX 7.2 Varying Postural Stabilization Requirements and Level of Difficulty

Base of Support
A wide-based stance is a common compensatory change in patients with decreased control. Postural control can be challenged by altering the BOS as follows:

- Progress from feet apart to feet close together to *tandem stance* (heel-toe position).
- Progress from bilateral UE support (e.g., parallel bars) to unilateral UE support (e.g., next to the treatment table) to no UE support.

Note: Light touch-down support (fingertip support) is preferred to holding on (e.g., grabbing onto parallel bars).

Support Surface
The type of support surface can influence postural alignment and control.

- A fixed support surface (e.g., tile floor) provides a stable initial base.
- Progress from standing on a fixed support surface to standing on a carpet, dense foam pad, or mobile surface (e.g., inflated disc, foam roller, wobble board).

Sensory Inputs
Sensory support and modification can influence postural alignment and control.

- Somatosensory cues are maximized by having the patient barefoot or wearing flexible-sole shoes.
- Somatosensory inputs can be varied to increase difficulty: Progress from both feet in contact with a fixed support surface (tile floor) to feet positioned on a soft compliant surface (e.g., dense foam, inflatable dome disc) to standing on a moving platform.
- Visual inputs can be varied to increase difficulty in maintaining standing: Progress from eyes open (EO) to eyes closed (EC).
- Visual cues and perceptual awareness of proper alignment can be assisted by using a mirror; a vertical line can be placed on the mirror; the patient can wear a shirt with a vertical line drawn or taped on the front to align with line on the mirror.
- The role of vestibular inputs can be increased by standing on foam with EC.

which the patient performs two tasks simultaneously (e.g., the patient is required to stand without UE support and carry on a conversation, read aloud, pour water from a pitcher into a glass, or bounce a ball).

Ø **Red Flag:** Training with mirrors may be contraindicated for patients with visual-perceptual spatial deficits (e.g., some patients with stroke or brain injury).

Strategies to Ensure Safety

Patients who are unstable in standing are likely to have heightened anxiety and a fear of falling. It is important for the therapist to demonstrate the ability to control for instability and falls in order to instill patient confidence. General safety tips are presented in Box 7.3.

Clinical Note: Light touch-down (fingertip) support is preferrable as it puts greater demands on the postural support system (i.e., trunk and LEs). Grasping and pulling on objects (e.g., parallel bars) decrease the demands on the postural support system and provide compensatory control using the UEs. If progression is planned to walking using an assistive device such as a walker or cane, practice in pulling will not transfer well to the control needed for using the devices.

Instructions and Verbal Cueing

The therapist should instruct the patient in the correct standing posture and demonstrate the position in order to provide an accurate *reference of correctness*. It is important to focus the patient's attention on key task elements and improve overall sensory awareness of the correct standing posture

and position in space (intrinsic feedback). Suggested verbal instructions and cueing are presented in Box 7.4.

Augmented feedback (e.g., tapping, light resistance, and verbal cueing) should focus attention on *key errors* (those errors that, when corrected, result in considerable improvement of performance, allowing other task elements to then be performed correctly). Slowed responses of some muscles may result in inadequate responses or falls. Tactile and proprioceptive cues can be used to call attention to missing elements. For example, tapping on a weak quadriceps can be used to assist the patient in generating effective contraction to stabilize the knee during standing. Augmented feedback should also emphasize positive aspects of performance, providing reinforcement and enhancing motivation.

Interventions to Improve Control in Modified Plantigrade

Modified plantigrade is an early standing posture that involves four-limb weightbearing (UEs and LEs). The patient stands next to a treatment table with both shoulders flexed (45 to 70 degrees), elbows extended, hands flat on the treatment table and weightbearing, and feet in symmetrical stance position (Fig. 7.11). The hips are flexed and the knees extended; the ankles are dorsiflexed. This creates a stable posture with a wide BOS and a high COM. The BOS and the degree of UE weightbearing can be increased or decreased by varying the distance the patient is standing from the table. The patient need not demonstrate complete knee extensor control required for upright standing in modified plantigrade, as the position of the COM is in front of the weightbearing line. This creates an extension moment at the knee, aiding weak extensors. As control develops, the patient can progress from flat hand to fingertip support and from bilateral to unilateral UE support to free standing. The LEs can be progressed from a symmetrical stance to a step position (Fig. 7.12). An alternative arm position is placing both hands on a ball (less stable surface) to increase the challenge (Fig. 7.13). This position increases the required

---

BOX 7.3 General Safety Considerations

- Initial early standing may require support devices, such as a standing frame or a frame with a body weight support (BWS) harness. A predetermined percentage of body weight is supported by the BWS device. As control is achieved, the percentage of weight support is decreased (e.g., 30 percent support to 20 percent support to 10 percent support to no support).
- Activities can progress to modified support standing with the use of parallel bars or by standing next to a treatment table using *light fingertip, touch-down support*. The patient can also stand with his or her back to the wall or positioned in a corner (corner standing).
- Gait (guarding) belts should be used as necessary for the patient who is at risk for falls. LE splints or orthoses may be necessary to stablize the position of a limb.
- Collaborative treatments (co-treat sessions) with two or more professionals may be necessary for very involved patients (e.g., the patient with brain injury and poor standing control).
- The patient should be instructed in safely getting on and off any equipment to be used during balance activities (e.g., wobble board, foam, inflated disc, or ball).

BOX 7.4 General Verbal Instructions and Cues

- *"Stand tall, hold your head up, and keep your chin tucked with your ears over your shoulders."*
- *"Look up and focus on the target directly in front of you."*
- *"Keep your back straight with shoulders over your hips and hips over your feet."*
- *"Tuck your stomach muscles in and flatten your stomach."*
- *"Keep your weight equally distributed over both feet."*
- *"Breathe normally and hold this posture as steady as you can."*
- *"Imagine you are a soldier standing guard at the Tomb of the Unkown Soldier; stand tall and on guard."*

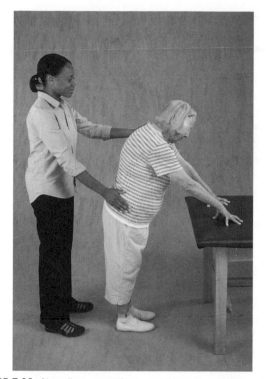

FIGURE 7.11 Standing, modified plantigrade, holding with the LEs in a symmetrical position and the UEs using tabletop fingertip support. The therapist is applying resistance to the upper trunk and pelvis using the technique of stabilizing reversals.

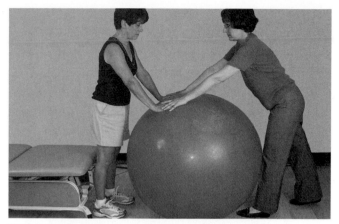

FIGURE 7.13 Standing, modified plantigrade, with both hands resting lightly on a large ball.

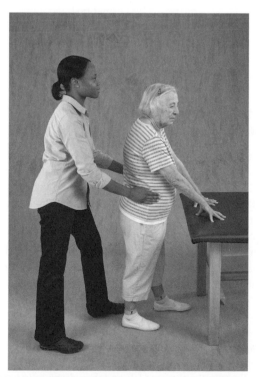

FIGURE 7.12 Standing, modified plantigrade, holding with the LEs in a step position and the UEs using tabletop fingertip support. The therapist is applying resistance to the pelvis using the technique of stabilizing reversals.

shoulder flexion ROM and weight borne on the LEs. Unilateral UE weightbearing can also be accomplished by positioning the patient sideways next to a treatment table or a wall with the shoulder in abduction.

Clinical Note: For patients who demonstrate UE flexor hypertonicity (e.g., the patient with traumatic brain injury [TBI] or stroke), plantigrade is a better choice for early standing compared to standing in the parallel bars and pulling on the bars. Pulling encourages increased flexor tone, while plantigrade promotes UE extension and weightbearing. The plantigrade position combines LE muscles in an out-of-synergy pattern (the hips are flexed with the knees extended). Thus it is a useful treatment activity for the patient with stroke who demonstrates strong abnormal LE synergies.

Stability (static postural control) is necessary for prolonged maintenance of upright standing. Important factors when examining stability control include the ability to maintain correct alignment with minimal postural sway (maintained center of alignment), and the ability to maintain the posture for prolonged times.

Modified Plantigrade, Holding, Stabilizing Reversals

The patient is asked to move in alternating directions while the therapist applies resistance, preventing motion. The therapist's manual contacts can be placed on the pelvis (see Fig. 7.12), on the pelvis and contralateral upper trunk (see Fig. 7.11), or on the upper trunk bilaterally. Resistance is applied first in one direction and then the other (anterior/posterior, medial/lateral, or on the diagonal with the LEs in the step position) (Fig. 7.14). The position of the therapist will vary according to direction of the line of force applied. Resistance is built up gradually from very light resistance to the patient's maximum. The contraction is maintained for several counts. Light approximation can be given to the top of the shoulders or the pelvis to increase stabilizing responses.

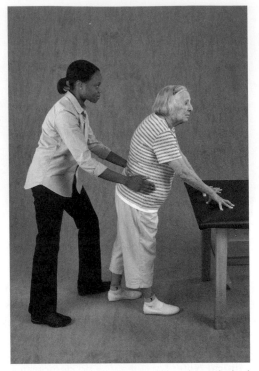

FIGURE 7.14 Standing, modified plantigrade, anterior/posterior weight shifts with the LEs in step position and the UEs using tabletop fingertip support. The therapist is applying resistance to the pelvis using the technique of dynamic reversals (both hands forward to resist the forward weight shift; both hands back to resist the backward weight shift).

Verbal cues include: *"Push against my hands, hold, don't let me push you backward, hold."* The therapist must then give a transitional command, *"Now, don't let me pull you forward,"* before sliding the hands to resist the opposite muscles and ask for a *"Hold"*; this allows the patient the opportunity to make appropriate anticipatory postural adjustments.

Modified Plantigrade, Holding, Rhythmic Stabilization

The patient is asked to hold the plantigrade position while the therapist stands behind and applies resistance to the trunk. In rhythmic stabilization, one hand is placed on the posterior pelvis on one side, pushing forward, while the other hand is on the anterior contralateral upper trunk, pulling backward. The verbal cue is *"Don't let me move you, hold, hold; now don't let me move you the other way."*

Outcomes
Motor control goal: Stability (static postural control).
Functional skill achieved: The patient is able to maintain upright standing with UE support independently with minimal sway and no loss of balance.

Modified Plantigrade, Active Weight Shifts

Controlled mobility (dynamic postural control) is necessary for moving in a posture (e.g., weight shifting) or moving the limbs (e.g., UE or LE movements) while maintaing postural stability. These movements produce disturbances of the COM and require ongoing postural adjustments in order to maintain upright standing. Initially, the patient's attention is directed to the key task elements required for successful postural adjustments and movement. With increased practice, the postural adjustments become more automatic.

Weight-shifting activities forward and backward in plantigrade can be used to increase ROM; these activities may be ideal for patients who are anxious about ROM exercises. Improved ROM in shoulder flexion can be achieved by shifting the weight backward (hands remain fixed on the table) by positioning the feet farther away from the treatment table. Improved ROM in ankle dorsiflexion can be achieved by weight shifts forward. Weight shifts with the patient facing a corner, each hand on adjacent walls, can be used to improve ROM of upper trunk and shoulder flexors (e.g., in the patient with a functional dorsal kyphosis and forward shoulders). Weight shifts can be combined with UE *wall push-ups* to increase the strength of the elbow extensors.

The patient actively shifts weight first forward (increasing loading on the UEs) and then backward (increasing loading on the LEs). Weight shifts can also be performed from side to side (medial/lateral shifts) with the LEs in a symmetrical stance, or diagonally forward and backward with the LEs in a step position (see Fig. 7.14). Active reaching activities can be used to promote weight shifting in all directions or in the direction of an instability (e.g., the patient with stroke). The therapist provides a target (*"Reach out and touch my hand"*) or uses a functional task like cone stacking to promote reaching. The patient can also put both hands on a ball placed on top of a flat treatment table (Fig. 7.15). The patient moves the ball from side to side, forward and backward, or diagonally forward and backward.

Modified Plantigrade, Weight Shifts, Dynamic Reversals

The therapist is standing at the patient's side for medial/lateral shifts and behind the patient for anterior/posterior shifts. Manual contacts may be placed on the pelvis, the pelvis/contralateral upper trunk, or bilaterally on the upper trunk. The movements are guided for a few repetitions to ensure that the patient knows the movements expected. Movements are then lightly resisted. The therapist alternates hand placement, resisting the movements first in one direction and then the other. Smooth reversals of antagonists are facilitated by well-timed verbal cues, such as *"Pull away from me, now, push back toward me."*

Variations in weight shifting include diagonal weight shifts with feet in step position (one foot forward of the other). Resistance is applied to the pelvis as the patient weight shifts diagonally onto the forward LE and then diagonally backward onto the other LE (Fig. 7.16). The verbal cue is *"Shift forward and away from me; now shift back and toward me."*

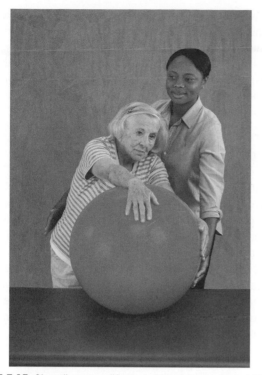

FIGURE 7.15 Standing, modified plantigrade, weight shifts with the LEs in a symmetrical position and the UEs supported by a ball placed on the treatment table. The patient moves the ball (forward and backward, side to side) while the therapist provides verbal cues and guarding.

Once control is achieved in diagonal shifts, focus is directed toward pelvic rotation. The patient is instructed to shift weight diagonally onto the forward LE while rotating the pelvis forward on the opposite side; then the weight is shifted diagonally backward while the pelvis is rotated backward. The therapist resists the motion at the pelvis (Fig. 7.17). This activity is a lead-up to stepping. The verbal cue is *"Shift forward and twist; now shift backward and twist."*

If the elbows flex, the upper trunk may also move forward as the pelvis rotates forward, producing an undesirable ipsilateral trunk rotation pattern. The therapist can isolate the pelvic motion by instructing the patient to keep both elbows fully extended.

Modified Plantigrade, Stepping, Dynamic Reversals

While in modified plantigrade, the patient can progress to taking a step forward with the dynamic limb while weight-shifting diagonally forward. The therapist maintains manual contacts on the pelvis to facilitate the accompanying pelvic rotation. The verbal cue is *"Shift forward and step; now shift backward and step."*

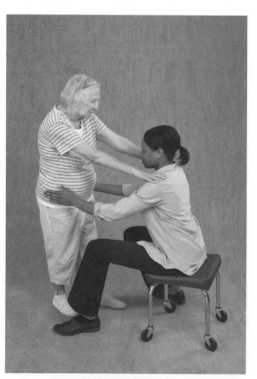

FIGURE 7.16 Modified plantigrade, diagonal weight shifts with the LEs in step position and the UEs using light touch-down support on the therapist's shoulders. The patient moves diagonally forward and over the more advanced left foot. The therapist provides resistance to the pelvis using the technique of dynamic reversals.

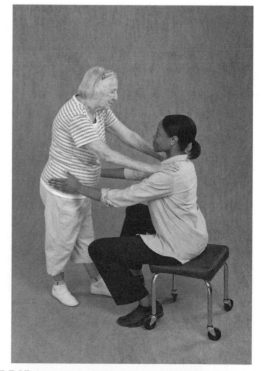

FIGURE 7.17 Modified plantigrade, diagonal weight shifts with pelvic rotation, LEs in step position, and the UEs using light touch-down support on the therapist's shoulders. The patient moves diagonally forward over the more advanced left foot while rotating the pelvis forward on the right. The therapist provides resistance to the pelvis using the technique of dynamic reversals.

Modified Plantigrade, UE PNF Patterns: D2 Flexion (D2F) and D2 Extension (D2E)

The patient is in modified plantigrade position with the one UE weightbearing near the end of the treatment table. For D2F, the dynamic limb is initially positioned in extension, adduction, and internal rotation with the hand of the dynamic limb positioned across the body toward the opposite hip with the hand closed and thumb facing down (Fig. 7.18A). The patient is instructed to open the hand, turn, and lift the hand up and out (Fig. 7.18B). For D2E, the patient closes the hand, turns, and pulls the hand down and across the body. The patient is instructed to follow the movements of the UE by looking at the hand. This encourages head and neck rotation. The therapist provides light resistance to the UE as it moves through the pattern. Verbal cues include *"Open your hand, turn, and lift it up and out"* (D2F) and *"Squeeze my hand, turn, and pull down and across your body"* (D2E).

A lightweight cuff can also be used to provide resistance during active movements. When using resistance, the level is determined by the ability of the static limbs and trunk to stabilize and maintain the plantigrade posture, and not by the strength of the dynamic limb.

Outcomes

Motor control goal: Improved controlled mobility (dynamic stability control).

Functional skills achieved: The patient is able to maintain standing with UE support during weight shifts and all voluntary limb movements with no loss of balance or falls. The patient is able to step independently with no loss of balance or falls, preparatory for independent locomotion.

Interventions to Improve Control in Standing

The patient is standing, with equal weight on both LEs. The feet are positioned parallel and slightly apart (a symmetrical stance position); knees should be extended or in slight flexion, not hyperextended. The pelvis is in neutral position. An alternative standing position is with one foot slightly advanced of the other in a step position. An elastic resistive band can be placed around the thighs (the LEs in a symmetrical stance position) to increase the proprioceptive input and promote pelvic stabilization by the lateral hip muscles (gluteus medius and minimus).

Clinical Note: Knee instability in which the knee buckles due to quadriceps weakness can be managed initially by having the patient wear a knee immobilizer splint. The patient can also practice standing on an inclined surface facing forward. The forward tilt of the body and anterior displacement of the COM provide a

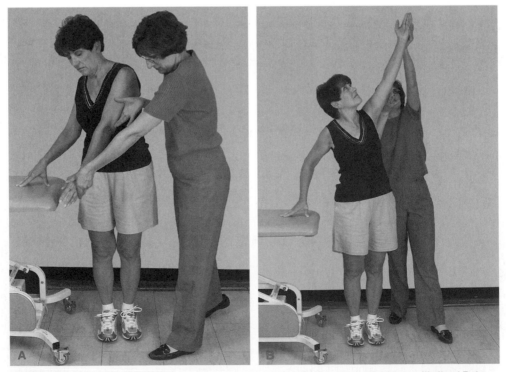

FIGURE 7.18 Standing, modified plantigrade, PNF UE D2 flexion and extension with the LEs in a symmetrical position and light fingertip support with one hand. The patient **(A)** begins with the dynamic limb in extension, adduction, and internal rotation with hand closed and **(B)** moves into flexion, abduction, and external rotation with hand open. The therapist provides resistance to the dynamic UE using the technique of dynamic reversals.

posteriorly directed moment (force) at the knee, helping to stabilize it in extension.

Standing, Holding, Stabilizing Reversals

The patient is asked to move, allowing only limited ROM progressing to holding the position while the therapist applies resistance to the trunk. The therapist's manual contacts may be placed on the pelvis, the pelvis and contralateral upper trunk (Fig. 7.19), or the upper trunk bilaterally. Resistance is applied first in one direction and then the other (anterior/posterior, medial/lateral, or on the diagonal with the LEs in the step position). The position of the therapist will vary according to the direction of the line of force applied. Resistance is built up gradually from very light resistance to the patient's maximum. The isometric contraction is maintained for several counts. Light approximation can be given to the tops of the shoulders or the pelvis to increase stabilizing responses. Verbal cues include *"Push against my hands, now hold. Don't let me push you backward, hold."* The therapist must then give a transitional command, *"Now don't let me pull you forward,"* before sliding the hands to resist the opposite muscles and asking for a *"Hold"*; this allows the patient the opportunity to make appropriate anticipatory postural adjustments.

Standing, Holding, Rhythmic Stabilization

In rhythmic stabilization, the patient holds the symmetrical standing position while the therapist applies resistance to the trunk. One hand is placed on the posterior pelvis on one side pulling forward, while the other hand is on the anterior contralateral upper trunk, pushing backward (Fig. 7.20). The verbal cue is *"Don't let me move you (twist you)—hold, hold; now don't let me move you (twist you) the other way, hold."*

Clinical Note: Interventions to promote stability are important lead-up skills for many ADL (both basic [BADL] and instrumental [IADL]) typically performed in the standing position, such as brushing teeth, combing hair, cooking, cleaning, and so forth. Stabilization control in standing is also an important lead-up activity for unilateral stance and bipedal gait.

Outcomes
Motor control goal: Stability (static postural control).
Functional skill achieved: The patient is able to maintain standing independently with minimal sway and no loss of balance for all ADL.

Standing, Active Weight Shifts

The patient is encouraged to actively weight shift forward and backward (anterior/posterior shifts) and from side to side (medial/lateral shifts) with the LEs in a symmetrical stance position. In a step position, the patient can perform forward and backward diagonal weight shifts, simulating normal weight transfer during gait. Reeducation of LOS is one of the first goals in treatment. The patient is encouraged

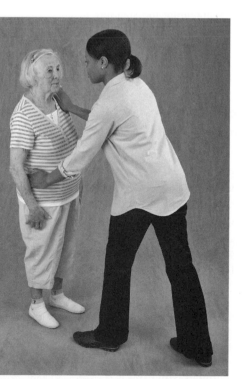

FIGURE 7.19 Standing, holding with the LEs in a symmetrical position. The therapist is applying resistance to the upper trunk and pelvis using the technique of stabilizing reversals (both hands pushing back).

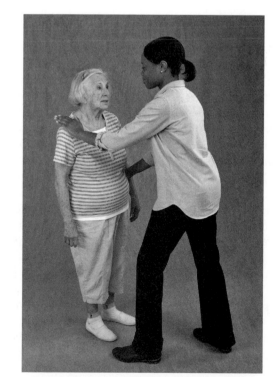

FIGURE 7.20 Standing, holding with the LEs in a symmetrical position. The therapist is applying resistance to the upper trunk and pelvis using the technique of rhythmic stabilization (the hand on the upper trunk is pushing back, while the hand on the pelvis is pulling forward).

to shift weight as far as possible in any one direction without losing balance and then to return to the midline position. Initially, weight shifts are small range but gradually the range is increased (moving through *increments of range*).

Clinical Note: Patients with ataxia (e.g., primary cerebellar pathology) exhibit too much movement and have difficulty holding steady in a posture (maintaining stability). Initially, weight shifts are large and then are progressed during treatment to smaller and smaller ranges (moving through *decrements of range*) to finally holding steady.

Standing, Weight Shifting, Dynamic Reversals

The therapist stands at the patient's side for medial/lateral shifts and either in front of or behind for anterior/posterior shifts. Manual contacts are placed on the pelvis or on the pelvis and contralateral upper trunk. The movement is guided for a few repetitions to ensure that the patient knows the movements expected. Movements are then lightly resisted. The therapist alternates hand placement, resisting the movements first in one direction and then the other. Smooth reversals of antagonists are facilitated by well-timed verbal cues, such as *"Pull away from me; now push back toward me."*

A hold may be added in one or both directions if the patient demonstrates difficulty moving in one direction. The hold is a momentary pause (held for one count); the antagonist contraction is then resisted. The verbal cue is *"Pull away from me, hold; now push back toward me."*

The patient can also perform diagonal weight shifts with the LEs in step position (one foot forward of the other). The therapist is diagonally in front of the patient, either sitting on a stool or standing. Manual contacts are on the anterior or posterior pelvis. Resistance is applied to the pelvis as the patient shifts weight diagonally forward over the limb in front and then diagonally backward over the opposite limb. The verbal cue is *"Shift forward and toward me; now shift backward and away from me."*

Once control is achieved in diagonal shifts, the patient is instructed to shift weight diagonally forward onto the forward limb (step position) while rotating the pelvis forward on the opposite side. Weight is then shifted diagonally backward while the pelvis is rotated backward. The therapist resists the motion at the pelvis. The verbal cue is *"Shift forward and twist; now shift backward and twist."*

The upper trunk may move forward on the same side as the pelvis rotates forward, producing an undesirable ipsilateral trunk rotation pattern. The therapist can isolate the pelvic motion by providing verbal or manual cues. The patient is instructed to hold the UEs in front with the shoulders flexed, elbows extended, and the hands clasped, or the hands can be lightly supported on the therapist's shoulders to stabilize the upper trunk motion (see Fig. 7.17). Verbal cues include: *"Clasp your hands and hold your arms directly in front of you. Keep them forward; don't let them move from*

side to side. Now shift forward and twist. Now shift back and twist."

Standing, Active Limb Movements

Active movements of the UEs or LEs can be used to challenge dynamic stability control and balance. Postural adjustments are required during each and every limb movement. Limb movements can be performed individually or in combination (bilateral symmetrical or reciprocal UE movements). Progression is to increased range and increased time on task. For example, during each of 10 repetitions, the patient holds the limb position for three counts and progresses to holding for five counts. One of the major benefits of this activity is that the patient focuses full attention on movement of the limbs and the task challenges imposed; postural control to maintain standing is largely automatic. Box 7.5 provides examples of activities involving dynamic limb movements in standing.

Clinical Note: If the patient is unable to maintain postural control during voluntary limb movements, it may be an indication that conscious control (cognitive monitoring) is still required. This is a characteristic finding in the patient with primary cerebellar damage. Automatic (nonconscious) control of posture is very difficult or impossible while compensatory cognitive monitoring makes some degree of control possible.

Standing, Single-Limb Stance

The patient stands on one LE and lifts the other off the ground, maintaining the standing position using single-limb stance. The patient is instructed to maintain the pelvis level. A pelvis that drops on the side of the dynamic limb is indicative of hip abductor weakness on the opposite (static limb) side (positive Trendelenburg).

Standing, Single-Limb Stance With Abduction

This is an advanced stabilization activity in which the patient stands sideways next to a wall about 4 inches (10 cm) from the wall (the trunk is not allowed to contact the wall). The LE closest to the wall becomes the dynamic limb, while the other LE is the support limb. The patient flexes the knee while maintaining hip extension and abducts the dynamic limb, pushing the knee against the wall. The static limb maintains the upright posture during unilateral stance with the knee extended (Fig. 7.23). Both groups of abductors are working strongly to push the knee against the wall on the dynamic side and to maintain single-limb stance position on the static side. Overflow from one side to the other is strong. This can also be done using a small ball between the knee and the wall.

Clinical Note: This is a useful activity for the patient with hip abductor weakness and Trendelenburg gait pattern (e.g., the patient with stroke). Initially the weaker limb is the dynamic limb. As control develops,

(text continues on page 178)

BOX 7.5 Examples of Dynamic Limb Movements in Standing

Upper Extremities

- **Lifts:** The patient raises one or both UEs with shoulders flexed and elbows extended to the forward or side horizontal position or overhead; hands can be clasped together for forward lifts.
- **Reaches:** The patient reaches forward or sideways to a target (*"Reach out and touch my hand"*) or reaches forward to pick up and place objects (i.e., cone stacking or bean bag toss) (Fig. 7.21).
- **Floor touches:** The patient reaches down to touch the floor or pick an object up off the floor.
- **Reaches and turns:** The patient lifts a ball up with both hands, turns, and moves the ball diagonally up and across the body (Fig. 7.22) (the size and weight of the ball can be varied).

Lower Extremities

- **Lifts:** The patient flexes the hip and knee of one LE and then lowers; side steps (abduction of the hip with knee extension), or extends the hip with the knee flexed.

- **Marching in place:** The patient alternately raises one LE up (the hip and knee flex) and then the other, marching in place; this activity can be combined with reciprocal arm swings or head turns.
- **Toe-offs and heel-offs:** The patient raises both toes off the floor, moving the weight backward onto both heels; the patient raises both heels off the floor, moving the weight forward onto the toes and balls of the feet.
- **Foot drawing:** The patient raises one foot off the floor (the hip flexes with the knee extended) and performs toe circles or writes the letters of the alphabet using the great toe as a "pencil."
- **Foot slides:** The patient places one foot on a towel and slides the towel forward and backward, side to side, or in circles. The patient can also place the foot on a small ball and roll the ball in all directions (the size of the ball can be varied).
- **Ball activities:** The patient stops a rolling ball with one foot or kicks the ball as it is rolled toward him or her.

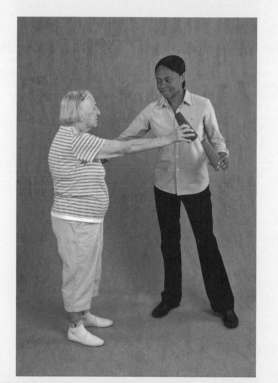

FIGURE 7.21 Standing, reaching with the LEs in a symmetrical position. The patient reaches forward with the right UE and places the cone on the target cone held in front (cone stacking task). The therapist holds the target cone in front of the patient. Target location can be varied to encourage weight shifting and reaching to one side or the other.

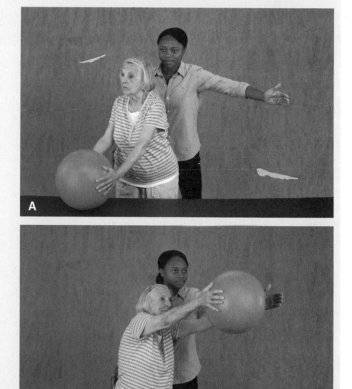

FIGURE 7.22 Standing, diagonal lifting with head and trunk rotation. **(A)** The patient picks up the small ball with both hands and **(B)** lifts the ball up and across to the left. The therapist provides the target and verbal cues to maximize head and trunk rotation.

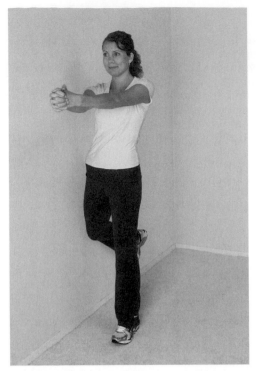

FIGURE 7.23 Standing, single-limb stance, limb abduction. The patient stands sideways next to a wall on one limb and lifts the other limb into hip extension with knee flexion. The dynamic limb is abducted with the knee pushing against the wall. The UEs are held with shoulders flexed, elbows extended, and hands clasped together (hands-clasped position). The therapist instructs the patient to push as hard as possible into the wall. The patient is not allowed to lean on the wall (no contact of the wall with the shoulder or hip is allowed).

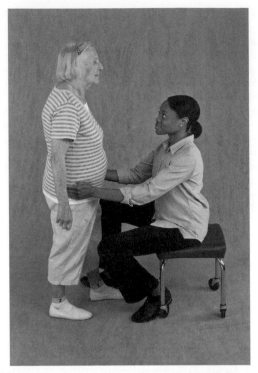

FIGURE 7.24 Standing, stepping. The patient practices stepping forward and backward with the dynamic limb; the static (support) limb does not change position. The therapist provides resistance with both hands on the pelvis using the technique of dynamic reversals. Sitting on a rolling stool allows the therapist to be positioned at pelvic height.

the support limb is reversed so that the weaker limb is used for single-limb stance. In the latter situation, the weaker limb is required to support most of the weight of the body, while in the former, only the weight of the limb must be supported.

Red Flag: The patient should not be allowed to flex the hip with knee flexion on the dynamic limb pushing into the wall. This permits substitution of the tensor fascia lata muscle for the gluteus medius (targeted muscle).

Standing, Stepping

This activity is initiated with the LEs in step position. The patient shifts weight diagonally forward over the anterior support limb (stance limb) and takes a step forward with the dynamic (swing) limb (Fig. 7.24). The movements are then reversed; the patient takes a step backward using the same dynamic limb. Lateral side steps and crossed steps can also be practiced (Fig. 7.25). Footprint or other markers on the floor can be used to increase the step length and improve the accuracy of stepping movements (Fig. 7.26). Verbal cues include: *"Shift your weight over onto your right (or left) foot. Now step forward with your left foot"* and *"Now shift back over your right foot and step back."*

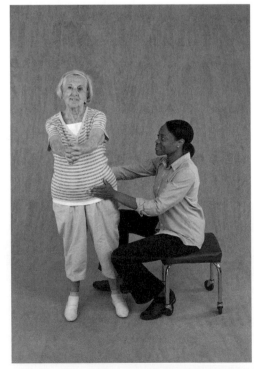

FIGURE 7.25 Standing, side-stepping. The patient practices stepping out to the side and back with the dynamic limb; the static (support) limb does not change position. The therapist provides resistance with both hands on the pelvis.

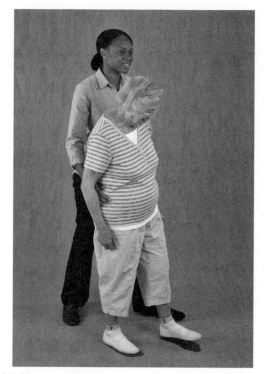

FIGURE 7.26 Standing, stepping. The patient practices active stepping using footprint floor markers.

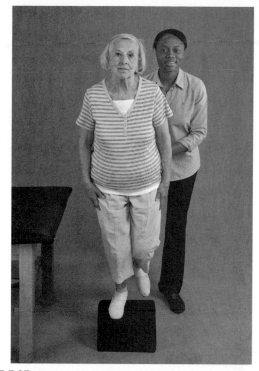

FIGURE 7.27 Standing, forward step-ups. The patient steps up onto a 4-in. (10-cm) step positioned in front; the foot is then returned to the start position (symmetrical stance position). The therapist provides verbal cueing and guarding.

The patient can also be instructed to place one foot up on a step positioned directly in front of the patient (Fig. 7.27). This variation requires increased hip and knee flexion of the dynamic limb. Lateral or side step-ups can also be practiced (Fig. 7.28). The height of the step can be varied from a low of 4 inches (10 cm) to a normal step height of 7 inches (18 cm). Verbal cues are *"Shift your weight over onto your right (or left) foot. Now place your left foot up on the step. Now bring it down."*

Stepping, Dynamic Reversals

The therapist is in front of the patient, either sitting on a rolling stool or standing. Manual contacts are on the pelvis. The therapist applies light stretch and resistance to facilitate forward pelvic rotation as the swing limb moves forward and backward. This is a useful activity to promote improved rotation of the pelvis during stepping. The verbal cue is *"Shift forward and step; now shift backward and step."*

Light resistance can also be provided by the therapist standing behind the patient using an elastic resistive band to provide resistance to the forward step (Fig. 7.29). Side-stepping can be resisted manually (dynamic reversals) or using an elastic resistive band, with the therapist positioned to the side of the patient (Fig. 7.30).

Standing, Partial Wall Squats

The patient stands with the back against a wall, with feet about 4 inches (10 cm) from the wall. The patient is instructed

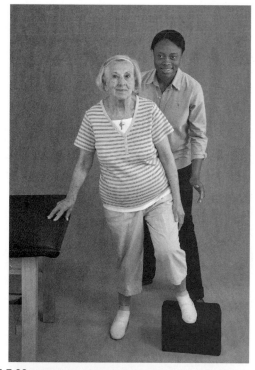

FIGURE 7.28 Standing, lateral step-ups. The patient steps up onto a 4-in. (10-cm) step positioned to her left side; the foot is then returned to the start position (symmetrical stance position). Light touch-down support of one hand is necessary. The therapist provides verbal cueing and guarding.

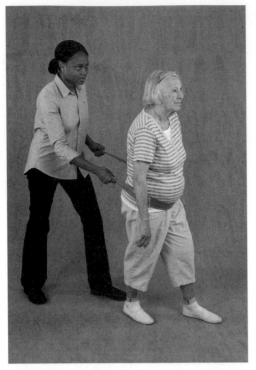

FIGURE 7.29 *Standing, resisted stepping. The patient steps forward against resistance and then steps back. The therapist provides resistance using an elastic resistive band positioned around the patient's pelvis.*

to bend both knees while sliding the back down the wall. Movement is restricted to partial range; the patient is instructed to stop when no longer able to see the tips of the toes (knees are not allowed to move forward in advance of the toes). The hips are maintained in neutral rotation to ensure proper patellar tracking. The pelvis is also maintained in neutral.

Clinical Note: Partial squats should be performed with a slight posterior pelvic tilt in the presence of low back pain.

The patient can also stand with the back supported by a medium-sized ball placed in the lumbar region; the feet are positioned directly underneath the body, with the trunk upright. The ball is resting on the wall. As the patient moves down into the partial squat position, the movement is facilitated by the ball rolling upward (Fig. 7.31). The correct size ball also helps to maintain a normal lumbar curve.

Clinical Notes: Partial wall squats are an important activity for the patient with quadriceps weakness. The patient is required to maintain control during both eccentric (lowering) contraction and concentric (raising) contractions. The patient is instructed not to

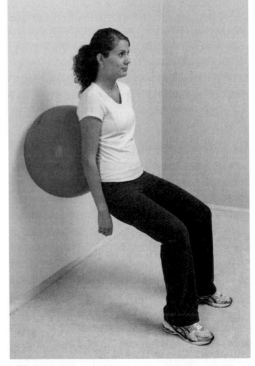

FIGURE 7.31 *Standing, partial wall squats. The patient stands with both feet about 2 ft (0.6 m) from the wall, hip-width apart. A ball is placed between the wall and the patient's low back. The patient leans back against the ball and slowly lowers, bending both knees. The patient is cautioned not to allow the knees to advance in front of the toes. The patient holds the position for 2 to 3 seconds and then slowly returns to standing. The therapist provides verbal instructions and guarding.*

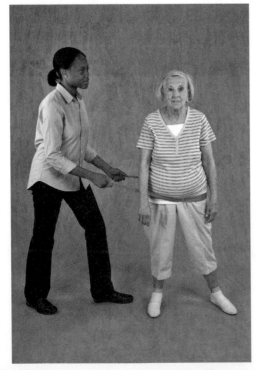

FIGURE 7.30 *Standing, resisted side-stepping. The patient steps out to the side against resistance and then steps back. The therapist provides resistance using an elastic resistance band positioned around the patient's pelvis.*

move the knee into hyperextension. A small towel roll or ball can be placed between the knees. The patient is instructed to hold the towel roll in position by squeezing both knees together during the squat. This enhances contraction of the vastus medialis and improves patellar tracking. An elastic resistive band placed around the thighs can be used to increase the stabilizing activity of the hip abductors during partial wall squats. Partial wall squats are an important lead-up activity for independent sit-to-stand transfers and stair climbing. Bilateral partial squats can be progressed to unilateral (single-limb) partial squats.

Standing, Lunges

The patient stands with feet hip-width apart and steps forward about 2 feet (0.6 m) with the dynamic limb, allowing the heel of the static limb to lift off the ground. The patient lowers into a lunge position by partially flexing the knee and keeping the knee directly over the foot (*partial lunge*) (Fig. 7.32). The position is held for 2 or 3 seconds, and then the patient pushes back up into standing. The trunk is maintained upright with the hips in neutral position. If the patient bends forward during the activity (flexes the trunk), he or she can be instructed to hold a dowel behind the back as a reminder to keep the trunk upright (Fig. 7.33). Partial lunges with the foot of the

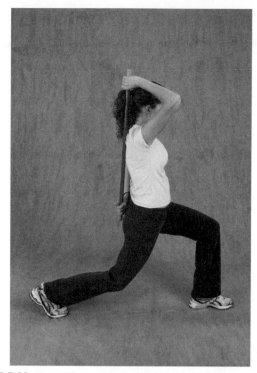

FIGURE 7.33 Standing, partial lunge. The patient performs a partial lunge holding onto a dowel positioned horizontally on the back. The dowel provides a cue to maintain the back straight during the partial lunge, preventing a forward trunk bend.

dynamic limb placed on a foam pad or inflated dome cushion increase the difficulty of the activity. Lunges are another activity in which the patient is required to maintain control during both eccentric (lowering) contraction and concentric (raising) contractions.

Partial lunges can progress to *full lunges,* in which the patient comes down onto one knee and then pushes back up into standing (Fig. 7.34). Wide-stance, sideways partial lunges can also be performed. The patient steps out to the side, bending the knee on the dynamic limb and lowering the body down. The patient then pushes back up and moves the dynamic foot back into symmetrical standing.

Floor-to-Standing Transfers

Floor-to-standing transfers should be practiced by all patients in preparation for recovery should a fall occur. Functional skills acquired during earlier movement transitions (supine to side-sit, side-sit to quadruped, quadruped to kneeling, kneeling to half-kneeling, and half-kneeling to standing) provide the building blocks (lead-up skills) for a successful floor-to-standing transfer. This movement transition can be accomplished by having the patient practice moving into quadruped, then kneeling, half-kneeling, and finally standing. The patient uses both UEs for support and the forward LE to push up into standing (Fig. 7.35).

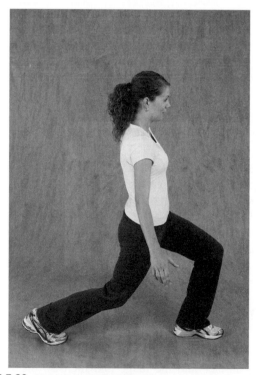

FIGURE 7.32 Standing, partial lunge. The patient stands with feet hip-width apart. The patient steps forward about 2 ft (0.6 m) with the left leg, allowing the right heel to lift off the ground and the left LE to slowly lower the body into a partial lunge position. The position is held for 2 to 3 seconds; then the patient slowly pushes back with the left LE and returns to standing. The therapist provides verbal instructions and guarding.

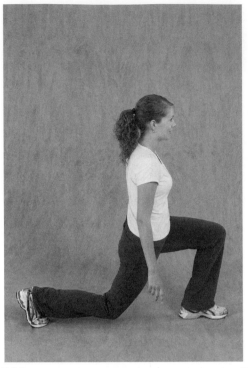

FIGURE 7.34 Standing, full lunge. The patient stands with feet hip-width apart. The patient steps forward about 2 ft (0.6 m) with the left LE, allowing the right heel to lift off the ground as the right knee is slowly lowered to the floor (half-kneeling position). The position is held for 2 to 3 seconds and then the patient slowly pushes back to standing with the left LE. The therapist provides verbal instructions and guarding.

Outcomes

Motor control goal: Controlled mobility (dynamic stability control).

Functional skills achieved: The patient is able to maintain standing during weight shifts and voluntary limb movements with no loss of balance or falls. The patient is able to step independently in all directions with no loss of balance or falls, preparatory for independent locomotion.

Interventions to Improve Balance Control

The therapist focuses on obtaining the correct neuromuscular synergies in response to balance challenges. Progression is from voluntary movements (anticipatory control) to automatic movements (reactive control).

Promoting Ankle Strategies

Small shifts in COM alignment or slow sway movements result in activation of an ankle strategy. The patient is instructed to sway gently forward and backward and then return to centered alignment using ankle motions (dorsiflexion or plantarflexion). The trunk and hips move as one unit, with the axis of motion at the ankles. Thus flexion and extension movements at the hips are not permitted. Slow verbal cues can be

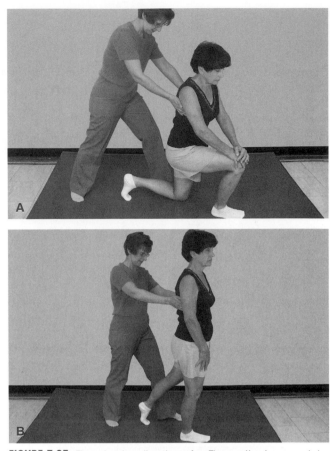

FIGURE 7.35 Floor-to-standing transfer. The patient moves into half-kneeling and places both hands on the front knee. From there the patient shifts forward and over the foot, pushes off with both hands, and stands up. **(A)** The therapist can assist by holding onto the patient's upper trunk (the therapist stands behind the patient). **(B)** The patient moves into the standing position.

used initially to pace the movements. Gentle perturbations applied at the hips or shoulders can also be used to activate ankle strategies. A small displacement backward activates dorsiflexors and a forward weight shift, while a small displacement forward activates plantarflexors and a backward weight shift. Wobble boards and foam rollers can also be used to activate ankle synergies. Standing on a wobble board (rocker board) and gently rocking the board forward and backward stimulate ankle actions. Small weight shifts performed while standing on a split foam roller (flat side up) can also be used to activate ankle synergies (Fig. 7.36).

Promoting Hip Strategies

Larger shifts in COM alignment or faster sway movements result in activation of a hip strategy. The patient is instructed to sway farther into the range and increase the speed of sway. Hip flexors or extensors serve to realign the COM within the BOS. Thus the upper trunk is moving opposite the direction of the lower body, with the axis of motion occurring at the hips. Stepping is discouraged.

Moderate perturbations applied at the hips or larger faster tilts on a wobble board can also be used to stimulate

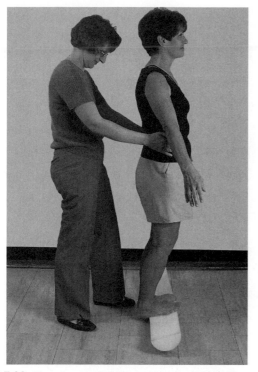

FIGURE 7.36 Standing, activating ankle strategies. The patient stands on a split foam roller, flat side up. The therapist instructs the patient to tilt the roller backward and forward, moving from a heels-down position to a toes-down position.

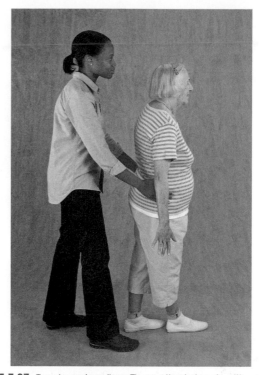

FIGURE 7.37 Tandem standing. The patient stands with one foot positioned in heel-toe position, directly in front of the other, with eyes open. The activity can be progressed to tandem standing with EC (sharpened Romberg postion). Tandem standing activates medial-lateral hip strategies. The therapist provides verbal cueing and contact guarding.

anterior-posterior hip strategies. Standing on a split foam roller (flat side down) can be used to produce larger weight shifts and hip strategies, as can standing on a foam cushion, especially with eyes closed (EC).

Medial-lateral adjustments in the COM are accomplished mainly by hip strategies. Tandem standing (heel-toe position) on the floor (Fig. 7.37), tandem standing on a split foam roller, or standing lengthwise on a roller can be used to promote medial-lateral hip strategies.

Standing on a foam roller can be initiated using the support of two poles with progression to a single pole (Fig. 7.38A) and then progression to standing on the foam roller with no UE support (Fig. 7.38B).

Promoting Stepping Strategies

Larger shifts in which the COM exceeds the LOS result in activation of *stepping strategies.* The patient practices leaning forward until the COM exceeds the BOS. This requires the patient to step forward to prevent a fall. Increased backward lean will result in a backward step, while increased sideward lean will result in a side step or crossed step. The patient then takes a return step to centered alignment. Stepping should be practiced in all directions, progressing from small steps to wider and wider steps. A circle can be drawn on the floor around the patient to encourage symmetry of stepping responses in all directions. An elastic resistive band applied around the hips and held by the therapist can also be used to provide a perturbation challenge. The patient is instructed to

lean forward (or backward or sideward) against the resistance (Fig. 7.39A). The therapist then suddenly releases the resistance (release maneuver) while still holding the band and guarding to protect against a fall. The patient is instructed to take a reactive step to maintain balance (Fig. 7.39B).

Promoting Balance Control Using Manual Perturbations

The therapist applies small, quick perturbations forward or backward (sternal nudge or pull), displacing the patient's COM in relation to the BOS. The patient responds with a counter movement to maintain balance. The challenges should be appropriate for the patient's range and speed of control. Progression is to varying the direction of the displacements (e.g., lateral, diagonal). Excessive perturbations such as vigorous pushes or shoves are not appropriate. Initially with patients who lack stability control, the patient can be informed of the direction of the perturbation *("Don't let me push you backward").* This assists the patient in readiness, engaging anticipatory postural control mechanisms. As control improves, the therapist progresses to using unexpected perturbations, emphasizing reactive, involuntary postural strategies. The patient is instructed to *"Maintain your standing balance at all times."* The BOS can also be varied to increase or decrease the difficulty (wide BOS to narrow BOS). Altering the support surface to foam can also increase the likelihood of a stepping strategy, especially with EC.

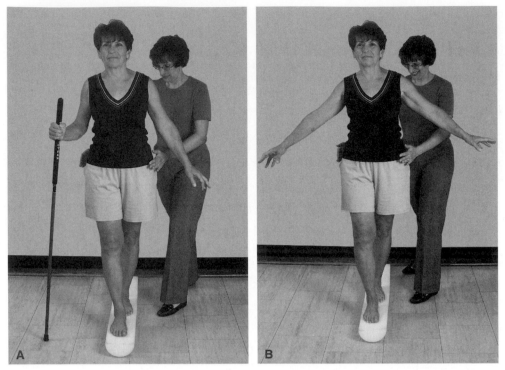

FIGURE 7.38 Tandem standing on foam roller. **(A)** The patient stands on a single foam roller, flat side up, with the support of one pole. **(B)** Progression is to tandem standing on a split foam roller with no UE support. Note the guard position of the patient's UEs. The therapist provides verbal cues and close guarding.

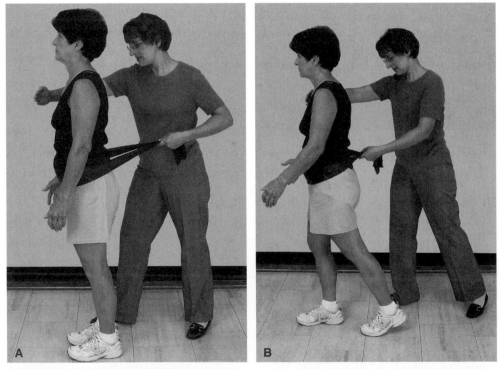

FIGURE 7.39 Standing, release maneuver activating stepping strategies. The patient stands in a symmetrical foot position. **(A)** The therapist places a resistive band around the patient's pelvis and provides tension, while the patient is instructed to lean into the band. **(B)** The therapist then provides a quick release of band tension, which requires the patient to take a reactive step forward to keep from falling. The therapist keeps one hand in front of the patient for guarding purposes and holds the band with the other hand.

Manual perturbations prepare the patient for unexpected challenges to balance (force displacements) that may occur in everyday life (e.g., standing and walking in crowded situations). The therapist should use appropriate safety precautions, carefully guarding to prevent falls in patients with delayed stepping responses.

Promoting Balance Control Using Mobile and Compliant Surfaces

Wobble Board

The patient stands on a wobble board (rocker board) and practices maintaining a centered balance position (the wobble board is not allowed to touch down on any side). The patient then practices self-initiated tilts (e.g., toe to heel, side to side, and rotations—clockwise and then counterclockwise), first with touch-down contact of the board with the ground and then with no touch-down. The patient can use light touch-down support with fingertips on a wall or table. Alternatively, poles can be used for additional stability. The foot position (BOS) or type of board can be varied to increase or decrease the level of difficulty. A limited-motion board provides bidirectional challenges (Fig. 7.40); a dome board provides multidirectional challenges (Fig. 7.41). The profile of a domed-bottom board can be varied from low dome to high dome to increase the excursion and difficulty. Advanced activities include single-limb

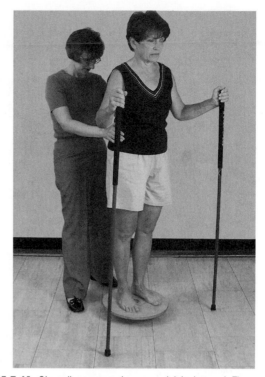

FIGURE 7.41 Standing on a dome wobble board. The patient stands centered on a multidirectional, dome wobble board, using two poles for support. The therapist instructs the patient to tilt the board backward and forward, side to side, or in circles. The dome board is more unstable than a bidirectional board; a low-dome board is more stable than a high-dome board. The therapist provides verbal cues and guarding.

stance and balloon tapping or catching and throwing a ball. The therapist should use appropriate safety precautions, guarding to prevent falls. See Appendix A for equipment sources.

Red Flag: These devices are inherently unstable. Gradual progression is indicated (e.g., from bidirectional board to low-dome board to high-dome board). The patient should be instructed to use caution when getting on and off the board and utilize support as needed. The feet should be positioned on the board using a wide stance, centrally located over the board. The area surrounding the board should be kept free of obstacles in case the patient needs to step off quickly. Finally, the patient should be instructed to keep his or her eyes focused directly in front on a target (looking down at the feet or the board may lead to loss of balance).

Foam Rollers

The patient can practice standing in neutral position on split foam rollers. For greatest stability, intially the flat sides are face down and the patient stands on two rollers with bilateral pole support (Fig. 7.42A). The activity can be progressed to standing with no pole support (Fig. 7.42B). As standing control improves, the flat side can be positioned face up to provide a mobile surface. The patient stands with support poles (Fig. 7.43A) progressiong to no pole support (Fig. 7.43B). Advanced activities include arm raises, head

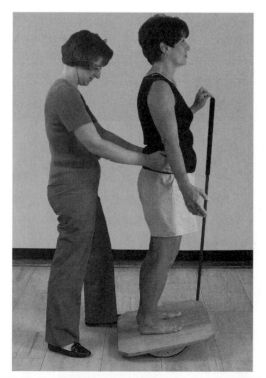

FIGURE 7.40 Standing on a wobble board. The patient stands centered on a bidirectional board, using one pole for support. The therapist instructs the patient to tilt the board backward and forward, moving from heels-down to toes-down position (activating ankle dorsiflexors and plantarflexors). The patient can also turn sideways, moving the board from side down to opposite side down positions (activating medial-lateral ankle muscles). The therapist provides verbal cues and guarding.

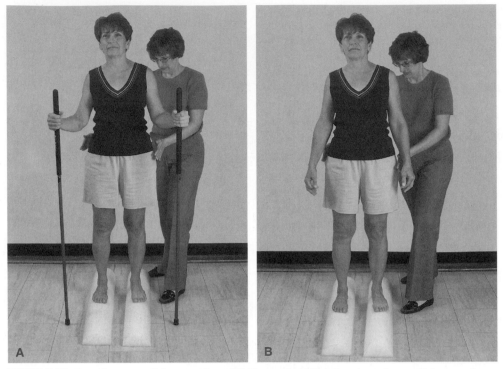

FIGURE 7.42 Standing on split foam rollers. **(A)** The patient first stands on two split foam rollers with the flat side down and holds support poles. **(B)** The activity is progressed to standing with no poles. The therapist provides verbal cues and guarding.

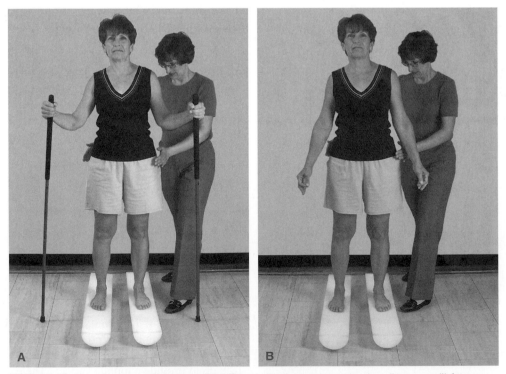

FIGURE 7.43 Standing on split foam rollers. The patient progresses to standing on split foam rollers, flat side up, **(A)** first with support poles and **(B)** then with no poles. This provides a more dynamic challenge to balance. The therapist provides verbal cueing and guarding.

and trunk rotations, catching and throwing a ball, and mini-squats. The therapist should use appropriate safety precautions, guarding to prevent falls.

Inflated Disc or Foam Pad

The patient can practice standing on a compliant surface such as an inflated disc (Dyna-Disc®, BOSU Balance Trainer®) (Fig. 7.44) or a closed cell foam pad (Airex Balance Pad®) (Fig. 7.45). The soft compliant surface requires continual adjustments by postural muscles (primarily foot/ankle muscles) to achieve stability on the device. Various activities can be performed while standing on the compliant surface (e.g., head turns, minisquats, bouncing compressions, single-leg stance [Fig. 7.46], marching, and throwing and catching a ball). Standing with EC significantly increases the level of difficulty and postural instability. EC eliminates visual support for balance; when EC is combined with already reduced somatosensory supports, the patient is left dependent on vestibular inputs for balance. See Appendix A for equipment sources.

Ball Activities

The patient stands with one foot flat on the floor and the other placed on a small ball. The patient actively rolls the ball (forward, backward, in circles) while maintaining upright balance using a single-limb stance. The therapist stands in front of the patient and guards as needed. The therapist can also stand in a mirror-image position with one foot placed on the same small ball. The therapist's foot is used to move the ball and stimulate reactive balance challenges for

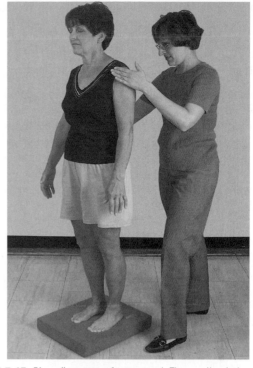

FIGURE 7.45 Standing on a foam pad. The patient stands on a dense foam pad with normal stance width. Balance is challenged by moving from EO to EC. The therapist provides verbal cueing and guarding.

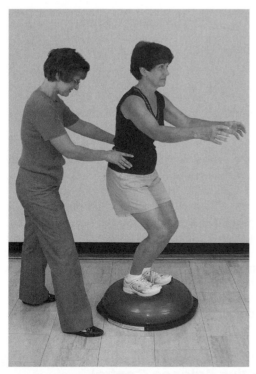

FIGURE 7.44 Standing on an inflated disc. The patient stands on an inflated dome (BOSU Trainer®) and performs minisquats. The therapist provides verbal cues and guarding.

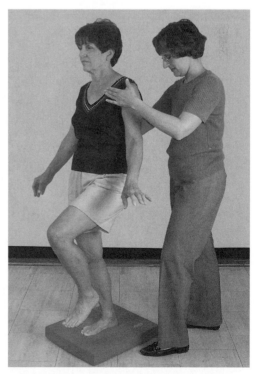

FIGURE 7.46 Marching on a foam pad. The patient stands on a dense foam pad, with EO progressing to EC. The patient performs alternating hip and knee flexion, marching in place. The therapist provides verbal cues and guarding.

the patient. Both the therapist and the patient can hold onto a wand for added stabilization (Fig. 7.47).

Promoting Balance Control Using Force-Platform Biofeedback

Force-platform biofeedback training devices (e.g., Biodex Balance System SD® [Fig. 7.48] or NeuroCom Balance Master®) can be used to provide center of pressure (COP) biofeedback. The weight on each foot is computed and converted into visual feedback regarding the locus and movement of the patient's COP. A computer provides data analysis and training modes using an interactive format. These devices can be used to improve postural symmetry (percent weightbearing and weight-shift training), postural stability (steadiness), LOS (total excursion), and postural sway movements (shaped and modified to enhance symmetry and steadiness).

Clinical Notes: Force-platform biofeedback is an effective training device for patients who demonstrate asymmetrical weightbearing. For example, the patient recovering from stroke typically stands with more weight on the less affected limb and needs to be instructed to shift weight toward the more affected side to assume a symmetrical stance position. COP biofeedback can be effective in improving symmetrical alignment.

Problems in force generation, producing either too much force (hypermetria) or too little force (hypometria),

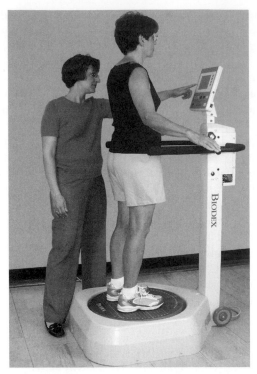

FIGURE 7.48 Standing, balancing on a force platform. The patient stands on a Biodex Balance Machine®. The therapist can select from two testing/training protocols: postural stability and dynamic limits of stability. During *postural stability,* the patient attempts to keep the board steady with centered alignment, with varying levels of difficulty of board tilt (platform perturbation). The machine calibrates the time in balance and provides a Stability Index. During *limits of stability,* the patient maintains centered balance and then, on signal, tilts the board (moving the cursor) to a predetermined box (range) and then moves the cursor back to centered alignment. Information is provided about patient excursion and accuracy in varied directions (limits of stability). The therapist provides verbal cues to direct the patient's attention to the biofeedback information provided.

can also be improved with force-platform biofeedback. For example, the patient with Parkinson's disease who demonstrates hypometric responses can be encouraged to achieve larger and faster sway movements using COP biofeedback. The patient with cerebellar pathology who demonstrates hypermetric responses can be encouraged to achieve smaller and smaller sway movements.

Red Flag: Learning that occurs as a result of practice on these devices is task-specific and should not be expected to transfer automatically to functional balance tasks (e.g., improved performance on sit-to-stand transfers, walking, or stair climbing). The *specificity of training rule* applies here. Practice of the specific functional balance tasks is required if balance performance is to be improved.

Activities and Strategies for Improving Adaptive Balance Control

Adaptive balance control refers to the ability to modify or change balance responses based on changing conditions

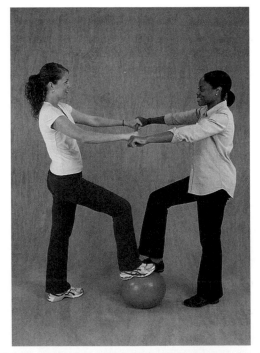

FIGURE 7.47 Single-limb standing: one foot on ball. The patient stands with one foot resting on a small ball positioned in front. The patient moves the ball (forward and back, side to side, and in circles) while balancing on the static limb. The therapist can also put one foot on the same ball (mirror-image position as shown) and move the ball, thereby requiring reactive balance strategies. Stability in a single-limb stance can be improved by having both the patient and the therapist hold onto a dowel.

(e.g., either task or environmental demands). These are sometimes referred to as *complex balance skills.* Interventions to promote adaptive balance control should therefore include a variety of challenges to balance, including task variations and environmental changes.

Task modifications should be gradual at the start, progressing to more significant challenges as control develops. In addition to general strategies for challenging standing control discussed in Box 7.2 (varying the BOS, the support surface, the use of UEs, and sensory inputs), the therapist can increase the challenge to balance control by manipulating the speed and range of the activity and by external pacing of the activity (using verbal cues [counting], manual cues [clapping], a metronome, or music with a consistent tempo [marching music]). Individual treatment sessions should combine some activities that are relatively easy for the patient with those that are more difficult. Effective practice schedules in which activity is

balanced with rest (distributed practice schedule) are indicated for most patients undergoing active rehabilitation and can improve patient responsiveness and overall performance. The patient should practice under close supervision at first and then progress to independent practice (e.g., HEP). An activity diary can be used to document practice sessions at home.

Environmental modifications should also be gradual at the start, progressing from a closed (fixed) environment with minimal distractions to a more open, variable (changing) environment. The patient practices first in the clinic environment (e.g., a quiet room or hallway, progressing to practice in a busy clinic gym). The patient then practices in simulated home, community, and work environments and finally in real-life environments (e.g., travel tests). Box 7.6 presents a comprehensive list of balance activities organized into three main groups: initial-level, intermediate-level, and advanced-level challenges.

BOX 7.6 Balance Activities Organized by Levels of Difficulty: Initial, Intermediate, and Advanced Challenges

Initial-Level Challenges to Balance
The following activities are appropriate for initial balance training for the patient with instability and significant disturbances in balance control.
Standing, back to the wall or corner standing, heels 4 inches (10 cm) from the wall; light touch-down support of both hands as needed:

• Maintained standing: Posture aligned to the wall, shoulders and hips touching the wall, head erect
• Altered visual input: EO to EC
• Altered BOS: Feet apart to feet together

Standing on the floor near the support surface (treatment table, parallel bars, or chair); light touch-down support of both hands:

• Weight shifts: Slow controlled weight shifts in all directions
• Look-arounds: Head and trunk rotation
• Head tilts: Head up and down, side to side
• Heel rises: Active plantarflexion
• Toe-offs: Active dorsiflexion
• Unilateral weightbearing: Single-leg stands
• Hip circles: Pelvic clock

Intermediate-Level Challenges to Balance
Standing on the floor near the support surface; light touch-down support of one hand progressing to no UE support:

• Heel-offs and toe-offs
• Single-leg stands
• Marching in place
• Partial lunges
• Alter surface: Stand on foam near a support surface; light touch-down support of one hand progressing to no UE support
• Altered BOS: Feet apart to feet together
• Altered visual inputs: EO to EC

• Chair rises: Sit-to-stand transfers, using varied seat heights progressing from high to low
• Arm circles: Forward and backward (shoulders abducted with elbows extended)
• Trunk and head rotation: UEs are raised to side horizontal (shoulders abducted to 90 degrees); patient twists trunk around in one direction and then to the other; combine with head turns to the same direction
• Functional reach: UE extended to forward horizontal position (shoulders flexed to 90 degrees), patient leans as far forward as possible without taking a step (as in the Functional Reach Test); activity can then be repeated backward and side to side

Advanced-Level Challenges to Balance
Standing on the floor with no UE support:

• Tandem stance (heel-toe position): EO progressing to EC (sharpened Romberg position)
• Single-leg stance
• Partial squats: Lifting an object off the floor
• Tracing the letters of the alphabet on the floor with great toe
• Kicking a ball
• Bouncing a ball
• Catching or throwing a ball: The weight and size of the ball can be varied
• Hitting (batting) a balloon
• Hitting a foam ball with a paddle
• Games that involve stooping and/or aiming: Bowling, shuffleboard, balloon volleyball
• Lunges to the full half-kneeling position
• Floor-to-standing transfers

Standing on a foam surface with no UE support:

• Tandem stance: EO progressing to EC
• Single-limb stance

Interventions to Improve Sensory Control of Balance

A complete sensory examination (somatosensory, visual, and vestibular) is necessary to determine which sensory systems are intact, which are disordered, and which are absent. CNS sensory integration mechanisms should also be examined (e.g., Clinical Test for Sensory Integration in Balance [CTSIB] or modified CTSIB). Intervention focuses on improving the function of individual systems and the interaction among systems.

Somatosensory Challenges

The patient stands on a firm, flat surface (floor) with reduced or compromised visual inputs, thereby increasing reliance on somatosensory inputs. Progression is to gradually increase the difficulty of the balance challenge while maintaining reliance on somatosensory inputs. This can be accomplished with the following activities and strategies:

- Standing, eyes open (EO) to EC
- Standing, full lighting to reduced lighting to dark room
- Standing, EO wearing lenses that reduce or distort vision (petroleum-coated goggles)
- Standing, with eyes engaged with a reading activity (a printed card held in front)
- Standing, with eyes reading a card held against a busy checkerboard pattern
- Marching in place, EC

Visual Challenges

The patient stands with reduced or compromised somatosensory inputs, thereby increasing the reliance on visual inputs. The patient should initially be instructed to keep the eyes focused on a stationary target directly in front of the patient. Progression is to increasing difficulty of the balance challenge while maintaining reliance on visual inputs.

This can be accomplished with the following activities and strategies:

- Standing on a compliant surface, EO; progressing from carpet (low pile to high pile) to foam cushion (firm density) of varying height (2 to 5 in. [5 to 12 cm])
- Standing on a moving surface (wobble board or foam roller), EO
- Marching in place on foam, EO

Vestibular Challenges

The patient stands with reduced or compromised visual and somatosensory inputs, thereby increasing the reliance on vestibular inputs. This is sometimes referred to as a *sensory conflict situation,* requiring resolution of the conflict by the vestibular system. This can be accomplished with the following activities and strategies:

- Standing on foam, EC
- Standing on foam with eyes engaged in reading task

- Standing on foam with vision distorted (petroleum-coated goggles)
- Tandem standing on foam, EC
- Marching in place on foam, EC

Compensatory Training

When significant postural and balance activity limitations persist, compensatory strategies are necessary to ensure patient safety. Cognitive strategies can be taught to substitute for missing automatic postural control. Sensory substitution strategies emphasize the use of more stable, reliable sensory inputs for balance. Assistive devices may be indicated to ensure patient safety and to prevent a fall. Compensatory balance strategies are presented in Box 7.7.

Clincial Note: If more than one sensory system is impaired, as in the patient with diabetes who has peripheral neuropathy as well as retinopathy, sensory compensatory strategies are generally inadequate. Some balance activity limitations will be evident.

Outcomes

Motor control goal: Improvement in all aspects of balance performance (anticipatory, reactive, and adaptive).

Functional skills achieved: The patient demonstrates appropriate functional balance during standing for all activities without loss of balance or falls.

Student Practice Activities in Standing

Sound clinical decision-making will guide identification of the most appropriate activities and techniques for an individual patient. Many of these interventions will provide the foundation for developing home management strategies to improve function. Although some of the interventions described clearly require the skilled intervention of a physical therapist, many can be modified or adapted for inclusion in an HEP for use by the patient (self-management strategies), family members, or other individuals participating in the patient's care.

Student practice activities provide an opportunity to share knowledge and skills as well as to confirm or clarify understanding of the treatment interventions. Each student in a group will contribute his or her understanding of, or questions about, the strategy, technique, or activity being discussed and demonstrated. Dialogue should continue until a consensus of understanding is reached.

Box 7.8 presents student practice activities focusing on the task analysis of standing. Box 7.9 presents student practice activities focusing on interventions to improve standing and standing balance control.

BOX 7.7 Compensatory Balance Strategies

The patient is taught to do the following:

- Widen the BOS when turning or sitting down
- Widen the BOS in the direction of an expected force (e.g., step position)
- Lower the COM when greater stability is needed (e.g., crouching when a threat to balance is imminent)
- Wear comfortable, well-fitting shoes with rubber soles for better friction and gripping (e.g., athletic shoes)
- Use light touch-down support as needed to increase somatosensory inputs and stability
- Use an assistive device as needed (e.g., a cane or walker) to provide support for standing
- Use a vertical or slant cane to increase somatosensory inputs from the hand

- Rely on intact senses, heightening patient awareness of available senses
- Use an augmented feedback device (e.g., auditory signals from a limb-load monitor or biofeedback cane) to provide additional sensory feedback information
- Recognize potentially dangerous environmental factors (e.g., low light or high glare for the patient who relies heavily on vision)
- Focus vision on a stationary visual target rather than a moving target
- Minimize head movements during more difficult balance tasks requiring vestibular inputs (sensory conflict situations)

BOX 7.8 STUDENT PRACTICE ACTIVITY: TASK ANALYSIS IN STANDING

OBJECTIVE: To analyze standing posture of healthy individuals.

EQUIPMENT NEEDS: Foam cushions and wobble boards (bidirectional and multidirectional [dome]).

PROCEDURE: Work in groups of two or three. Begin by having each person in the group stand in a symmetrical stance position, with feet apart and shoes and socks off. Then have each person stand with feet together, in tandem (heel-toe position); repeat on dense foam. In each condition, have the person begin with EO and progress to EC. Then have each person practice weight shifts to the LOS in all positions and conditions (feet apart, feet together, feet in tandem position while standing on the floor and on foam). Finally have each person stand on a wobble board, using both bidirectional and multidirectional (dome) boards. Have each person practice standing centered on the board (no tilts); then have each person practice slow tilts to each side.

OBSERVE AND DOCUMENT: Using the following questions to guide your analysis, observe and record the variations and similarities among the different standing patterns represented in your group.

- ▲ What is the person's normal standing alignment?
- ▲ What changes are noted between normal, feet together, tandem, on foam positions? EO to EC? Position of UEs?
- ▲ During weight shifts exploring the LOS, are the shifts symmetrical in each direction?
- ▲ During standing on a wobble board, how successful is the person at maintaining centered alignment on the board (no touch-down)? What are the positions of the UEs?
- ▲ What types of pathology/impairments might affect a patient's ability to achieve or maintain standing?
- ▲ What compensatory strategies might be necessary?
- ▲ What environmental factors might constrain or impair standing?
- ▲ What modifications are needed?

BOX 7.9 STUDENT PRACTICE ACTIVITY: INTERVENTIONS TO IMPROVE STANDING AND STANDING BALANCE CONTROL

OBJECTIVE: Sharing skill in the application and knowledge of strategies to promote improved standing.

EQUIPMENT NEEDS: Wobble boards (bidirectional and multidirectional dome), split foam rollers, inflated domes, poles, small balls (inflated and weighted), stacking cones, treatment table, water bottle and drinking cup, and force platform training device.

DIRECTIONS: Work in groups of three to four students. Below is an outline to guide practice, titled Activities

and Techniques to Improve Standing and Standing Balance Control. Members of the group will assume different roles (described below) and will rotate roles each time the group progresses to a new item in the outline.

- ▲ One person assumes the role of therapist (for demonstrations) and participates in discussion.
- ▲ One person serves as the subject/patient (for demonstrations) and participates in discussion.

(box continues on page 192)

BOX 7.9 STUDENT PRACTICE ACTIVITY: INTERVENTIONS TO IMPROVE STANDING AND STANDING BALANCE CONTROL (continued)

▲ The remaining members participate in task analysis of the activity and discussion. Following the demonstration, members should provide supportive and corrective feedback. One member of this group should be designated as a "fact checker" to return to the text content to confirm elements of the discussion (if needed) or if agreement cannot be reached.

Thinking aloud, brainstorming, and sharing thoughts should be continuous throughout this activity! As each item in the section outline is considered, the following should ensue:

1. An initial discussion of the *activity,* including patient and therapist positioning. Also considered here should be positional changes to enhance the activity (e.g., prepositioning a limb, altering the BOS, and so forth).
2. An initial discussion of the *technique,* including its description, indication(s) for use, therapist hand placements (manual contacts), and verbal cues.
3. A *demonstration* of the activity and application of the technique by the designated therapist and subject/patient. Discussion is limited during the demonstration, with constructive comments provided following the demonstration. All group members should provide supportive and corrective feedback, providing recommendations and suggestions for improvement. Particularly important is a discussion of strategies to make the activity either *more* or *less* challenging for the patient/subject.
4. If any member of the group feels he or she requires additional practice with the activity and technique, time should be allocated to accommodate the request.

Activities and Techniques to Improve Standing and Standing Balance Control

▲ Modified Plantigrade, Holding
 • Stabilizing reversals
 • Rhythmic stabilization
▲ Modified Plantigrade, Weight Shifts
 • Weight shifts, dynamic reversals: side to side, forward-backward, diagonal, diagonal with pelvic rotation
▲ Modified Plantigrade, Limb Movements
 • Reaching (cone stacking)
 • PNF UE D2 flexion and extension, dynamic reversals
▲ Standing, Holding
 • Stabilizing reversals
 • Rhythmic stabilization

▲ Standing, Weight Shifts
 • Weight shifts, dynamic reversals: side to side, forward backward, diagonal, diagonal with pelvic rotation
▲ Standing, Dynamic Limb Movements
 • UE lifts, LE lifts, marching, toe-offs, heel-offs, foot drawing, foot slides
 • Reaching, cone stacking
 • Single limb stance (active abduction into wall)
 • Partial wall squats (with ball)
▲ Standing, Stepping, Dynamic Reversals (forward-backward)
▲ Standing Lunges (partial, full, multidirectional)
▲ Floor-to-Standing Transfers
▲ Standing, Manual Perturbations
▲ Standing on Foam
 • EO to EC
 • Wide BOS to tandem stance to sharpened tandem to single limb stance
 • Minisquats
▲ Standing on Wobble Boards
 • Centered standing, bidirectional to multidirectional boards
 • Touch down, circles (clockwise, counterclockwise)
▲ Standing on Foam Rollers
 • Double to single rollers, flat side down to flat side up
▲ Standing on Inflated Dome (BOSO®)
 • Head and trunk turns
 • Minisquats
 • Double to single leg stance
 • Marching
 • UE activities: overhead lifts
 • Step-ups onto dome
▲ Standing, Ball Activities
 • Catching and throwing ball (inflated ball, weighted ball)
 • Batting a balloon; kicking a ball
 • Standing with one foot on a small ball and moving the ball (forward-backward, circles)
▲ Standing, Dual Task Activities
 • Pouring a glass of water from a pitcher
 • Counting backwards by 7 from 100
▲ Standing, Force Platform Training
 • Biofeedback training to improve centered alignment, LOS

SUMMARY

This chapter presented the foundational requirements of standing and standing balance control. Overall strategies to improve standing function focused on stability, controlled mobility, and balance skills. The level of challenge during standing may be modified by manipulating both the activity (task) and the environment. A variety of exercise interventions and progressions to enhance standing control were discussed. Multisensory training strategies focusing on modifiying somatosensory, visual, and vestibular influence on balance were also addressed. Finally, compensatory and safety strategies were discussed.

Equipment Sources

Balance Master®
NeuroCom International, Inc.
9570 SE Lawnfield Road
Clackamas, OR 97015
www.onbalance.com
800.767.6744

Balls
Ball Dynamics International, LLC
14215 Mead Street
Longmont, CO 80504
www.fitball.com
800.752.2255

Balls, Wobble Boards, Inflatable Discs, Foam Pads, and Rollers
Orthopedic Physical Therapy Products (OPTP)
3800 Annapolis Lane
Minneapolis, MN 55447
www.optp.com
800.367.7393

Biodex Balance System SD®
Biodex Medical Systems, Inc.
20 Ramsay Road
Shirley, NY 11967-4704
www.biodex.com
800.224.6339

BOSU Balance Trainer®
BOSU Fitness, LLC
3434 Midway Drive
San Diego, CA 92110
www.BOSU.com

Elastic Resistance Bands and Balls
Thera-Band®/Hygenic Performance Health
1245 Home Avenue
Akron, OH 44310-2575
www.thcra-band.com
800.321.2135

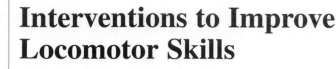

Interventions to Improve Locomotor Skills

THOMAS J. SCHMITZ, PT, PHD

"*Gait* is the manner in which a person walks, characterized by rhythm, cadence, step, stride, and speed. *Locomotion* is the ability to move from one place to another."
—*Guide to Physical Therapist Practice*[1](p64)

Human locomotion is a foundational component of independent function; it represents the final and highest level of motor control (skill). It involves highly coordinated movements that allow for adaptability to task demands and interaction with the environment. It is also a skill commonly affected by impairments and activity limitations. The result is that enhanced locomotor skill is an expected outcome for many patients seeking physical therapy intervention. The *Guide to Physical Therapist Practice*[1] includes elements of gait and locomotor training as an intervention category within each of the four preferred practice patterns.

This chapter focuses on interventions to improve locomotion. The foundational elements of successful human locomotion include: (1) the appropriate strength and control of the lower extremities (LEs) and trunk to support body mass; (2) the ability to generate locomotor rhythm; (3) dynamic balance control (the ability to maintain stability and orientation with the center of mass [COM] over the base of support [BOS] while parts of the body are in motion); (4) the propulsion of the body in the intended direction; and (5) the adaptability of locomotor responses to changing task and environmental demands.

Development of a plan of care (POC) to enhance gait and locomotor skills requires knowledge of the presenting pathology, the patient's weightbearing status, and impairments and activity limitations that affect movement. Although identification of specific tests and measures is based on the history and systems review, there are several examination areas of consistent importance to gait and locomotion. These include postural alignment and balance control, joint integrity and mobility, motor function (motor control and motor learning), muscle performance (strength, power, endurance), and range of motion (ROM). Examination of sensory function includes central sensory integration (the ability of the brain to organize, interpret, and use sensory information) and utilization of sensory cues for locomotor control. Another important consideration is the patient's ability to safely adapt or modify locomotor responses relative to changing task and environmental demands.

Gait: Cycle and Terminology

Gait Cycle

The *gait cycle* is the largest element used to describe human gait. It is divided into two phases: swing and stance, with two periods of double support. The *swing phase* is the portion of the cycle when the limb is off the ground and moving forward (or backward) to take a step (40 percent of the cycle). The *stance phase* is the portion of the cycle when the foot is in contact with the ground (60 percent of the cycle). The term *double support time* refers to the period when both feet are simultaneously in contact with the ground as weight is transferred from one foot to the other.

Gait Terminology

Traditional terminology subdivides the phases of the gait cycle as follows: (1) stance components include *heel strike, footflat, midstance, heel-off,* and *toe-off;* and (2) swing includes *acceleration, midswing,* and *deceleration.* The Los Amigos Research and Education Institute, Inc. (LAREI), of Rancho Los Amigos National Rehabilitation Center has developed different terminology that subdivides the phases of the gait cycle as follows: stance includes *initial contact, loading response, midstance, terminal stance,* and *preswing;* and swing includes *initial swing, midswing,* and *terminal swing.*[2] A comparison of the two sets of terminology is presented in Table 8.1 together with the normal muscle activation patterns that occur within each phase of gait. Table 8.2 presents common terminology used to describe the various parameters of gait.

Task Analysis

Recall that task analysis informs the therapist about the link between abnormal movement (patient-selected gait and locomotor strategies) and underlying impairments (e.g., diminished strength or ROM). The information helps identify the need for additional examination procedures and directs and guides the selection of interventions. Task analysis involving gait (e.g., observational gait analysis [OGA]) is perhaps the most common form of task analysis conducted by physical therapists. Although there are many approaches to gait analysis, the most common method used to organize and structure the OGA is most likely the Rancho Los Amigos Observational Gait Analysis system.[2]

Critical to performing a gait analysis is knowledge of the normal kinematics and kinetics of human gait. This requires the ability to deconstruct normal gait into its component skills and variables to establish a normative reference

TABLE 8.1 Overview of Gait Terminology and Normal Muscle Activation Patterns

Stance Phase		
Traditional	**Rancho Los Amigos**	**Muscle Activation Pattern**
Heel strike: The beginning of the stance phase when the heel contacts the ground (the same as initial contact).	***Initial contact:*** The beginning of the stance phase when the heel or another part of the foot contacts the ground.	Quadriceps active at heel strike through early stance to control small amount of knee flexion for shock absorption; pretibial group acts eccentrically to oppose plantarflexion moment and prevent foot slap.
Foot flat: Occurs immediately following heel strike, when the sole of the foot contacts the floor. (This event occurs during the loading response.)	***Loading response:*** The portion of the first double support period of the stance phase from initial contact until the contralateral extremity leaves the ground.	The gastrocnemius-soleus muscles are active from foot flat through midstance to eccentrically control forward tibial advancement.
Midstance: The point at which the body passes directly over the reference extremity.	***Midstance:*** The portion of the single-limb support stance phase that begins when the contralateral extremity leaves the ground and ends when the body is directly over the supporting limb.	The hip, knee, and ankle extensors are active throughout the stance phase to oppose antigravity forces and stabilize the limb; hip extensors control forward motion of the trunk; hip abductors stabilize the pelvis during unilateral stance; plantarflexors propel the body forward.
Heel-off: The point following midstance at which time the heel of the reference extremity leaves the ground. (Heel-off occurs prior to terminal stance.)	***Terminal stance:*** The last portion of the single-limb support stance phase that begins with heel rise and continues until the contralateral extremity contacts the ground.	Peak activity of the plantarflexors occurs just after heel-off, to push off and generate forward propulsion of the body.
Toe off: The point following heel-off when only the toe of the reference extremity is in contact with the ground.	***Preswing:*** The portion of the stance phase that begins the second double support period from the initial contact of the contralateral extremity to lift off of the reference extremity.	Hip and knee extensors (hamstrings and quadriceps) contribute to forward propulsion with a brief burst of activity.
Swing Phase		
Traditional	**Rancho Los Amigos**	**Muscle Activation Pattern**
Acceleration: The portion of the swing phase beginning from the moment the toe of the reference extremity leaves the ground to the point when the reference extremity is directly under the body.	***Initial swing:*** The portion of the swing phase from the point when the reference extremity leaves the ground to maximum knee flexion of the same extremity.	Forward acceleration of the limb during early swing is achieved through the action of the quadriceps; by midswing the quadriceps are silent and pendular motion is in effect; hip flexors (the iliopsoas) aid in forward limb propulsion.
Midswing: The portion of the swing phase when the reference extremity passes directly below the body. Midswing extends from the end of acceleration to the beginning of deceleration.	***Midswing:*** The portion of the swing phase from maximum knee flexion of the reference extremity to a vertical tibial position.	Foot clearance is achieved by contraction of the hip and knee flexors and the ankle dorsiflexors.

(table continues on page 196)

TABLE 8.1 Overview of Gait Terminology and Normal Muscle Activation Patterns *(continued)*

	Stance Phase	
Traditional	Rancho Los Amigos	Muscle Activation Pattern
Deceleration: The portion of the swing phase when the reference extremity is decelerating in preparation for heel strike.	***Terminal swing:*** The portion of the swing phase from a vertical position of the tibia of the reference extremity to just prior to initial contact.	The hamstrings act during late swing to decelerate the limb in preparation for heel strike; the quadriceps and ankle dorsiflexors become active in late swing to prepare for heel strike.

Adapted from Norkin, CC: Examination of Gait. In O'Sullivan, SB, and Schmitz, TJ (eds): Physical Rehabilitation, ed 5, FA Davis, Philadelphia, 2007, p 317, with permission.

TABLE 8.2 Common Gait Terminology

Acceleration	The rate of change of velocity with respect to time.
Cadence	Normal cadence is the number of steps taken per unit of time; the normal range for cadence is 91 to 138 steps per minute. Increased cadence is accompanied by a shorter step length and decreased duration of the period of double support. Running occurs when the period of double support disappears, typically at a cadence of 180 steps per minute.
Double Support Time	The time period of the gait cycle when both lower extremities are in contact with the supporting surface (double support); measured in seconds.
Foot Angle (degree of toe-out or toe-in)	Degree of toe-out or toe-in; the angle of foot placement with respect to the line of progression; measured in degrees. *Note*: Increased foot angle (turning the foot outward) is often associated with decreased postural stability.
Rhythm	Consistency of gait cycle duration (stride time) from one stride to the next.
Stance Time	The duration of the stance phase of one extremity in the gait cycle.
Single-Limb Time	The time period of the gait cycle when only one limb is in contact with the floor or other support surface.
Step Length	The linear distance between the point of heel strike of one extremity and the point of heel strike of the opposite extremity (in centimeters or meters).
Step Time	The number of seconds that elapse during a single (one) step.
Step Width	The distance between feet (base of support), measured from one heel to the same point on the opposite heel; normal step width ranges between 1 inch (2.5 cm) and 5 inches (12.5 cm). Step width increases as stability demands rise (for example, in older adults or very young children).
Stride Length	The linear distance between two consecutive points of foot contact (preferably heel strike) of the same extremity (in centimeters or meters).
Stride Time	The number of seconds that elapse during one stride (one complete gait cycle).
Stride Width	The side-to-side distance between the two feet. Step width is increased with instability.
Swing Time	The duration of the swing phase of one extremity in the gait cycle.
Velocity (speed)	Also called walking speed, the distance covered per unit of time (meters/second). Average walking speed is 2.2 to 2.8 mph [0.98 to 1.3 m/s].* Speed is increased by lengthening stride. Speed or velocity is affected by physical characteristics such as height, weight, and gender; it decreases with age, physical disability, and so forth.

*Some estimates of average walking speed are higher (e.g., 3.5 to 4 mph [1.6 to 1.8 m/s]).

for movement patterns and joint positions. Therapists typically acquire this skill by performing repeated OGA of normal subjects using a segmental approach beginning with the foot/ankle and moving up to the knee, hip, pelvis, and trunk. Once established, the normative reference provides the basis for identification of deviations from the norm. For a comprehensive handling of gait analysis including gait variables and common gait deviations, the reader is referred to the work of Norkin.[3]

Although the following list is not all-inclusive, data from the gait analysis assist the therapist with[1,3]:

- Identifying patient gait characteristics that deviate from a normative reference as well as their possible causes. Box 8.1 presents some of the more common gait deviations as well as their possible causes.
- Establishing the physical therapy diagnosis and prognosis (the predicted level of improvement).

- Developing an appropriate POC to address gait impairments.
- Determining the need for assistive, adaptive, or protective equipment and orthotic or prosthetic devices.
- Examining the effectiveness and fit of the devices or equipment selected.
- Promoting improved function.

Walking: Interventions, Outcomes, and Management Strategies

Prerequisite Requirements

The foundational prerequisite requirements for the initiation of interventions to improve locomotor skills include appropriate weightbearing status, musculoskeletal (postural) alignment, ROM, muscle performance (strength, power, and endurance),

---

BOX 8.1 Common Gait Deviations

Trunk, Pelvis, and Hip: Stance Phase
Common gait deviations involving the trunk, pelvis, and hip that occur during the stance phase include the following:

- *Lateral trunk bending*—the result of gluteus medius weakness; bending occurs to the same side as the weakness.
- *Trendelenburg gait*—the pelvis drops on the contralateral side of a weak gluteus medius; a compensatory strategy is lateral trunk bending.
- *Backward trunk lean*—the result of a weak gluteus maximus; the patient also has difficulty going up stairs or ramps.
- *Forward trunk lean*—the result of weak quadriceps (the forward trunk lean decreases the flexor moment at the knee); may also be associated with hip and knee flexion contractures.
- *Excessive hip flexion*—the result of weak hip extensors or tight hip and/or knee flexors.
- *Limited hip extension*—the result of tight or spastic hip flexors.
- *Limited hip flexion*—the result of weak hip flexors or tight extensors.
- *Antalgic gait* (painful gait)—stance time is abbreviated on the painful limb, resulting in an uneven gait pattern (limping); the uninvolved limb has a shortened step length, since it must bear weight sooner than normal.

Knee: Stance Phase
Common gait deviations involving the knee during the stance phase include the following:

- *Excessive knee flexion*—the result of weak quadriceps (the knee wobbles or buckles) or knee flexor contractures; the patient also has difficulty going down

stairs or ramps; forward trunk bending can compensate for weak quadriceps.
- *Hyperextension*—the result of weak quadriceps, plantarflexion contracture, or extensor spasticity (quadriceps and/or plantarflexors).

Foot/Ankle: Stance Phase
Common gait deviations involving the ankle/foot during the stance phase include the following:

- *Toes first*—at initial contact, the toes touch the floor first—the result of weak dorsiflexors, spastic or tight plantarflexors; toes first may also be due to a shortened LE (leg-length discrepancy), a painful heel, or a positive support reflex.
- *Foot slap*—the foot makes floor contact with an audible slap—the result of weak dorsiflexors or hypotonia; the slap is compensated for with a *steppage gait*.
- *Foot flat*—the entire foot contacts the ground—the result of weak dorsiflexors, limited range of motion, or an immature gait pattern.
- *Excessive dorsiflexion with uncontrolled forward motion of the tibia*—the result of weak plantarflexors.
- *Excessive plantarflexion* (equinus gait)—the heel does not touch the ground—the result of spasticity or contracture of the plantarflexors; eccentric contraction is poor, as in tibia advancement.
- *Varus foot*—at foot contact, the lateral side of the foot touches first; the foot may remain in varus throughout the stance phase—the result of spastic anterior tibialis or weak peroneals.
- *Claw toes*—the result of spastic toe flexors, possibly a plantar grasp reflex.
- *Inadequate push-off*—the result of weak plantarflexors, decreased range of motion, or pain in the forefoot.

(box continues on page 198)

BOX 8.1 Common Gait Deviations (continued)

Trunk, Pelvis, and Hip: Swing Phase

Common gait deviations involving the trunk, pelvis, and hip that occur during the swing phase include the following:

- *Insufficient forward pelvic rotation* (pelvic retraction)—the result of weak abdominal muscles and/or weak hip flexor muscles (for example, in the patient with stroke).
- *Insufficient hip and knee flexion*—the result of weak hip and knee flexors or strong extensor spasticity, resulting in an inability to lift the LE and move it forward.
- *Circumducted gait:* the LE swings out to the side (abduction/external rotation followed by adduction/internal rotation)—the result of weak hip and knee flexors.
- *Hip hiking* (quadratus lumborum action)—a compensatory response for weak hip and knee flexors, or extensor spasticity.
- *Excessive hip and knee flexion* (steppage gait)—a compensatory response to a shorten contralateral lower limb or the result of same side dorsiflexor weakness (e.g., resulting from neuritis of the peroneal nerve in the patient with diabetes).
- *Abnormal synergistic activity or spasticity* (e.g., the patient with stroke):
  - Use of a strong flexor synergy pattern—excessive abduction with hip and knee flexion.
  - Use of a strong extension synergy pattern—excessive adduction with hip and knee extension and ankle plantarflexion (scissoring); more commonly seen.

- *Decreased amplitude in trunk and pelvic rotation*—seen in the elderly and characteristic of several known neurological disorders (e.g., the patient with stroke or Parkinson's disease).

Knee: Swing Phase

Common gait deviations involving the knee that occur during the swing phase include the following:

- *Insufficient knee flexion*—the result of extensor spasticity, pain, decreased range of motion, or weak hamstrings.
- *Excessive knee flexion*—the result of flexor spasticity; flexor withdrawal reflex.

Foot/Ankle: Swing Phase

Common gait deviations involving the ankle and foot that occur during the swing phase include the following:

- *Foot-drop* (equinus)—the result of weak or delayed contraction of the dorsiflexors or spastic plantarflexors.
- *Varus or inverted foot*—the result of spastic invertors (anterior tibialis), weak peroneals, or an abnormal synergistic pattern (e.g., in the patient with stroke).
- *Equinovarus*—the result of spasticity of the posterior tibialis and/or gastrocnemius/soleus; or structural deformity (club foot).

---

motor function, balance, and static and dynamic standing control. Many of these prerequisites are dependent on intact neuromuscular synergies (necessary for static and dynamic control), intact sensory (somatosensory, visual, and vestibular) systems, and intact central nervous system (CNS) sensory integration mechanisms. Also required is the ability to safely stand while engaged in upper extremity (UE) functional movements (e.g., reaching) under varying environmental demands (dual-task activity).

Activity: Walking Forward and Backward

The patient practices walking forward and backward as a progression from stepping in place (standing and stepping). The therapist focuses on appropriate timing and sequencing, beginning with the weight shift diagonally forward or backward onto the stance limb and pelvic rotation with advancement of the swing limb. It is important to ensure that knee extension (not hyperextension) occurs with hip flexion during forward progression and that knee flexion occurs with hip extension during backward progression. The movements are repeated to allow for a continuous movement sequence.

Manual contacts can be used to guide movements and facilitate missing elements. For example, the therapist can facilitate forward pelvic rotation during swing by placing the hands on the anterior pelvis. This is an effective strategy for managing a retracted and elevated pelvis, a problem that exists for many patients with LE spasticity. For backward progression, the therapist's hand can be placed posteriorly over the gluteal muscles to facilitate hip extension and weight acceptance on the stance limb. This also helps to prevent the knee on the stance limb from hyperextending.

Verbal Cues for Walking Forward and Backward

Forward progression: *"Shift forward, and step, step, step."* Backward progression: *"Shift backward, and step, step, step."*

To progress the activity of walking forward and backward, the therapist can do the following:

- Alter the level of assistance or supervision by progressing from walking next to parallel bars or a wall to unassisted walking.
- Increase the step length from initially reduced to normal.
- Change the speed of walking from reduced to normal to increased. This can include both treadmill and overground walking.

Clinical Note: As the speed of walking increases, so do the requirements for timing and control. In general, older adults will demonstrate reduced walking speed compared to younger adults.

- Modify the BOS from feet apart (wide base) to normal to feet close together (narrow base) to tandem walking (heel-to-toe pattern).
- Vary the acceleration or deceleration by having the patient practice stopping and starting or turning on cue.
- Include dual-task walking, such as walking and talking, walking and turning the head (right or left and up or down), and walking and bouncing a ball.
- Alter the environment by (1) varying the walking surface from flat to carpeted to irregular (outdoors); (2) including anticipatory timing demands, such as the time required to cross a street at a stoplight; and (3) including goal-directed leisure or occupational requirements (return-to-work skills).

Clinical Notes: In the presence of UE flexor spasticity, tone may be reduced by muscle elongation and sustained stretch using an inhibitory pattern. Initially, the therapist slowly moves the limb into the lengthened range while gently rotating (rocking) the limb back and forth (rhythmic rotation). Once full range is gained, the therapist maintains the elongated position using an inhibitory pattern in which the shoulder is extended, abducted, and externally rotated with the elbow, wrist, and fingers extended.

Upright or vertical alignment with adequate control of head/trunk extension is important for postural alignment and balance during walking. Shortening of hip and knee flexors and hip extensor weakness should be addressed in the POC. The patient who demonstrates a kyphotic posture and looks continually down at the feet should be instructed to *"Look up"* at a target (placed directly in front of the patient). Vertical walking poles can also be used to assist upright posture while walking.

Techniques and Verbal Cues

Resisted Progression

This is an ideal technique to facilitate lower trunk and pelvic motion. The therapist is positioned standing either in front of (Fig. 8.1A) or behind (Fig. 8.1B) the patient. An alternative position for the therapist is sitting on a rolling stool. As the patient moves forward, the therapist also moves in a reverse or mirror-image of the patient's movements. The therapist provides maintained resistance to the forward or backward progression by placing both hands on the pelvis. Resistance should be light (facilitatory) to encourage proper timing of the pelvic movements. Approximation can be applied down through the top of the pelvis to promote stabilizing responses as weight is taken on the stance limb. A stretch to the pelvic rotators can be added as needed to facilitate the initiation of the pelvic motion. An alternative position for manual contacts is on the pelvis and contralateral shoulder.

Verbal Cues for Resisted Progression, Walking Forward and Backward

Overall timing of locomotion can be facilitated with appropriate verbal cues. Forward progression: *"On three, I want you to step forward, beginning with your right leg. One, two, three and step, step, step."* Backward progression: *"On three, I want you to step backward, beginning with your left leg. One, two, three and step, step, step."*

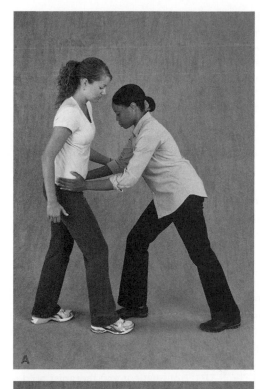

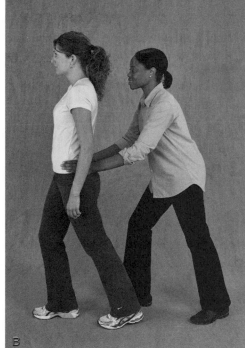

FIGURE 8.1 Using the technique of resisted progression, manual contacts are on the pelvis as the patient moves both **(A)** forward and **(B)** backward. Stretch, approximation, and light resistance are applied manually to facilitate lower trunk and pelvic motion.

Ø **Red Flag:** Problems can arise if the therapist's movements are not synchronized with the patient's. The pacing of the activity is dependent on the timing of the therapist's verbal cues. Movements can become uncoordinated or out of synchronization if the manual resistance on the pelvis is too great. The patient will feel as if he or she is "walking uphill" and may respond with exaggerated movements of the trunk (e.g., forward head and trunk flexion). This defeats the overall purposes of facilitated walking—that is, to improve timing and sequencing of gait and to decrease effort.

Comments

- For the application of resisted progression during forward and backward walking, resistance may also be applied using an elastic resistive band wrapped around the patient's pelvis. The therapist holds the resistive band either from behind as the patient moves forward (Fig. 8.2A) or from the front as the patient moves backward (Fig. 8.2B).
- To promote reciprocal arm swing and trunk counterrotation, two wooden poles (dowels) may be used. The therapist is positioned either behind as the patient walks forward (Fig. 8.3A) or in front as the patient walks backward (Fig. 8.3B). Both patient and therapist hold onto the poles. The therapist is then able to assist in sequencing the arm swings and guide trunk counterrotation during forward and backward progressions. Similarly, reciprocal arm swing and trunk counterrotation can be promoted using elastic resistive bands and application of light resistance (this activity requires two resistive bands of approximately the same length). The ends of the bands are held bilaterally by both patient and therapist, allowing the therapist to assist and guide movement as well as apply light facilitatory resistance. This is a particularly useful activity for patients with Parkinson's disease who frequently demonstrate reduced trunk rotation and arm swing.

Outcomes

Motor control goal: Skill.

Functional skill achieved: The patient is able to ambulate independently with appropriate timing and sequencing of movement components.

Indications Indications include impaired timing and sequencing of locomotor movement components.

Activity: Walking, Side-Stepping

Techniques and Verbal Cues

Resisted Progression

The patient practices walking sideways. The side-step involves abduction and placement of the dynamic limb to the side (Fig. 8.4A). The remaining limb is then moved parallel to the first *("Step together")*. Abductors are active on both the dynamic limb (to move the limb) and the static limb (to keep the pelvis level). For the application of resisted progression, the therapist is positioned (with a wide BOS) at

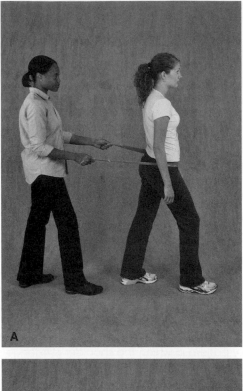

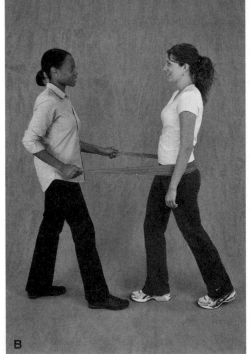

FIGURE 8.2 During **(A)** forward and **(B)** backward walking progressions, resistance may be applied using an elastic resistive band wrapped around the patient's pelvis.

the side of the patient's abducting limb. Manual resistance is applied on the lateral aspect of the pelvis on the side of the abducting limb. The therapist may also apply resistance by standing on the stance side and holding an elastic resistive band wrapped around the lateral aspect of the pelvis on the abducting side. The therapist is positioned on the side opposite the abducting limb (Fig. 8.4B).

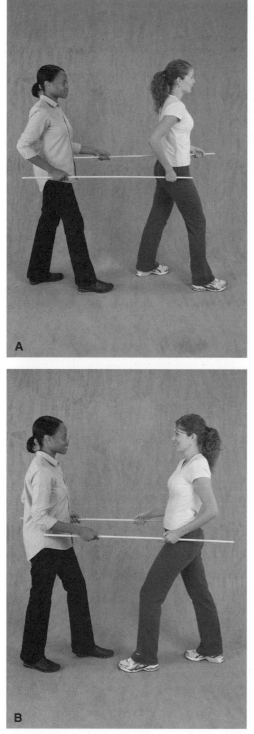

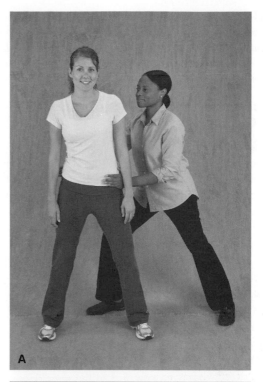

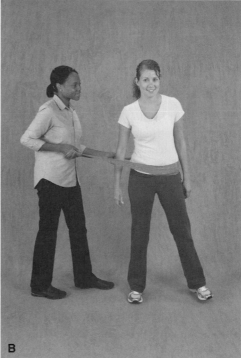

FIGURE 8.3 Wooden dowels held by both the patient and the therapist can be used to promote reciprocal arm swing and trunk counterrotation in either a **(A)** forward or **(B)** backward progression. This allows the therapist to assist in sequencing and guiding arm swing and trunk counterrotation.

FIGURE 8.4 Walking, side-stepping, resisted progression. *Not shown:* The patient is in a comfortable stance position to begin side-stepping. **(A)** The patient side-steps by moving the left LE into abduction. *Not shown:* The patient then moves the right LE parallel to the left (step together). **(B)** Resisted progression can also be implemented using a resistive band wrapped around the lateral aspect of the pelvis on the abducting side.

Verbal Cues for Walking, Side-Stepping, Resisted Progression
"On three, step out to the side, beginning with your left leg, and then step together with the opposite leg. And again, step out to side; then step together."

Activity: Walking, Side-Stepping and Crossed-Stepping

Strategies and Verbal Cues
Side-stepping involves abduction of the leading dynamic limb with foot placement followed by movement of the remaining limb to a parallel position with the first (a symmetrical stance). Emphasis should be placed on keeping the pelvis level. Following the initial side-step (Fig. 8.5A), crossed-stepping involves moving the opposite leg up, across, and in front of the original side-step leg (Fig. 8.5B). The movements are then repeated to allow for a continuous movement sequence. The therapist is positioned behind the patient. Movements can be guided and facilitated using manual contacts on the pelvis. A progression can then be made to the application of resistance (resisted progression) with manual contacts on the pelvis and thigh.

Verbal Cues for Walking, Side-Stepping and Crossed-Stepping
"On three, step out to the side, beginning with your left leg; then step up and across with the right leg. And again, step out to the side and up and across."

Outcomes
Motor control goal: Skill.
Functional skill achieved: The patient is able to walk sideways independently with appropriate timing and sequencing of movement components (required for movement in confined areas).

Indications Hip abductor weakness is an indication. These activities facilitate the protective side-steps (stepping strategy) needed to regain balance.

Activity: Walking, Braiding

Strategies and Verbal Cues
The patient begins with a side-step (Fig. 8.6A), followed by a crossed-step up and across in front (Fig. 8.6B) (the LE moves in a PNF LE D1F pattern). This sequence is followed by another side-step (Fig. 8.6C), then a crossed-step backward and behind the first limb (Fig. 8.6D) (the LE moves in a PNF LE D2E pattern). The movements are repeated to allow for a continuous movement sequence. The therapist is behind the patient in a guard position.

    Braiding is a highly coordinated sequence that is difficult for many patients to learn. The therapist can facilitate learning by standing in front of the patient and modeling the desired steps. Initially, the patient may require light touch-down support of both hands in modified plantigrade position (supported standing). A treatment table, the outside of the

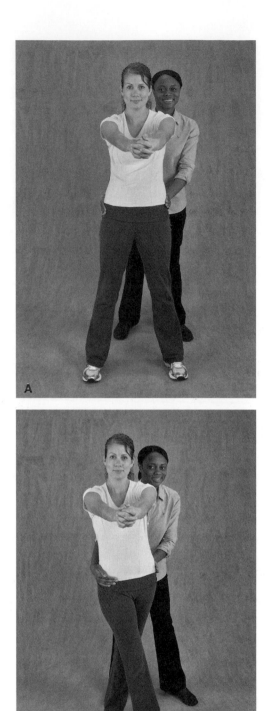

FIGURE 8.5 Walking, side-stepping and crossed-stepping. *Not shown:* To begin, the patient is in a comfortable stance position. **(A)** The left leading LE is abducted with foot placement (side-step). **(B)** The right LE is then moved up and over the opposite limb (crossed-step).

parallel bars (or oval parallel bars), or a wall can be used as the support surface.

    Alternatively, touch-down support can be provided by having the therapist place both hands directly in front, with the elbows flexed and forearms supinated, and having the

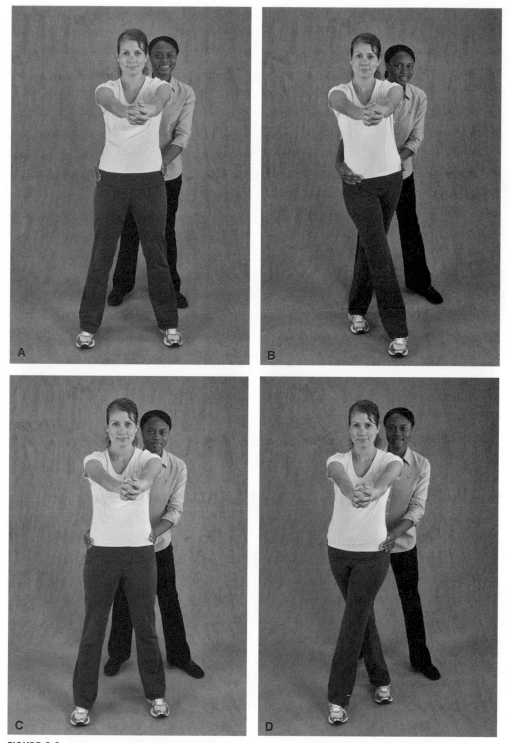

FIGURE 8.6 Walking, braiding. *Not shown:* To begin, the patient is in a comfortable stance position. **(A)** The patient side-steps with the left LE. **(B)** The right LE is then crossed up and over in front. **(C)** The left LE side-steps. **(D)** The right LE then cross-steps back and behind.

patient lightly place his or her hands on top of the therapist's hands. A wooden dowel held horizontally by both the therapist and patient can also be used to provide support (Fig. 8.7). For these activities, the patient and therapist face each other and move in unison.

Verbal Cues for Walking, Braiding

"Step out to the side; now step up and across; step out to the side; now step back and behind." Verbal cues should be well timed to ensure a continuous movement sequence.

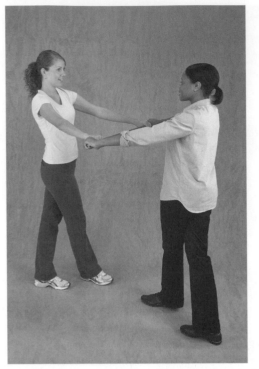

FIGURE 8.7 Walking, braiding. Support can be provided using a wooden dowel held horizontally by both the patient and the therapist. The patient and therapist face each other and move together.

Resisted Progression

The therapist is behind the patient, standing slightly to the side in the direction of the movement. As the patient moves sideward in braiding, the therapist moves in the same sequence and timing with the patient. The therapist provides maintained resistance to the sideward progression by placing one hand on the side of the pelvis. The other hand alternates, first on the anterior pelvis resisting the forward pelvic motion and crossed-step in front. It then moves to the posterior pelvis to resist the backward pelvic motion and crossed-step behind. Resistance should be light (facilitatory) to encourage proper timing of the pelvic movements. If needed, a quick stretch to the pelvic rotators can be added to facilitate the initiation of the pelvic motion.

Outcomes

Motor control goal: Skill.

Functional skill achieved: The patient ambulates independently using complex stepping patterns.

Indications Resisted progression can be used to facilitate lower trunk rotation and LE patterns in combination with upright postural control as well as to promote protective stepping strategies for balance.

Activity: Stair Climbing

Prerequisite Requirements

Important lead-up activities for stair climbing include: bridging, sit-to-stand transfers, kneeling-to-heel-sitting transitions, partial squats, and stepping activities.

Strategies and Verbal Cues

Normal stair climbing involves a step-over-step pattern. The patient transfers weight onto the stance limb and lifts the dynamic limb up and onto the step. Weight is then transferred onto this limb as it extends and moves the body up and onto the step. Quadriceps and gastrocnemius activity powers the elevation of the body. Walking down stairs involves a similar weight transfer onto the stance limb with an accompanying eccentric contraction of hip and knee extensors to lower the body to the next step. Weight is then transferred onto this limb as it extends and accepts weight. The patient needs to shift weight diagonally forward over the stepping limb. The therapist should watch for, and prevent, excessive trunk bending. The sequence is repeated to allow for completion of a set of steps. UE support using a handrail is typically needed during early stair climbing training to steady the body. The patient should not be allowed to pull the body up the stairs. Progression should be from light touch-down support to no UE support.

Verbal Cues for Walking, Stair Climbing

"Alternate shifting weight over one leg and stepping with the other. Now, shift and step up, shift and step up again."

For some patients, stepping practice will be indicated prior to stair climbing. Initial practice can be accomplished using a low-rise step (4 in. [10 cm]) placed in front of the patient with progression to higher steps and finally to a normal-rise step (7 in. [17.5 cm]) (Fig. 8.8). Commercially available small interlocking aerobic steps are effective for this purpose. This activity requires diagonal weight shifts toward the support limb to free the dynamic limb for placement on the step. The therapist provides assistance as needed. Assistance with the diagonal weight shifts may be required and can be accomplished by manual contacts placed on the patient's pelvis.

Clinical Note: Having the patient clasp both hands together with shoulder flexion and elbow extension may be helpful in initially facilitating forward weight transfer (this positioning is also effective for inhibiting UE spasticity). In addition, knee extensors may require assistance. The therapist can guide and assist extension using a manual contact directly over the lower thigh and pressing downward over the quadriceps. During descent, the therapist can guide the correct foot placement and again provide stimulation over the quadriceps.

Outcomes

Motor control goal: Skill.

Functional skills achieved: The patient ambulates independently up and down stairs and ambulates independently in the community up and down curbs.

Indications

An indication is the impaired ability to transfer weight onto the stance limb and simultaneously lift the opposite dynamic limb up and onto a step.

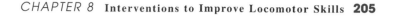

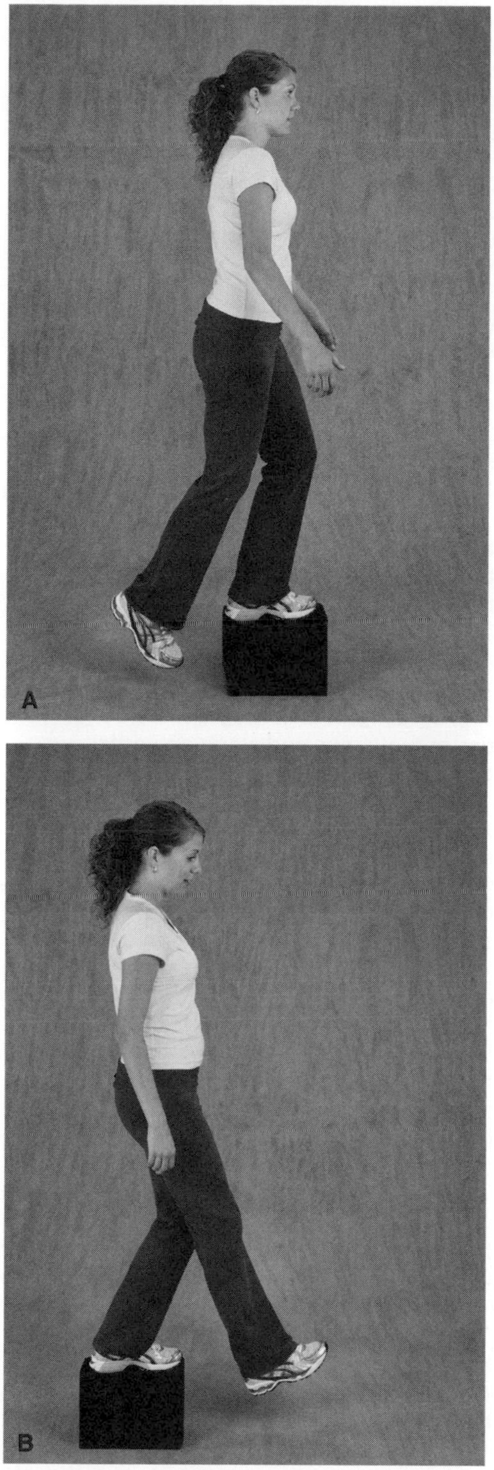

FIGURE 8.8 Step-ups and step-downs. Initial practice in preparation for stair climbing can be accomplished using a step placed directly in front of the patient. *Not shown:* To begin, the patient is in a comfortable stance position. **(A)** The patient then weight shifts laterally toward the support limb and places the dynamic left limb on the step. This is followed by the right limb moving up to the step. *Not shown:* Both feet are now positioned on the step. **(B)** The patient again weight shifts toward the support limb and steps down, leading with the right limb. A progression is to stepping up and down without the interval of double support (i.e., both feet on the step).

Clinical Note: Marked weakness of hip and knee extensors and ankle plantarflexors may preclude stair climbing until adequate gains in strength are achieved.

Strategies for Varying Locomotor Task Demands

Locomotion is an automatic postural activity. Neural control originates from subcortical and spinal centers (spinal pattern generators). The cerebellum and cortex adapt locomotion to specific task demands and environmental changes and correct motor patterns. Later-stage locomotor intervention strategies using distracters such as ongoing conversation or dual-task activities can provide confirmation of a developing level of autonomous control.

Varying locomotor task demands is also critical to establishing adaptability and *resistance to contextual change.* This refers to the patient's ability to maintain the same quality of locomotor skills with task variations or in new or altered environments. For example, a patient who has learned a new locomotor skill in one environment (e.g., walking on indoor level surfaces with a cane) can apply the skill in different environmental contexts (e.g., walking in a shopping mall or on outdoor surfaces). Since learning is task- and environment-specific, practice should include high levels of variation in both task demands and the environments in which they are practiced. Examples of strategies to vary locomotor task demands follow; additional examples are presented in Box 8.2. Box 8.3 offers sample strategies for varying environmental demands.

- Walking with cues for head turns, such as *"Look right," "Look left," "Look up,"* and *"Look down"* (Fig. 8.9)
- Walking with cues for speed changes, such as *"Walk slow"* and *"Walk fast"*
- Walking with cues for directional changes and abrupt starts and stops, such as *"Turn right," "Turn left," "Pivot 360 degrees," "Stop,"* and *"Start"*
- Walking with an external pacing device such as a metronome or personal listening device using marching music to increase speed and improve rhythm
- Walking on varied indoor surfaces, such as tile, wood flooring, and carpeting; difficulty can be increased by having the patient step on and off inflatable discs or foam pads placed strategically on the floor (Fig. 8.10)
- Walking through an obstacle course, over and around obstacles (Fig. 8.11), or over a floor grid to improve foot placement
- Dual-task activities such as the following:
  - Walking while engaged in a conversation (Walkie-Talkie test) or a cognitive task (e.g., counting backward by 7s from 100)
  - Walking while holding a ball and moving it side to side with outstretched arms (Fig. 8.12)
  - Walking while holding a tray or carrying a grocery bag or laundry basket
  - Walking while catching and throwing a lightly weighted ball or balloon

(text continues on page 208)

BOX 8.2 Strategies for Varying Locomotor Task Demands

Upright Postural Alignment
- Practice walking upright; the therapist assists the patient in vertical trunk posture using manual and verbal cues, such as *"Look up and stand tall."*
- Use long poles or a body weight support harness to promote upright alignment and reduce UE support, forward head, and flexed trunk position (common with the use of an assistive device such as a walker).
- Progress UE support provided by assistive device to light touch-down support, then to use of a pole or wall for support as needed, and finally to no support.

Foot Placement/Toe Clearance
- Practice heel-toe initial contact using verbal cues such as *"Step with heels first."*
- Practice high-step marching in place and then high-step walking accompanied by marching music.
- Practice walking with even steps using footprints attached to the floor.
- Practice increasing step length and/or step width using footprints or a floor grid.
- Practice walking with altered BOS; progressing from wide base (8 to 12 in. [20 to 30 cm] apart) to narrow base (2 in. [5 cm] apart) to tandem (heel-to-toe).
- Practice step-to-walking (i.e., take a long step with one limb and then bring the opposite limb even with the first on the next step).
- Practice walking on a 3-inch (8-cm) wide line taped to the floor, on a split half-foam roller, or low balance beam.

Single- and Double-Limb Support
- Practice controlled lateral and diagonal weight shifts.
- Combine diagonal weight shifts with pelvic rotation movements and stepping forward and backward.

Forward Progression and Push-off
- Practice toe rises (heel-offs) in stance; progress to toe-walking.
- Practice heel-rises (toe offs) in stance; progress to heel-walking.
- Practice forceful push-off on cue during walking.
- Practice alternating between heel-walking and toe-walking (i.e., walk a certain number of steps on heels and then the same number on toes).

Walking Against Resistance
- Practice walking against manual resistance using resisted progression.
- Practice walking against resistance from an elastic resistive band around the pelvis.
- Practice pool walking (ideal initial supportive environment for patients with ataxia).

Trunk Counterrotation and Arm Swing
- Practice walking with exaggerated arm swings.
- Practice walking with long poles; the therapist is behind and holds one end of the poles; the patient is in front and holds the other end of the poles.

Walking Sideward
- Practice walking using lateral side-steps, with resisted progression (manual and elastic resistive bands).
- Practice walking using crossed-steps and side-steps.
- Practice walking using braiding.

Walking Backward
- Practice walking backward (retro-walking).
- Practice large backward steps (exaggerated knee flexion in combination with hip extension).

Step-Ups/Step-Downs
- Practice stepping up and stepping down; vary the step height, progressing from low (4 in. [10 cm]) to high (8 in. [20 cm]).
- Practice lateral step-ups.
- Practice forward step-ups.
- Practice stepping onto and off of varied surfaces (e.g., foam pad, half-foam roller, inflatable disc, BOSU® Balance Trainer).

Stopping, Starting, and Turning on Cue
- Practice abrupt stops and starts on verbal cue.
- Practice turns on verbal cue, progressing from a quarter turn to half turn to full turn; progress from wide-base to narrow-base turns.
- Practice figure-8 turns.

Visual Input
- Practice walking alternating between eyes open (EO) and eyes closed (EC); three steps with EO and then three steps with EC.

Head Movements
- Practice walking with alternating head movements; alternate between taking three steps with head to the right and then three steps with head to the left.
- Practice walking with varying head movements on verbal cues, such as *"Look right,"* *"Look left,"* *"Look down,"* and *"Look up."*
- Practice walking with diagonal head movements on verbal cues, such as *"Look over your right shoulder"* and *"Look down toward your left hip."*

Timed Walking, Increasing Speed and Locomotor Rhythm
- Practice walking at a self-selected comfortable speed and then increasing speed to fast walking.
- Use pacing cues to vary speed, such as *"Walk slow"* and *"Walk fast."*
- Use a metronome or brisk marching music to increase speed and improve locomotor rhythm.
- Practice alternating short bursts of fast walking (on verbal cue) with walking at a comfortable speed.

BOX 8.2 Strategies for Varying Locomotor Task Demands (continued)

Duration of Walking
• Progress to longer distances with fewer rest intervals.

Dual-Task Walking
• Walk and talk.
• Walk and count by 3s.
• Walk and bounce or toss a ball or carry a tray.

Compensatory Responses to Unexpected Perturbations
• Change the speed of the treadmill, or stop and start the treadmill while the patient is walking on it.
• Practice resisted forward progression using an elastic resistive band with unexpected release of resistance.
• Practice walking while recovering from small external perturbations given manually.

BOX 8.3 Strategies for Varying Environmental Demands

Walking Surfaces
• Practice walking on a variety of indoor and outdoor surfaces.
  • Indoor surfaces: tile, linoleum, low- and high-pile carpet, and hardwood and laminate flooring
  • Outdoor surfaces: sidewalks, concrete, gravel, asphalt, and grassy terrains

Stair Climbing
• Practice stair climbing using a handrail; progress to stair climbing without the use of a handrail.
• Practice stair climbing one step at a time; progress to step over step; alter requirements for step height and number of steps.

Obstacles
• Practice walking while avoiding or contending with obstacles in the environment such as the following:
  • Walking over and around a static obstacle course created with objects of varying heights and widths (e.g., step stool, chair, cans, yardstick, stacking cones, books, and so forth); altering requirements for foot clearance, step length, step time, and walking speed
  • Walking with dynamic (moving) obstacles in the path (e.g., revolving door, elevator, or escalator)
  • Walking on varying paths (e.g., changing environment)
  • Walking with two individuals navigating the same obstacle course (collision avoidance)

Slopes or Ramps
• Practice walking on ramps and slopes of varying heights.
  • Gradual incline: using smaller steps
  • Steep incline: smaller steps using a diagonal, zigzag pattern (step length decreases with increasing slope)
• Requirements for navigating slopes or ramps include the following:
  • Descent is associated with increased knee flexion (stance) and increased ankle and hip motions (swing);

during descent, peak moments and powers are higher at the knees.
  • Ascent is associated with decreased speed, cadence, and step length.

Open Environments
• Practice walking in busy, open, community environments (e.g., a busy hallway, hospital lobby, shopping mall, or grocery store).
• Practice finding solutions to real-life functional problems, such as the following:
  • Pushing or pulling open doors
  • Pushing a grocery cart
  • Car transfers: getting into and out of a car
  • Getting on and off a bus or other public transportation vehicle
  • Carrying a bag of groceries
• Practice walking and traversing unfamiliar routes and unfamiliar places.
• Practice stepping up and down curbs.

Time Requirements
• Practice walking with anticipatory timing requirements, such as the following:
  • Crossing at a stoplight
  • Moving on and off moving walkways
  • Moving on and off an escalator
  • Walking through automatic revolving doors

Visual Conditions
• Practice walking in varying visual conditions, such as the following:
  • Full lighting with progression to reduced and low lighting
  • With dark glasses to alter visual conditions
  • Varied lighting conditions (e.g., outside to inside lighting)

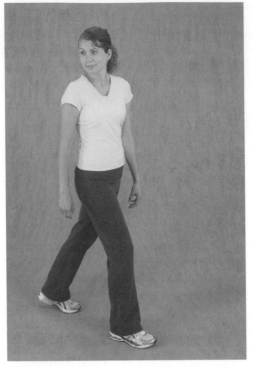

FIGURE 8.9 Walking with head turns to the left and right on verbal cues (in this example, the head is turned toward the right). A variation is to have the patient look up and down while walking.

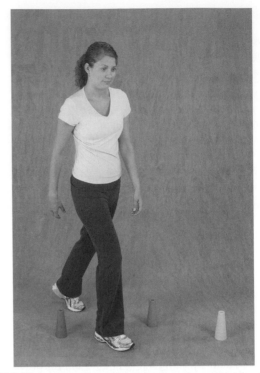

FIGURE 8.11 Walking through obstacles placed on the floor. An obstacle course can be created using a variety of common objects. In this example, the course was created using stacking cones.

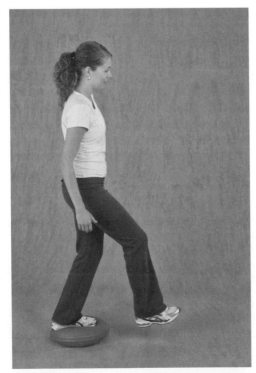

FIGURE 8.10 The walking surface can be altered by the tactical placement of inflatable discs on the floor. The patient steps up onto the disc with one limb and uses the opposite limb to step beyond the disc and make contact with the floor surface.

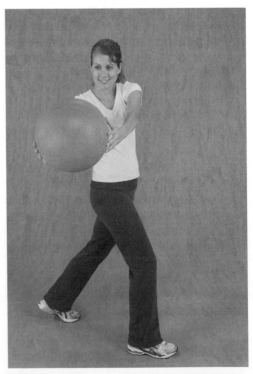

FIGURE 8.12 Dual-task locomotor activity. With the shoulders flexed to approximately 90 degrees and the elbows extended, the patient moves the ball from side to side while walking.

- Walking while bouncing a ball
- Walking while pushing and pulling loads (e.g., a grocery cart)
- Walking through doorways and opening and closing doors
- Walking and stopping to pick an object up off the floor
- Walking increased distances that simulate community distances (e.g., 1,200 ft [366 m]) or increased times that simulate the times needed for crosswalks (e.g., approximately 2.62 ft/sec [0.8 m/sec] for a 40-ft [12-m] crosswalk)
- Walking outdoors under different conditions (e.g., terrain, illumination, and weather) or in busy, noisy environments (e.g., busy hallways or clinic entrances and shopping malls).
- Walking while practicing recovery strategies, such as stops or starts on a treadmill

Clinical Notes: The level of task difficulty is increased considerably by adding a second task (*dual-task activity*) such as catching and throwing a weighted ball or walking while carrying a tray that holds a glass of water. Initially, such activities require constant cognitive monitoring; they may be mentally fatiguing and prone to errors when the patient becomes distracted. To begin, a closed environment is most effective. The patient should be guarded cautiously during the introduction of new or novel dynamic locomotor tasks; a gait belt or an overhead harness may be warranted to ensure patient safety. Most important, careful observance of safety precautions will improve patient confidence and trust in the therapist's ability to provide safe treatment.

Body Weight Support and Treadmill Training

The use of a body weight support (BWS) system and a treadmill (TM) combined with verbal and manual guidance from the therapist is an important intervention for improving locomotor skills. The desired amount of body weight is supported through a trunk harness donned by the patient that attaches to an overhead suspension system; the system's wheeled-base (locking casters) allows positioning of the unit over a TM. The unit can then be moved away from the TM for progression to overground locomotion. As a safety strategy, the suspension system may also be used without actually supporting body weight (the patient supports full body weight). This provides a safe and effective environment for the patient and therapist to focus on improving locomotor skills without undue attention devoted to preventing falls.

Locomotion is an automatic postural activity. Unique to the combined use of BWS and a TM is the ability to facilitate automatic locomotion using intensive task-oriented practice. Neural control of locomotion arises from subcortical and spinal centers (spinal pattern generators [SPGs]). As such, reciprocal locomotor patterns can be produced at the spinal cord level in the absence of supraspinal input.[4] This is a central tenet supporting the use of this approach. The constant speed of the TM (speed of walking is controlled) provides rhythmic input that helps to reestablish or reinforce coordinated reciprocal LE locomotor patterns. Of critical importance to successful outcomes early on is the *hands-on* role of physical therapists and physical therapist assistants (trainers). For example, during the stance phase of gait, the foot moves smoothly through initial contact, loading response, midstance, terminal stance, and preswing. If motor function impairments prevent these normal transitions during TM walking, peripheral sensory input to the SPGs will be incorrect and normal locomotor patterns will not be reestablished. Such circumstances require a trainer to sit next to the TM (on the side of weakness) and, using manual contacts on the foot and lower leg, repeatedly guide the patient's foot through the correct sequence of movements and foot placements required during stance. A second therapist can also stand behind the patient and assist the pelvic motions to initiate stepping using both hands positioned on the patient's pelvis.

Conventional gait training typically incorporates a *parts-to-whole* practice strategy. This requires considerable time to accomplish component lead-up skills such as static and dynamic balance control, weight shifting, stepping strategies, and so forth. The early use of parallel bars and assistive devices can produce undesirable compensatory patterns such as a forwardly flexed posture, asymmetry, and substitution of the UEs for impaired LE function. These patterns are often difficult to change later on. In addition, considerable demands are placed on both the patient and the therapist to ensure that static and dynamic stability is maintained. This may negatively affect the amount of time actually spent on locomotor training.[5] In contrast, training using BWS and a TM focuses on the facilitation of automatic walking movements using a *whole-task* practice strategy. The support of the patient's body weight with a BWS system allows training to begin well before the patient acquires all the component lead-up skills required of more traditional gait training approaches. The TM speed provides a rhythmic input that reinforces the manually guided reciprocal movements of the limbs through each phase of the gait cycle. This continues until the patient is able to participate in generating the reciprocal stepping patterns before a progression is introduced.[6]

The importance of sensory input through manual guidance provided by the trainers cannot be overemphasized. The BWS system and TM allow access to the patient's hips, pelvis, and LEs to manually assist, guide, or adjust locomotor rhythm, limb placement, weight shifts, and symmetry. Guided movements are coordinated to simulate a normal gait, and ensure that upright posture and balance are maintained. The sensory input (e.g., joint proprioceptors of hip, knee, and ankle; pressure receptors of foot) from appropriately timed manually assisted limb movements promotes function-induced recovery.[4,7] This sensory input provides spinal level *facilitation* and *inhibition* of flexor-extensor motor neuron pools at the appropriate time in the gait cycle.[8]

BOX 8.4 Benefits of Body Weight Support (BWS) and a Treadmill (TM) to Improve Locomotor Skill

- Locomotor interventions may be implemented earlier in the episode of care (compared to more conventional approaches).
- Loading of the UEs is minimized or eliminated owing to maximal loading of the LEs.
- LE loading can be varied based on the patient's ability to support weight.
- Compensatory movement strategies are reduced or eliminated.
- Learned nonuse may be eliminated secondary to weightbearing and "forced" stepping movements of more involved segments.
- Normal gait kinematics and phase relationships of the full gait cycle are promoted (e.g., limb loading in midstance; unweighting and stepping during swing).
- The fear of falling is reduced or eliminated.

- Inter- and intra-limb locomotor timing and rhythm can be promoted without the demands of supporting the full body weight.
- Rhythmic input from the constant speed of the TM helps to reestablish or reinforce coordinated reciprocal LE patterns.
- Using greater BWS and low TM velocity, gait deviations may be addressed early.
- Dynamic balance training can be practiced by decreasing BWS and increasing the TM speed.
- Sensory inputs facilitate muscle activation.
- Coordinated kinematics of the trunk, pelvis, and limbs specific to the locomotor task are promoted.
- Walking speed and distance improve.
- Muscular and cardiovascular endurance improves.

Box 8.4 provides an overview of the benefits associated with use of BWS and a TM to improve locomotor skills.

BWS and TM Training: Management Strategies

Although specific training protocols have not been definitively established, sufficient information is available to provide general guidelines for using BWS and TM locomotor training.[4-8;9-13]

- To begin, the patient is assisted with donning a trunk harness that includes adjustable straps attached to an overhead BWS suspension system. The BWS unit is positioned over a TM, providing trainer access to the trunk/pelvis, hips, knees, and ankle/foot. If patient involvement is bilateral, trainers will need to be positioned on both sides of the TM.
- The BWS system supports a portion of the patient's body weight (e.g., starting at 40 percent with progressions to 30 percent, 20 percent, 10 percent, and then no BWS). Decreasing the amount of body weight supported is an important measure of progression.
- Increasing the TM *speed* is another important measure of progression. Initially, slow TM speeds are used (e.g., 0.52 mph [0.23 m/s]); then the speed is gradually increased as the patient's locomotor skills improve (e.g., to 0.95 mph [0.42 m/s]).
- Total locomotor training time recommendations range from 30 to 60 minutes with intervening rest intervals. Duration is increased gradually. On average, the patient training is intense (e.g., 5 days per week for 6 to 12 weeks). With severe involvement, however, initial training bouts may be as short as 3 minutes with 5-minute rest intervals.[6]
- Once locomotor training in initiated, trainers provide manual assistance to normalize gait. With unilateral involvement, for example, one trainer may provide assistance with foot placement while another trainer assists at the trunk and pelvis to promote upright posture and

pelvic rotation. In the presence of muscle weakness, poor balance, or other impairments, the physical therapist must determine whether the patient's walking strategies are effective, what elements are consistent with the task of walking and should be promoted, and what elements are inconsistent that need to be modified or eliminated. Decreasing the amount of *manual assistance* provided is another important measure of progression.

- Parameters are established for the percentage of body weight supported, the TM speed, the duration of training bouts and rest intervals, and the amount and location of manual assistance. A determination of the specific strategies to be used is also required (Box 8.5). In the planning of treatment parameters, the following foundational principles are considered:
  - LE weightbearing should be maximized while UE support is minimized.
  - Sensory cues and input via appropriate handling techniques should be optimized to ensure the desired or most favorable stepping pattern (assisted by trainers).
  - Normal walking kinematics should be promoted, with emphasis on trunk, pelvis, and limb movements.
  - Recovery should be maximized and compensatory movements minimized or eliminated.
  - Manual assistance is limited to only that which is essential for accomplishing the desired movement.
- As reciprocal patterns of movement begin to develop, locomotor training is progressed by reducing the amount of body weight supported, increasing the TM speed, and reducing the amount of manual guidance. Progression continues until the patient is walking independently supporting full body weight at a speed of 1.0 mph (0.44 m/s).[6]
- Locomotor training using BWS is continued by progressing to overground walking. When the casters are unlocked, the BWS unit becomes mobile and can be moved away from the TM for use on overground surfaces.

BOX 8.5 Strategies for Locomotor Training Using Body Weight Support (BWS) and a Treadmill (TM)

Standing Training
- Initially, a determination is made of how much body weight the patient's LEs can support.
- The goal is to decrease BWS to the lowest amount possible.
- Maximum unweighting (e.g., 30 to 40 percent) is progressed to reduced amounts of body weight supported (e.g., 20 to 10 percent BWS with progression to full LE weightbearing with no BWS).
- The use of the hands and UEs for balance is discouraged; upright posture is promoted (forward lean avoided).

Step Training
- Manual assistance and verbal cues are provided by trainers to control and assist pelvic rotation and hip, knee, and foot motions.
- Focus is on rhythmic stepping, toe clearance, step length, and foot placement.
- The goal is to reestablish a kinematically correct stepping pattern at the lowest possible BWS and at normal walking speed (2.2 to 2.8 mph [0.98 to 1.3 m/s]).
- Based on clinical presentation, manual assistance is provided to one or both LEs.

Step Adaptability Training
- This training begins with greater BWS at a slower speed, with progression toward independence.
- The TM speed is gradually increased based on the patient's tolerance.

- The TM slope is gradually increased to challenge step adaptability.
- The duration of walking is gradually increased with each training bout.

Overground Walking Training
- A determination is made of patient carryover of locomotor skills from TM using BWS to overground progression without BWS.
- An examination is performed to determine the level of performance in transfers, bed mobility, standing, and walking without the use of assistive devices, orthotics, or compensatory strategies.
- The BWS harness may be indicated initially, with progression to no harness.
- Emphasis is placed on an even stride and step length.
- Physical assistance and verbal cues are provided as needed.

Community Integration
- An examination is performed to determine the level of performance in the home and community environments.
- Emphasis is placed on ensuring safety and independence (the least restrictive assistive device is selected).
- Emphasis is on increased weightbearing and locomotor timing and rhythm.

Elimination of the rhythmic steady-state input from the TM causes the overground walking speed to be initially reduced. The BWS unit is manually moved by the trainers to keep pace with the patient's forward progression. The use of an assistive device may be introduced during BWS overground walking. The same parameters continue to be used to monitor progress: adjusting *body weight, speed*, and *manual assistance*.
- Last, the patient is progressed to overground walking without an assistive device and without BWS. It should be noted that the desired walking speed will vary based on the demands of the environment the patient will be negotiating. For example, functional speeds required for community ambulation (normal healthy population) average 2.8 mph (1.3 m/s).[14]

Appendix A presents an overview of locomotor training with application to patients with spinal cord injury (SCI); the information provides the framework for Case Study 3.

Student Practice Activities

Sound clinical decision-making will help identify the most appropriate activities and techniques to improve locomotor skills for an individual patient. Student practice activities provide an opportunity to share knowledge and skills as well as to confirm or clarify understanding of the treatment interventions. Each student in a group contributes his or her understanding of, or questions about, the strategy, technique, or activity, and participates in the activity being discussed. Dialogue should continue until a consensus of understanding is reached. Box 8.6 Student Practice Activity presents activities that focus on interventions and management strategies to improve locomotor skills.

BOX 8.6 STUDENT PRACTICE ACTIVITY: INTERVENTIONS AND MANAGEMENT STRATEGIES TO IMPROVE LOCOMOTION

OBJECTIVE: Sharing skill in the application and knowledge of treatment interventions to enhance locomotion.

EQUIPMENT NEEDS: Step stool, ball, inflated disc, two poles, two elastic resistive bands, a treadmill, and several common objects to create an obstacle course (e.g., staking cones, plastic cups, books, soup cans, and so forth).

STUDENT GROUP SIZE: Four to six students.

DIRECTIONS: Divide into pairs, with one person serving as the patient/subject and the other functioning as the therapist (reverse roles prior to addressing the guiding questions).

1. **Practice walking forward and backward.** Direct the patient/subject to practice walking forward and backward as the therapist guards and directs the activities. Complete the following activities:
   * Increase the step length from initially reduced to normal.
   * Change the speed of walking from slow to normal to fast; progress to treadmill walking (if available).
   * Modify the BOS from feet apart (wide base) to normal to feet close together (narrow base) to tandem walking (heel-to-toe pattern).
   * Vary the acceleration or deceleration by having the patient/subject practice stopping and starting or turning on cue.
   * Practice dual-task walking, such as walking and counting backward by 7s from 100, walking and turning the head left or right and up or down on cue, and walking and bouncing a ball.
   * Vary the walking surface from flat to on and off foam to irregular (outdoors).
   * Using an elastic resistive band, practice both forward and backward resisted progressions. Depending on the direction of movement, the therapist stands either in front of or behind the patient holding the ends of the band.
   * Practice walking forward and backward on a treadmill, and practice walking with stops and starts of the treatmill.
   * Practice walking through an obstacle course.

Guiding Questions

With consideration of the variations in locomotor tasks just practiced:

▲ What did you learn about changes in postural stability demands with each activity?
▲ What activities provided the *greatest* and *least* challenges to postural stability?
▲ Compare and contrast the rhythmic stepping patterns used during forward versus backward walking. What differences did you notice?
▲ As the speed of walking was reduced and increased, what changes occurred in the requirements for timing and control?
▲ Multiple muscle groups are active in alternating between forward and backward walking. Differentiate

between the muscles that contribute to dynamic limb advancement (swing phase) during forward versus backward progressions.

▲ What insights did the activities provide that can be applied clinically?
▲ Describe the importance of synchronizing the therapist's movements with those of the patient's during resisted progression. How is pacing of the activity maintained?
▲ What strategies can be used to assist in sequencing arm swings and promoting trunk counterrotation during forward and backward progressions?
▲ How did walking on a TM affect locomotor rhythm?
▲ Did the level of task difficulty change by adding a second task (*dual-task activity*)? What impact did the dual task have on cognitive monitoring? Was the quality of performance affected by the addition of a second task?

2. **Practice walking, side-stepping.** Direct the patient/subject to side-step by abducting and placement of the dynamic limb to the side; the remaining limb is then moved parallel to the first. Complete the following activities:
   * Practice active side-stepping in each direction.
   * Apply resisted progression in side-stepping using an elastic resistive band (around the lateral aspect of the pelvis on the abducting side).
   * Change the speed of side-stepping from reduced to normal to increased.
   * Practice side-stepping on a treadmill.

Guiding Questions

▲ What are the functional implications of side-stepping?
▲ During side-stepping, what action is provided by the hip abductors on the dynamic limb? On the static limb?
▲ As the speed of walking was reduced and increased, what changes occurred in the requirements for timing and control?
▲ What changes in timing and rhythm occurred during side-stepping on the TM?

3. **Practice walking, side-stepping and crossed-stepping.** Instruct the patient/subject to abduct the leading dynamic limb with foot placement followed by movement of the remaining limb to a parallel position with the first (a symmetrical stance) and then crossed-step by moving the opposite leg up, across, and in front of the original side-step limb. Complete the following activities:
   * Practice active side-stepping and crossed-stepping in each direction.
   * Apply resisted progression in side-stepping and crossed-stepping using manual resistance.
   * Alter the speed of side-stepping and crossed-stepping from reduced to normal to increased.

Guiding Questions

▲ What are the clinical indications for the use of side-stepping and crossed-stepping?

BOX 8.6 STUDENT PRACTICE ACTIVITY: INTERVENTIONS AND MANAGEMENT STRATEGIES TO IMPROVE LOCOMOTION (continued)

▲ As the speed of side-stepping and crossed-stepping was altered, what changes occurred?

4. **Practice walking, braiding.** Direct the patient to begin with a side-step and follow with a crossed-step up and over in front (PNF LE D1F pattern), then a side-step, and then a crossed-step backward and behind the first limb (PNF LE D2E pattern). Complete the following activities:
   • Practice active braiding in each direction.
   • Apply resisted progression in braiding using manual resistance.

Guiding Questions

▲ Braiding is a challenging sequence to learn for many patients. How can the therapist facilitate the learning of this new skill?
▲ What therapeutic goal(s) can be addressed using braiding?

5. *Directions:* Working in a small group, respond to the following:
   • Describe strategies for varying locomotor task demands during training.
   • Describe strategies for varying environmental demands during training.
   • What are the prerequisite requirements for the initiation of stair climbing?
   • Describe the rationale for locomotor training using BWS and a TM. What benefits are associated with this approach?

SUMMARY

Improving or reestablishing locomotor skills is often the highest priority for patients seeking skilled physical therapy intervention. Locomotion is an essential function that supports and enhances effective interaction with the environment. It represents the highest level of motor control (skill) and requires the integrated function of many interacting systems. The foundational requirements of walking include: support of body weight, locomotor rhythm, dynamic balance, propulsion of the body in the desired direction, and the ability to adapt to changing task and environmental demands. Establishing an effective POC to improve locomotor skills requires a comprehensive gait analysis, including gait variables and common gait deviations as well as knowledge of the impairments and activity limitations that affect movement. An important focus of intervention is promoting adaptation skills through variations in both locomotor task and environmental demands. The documented benefits of using BWS and a TM to improve locomotion support its expanding clinical applications. Finally, the therapist must consider the demands of the patient's home, community, and work environment to achieve successful outcomes.

REFERENCES

1. American Physical Therapy Association. Guide to Physical Therapist Practice, ed 2. Phys Ther 81:9, 2001 (revised June 2003).
2. Pathokinesiology Service and Physical Therapy Department. Observational Gait Analysis Handbook. Los Amigos Research and Education Institute, Inc., Downey, CA, 2001.
3. Norkin, CC. Examination of gait. In O'Sullivan, SB, and Schmitz, TJ (eds): Physical Rehabilitation, ed 5. FA Davis, Philadelphia, 2007, p 317.
4. Field-Fote, EC. Spinal cord control of movement: Implications for locomotor rehabilitation following spinal cord injury. Phys Ther 80(5):477, 2000.
5. Brown, TH, Mount, J, Rouland, BL, et al. Body weight-supported treadmill training versus conventional gait training for people with chronic traumatic brain injury. J Head Trauma Rehabil 20(5):402, 2005.
6. Seif-Naraghi, AH, and Herman, RM. A novel method for locomotion training. J Head Trauma Rehabil 14(2):146, 1999.
7. Visintin, M, and Barbeau, H. The effects of body weight support on the locomotor pattern of spastic paretic patients. Can J Neurol Sci 16:315, 1989.
8. Kosak, MC, and Reding, MJ. Comparison of partial body weight-supported treadmill gait training versus aggressive bracing assisted walking post stroke. Neurorehabil Neural Repair 14(1):13, 2000.
9. Moseley, AM, Stark, A, Cameron, ID, et al. Treadmill training and body weight support for walking after stroke [update of Cochrane Database Syst Rev 2003 (3):CD002840], Cochrane Database Syst Rev 2005 (4):CD002840. Available at: http://www.thechochranelibrary.com. Accessed May 9, 2009.
10. Foley, N, Teasell, R, and Bhogal, S. Evidence-based review of stroke rehabilitation: Mobility and the lower extremity. Canadian Stroke Network, 2006. Available at: http://www.ebrsr.com/modules/modules9.pdf. Accessed May 9, 2009.
11. Salbach, NM, Mayo, NE, Wood-Dauphinee, S, et al. A task-oriented intervention enhances walking distance and speed in the first year post stroke: A randomized controlled trial. Clin Rehabil 18(5):509, 2004.
12. Sullivan, KJ, Knowlton, BJ, and Dobkin, BH. Step training with body weight support: Effect of treadmill speed and practice paradigms on poststroke locomotor recovery. Arch Phys Med Rehabil 83:683, 2002.
13. Sullivan, K, Brown, DA, Klassen, T, et al. Effects of task-specific locomotor and strength training in adults who were ambulatory after stroke: Results of the STEPS randomized clinical trial. Phys Ther 87:1580, 2007.
14. Perry, J, Garrett, M, Gronley, JK, et al. Classification of walking handicap in the stroke population. Stroke 26:982, 1995.

Brief Overview of Locomotor Training Using a Body Weight Support System and a Treadmill (Case Study 3)

Elizabeth Ardolino, PT, MS,[1] Elizabeth Watson, PT, DPT, NCS,[1] Andrea Behrman, PT, PhD,[2] Susan Harkema, PhD,[3] Mary Schmidt-Read, PT, DPT, MS[1]

Conventional gait-training interventions after spinal cord injury (SCI) focus on increasing independence by using compensatory methods to address deficits in strength, motor control, balance, and sensation. Typical gait-training goals for patients with SCI address compensation for paresis or paralysis using braces and assistive devices. Locomotor training (LT) using a body weight support (BWS) system and a treadmill (TM) is a relatively new form of physical therapy treatment based on the activity-dependent plasticity and motor learning capacity of the spinal cord.[1-3]

A network of spinal interneurons process and integrate both ascending sensory input and descending supraspinal input to generate the motor output of walking.[4] With diminished supraspinal drive after incomplete SCI, LT targets the promotion of locomotor-specific input to the neural axis to promote locomotor output below the level of the lesion.[5] Intense repetitive and task-specific practice of walking (through LT) is aimed at fostering neurological recovery of balance and gait as well as improving the overall health and quality of life for patients with SCI and other neurological disorders.

LT is based on the following four principles[6]:

1. **Maximize LE weightbearing.** Patients are encouraged to bear as much body weight on the LEs as often as possible, while decreasing the amount of weightbearing through their UEs.
2. **Optimize the use of sensory cues.** LT utilizes appropriate manual facilitation from therapists to optimize the quality of the stepping pattern, while walking at or near preinjury walking speeds.
3. **Optimize kinematics for each motor task.** LT focuses on upright posture, proper pelvic rotation, and appropriate inter-limb coordination for walking. Patients initiate stepping by beginning in a stride position, with hip extension of the trailing limb. Emphasis is placed on the use of standard kinematics for sit-to-stand transitions, standing, and other tasks.

4. **Maximize recovery and minimize compensation.** Patients are assisted, when needed, to perform movements using typical spatial-temporal components to accomplish a task. Performance of tasks using compensatory strategies (i.e., momentum and leverage) is minimized. Patients attempt to accomplish a task while using the least restrictive assistive devices, without orthoses, and as little physical assistance as possible.

LT using a BWS system and a TM consists of three main components: *step training, overground examination,* and *community integration.*

Step Training

The *step training* environment includes a BWS system placed over a TM, with physical therapists and physical therapist assistants (trainers) providing hands-on manual assistance. The BWS system and the TM provide an ideal environment for safe practice of the task of walking. Step training consists of four components: *stand retraining, stand adaptability, step retraining,* and *step adaptability.*

- **Stand retraining.** The purpose of stand retraining is to examine how much body weight the patient's LEs can support. The goal is to decrease the body weight support to the lowest amount possible, with the trainers (who have undergone specific training in the techniques of LT) providing as much assistance as needed for the patient to maintain an appropriate upright standing posture.
- **Stand adaptability.** The purpose of stand adaptability is to examine the body weight parameters necessary to maintain independence at different body segments (e.g., trunk, pelvis, right knee, left knee, right ankle, left ankle) during both static and dynamic standing.
- **Step retraining.** The purpose of step retraining is to retrain the nervous system's ability to walk by establishing a kinematically correct stepping pattern at the lowest possible amount of BWS and at normal walking speed (2.2 to 2.8 mph [0.98 to 1.3 m/s]).
- **Step adaptability.** The purpose of step adaptability is to promote independent control of each body segment for the task of walking. Initially, the patient will require more

[1] Magee Rehabilitation Hospital, Philadelphia, PA 19006
[2] College of Public Health and Health Professions, University of Florida
[3] Department of Neurological Surgery, University of Kentucky

BWS at a slower speed, with gradual progression to less BWS and faster speeds until independence is achieved.

Overground Examination

The purpose of the *overground examination* is to determine the carryover of skills acquired during step training on the TM to the overground progression without BWS. In this component, the therapist examines the patient's ability to perform functional mobility, such as transfers, bed mobility, standing, and ambulation, without the use of assistive devices, braces, or compensations. Goals for the next step training session and for community integration are identified based on the overground performance. The therapist and patient identify the factor(s) limiting successful independent ambulation and then use the information to establish new training goals.

Community Integration

Community integration focuses on the application of LT principles in the patient's home and community environment. The therapist selects the least restrictive assistive device that allows safe and independent standing and walking. The goal is to increase the amount of weightbearing in more open environments.

A typical LT session is 90 minutes, with a goal of 60 minutes of weightbearing with BWS. At least 20 of these minutes should be focused on step retraining at a normal walking speed. Because the ultimate goal of LT is to promote maximal recovery of the nervous system, patients often require an extended course of treatment as compared to more conventional outpatient episodes of care. It is not unusual for patients to need in excess of 40 sessions of LT. Following discharge, patients typically start by attending LT out-patient sessions five times per week and then, as they advance, progress down to four and then three times per week.

APPENDIX A REFERENCES

1. Barbeau, H, Wainberg, M, and Finch, L. Description and application of a system for locomotor rehabilitation. Med Biol Eng Comput 25:341, 1987.
2. Barbeau, H, and Blunt, R. A novel interactive locomotor approach using body weight support to retrain gait in spastic paretic subjects. In Wernig, A (ed): Plasticity of Motorneuronal Connections. Restorative Neurology, Vol. 5. Elsevier, Amsterdam, The Netherlands, 1991, p 461.
3. Barbeau, H, Nadeau, S, and Garneau, C. Physical determinants, emerging concepts, and training approaches in gait of individuals with spinal cord injury. J Neurotrauma 23(3–4):571 (review), 2006.
4. Harkema, SJ. Plasticity of interneuronal networks of the functionally isolated human spinal cord. Brain Res Rev 57(1):255, 2008.
5. Edgerton, VR, Niranjala, JK, Tillakaratne, AJ, et al. Plasticity of the spinal neural circuitry after injury. Annu Rev Neurosci 27:145, 2004.
6. Behrman, AL, Lawless-Dixon, AR, Davis, SB, et al. Locomotor training progression and outcomes after incomplete spinal cord injury. Phys Ther 85:1356, 2005.

Interventions to Improve Upper Extremity Skills

SHARON A. GUTMAN, PhD, OTR, AND
MARIANNE MORTERA, PhD, OTR

This chapter is written from the perspective of the practicing occupational therapist and addresses how impairments of the upper extremity (UE) are treated within the context of daily living skills. This chapter is designed to provide the physical therapist with information to (1) provide effective interventions to improve UE function, (2) understand the unique contributions of the occupational therapist in UE functional skill training, and (3) communicate with occupational therapy colleagues concerning comprehensive interdisciplinary patient management.

Task Analysis Guidelines

Prior to treatment planning, the therapist performs a task or activity analysis. Activity analysis is the breakdown of activities into their component parts in order to understand the demands of the activity and identify patient deficits that hinder successful participation in the activity (Box 9.1). Therapists consider three primary components in the activity analysis process: patient performance components, activity demands, and environmental factors. *Patient performance components* refer to the skills necessary to participate in the activity and are further broken down into the following skill

categories: *sensory, perceptual, neurological, musculoskeletal, cognitive,* and *psychosocial.* This chapter focuses on the neurological and musculoskeletal skills needed to perform basic activities of daily living (BADL).

Activity demands refer to the requirements embedded in each step of the activity. *Environmental factors* are the physical characteristics of the environment that may impede or promote performance as well as the social and/or cultural values and beliefs that may influence a patient's ability and desire to perform specific ADL. Once an analysis of all three areas is complete, the therapist can modify the activity and/or the environment to enhance the patient's ability to participate in specific ADL. To improve patient performance, therapists can also use specific interventions designed to enhance the patient's neurological and/or musculoskeletal function.

Activity Analysis of Self-Feeding

Below is an example of an abbreviated activity analysis process. The example illustrates how the activity of self-feeding is analyzed with respect to neurological and musculoskeletal performance components of the UE, activity demands, and environmental factors.

BOX 9.1 The Process of Activity Analysis

Patient Performance Components
- Sensory
- Perceptual
- Neurological
- Musculoskeletal
- Cognitive
- Psychosocial

The therapist asks: "*What are the sensory, perceptual, neurological, musculoskeletal, cognitive, and perceptual impairments that are limiting the patient's performance in a specific ADL?*"

Activity Demands
- Specific steps of the activity (requirements embedded in each step of the activity)
- Functional requirements needed to complete the activity

The therapist asks: "*What are the specific steps of the activity? What specific functional requirements are needed to perform the activity? Does the patient have the performance components needed to successfully participate in the activity?*"

Environmental Considerations
- Physical
- Sociocultural

The therapist asks: "*What are the physical characteristics of the environment that may obstruct the patient's performance? What social and/or cultural values and beliefs does the patient have that may impede his or her ability to participate in the activity?*"
Analysis of the above allows the therapist to modify the activity and the environment to improve the patient's performance in specific activities of daily living.

Neurological and Musculoskeletal Performance Components of Self-Feeding

The following are required performance components or *lead-up skills* to the actual activity of self-feeding.

- **Trunk postural stability.** Appropriate upper and lower trunk stability (i.e., upper trunk extension and abdominal support) is essential to maintain an upright seated position (Fig. 9.1). A neutral position or slight anterior tilt of pelvis and hip abduction enhance lower trunk stability. An upright seated position is necessary for normal UE movement patterns to occur as well as to prevent aspiration of food items.

- **Shoulder stability and mobility.** Cocontraction of the shoulder girdle muscles is needed to support distal UE movement in space during reaching activities, as in reaching for and retrieving utensils and food items (Fig. 9.2).

- **Elbow stability and mobility.** Cocontraction of the elbow musculature to support distal UE movement in space during reaching is also a required lead-up skill (Fig. 9.3). For example, elbow stability is needed to grasp a drinking glass securely. Elbow flexion and extension are needed to bring the glass to the mouth and back to the table.

- **Wrist stability and mobility.** The ability to maintain the wrist in a neutral or extended position to allow for grasp and prehension patterns (described below) is required (Fig. 9.4). For example, maintenance of the wrist in an extended position (approximately 20 to 30 degrees of wrist extension) is required to grasp a milk container and pour the liquid into a glass.

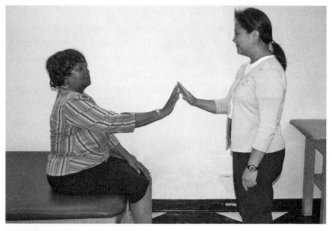

FIGURE 9.2 Shoulder stability and mobility are lead-up skills for self-feeding required for reaching and retrieving utensils and food items. Here the patient practices reaching using the therapist's hand as a target.

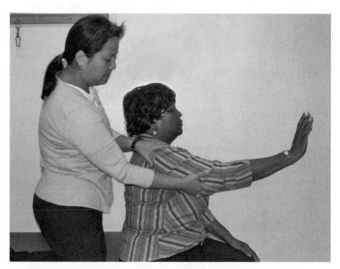

FIGURE 9.3 Elbow stability and mobility are necessary to support distal UE movement in space; they are lead-up skills for self-feeding.

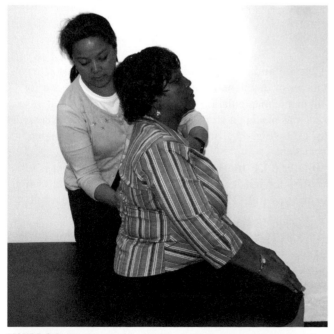

FIGURE 9.1 Postural trunk stability is a necessary lead-up skill for self-feeding. It allows for normal UE movement patterns to occur, and upright posture of head and trunk prevents aspiration of food items.

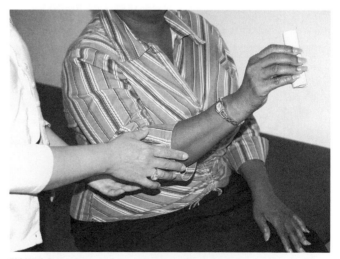

FIGURE 9.4 Wrist stability and mobility allow for grasp and prehension patterns required for self-feeding.

- **Gross grasp.** *Gross grasp* refers to a grip that places an object in contact with the palm and palmar surface of digits. Gross thumb and finger flexion and extension are needed to grasp and release larger food items (such as a sandwich) and drinking glasses (Fig. 9.5).
- **Prehension patterns.** *Prehension* refers to a hand position that allows for finger and thumb opposition and manipulation of objects. A variety of prehension patterns contribute to hand function and the execution of daily living skills. For example, with *palmar prehension* (also referred to as *three jaw chuck* or *tripod*), the thumb is in opposition to one or more fingers (e.g., the index and long fingers) as if picking up a small square object. *Lateral prehension* is between the thumb and the radial side of the index and long fingers, as if holding a key. Prehension patterns are required to hold smaller utensils, such as the thin stem of a fork (Fig. 9.6) or knife, the handle of a mug or teacup, a key (Fig. 9.7), and small food items such as pretzel nuggets (Fig. 9.8) or crackers.

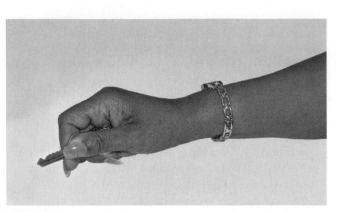

FIGURE 9.7 Palmar prehension pattern used to hold a key is a lead-up skill for self-feeding.

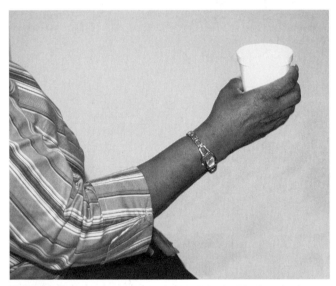

FIGURE 9.5 Gross grasp is required to take hold of and release larger food items and drinking glasses during self-feeding.

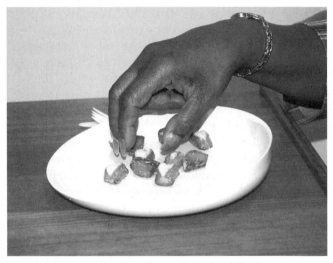

FIGURE 9.8 Lateral prehension pattern used to pick up pretzel nuggets is a lead-up skill for self-feeding.

- **Thumb and finger manipulation.** The fine motor movements of thumb and finger manipulation are needed for dynamic manipulation of small utensils and food items, such as placing a straw in a glass, tearing open sweetener packets (Fig. 9.9), and opening the plastic wrap on tea crackers.
- **Bilateral UE movement.** Bilateral UE movement is required for self-feeding skills, such as cutting food with a knife and fork (Fig. 9.10) and applying butter to a roll.

The UE functions needed for self-feeding are dependent on a progression of lead-up skills. These skills must be addressed in a specific sequence because each depends on a previous prerequisite skill in an ordered progression. Adequate trunk stability is a key prerequisite for all UE skills. Once trunk stability has been established, UE skills should be addressed in the following order:

- Shoulder stability and mobility
- Elbow stability and mobility
- Wrist stability and mobility

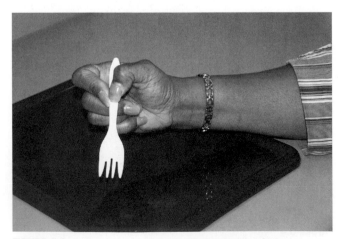

FIGURE 9.6 Prehension pattern is used to hold a fork.

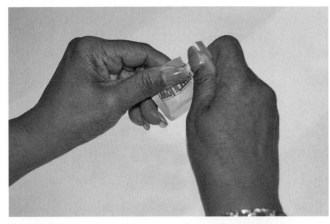

FIGURE 9.9 Thumb and finger manipulation used to open a sweetener packet is a lead-up skill for self-feeding.

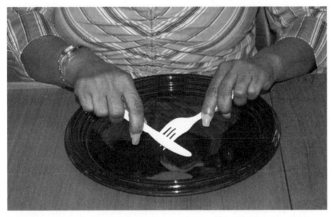

FIGURE 9.10 Bilateral UE movement used to hold an eating utensil in each hand is a lead-up skill for self-feeding.

- Gross grasp and prehension patterns
- Thumb and finger manipulation
- Bilateral UE movements

Most self-feeding skills require two-handed or bilateral manipulation. Bilateral UE integration is the highest skill level required for self-feeding and thus is the final skill addressed in the sequence.

Activity Demands of Self-Feeding: Steps of Self-Feeding

1. The patient must be seated upright at a table (or bed/lap tray) with meal, utensils, and drinking glass positioned in front. Adaptive equipment is used as needed. The pelvis and lower extremities (LEs) should be properly aligned to encourage a neutral position or slight anterior tilt of pelvis and hip abduction. Proper pelvic support is necessary for adequate upper body alignment during self-feeding (Fig. 9.11).
2. The UEs are positioned to encourage shoulder stabilization. Shoulder stabilization is necessary to facilitate the normal movement pattern of forward reach with elbow

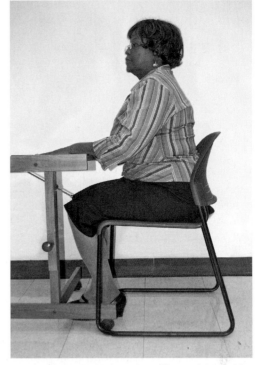

FIGURE 9.11 Upright seated posture. The pelvis and lower extremities should be properly aligned to encourage a neutral position or slight anterior tilt of pelvis and hip abduction.

extension and wrist stabilization so that functional distal hand movements can occur (Fig. 9.12).

3. Food is brought to the mouth via gross grasp (i.e., combined thumb and finger flexion) if finger foods are used (Fig. 9.13). If utensils are used, food is brought to the mouth using prehension patterns to grasp utensils. The normal movement pattern for gross grasp and prehension includes normal finger and thumb extension to release items.

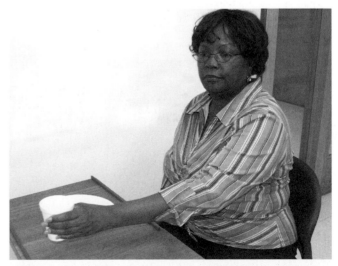

FIGURE 9.12 Shoulder stabilization facilitates the normal movement pattern of forward reach with elbow extension and wrist stabilization so that functional distal hand movements can occur.

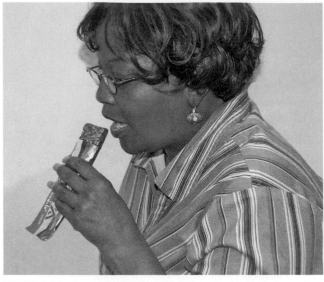

FIGURE 9.13 Food is brought to the mouth via gross grasp for finger feeding (finger foods). *Not shown:* When grasping utensils, prehension patterns are used.

4. The hand is brought back and forth from plate to mouth. Owing to the frequency and duration of this movement pattern in self-feeding (i.e., shoulder, elbow, and wrist stabilization against gravity), the patient's endurance and tolerance for this movement pattern must be monitored for fatigue.
5. Liquids are retrieved from the table using a gross grasp for cups and drinking glasses and prehension patterns for mugs with handles and teacups. These patterns allow liquids to be brought to the mouth and returned to the table (Fig. 9.14).
6. Two-handed cutting (Fig. 9.15) and manipulation of food require bilateral UE integration.

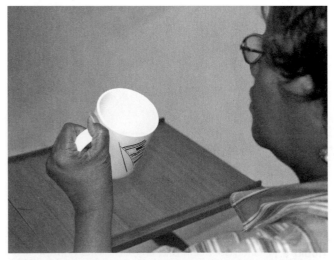

FIGURE 9.14 Liquids are retrieved from the table using gross grasp for glasses and prehension patterns for cups with handles.

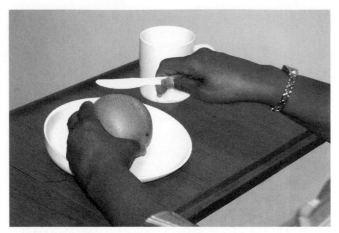

FIGURE 9.15 Bilateral UE integration is required for two-handed cutting and manipulation of foods. The patient holds the knife with one hand and handles the food item in the opposite hand.

Environmental (Physical) Factors

- The patient must be able to maintain an upright seated position in a chair, wheelchair, or bed.
- The table must be at the patient's mid-trunk level.
- The table surface must be large enough and sufficiently stable to accommodate food items, utensils, and the patient's UEs.
- All food items must be consistent with the patient's dietary, nutritional, religious, and social and cultural preferences and restrictions.

Treatment Strategies and Considerations

The following treatment approaches addressing UE function within the context of self-feeding will be described: *neuromuscular facilitation, Proprioceptive Neuromuscular Facilitation (PNF), compensatory training, motor learning,* and *modified constraint-induced therapy.* A discussion of each approach will describe how the therapist may use the intervention to facilitate UE function within the context of self-feeding. The therapist can also use these approaches to promote UE lead-up skills needed to perform BADL.

Therapists use and sequence the treatment approaches in varying combinations depending on patient needs and UE function. An important consideration when deciding when and how to use these approaches is whether the patient has appropriate UE voluntary movement. Patients who demonstrate sufficient recovery of voluntary movement may not benefit from neuromuscular facilitation or an intensive hands-on approach. Rather, such patients benefit more from direct engagement in ADL retraining. Neuromuscular facilitation and PNF are particularly useful for patients who require development or enhancement of lead-up skills (e.g., patients who demonstrate poor shoulder stabilization, reaching, pushing, grasp and prehension patterns, or patients with poor bilateral

UE use owing to movement patterns impaired by increased or decreased tone, weakness, and movement decomposition).

Neuromuscular Facilitation

Neuromuscular facilitation is an important intervention for the development of lead-up skills needed to perform self-feeding. Selected components of the intervention are described within the context of facilitating the following lead-up skills: *stabilization*, *reach*, and *grasp and prehension* patterns.

Stabilization

Joint approximation can be used to promote proximal shoulder stabilization via weightbearing activities. The patient is instructed to bear weight on the more affected UE, which is positioned in elbow extension and supported by the therapist (Fig. 9.16) or by another support surface (e.g., a platform mat). Approximation can be used to facilitate shoulder/scapular stabilizers and elbow extensors. Sufficient shoulder stability is required before the patient can achieve dynamic distal movement in space against gravity (required for all self-feeding skills).

Reach

Once shoulder stabilization is established, reaching is addressed. Reaching can be facilitated using active scapular protraction, shoulder flexion, and elbow extension. The patient is initially instructed to slide the UE (gravity minimized) along a tabletop surface in a forward direction as if reaching for a target food item (Fig. 9.17). When this skill is achieved, the patient can begin to practice the higher-level skill of reaching (against gravity) into space to grasp a glass

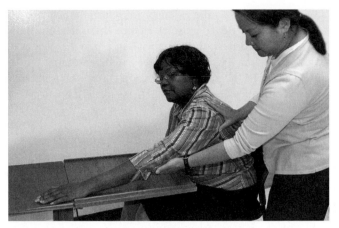

FIGURE 9.17 To facilitate reaching, the patient is instructed to slide the UE (with gravity minimized) along a tabletop as if reaching for a targeted food item.

or bread roll (Fig. 9.18). To facilitate agonist contraction of the anterior deltoid for forward reach, tapping over the muscle belly can be incorporated. Tapping elicits a quick stretch of these muscles. The muscle contraction that is generated, however, is short lasting. Therefore, resistance may be added to maintain muscle contraction. Once these lead-up skills have been performed, the therapist can guide the patient in the use of these skills to perform reaching movements in an actual self-feeding activity.

Grasp and Prehension

An important goal of neuromuscular facilitation is to reduce flexor spasticity and promote extension in patients with UE flexor synergy patterns. For these patients, reduced flexor spasticity in the wrist and fingers is required for grasp and prehension patterns. Functional grasp and prehension patterns involve voluntary active finger and thumb flexion and voluntary active finger, thumb, and wrist extension. Without voluntary grasp and prehension patterns, independence in self-feeding cannot be achieved. Wrist and finger extensors can be activated by tapping over the respective muscle

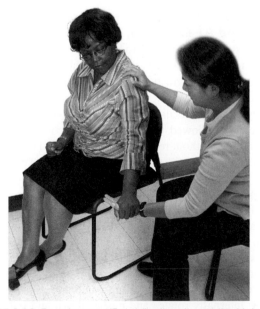

FIGURE 9.16 To enhance UE stabilization, the patient is instructed to bear weight on the more affected UE positioned in elbow extension on a support surface. Support is provided using manual contacts from the therapist. Alternatively, a treatment table or mat surface can be used to support the UE.

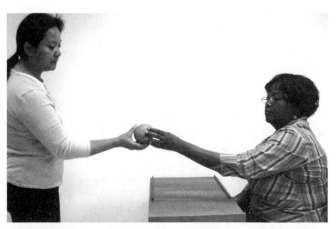

FIGURE 9.18 The patient practices reaching against gravity into space to grasp a food item.

bellies. Tapping over the extensor muscles is thought to inhibit the spastic flexor muscles.[1] Once these lead-up skills have been performed, the therapist can guide the patient to practice voluntary wrist and finger extension during a self-feeding task (e.g., grasp and release of a drinking glass or prehend and release small food items, such as a bread roll or tea cracker).

Clinical Note: When using neuromuscular facilitation techniques, therapists must consistently maintain an acute awareness of the patient's quality of UE movement. Compensatory movement patterns should be brought to the patient's attention, and verbal and manual cues should be used to help the patient correct abnormal movement patterns so they do not become learned habits. For example, when attempting forward reach, a patient may compensate with shoulder elevation and abduction rather than appropriate shoulder flexion and scapular protraction. Similarly, patients attempting distal movements may also exhibit excess shoulder movements. Such compensatory movement must be noted immediately and corrected. Correction should begin with verbal and manual cues to offer both auditory and proprioceptive feedback. As the patient begins to demonstrate learning, verbal cues (VCs) should be continued while manual cues are decreased. Eventually, VCs can also be diminished as the patient gains the ability to self-correct inappropriate movement patterns. Practice of desired normal movement patterns should begin with proximal musculature and progress distally as the patient's performance becomes more skilled. Eventually, the practice of both proximal and distal movement patterns can be combined (as they would be in functional activities).

Red Flag: The observation of abnormal movement patterns and the use of compensation strategies in place of appropriate movement may indicate that the patient has been challenged to perform a motor activity that is presently beyond his or her skill level. The range of motion (ROM) or the physical effort required for performing a specific shoulder, elbow, wrist, or hand movement may be too demanding for the patient and could inhibit his or her ability to practice and learn normal movement patterns. In these situations, the therapist should immediately intervene to modify the task to provide a therapeutic challenge that is more appropriate. The observation of increased spasticity in any muscle group is also an indication that the patient has been asked to perform an activity that is too demanding. In such cases, facilitation of one joint at a time and the use of gravity-minimized positions may help to decrease the challenge level of a particular activity.

Note: The student practice activities in this chapter are presented as short patient examples with accompanying guiding questions. Box 9.2 Student Practice Activity presents a patient example with application of neuromuscular facilitation.

Proprioceptive Neuromuscular Facilitation (PNF)

Like neuromuscular facilitation, PNF may also be used to promote the required lead-up skills to feeding (UE stabilization, reach, grasp, and prehension). Because normal movement patterns are made through a combined use of rotational and diagonal planes, PNF can be used to facilitate the normal movement patterns needed for functional activities. Bilteral UE PNF patterns that place demands on trunk control can facilitate the needed lead-up skills in preparation for self-feeding. PNF guiding principles call for a progression of activities within the stages of motor control: *mobility, stability, controlled mobility,* and *skill.* The following guidelines may be used to promote the lead-up skills needed for self-feeding.

Trunk Stabilization, Rhythmic Stabilization

Trunk stabilization is critical for adequate UE use. During feeding activities, patients must be able to use the trunk to lean forward while bringing food to the mouth and to use shoulder stability to facilitate reaching and hand-to-mouth patterns. Trunk stabilization may be enhanced through the PNF technique of *rhythmic stabilization.* Rhythmic stabilization uses isometric contractions against resistance (no motion occurs). To promote initial trunk stabilization using rhythmic stabilization, the patient is positioned sidelying. Resistance is applied simultaneously to the upper trunk flexors with one hand and to the lower trunk extensors with the opposite hand (Fig. 9.19). Repetitions of this technique should be performed in accordance with the patient's tolerance and fatigue level. The activity can be progressed to sitting with application of rhythmic stabilization.

Shoulder Stabilization, Upper Extremity PNF D1 Flexion and D1 Extension, Dynamic Reversals

Shoulder stability is critical to achieving functional reach using hand-to-mouth patterns; forearm and wrist stabilization is necessary for grasp and prehension of eating utensils and food items.

Dynamic reversals promote isotonic contractions in one direction followed by isotonic contractions in the reverse direction without relaxation. VCs are used to mark initiation of movement in the opposite direction. The patient may be positioned in supine (which provides good trunk support) or sitting. The patient is instructed to move into the UE D1 flexion (UE D1F) pattern against resistance, but only to midrange (Fig. 9.20). The shoulder externally rotates and pulls up and across the face, moving into shoulder adduction and flexion. The patient is asked to hold this position for approximately 3 seconds. The patient then moves into the UE D1 extension (UE D1E) pattern against resistance. The shoulder internally rotates and pushes down and out, moving into abduction and extension (Fig. 9.21). Resistance is gradually increased in both directions before the patient is asked to hold the position. The holding position may be

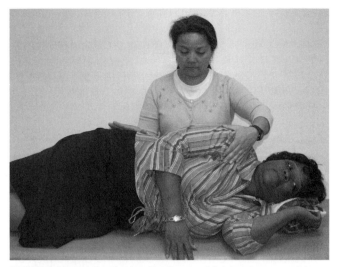

FIGURE 9.19 Rhythmic stabilization in sidelying to promote trunk stability. The patient is in sidelying while the therapist applies matched isometric resistance to the upper trunk flexors with one hand and matched resistance to the lower trunk extensors with the other hand. Resistance is applied simultaneously to opposing muscle groups (e.g., upper trunk flexors and lower trunk extensors, or upper trunk extensors and lower trunk flexors). Although no movement occurs, resistance is applied as if twisting or rotating the upper and lower trunk in opposite directions.

varied at different points in the joint range. Repetitions of dynamic reversals with a hold should be performed in accordance with the patient's tolerance and fatigue level.

Reach With Forearm Stabilization, UE PNF D1F and D1E, Dynamic Reversals

Once shoulder stabilization has been achieved, forearm stabilization during reaching activities should be addressed. In self-feeding, forearm stabilization is needed to support and

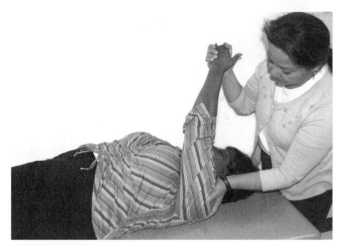

FIGURE 9.20 Supine, UE PNF D1 flexion, dynamic reversals. The patient moves into the D1F pattern to midrange while the therapist applies continuous resistance to isotonic contractions.

BOX 9.2 STUDENT PRACTICE ACTIVITY: PATIENT EXAMPLE—APPLICATION OF NEUROMUSCULAR FACILITATION

Mr. Goldman is an 84-year-old male who is 3 weeks status post a left cerebrovascular accident (CVA) resulting in right UE hemiparesis. The quality of right UE movement is characterized by minimal active shoulder movement, minimal active elbow and wrist movement, and minimal active finger, thumb, and wrist flexion and extension. There is evidence of a mild flexor synergy pattern against gravity. The patient also exhibits mild visual-spatial impairment and requires minimal VCs to attend to multiple-step activities.

Mr. Goldman was initially provided with weightbearing activities of the UE to facilitate cocontraction of the shoulder musculature and active elbow extension. In order to facilitate active shoulder and elbow movements for forward reaching, Mr. Goldman was provided with active-assistive exercises to decrease the effort needed to move against gravity. Once Mr. Goldman was able to independently support his shoulder and elbow within a minimal ROM, he was encouraged to practice grasp-release hand patterns requiring active wrist extension. When Mr. Goldman was able to demonstrate UE movement patterns with only a slight flexor synergistic overlay, he was offered a self-feeding task using a plastic fork to prehend and spear

lightweight, large food items. He practiced the hand-to-mouth pattern requiring shoulder stabilization with active distal movements several times, incorporating rest breaks as needed.

Guiding Questions

1. How can neuromuscular facilitation techniques be used in conjunction with a therapeutic exercise program? What would a therapeutic exercise program consist of? How would you teach Mr. Goldman's caregivers to carry out a therapeutic exercise program in his home environment? What contraindications should be noted? What are signs or red flags that caregivers should be alerted to when working with Mr. Goldman?
2. What specific lead-up skills would you use to facilitate trunk and postural control to encourage normal UE movement patterns?
3. What specific lead-up skills would you use to facilitate normal UE movement patterns of the shoulder, elbow, wrist, and hand?
4. How can the physical therapist and occupational therapist collaborate to enhance the relearning of normal movement patterns and increase independence in functional tasks such as self-feeding?

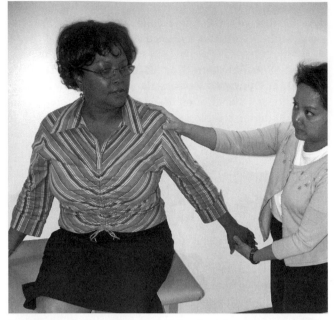

FIGURE 9.21 Sitting, UE PNF D1 extension, dynamic reversals. The patient moves into the D1E pattern while the therapist applies continuous resistance to isotonic contractions.

maintain the wrist in a position of slight extension (approximately 20 to 30 degrees). This prerequisite lead-up skill allows for the appropriate hand manipulation of food items and utensils. The patient is positioned in sitting. Dynamic reversals may be used to promote isotonic contractions of the UE agonists, followed by isotonic contractions of the UE antagonists performed with resistance. The UE D1F pattern in which the shoulder flexes, adducts, and externally rotates facilitates reach and hand-to-mouth patterns (this pattern is illustrated in Fig. 9.20 from a *supine* position). The patient is instructed to close the hand, wrist, and fingers and to pull the limb up and across the face so that the shoulder is adducted and flexed, with the elbow extended. The therapist should apply matched resistance (matched to the strength of the patient's contractions) to this UE D1F pattern. When the patient's UE is positioned near the end of its range, he or she is instructed to change direction into the UE D1E pattern. The patient is asked to open the hand and extend the fingers and wrist, with the shoulder internally rotated pushing down and out (see Fig. 9.21). The shoulder should now be in abduction and extension. The therapist should apply matched resistance to this UE D1E pattern. When these PNF patterns are reversed, movement should be smooth and continuous without relaxation and resistance maintained from one pattern into the opposite pattern.

Clinical Note: The therapist should continuously observe the quality of the patient's performance in desired movement patterns and then monitor and adjust the amount of matched resistance using manual and verbal cueing to correct abnormal postures and positioning. Manual contacts used as cues should be progressively

decreased as the patient is able to demonstrate more normal movement patterns. As manual contacts are decreased, verbal cueing continues but is progressively withdrawn as the patient is able to demonstrate self-correction of inappropriate movement patterns, replacing them with normal movements (or with movements approximating normal patterns).

Red Flag: The above PNF techniques are indicated only for patients who possess no less than minimal to moderate active movement and no more than minimal hypertonicity in the UE and trunk. If significant hypertonicity is noted, PNF techniques must be used with caution or may be contraindicated, as the application of resistance may increase hypertonicity and reduce the quality of the desired movement patterns. Evidence of pain should also be monitored during the application of gradual increments in resistance and during movement of a joint through its range.

Box 9.3 Student Practice Activity presents a patient example with application of PNF UE D1F and UE D1E patterns.

Compensatory Training

A compensatory training approach should be used when UE recovery is limited and ADL function must be promoted through adaptive methods. In the compensatory approach, the less affected UE and all preserved function of the more affected UE are used in the context of direct engagement in ADL retraining. Facilitation techniques are not used because significant return of further function is not expected. Selected adaptive devices can be used to substitute for the absence of foundational UE skills. For example, poor proximal shoulder stability can be addressed using a mobile arm support (described below). Splints designed to enhance wrist support can compensate for the absence of wrist extension, which is a necessary prerequisite skill for gross grasp and prehension. Built-up handles on utensils further aid gross grasp and prehension patterns.

Shoulder Stabilization

A mobile arm support (MAS) can be used to compensate for poor proximal shoulder stability (Fig. 9.22). The MAS attaches to the patient's wheelchair to support the shoulder, elbow, forearm, and wrist. It provides shoulder stabilization so that the distal UE is placed in a position of function to promote movements needed in self-feeding (i.e., bringing food items back and forth from mouth to plate).

Reaching

Shoulder stabilization and scapular protraction are prerequisite skills for reaching. Once shoulder stabilization and scapular protraction have been appropriately established through compensatory strategies (such as a MAS), shoulder forward reach and elbow extension in space can be facilitated to promote reaching patterns. The therapist should

BOX 9.3 STUDENT PRACTICE ACTIVITY: PATIENT EXAMPLE—APPLICATION OF PNF UE D1F AND UE D1E PATTERNS

Mrs. Wong is a 54-year-old female who is 12 weeks status post a right humeral fracture. She is able to demonstrate approximately 0 to 90 degrees of active right shoulder flexion and abduction. Moderate limitations in active internal and external rotation are also noted. UE patterns and dynamic reversals were used to promote isotonic contractions of shoulder agonists (i.e., shoulder flexion, adduction, and external rotation), followed by isotonic contractions of shoulder antagonists (i.e., shoulder extension, abduction, and internal rotation) performed with resistance. The therapist guided Mrs. Wong to move into the UE D1F pattern (shoulder adduction and flexion) and applied matched resistance. The patient was then instructed to change direction into the UE D1E pattern, moving the shoulder into abduction and extension against matched resistance. Providing resistance with UE PNF patterns can increase joint ROM and muscular strength in shoulder movements while incorporating the rotational and diagonal movements required in self-feeding (e.g., the hand-to-mouth feeding pattern). Once Mrs. Wong's shoulder ROM and muscular strength

increased, she was given a self-feeding activity to practice incorporating the combined UE movements needed to perform normal hand-to-mouth patterns.

Guiding Questions

1. How can the above methods be used in conjunction with a therapeutic exercise program? What would a therapeutic exercise program consist of? How would you teach Mrs. Wong's caregivers to carry out a therapeutic exercise program in her home environment? What are signs or red flags that caregivers should be alerted to when working with Mrs. Wong?
2. What additional lead-up skills would facilitate UE ROM and strength?
3. How can the physical therapist and occupational therapist collaborate to enhance relearning of normal movement patterns and increase independence in functional tasks such as self-feeding?
4. What contraindications should you consider when using PNF techniques for patients who have sustained a shoulder fracture?

---

instruct the patient to practice shoulder forward reach and elbow extension during the retrieval of food and in the context of hand-to-mouth patterns.

Grasp and Prehension

A MAS provides stabilization by compensating for weak proximal shoulder stability, supporting the shoulder in slight abduction and flexion. The MAS forearm trough supports the elbow, forearm, and wrist and facilitates forward reaching, which allows the movements needed for grasping and prehension. For patients who may experience distal return of musculature (e.g., peripheral nerve injury), a dorsal wrist support can be used to provide wrist stabilization (Fig. 9.23)

so that thumb and finger flexion can be achieved for gross grasp and prehension of utensils and food items. Once shoulder and wrist stabilization are established, the therapist should instruct the patient to practice gross grasp patterns. For example, the therapist may guide patient practice in grasping a small carton of milk and pouring it into a drinking glass. Patients who are not expected to experience distal return (e.g., those with spinal cord injury [SCI]) may still be candidates for dorsal wrist support, but adaptations to compensate for lost thumb and finger movements are indicated.

Grasp and prehension patterns can also be enhanced using built-up handles on utensils—an adaptive device that compensates for weakness and lack of isolated movement of

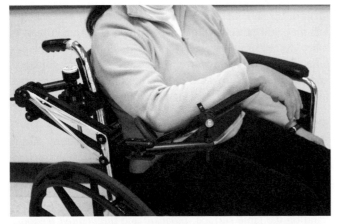

FIGURE 9.22 A mobile arm support can be used to compensate for weak proximal shoulder stability so that distal UE movements can occur.

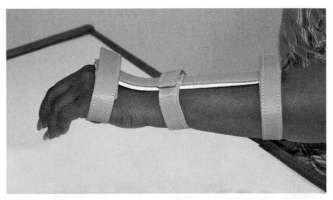

FIGURE 9.23 A dorsal wrist support can be used to provide wrist stabilization so that thumb and finger flexion can be achieved for gross grasp and prehension of utensils and food items.

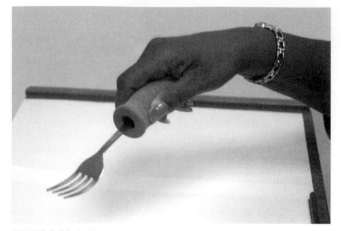

FIGURE 9.24 Built-up handles on utensils compensate for weakness and lack of isolated movement of the finger flexors.

the finger flexors (Fig. 9.24). A universal cuff—which can hold utensils when isolated finger movements are absent—can be applied to the palmar surface of the hand to compensate for absent finger and thumb movements (Fig. 9.25).

Bilateral UE Use

After the above prerequisite skills of shoulder stabilization, scapular protraction, shoulder forward reach, elbow extension, and grasp and prehension have been facilitated through compensation, bilateral UE use can be promoted through activities such as cutting with both hands or picking up a sandwich. The therapist should guide the patient in integrating both UEs within the context of an actual self-feeding activity.

Clinical Note: Many patients perceive adaptive equipment as a sign of disability. Although adaptive devices help patients compensate for lost motor function and can ultimately help them achieve a desired level of independence in self-feeding, many patients resist their use owing to fear and stigmatization. For some patients, the use of adaptive devices may represent an

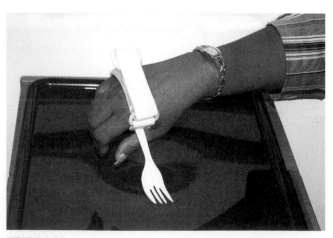

FIGURE 9.25 A universal cuff can compensate for absent finger and thumb movements.

admission that little or no further recovery is possible. Because of this perception, the use of adaptive devices must be presented to patients with gentleness and in accordance with their own readiness to accept their injury or illness. The introduction and presentation of self-feeding devices must emphasize the patient's ability to achieve independence in this BADL. Patients should be able to exercise their own freedom to decide whether they are emotionally able or ready to use self-feeding devices.

Red Flag: Research regarding the brain's neuroplasticity has demonstrated that motor recovery, in some patients, can occur several years following a neurological insult—long after further motor recovery was thought to be possible.[2] Thus, therapists must understand that the long-term use of adaptive equipment to compensate for poor motor recovery may prevent further potential return. Patients should be encouraged to use adaptive equipment to increase independence and ADL efficiency, but they should also be provided with a therapeutic exercise program to facilitate the potential return of desired muscle function in involved limbs.

Box 9.4 Student Practice Activity presents a patient example with application of compensatory training strategies.

Motor Learning

Motor learning is used with patients who are able to engage in repeated practice of desired skills and who can cognitively use feedback to modify movement errors. Motor learning relies heavily on actual practice, mental practice, and feedback. Rather than relying on facilitation techniques (e.g., neuromuscular facilitation and PNF) to improve lead-up skills needed for functional skill performance, motor learning is based on the theory that motor skills are best relearned when practice takes place within the context of the actual desired activity (activity- or task-specific training).

Thus, patients who are candidates for motor learning strategies should demonstrate some recovery of isolated movement of the shoulder, elbow, wrist, and/or hand. The patient's UE may still present with some weakness or impairment of tone. Motor learning is chiefly used to organize movement patterns (i.e., synergistic movement patterns). Cues, guidance, and feedback are provided to help the patient relearn normal movement patterns as they are practiced in actual activities.

Shoulder Stabilization and Reaching

Selected components of the UE movement pattern during feeding (i.e., shoulder stabilization, scapular protraction, shoulder forward reach, and elbow extension) should initially be addressed in isolation. The patient can be instructed to perform the motor pattern by reaching forward to place his or her hand on the table surface. *Intrinsic* and *augmented feedback* are used to help the patient understand what normal movement feels like. ***Intrinsic feedback*** provides proprioceptive

BOX 9.4 STUDENT PRACTICE ACTIVITY: PATIENT EXAMPLE—APPLICATION OF COMPENSATORY TRAINING STRATEGIES

Raphael is a 22-year-old male construction worker who is status post a C5 incomplete SCI sustained in a work-related accident. A MAS was used to compensate for weak proximal shoulder stability and to facilitate forward reaching during a self-feeding activity. It stabilized the shoulder against gravity and provided support to the elbow, forearm, and wrist. The MAS was positioned to facilitate elbow extension and the forearm to move with the assistance of gravity—to compensate for poor elbow extension. Since Raphael had minimal active elbow flexion, he could engage an eccentric contraction of the biceps to help control the speed of elbow extension. The use of a MAS to compensate for weak proximal stabilization also promoted distal movements (e.g., bringing food items back and forth from mouth to plate). Additionally, adaptive devices including a dorsal wrist support (Fig. 9.23) and a universal cuff (Fig. 9.25) were used to compensate for poor wrist extension and weak or absent grasp and prehension. Practicing the UE movement pattern of bringing food items back and forth from mouth to plate during an actual feeding activity also strengthened the musculature that may have been spared following Raphael's incomplete SCI. The use of compensatory devices is necessary to promote independence in feeding when patients do not otherwise have the physical capability needed for basic feeding skills. However, if there is evidence that motor return is occurring in the shoulder or other musculature, the use of compensatory devices may be diminished as the patient improves and is able to use his own muscle power for self-feeding and other functional activities.

Guiding Questions

1. What shoulder and elbow movements are preserved at a C5 spinal cord level? What movements are lost? How do you think such losses affect specific daily activities?
2. If you were Raphael's physical therapist, what type of therapeutic exercise program would you design to enhance his UE use? What specific exercises could be used to target the spared musculature at the C5 spinal cord level? How could your therapeutic exercise program support the occupational therapist's effort to help Raphael regain independence in self-feeding?
3. How can the physical therapist and occupational therapist collaborate to enhance potential return of the UE musculature in patients with incomplete spinal cord injuries?
4. How would you train Raphael's caregivers in the use of a home exercise program (HEP)?

---

and tactile information about the patient's own movement. For example, the patient can be instructed to use the less affected side to reinforce what normal movement feels like when spearing food with a utensil.

Augmented feedback provides information about the patient's movement patterns from external sources (e.g., VCs from the therapist and visual cues from observing one's own movement in a mirror). *Knowledge of performance* is a type of augmented feedback that provides information about the patient's performance of movement patterns. For example, the therapist may offer verbal feedback to the patient about the inappropriate use of shoulder elevation to compensate for impaired shoulder flexion during reaching. The therapist might also use a mirror to show the patient how he or she elevates the shoulder as a form of compensation for impaired shoulder flexion during reaching. *Knowledge of results* is another form of augmented feedback that provides information about the outcome of the movement pattern. For example, after repeated practice and feedback, the patient may be able to spear food with decreased shoulder elevation and increased shoulder flexion. Successfully reaching for and spearing food with a utensil (without excessive shoulder elevation) provide the patient with knowledge that the desired outcome was attained.

Grasp and Prehension

Once normal movement patterns of the shoulder and elbow have been achieved through motor learning principles, wrist stabilization to support grasp and prehension can be addressed using intrinsic feedback. For example, the patient can be instructed to place the less affected wrist in a position of stabilization while bringing a drinking glass toward the mouth. The patient is asked to observe what more normal proprioceptive feedback feels like in response to wrist stabilization. *Knowledge of performance* can provide augmented feedback about wrist stabilization through external sources. For example, a patient who lacks wrist stabilization may overcompensate with shoulder abduction. The therapist can use VCs and a mirror to help the patient understand that he or she is substituting shoulder abduction for wrist stabilization. Through VCs and the visual feedback of a mirror, the patient is guided to practice normal wrist stabilization patterns with increased wrist extension and reduced shoulder abduction. *Knowledge of results* is provided when the patient is able to reach for and grasp a drinking glass with normal shoulder stabilization, scapular protraction, shoulder forward reach, elbow extension, wrist stabilization, and finger/thumb grasp and prehension patterns.

Bilateral UE Use

Once normal shoulder, elbow, wrist, and finger/thumb movement patterns have been established, the patient can be guided in bilateral UE use. The patient can be instructed to practice bilateral integration by using the less affected UE to pour milk into a cereal bowl while using the more affected UE to stabilize the bowl. Intrinsic feedback can be highlighted by directing the patient's attention to the proprioceptive and tactile information that accompanies bilateral integration. Use of an object (e.g., the milk container) with the less involved UE provides proprioceptive information regarding the initial weight of the container, the changing weight of the milk container as the liquid is poured into the bowl, the change in forearm positions from neutral to pronated as the milk is poured from the container, and the maintenance of shoulder stabilization as the forearm pronates while pouring the milk. *Knowledge of performance* can then be attained when the patient pours the milk with the more affected limb. The therapist may use VCs to help the patient understand that he or she needs to bring the UE closer to midline (through shoulder adduction and elbow flexion) to pour the milk into the bowl instead of onto the table. Auditory cues of the milk as it hits the cereal (instead of the side of the bowl) can also serve as augmented feedback regarding the need to modify motor patterns. Finally, *knowledge of results*—for example, the milk spilling on the tabletop instead of on the cereal—can be used to help the patient correct motor errors until the desired movement pattern is achieved.

Practice

After a patient successfully demonstrates a desired movement pattern, he or she is asked to engage in constant or repeated practice of that movement pattern within the context of a specific activity.

• *Constant practice* involves a single motor skill that is rehearsed repeatedly until mastered. For example, a patient may practice palmar prehension with wrist extension to retrieve similar-sized food items presented on a plate positioned at midline.
• *Variable practice* involves the ability to modify motor patterns in accordance with the demands of a specific activity. Variable practice involves a higher-level skill than constant practice and should be addressed after constant practice has sufficiently been performed. For example, a patient is given a plate of food items having varied sizes and weights and is asked to retrieve each food item separately. The demands of this activity require the patient to modify grasp and prehension patterns in accordance with each food item, as it varies in weight and size.
• *Mental practice* is a form of practice in which the patient uses cognitive rehearsal to improve motor patterns, without actually attempting physical movement. For example, as a patient begins to practice desired movement patterns in therapy, the therapist may instruct the patient to spend 15 minutes in the afternoon and before bed mentally

rehearsing the performance of reaching to retrieve a glass using shoulder stabilization without elevation.

When using motor learning, therapists must be cautious to monitor patients' level of fatigue continuously, which will determine the duration of practice. Augmented feedback that addresses the primary senses (i.e., audition, vision, and sensation) should be provided to best meet patients' unique learning styles. Activities should first be practiced as selected segments. Once mastery of selected segments has been achieved, practice of the activity as a whole is recommended (i.e., parts-to-whole training).

Clinical Note: The type and amount of practice are important considerations for promoting motor learning principles. Research has shown that variable practice (in which the patient is asked to make rapid modifications of the skill to meet the changing demands of the task or environment) is better for retention and generalization of learning compared to constant practice (in which the patient is asked to repeatedly practice a single motor skill that does not change).[3] Therefore, movement patterns should be practiced using varied positions, heights, and ranges. The use of *massed practice* (in which the amount of rest time is less than the total practice time) versus *distributed practice* (in which the amount of rest time is equal to or greater than the total practice time) must also be considered. Massed practice may lead to decreased movement quality as patients become fatigued. A patient's tolerance and fatigue level must be continuously monitored to determine whether massed practiced can be tolerated or distributed practice must be initiated.

Red Flag: Because practice may easily fatigue a patient with compromised status, therapists must carefully observe for signs of muscular, cardiovascular, and mental fatigue. Fatigue may also lead to an increase in spasticity and, subsequently, a decrease in the quality of the desired movement patterns. The monitoring of heart rate, blood pressure, and oxygen saturation levels is indicated for patients with compromised cardiovascular status. Patients with minimal cognitive impairments may require frequent visual, verbal, and manual cueing to follow prescribed practice protocols. Consequently, generalization of learning may be difficult for such patients, and caregiver training should be initiated in addition to patient instruction. Progression from constant to variable practice is generally contraindicated for patients with severe cognitive impairment.

Box 9.5 Student Practice Activity presents a patient example with application of motor learning principles.

Modified Constraint-Induced Movement Therapy

Constraint-induced movement therapy (CIMT or CI therapy) is a treatment approach that improves use of the more

BOX 9.5 STUDENT PRACTICE ACTIVITY: PATIENT EXAMPLE—APPLICATION OF MOTOR LEARNING PRINCIPLES

Jake is an 18-year-old male who sustained a traumatic brain injury (TBI) in a motor vehicle accident. He presents with frontal lobe dysfunction marked by mild attention problems and decreased awareness of disability. Jake is able to follow two- or three-step directions with minimal verbal and visual cues. He exhibits overall weakness, however, and has moderate active movement in his right UE, including grasp and prehension. Jake currently appears to favor his left UE, although he is right-hand dominant.

Knowledge of performance was used to provide augmented feedback to Jake during the use of his right UE in self-feeding activities. *Augmented feedback* incorporated visual and VCs to provide information about his performance of UE movement patterns. Because Jake was using shoulder elevation to compensate for impaired shoulder flexion during reaching activities, he was provided with VCs to decrease excess shoulder elevation. The therapist initially addressed isolated shoulder movements to minimize the cognitive demands of simultaneously attending to prehension patterns (using a thin-stemmed fork). Jake was also provided with a mirror to visually cue him to recognize his use of shoulder elevation as a form of compensation for weak shoulder flexion during reaching.

Once Jake was able to perform reaching with appropriate scapular protraction and shoulder forward reach,

variable practice was used to enhance his hand-to-mouth feeding pattern. Jake was given a plate of food items that were positioned on different areas of the dish; he was then asked to grasp 1- to 2-inch (2.5 to 5 cm) foods that required him to vary his reach pattern. The demands of this activity required Jake to adjust his reach patterns depending on where each food item was positioned on the plate. *Knowledge of results* was attained once Jake was able to successfully reach for and grasp the different-sized food items while using a normal UE movement pattern.

Guiding Questions

1. What is important to consider when treating a patient who has both physical and cognitive deficits? What cognitive demands are required for self-feeding activities?
2. If you were Jake's physical therapist, how would you challenge Jake to enhance his UE control without using therapeutic activities that are too cognitively demanding?
3. What types of cues would best facilitate Jake's performance without causing him to become agitated?
4. How can the physical therapist and occupational therapist collaborate to enhance relearning of normal movement patterns and increase independence in functional tasks such as self-feeding?

affected extremity following a stroke. It includes intense task-specific practice with multiple treatment elements and is discussed fully in Chapter 10. Modified constraint-induced movement therapy (mCIMT) was developed to provide a less intense movement therapy protocol for patients with chronic stroke.[4] Modified CIMT combines half-hour-long structured functional practice sessions with restriction of the less affected UE 5 days a week for 5 hours, during a 10-week period.[5] Several randomized controlled studies have found that mCIMT effectively improved the use and function of the more affected UE in all stages of acquired brain injury recovery.[6-8] Patients who have used mCIMT also reported good adherence with decreased incidence of pain. Modified CIMT is intended to be used as an outpatient intervention and is reimbursable within the parameters of most managed care plans.[5]

mCIMT Protocol

Modified CIMT provides (1) repeated practice attempts that are known to facilitate skill acquisition, (2) purposeful specific practice, (3) a practice schedule that is safe and motivating for participants, and (4) active problem-solving to facilitate learning.

1. Treatment consists of 30 minutes of occupational therapy and 30 minutes of physical therapy, each three times per week for 10 weeks.
2. Occupational therapy focuses on use of the more affected limb in meaningful functional activities that provide opportunity for UE strengthening and control.
3. Physical therapy focuses on UE limb strengthening and stretching, dynamic standing balance, and gait activities.
4. Shaping—a principal derived from CIMT—is the use of small steps that progressively increase in difficulty. Shaping is used to slowly but steadily increase motor performance.
5. Shaping techniques, functional activities, and rest periods are alternated for approximately 5 minutes each during therapy.
6. The less affected UE is restrained every weekday for a 5-hour period in which patients must actively attempt to use their more affected UE during daily activities.
7. The less affected UE is restrained using a cotton sling with the hand placed in a meshed, polystyrene-filled mitt with hook and loop straps around the wrist.

8. A log is used to record periods of mCIMT in the patient's home; the log is also used to record the specific activities performed during restraint periods of the less affected UE.

Clinical Note: The primary therapeutic factor in both CIMT and mCIMT appears to be the repeated use of the more affected UE, which is theorized to induce cortical reorganization with accompanying functional improvements. Repeated functional practice using the more affected UE (as directed by the protocol) appears to overcome learned nonuse and improves function.

Red Flag: One shortcoming of both CIMT and mCIMT is that patients must demonstrate the minimum active range of motion (AROM) of distal extension in the more affected UE (see Table 10.1 in Chapter 10). Functional electrical stimulation (FES) has been shown to be an effective means to facilitate active wrist and finger extension in patients who fail to meet these criteria but demonstrate traces of motor unit activity in their more affected forearms.[9] It is important to identify such patients and attempt to activate distal UE extension through FES before determining that they are ineligible for mCIMT.

Box 9.6 Student Practice Activity presents a patient example with application of mCIMT.

SUMMARY

This chapter has addressed the basic requirements for UE function within the context of daily living skills. Task analysis guidelines were presented. Activity demands and suggested interventions were discussed for the tasks of self-feeding as well as the pre-feeding tasks of stabilization, reach, grasp, and prehension. The treatment approaches discussed included neuromuscular facilitation, proprioceptive neuromuscular facilitation, compensatory training, motor learning, and modified constraint-induced therapy.

BOX 9.6 STUDENT PRACTICE ACTIVITY: PATIENT EXAMPLE—APPLICATION OF MODIFIED CONSTRAINT-INDUCED MOVEMENT THERAPY

Mrs. Lopez is a 62-year-old female with a history of hypertension and type II diabetes. She is currently 6 weeks status post a right CVA with resultant left UE hemiparesis. The quality of left UE movement is characterized by moderate active shoulder movement; minimal active elbow and wrist movements; and moderate active finger, thumb, and wrist flexion/extension. On active movement, a moderate flexor synergy pattern emerges. Visual perception and cognition (specifically attention, recall, and basic problem-solving skills) are intact. Although the patient is left-hand dominant, she fails to use her left UE for ADL and requires moderate assistance for most functional self-care activities.

Mrs. Lopez received outpatient occupational therapy three times per week for 30-minute sessions over the course of 10 weeks. She chose two functional activities to address in therapy: self-feeding and donning clothing with moderate assistance. Therapy consisted of practicing feeding techniques for 5 minutes at a time during which hand-to-mouth patterns were incorporated while using the left hand to prehend a lightweight fork for spearing foods. The hand-to-mouth pattern was repeated three or four times per 30-minute session, leaving time for appropriate rest periods. Shaping was used to decrease compensatory movements (i.e., excess shoulder elevation and abduction) and increase normal movement patterns. In physical therapy, Mrs. Lopez practiced ambulating with a straight cane (progressing from her current use of a quad cane).

When Mrs. Lopez was at home, her less affected right UE was restrained for 5 hours each day during the performance of her routine daily activities (e.g., feeding, dressing, preparing light cold meals, and doing light dusting). The patient's spouse maintained a log of her activities performed while her right UE was restrained. He also assisted with all ADL tasks as needed and secured the UE mCIMT restraint device. After 10 weeks, Mrs. Lopez could independently use a left UE hand-to-mouth pattern to spear large food items with a lightweight fork. She also could independently don upper body garments, using both UEs and minimal assistance to don lower body garments.

Guiding Questions

1. If you were Mrs. Lopez's physical therapist, what lead-up skills would you select to facilitate normal UE movement patterns in preparation for self-feeding?
2. What type of HEP would you design for her? How would you train Mrs. Lopez's spouse to carry out the HEP? What red flags and contraindications should the spouse be informed of in order to best facilitate his wife's recovery?
3. How can the physical therapist and occupational therapist collaborate to enhance relearning of normal movement patterns and increase independence in functional tasks such as self-feeding?

REFERENCES

1. Carr, JH, and Shepherd, RB. Neurological Rehabilitation: Optimizing Motor Performance. Elsevier, New York, 1998.
2. Dobkin, BH. Rehabilitation after stroke. N Engl J Med 352(16):1677, 2005.
3. Shumway-Cook, A, and Woollacott, MH. Motor Control: Theory and Practical Applications, ed 2. Lippincott Williams & Wilkins, Philadelphia, 2001.
4. Page, S, Sisto, S, Johnston, M, et al. Modified constraint-induced therapy: A randomized, feasibility and efficacy study. J Rehabil Res Dev 38(5):583, 2001.
5. Page, SJ, and Hill-Hermann, V. Modified constraint-induced therapy: An efficacious outpatient therapy for persons with hemiparesis. Physical Disabilities Special Interest Section Quarterly of the American Occupational Therapy Association 30(4):1, 2007.
6. Page, S, Levine, P, and Leonard, A. Modified constraint-induced therapy in acute stroke: A randomized controlled pilot study. Neurorehabil Neural Repair 19(1):27, 2005.
7. Page, S, Sisto, S, Johnston, M, et al. Modified constraint-induced therapy after subacute stroke: A preliminary study. Neurorehabil Neural Repair 16(3):223, 2002.
8. Page, S, Sisto, S, Levine, P, et al. Efficacy of modified constraint-induced therapy in chronic stroke: A single blinded randomized controlled trial. Arch Phys Med Rehabil 85(1):14, 2004.
9. Page, S, and Levine, P. Back from the brink: Electromyography-triggered stimulation combined with modified constraint-induced movement therapy in chronic stroke. Arch Phys Med Rehabil 87(1): 27, 2006.

Constraint-Induced Movement Therapy

DAVID M. MORRIS, PT, PHD, AND EDWARD TAUB, PHD

Constraint-induced (CI) movement therapy, or CI therapy, involves a variety of intervention components used to promote increased use of a more impaired upper extremity (UE) both in the research laboratory and clinic setting and, most important, in the home.[1-9] The CI therapy protocol has its origins in basic animal research, conducted by one of us (Taub) concerning the influence on movement of the surgical abolition of sensation from a single forelimb in monkeys by dorsal rhizotomy. This series of deafferentation studies led Taub to propose a behavioral mechanism that can interfere with recovery from a neurological insult—*learned nonuse*.[10,11] In more recent years, a linked but separate mechanism, *use-dependent brain plasticity,* has also been proposed as partially responsible for producing positive outcomes from CI therapy.[12-19] Over the last 20 years, a substantial body of evidence has accumulated to support the efficacy of CI therapy for hemiparesis following chronic stroke —that is, more than 1 year post injury.[4,20] Evidence for efficacy includes results from an initial small, randomized controlled trial (RCT) of CI therapy in individuals with UE hemiparesis secondary to chronic stroke[1]; a larger placebo controlled trial in individuals of the same chronicity and level of impairment[21]; and a number of other studies.[2-9] There has also been a large, multisite randomized clinical trial in individuals with UE hemiparesis in the subacute phase of recovery—that is, 3 to 9 months post-stroke.[22-24] Positive findings regarding CI therapy after chronic stroke are also published in several studies from other laboratories employing within-subjects control procedures and numerous case studies.[25-28] Altogether more than 200 studies on the clinical effects of CI therapy have been published, all with positive results. Moreover, the most recent post-stroke clinical care guidelines, developed by a working group organized by the U.S. Department of Veterans Affairs and the U.S. Department of Defense, describe CI therapy as an intervention that has evidence of benefit for survivors of stroke with mild to moderate UE hemiparesis.[29]

Intervention: The CI Therapy Protocol

CI therapy is a "therapeutic package" consisting of a number of different components. Some of these intervention elements have been employed in neurorehabilitation before, usually as individual procedures and at a reduced intensity compared to CI therapy. The main novel features of CI therapy are: (1) the introduction of a number of techniques designed to promote the transfer of the therapeutic gains achieved in the clinic/ laboratory to the home environment, and (2) the combination of these treatment components and their application in a prescribed, integrated, and systematic manner. This involves many hours a day for a period of 2 or 3 consecutive weeks (depending on the severity of the initial deficit) to induce a patient to use a more impaired extremity. In the University of Alabama at Birmingham (UAB) CI Therapy Research Laboratory and Taub Training Clinic, patients are categorized according to their ability to achieve minimal movement criteria with the UE prior to treatment. To date, six categories, referred to as "grades," have been described (Table 10.1). The participant in Case Study 9 (Part III) exhibits movement that would be categorized as Grade 3.

CI therapy has evolved and undergone modification over the two decades of its existence. However, most of the original treatment elements remain part of the standard procedure. The present CI therapy protocol, as applied in our research and clinical settings, consists of three main elements and multiple components and subcomponents under each (Table 10.2).[1,7,9] These elements are: (1) practicing repetitive, task-oriented training of the more impaired UE for several hours a day for 10 or 15 consecutive weekdays (depending on the severity of the initial deficit); (2) applying a "transfer package" of adherence-enhancing behavioral methods designed to transfer gains made in the research laboratory or clinical setting to the patient's real-world environment; and (3) inducing the patient to use the more impaired UE during waking hours over the course of treatment, usually by restraining the less impaired UE in a protective safety mitt (Fig. 10.1). Each of the elements, along with component and subcomponent strategies, is described in the following sections.

Repetitive, Task-Oriented Training

On each of the weekdays during the intervention period, participants receive training, under supervision, for several hours each day. The original protocol called for 6 hours per day for this training. More recent studies indicate that a shorter daily training period (i.e., 3 hours per day) is as effective for certain groups of patients (i.e., Grades 2 and 3).[27,28] Two distinct training procedures are employed as patients practice functional task activities: *shaping* and *task practice*.

TABLE 10.1 Grade Criteria—Minimum Active Range of Motion and Motor Activity Log Scores

Impairment	Shoulder	Elbow	Wrist	Fingers	Thumb
Grade 2 (MAL < 2.5 for AOU and HW scale)	Flexion ≥ 45° and abduction ≥ 45°	Extension ≥ 20° from a 90° flexed starting position	Extension ≥ 20° from a fully flexed starting position	Extension of all MCP and IP (either PIP or DIP) joints ≥ 10°[a]	Extension or abduction of thumb ≥ 10°
Grade 3 (MAL < 2.5 for AOU and HW scale)	Flexion ≥ 45° and abduction ≥ 45°	Extension ≥ 20° from a 90° flexed starting position	Extension ≥ 10° from a fully flexed starting position	Extension ≥ 10° MCP and IP (either PIP or DIP) joints of at least two fingers[b]	Extension or abduction of thumb ≥ 10°
Grade 4 (MAL < 2.5 for AOU and HW scale)	Flexion ≥ 45° and abduction ≥ 45°	Extension ≥ 20° from a 90° flexed starting position	Extension ≥ 10° from a fully flexed starting position	Extension of at least two fingers > 0° and <10°[b]	Extension or abduction of thumb ≥ 10°
Grade 5 (MAL < 2.5 for AOU and HW scale)	At least one of the following: flexion ≥ 30°, abduction ≥ 30°, scaption ≥ 30°	Initiation[c] of both flexion and extension	Must be able to either initiate[c] extension of the wrist or initiate extension of one digit		

Each movement must be repeated three times in 1 minute. Grade 6 patients fall below the minimum Grade 5 criteria.

[a]Informally examined when picking up and dropping a tennis ball.

[b]Informally examined when picking up and dropping a washcloth.

[c]Initiation is defined for the purposes of criteria as minimal movement (i.e., below the level that can be measured reliably by a goniometer).

Abbreviations: AOU, Amount of Use Scale; HW, How Well Scale; IP, Interphalangeal; MAL, Motor Activity Log; MCP, Metacarpophalangeal; PIP, Proximal Interphalangeal.

Note: The Motor Activity log that includes the Amount of Use Scale and the How Well Scale is discussed later in the chapter under "Adherence-Enhancing Behavioral Subcomponents."

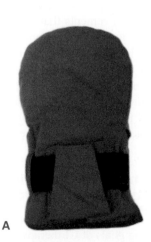
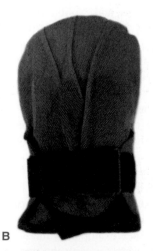

FIGURE 10.1 A protective safety mitt is used to restrain the more affected UE during CI therapy intervention: **(A)** palmar view; **(B)** dorsal view.

TABLE 10.2 Components and Subcomponents of the CI Therapy Protocol

Repetitive, Task-Oriented Training

- Shaping
- Task practice

Adherence-Enhancing Behavioral Strategies (i.e., Transfer Package)

- Daily administration of the Motor Activity Log (MAL)
- Home diary
- Problem-solving to overcome apparent barriers to the use of the more affected UE in real-world situations
- Behavioral contract
- Caregiver contract
- Home skill assignment
- Home practice
- Daily schedule
- Weekly phone calls for the first month after treatment to administer the MAL and problem-solve

Constraining (Encouraging) the Use of the More Affected UE

- Mitt restraint of the less affected UE
- Any method to continually remind the participant to use the more affected UE

Shaping

Shaping is a training method based on the principles of behavioral training.[30-33] In this approach, a motor or behavioral objective is approached in small steps by "successive approximations"; for example, the task can be made more difficult in accordance with a participant's motor capabilities, or the requirement for speed of performance can be progressively increased. Each functional activity is practiced for a set of ten 30-second trials, and explicit, immediate feedback is provided regarding the participant's performance after each trial.[33] When the level of difficulty of a shaping task is increased, the progression parameter selected for change should relate to the participant's movement problems. For example, if the participant's most significant movement deficits are with thumb and finger dexterity and an object-flipping task is used, the difficulty of the task would be increased by making the object progressively smaller if the movement problem was in thumb and finger flexion and adduction (i.e., making a pincer grasp). In contrast, if the movement problem involved thumb and finger extension and abduction (i.e., releasing a pincer grasp), the difficulty of the task would be increased by making the object progressively larger. As another example, if there is a significant deficit in elbow extension (as with the participant in Case Study 9 [Part III]) and a pointing or reaching task is used,

the shaping progression might involve placing the target object at increasing distances from the participant.

The shaping task is typically made progressively more difficult as the participant improves in performance. Generally, only one shaping progression parameter at a time should be varied. However, for higher functioning patients, more than one progression parameter may be changed if the trainer (physical therapist) believes that a participant would benefit from varying a second parameter at the same time as the first. The amount of difficulty increase should be such that it is likely that the participant will be able to accomplish the task, though with effort. This often makes it possible to achieve a given objective that might not be attainable if several large increments in motor performance were required. Another advantage of this approach is that it avoids excessive participant frustration, assuring continued motivation to engage in the training. Figures 10.2 and 10.3 illustrate two different levels of complexity for selected shaping tasks.

Task Practice

Task practice is another, less structured, repetitive task-oriented training procedure. It involves functionally based activities performed continuously for a period of 15 to 20 minutes (e.g., wrapping a present or writing). The tasks are not designed to be carried out as individual trials of discrete movements. In successive periods of task practice, the spatial requirements of activities or other parameters (such as duration) can be changed to require more demanding control of limb segments for task completion. Global feedback about overall performance (knowledge of results) is provided at the end of the 15- to 20-minute period. Figure 10.4 shows a shaping task in the earlier and later stages of execution.

Progression of Shaping Tasks

A large bank of tasks has been created for each type of training procedure. Therapists are encouraged to provide four forms of interaction during the shaping and task practice activities. Table 10.3 provides a description of these modes of interaction and guidelines for applying them. Training tasks are selected for each patient, considering: (1) the specific joint movements that exhibit the most pronounced deficits, (2) the joint movements believed to have the greatest potential for improvement, and (3) patient preference among tasks that have similar potential for producing specific improvement. Frequent rest intervals are provided throughout the training day, and the intensity of training (i.e., the number of trials per hour [shaping] or the amount of time spent on each training procedure [task practice]) is recorded.

Adherence-Enhancing Behavioral Methods to Increase Transfer to the Life Situation (Transfer Package)

One of the overriding goals of CI therapy is to transfer gains made in the research or clinical setting to the participant's real-world environment (e.g., home and community settings).

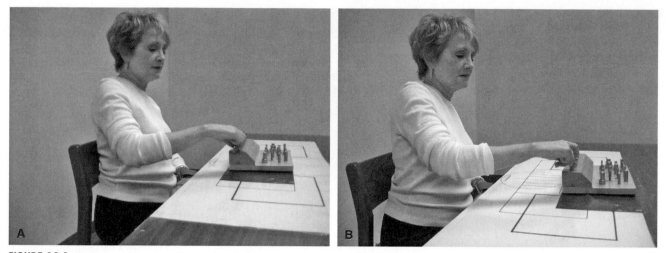

FIGURE 10.2 Participant is executing a shaping task involving unscrewing a nut from a bolt **(A)** at a lower level of complexity with the bolt placed closer to participant, and **(B)** at a higher level of complexity with the bolt placed farther away.

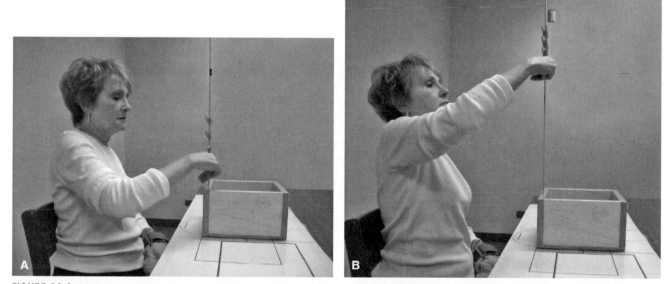

FIGURE 10.3 Participant is executing a shaping task involving removing clothespins from a horizontally positioned wooden stick **(A)** at a lower level of complexity with the clothespins placed low on the stick, and **(B)** at a higher level of complexity with the clothespins placed high on the stick.

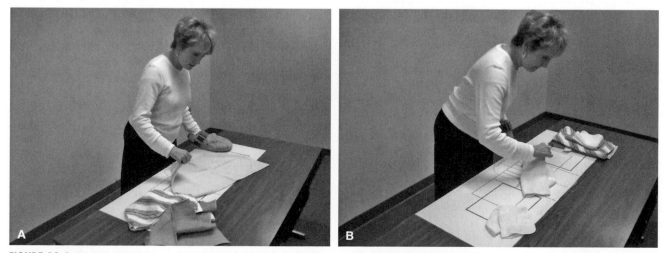

FIGURE 10.4 Participant is executing a task practice activity involving folding towels and stacking them during **(A)** early and **(B)** later stages of execution.

TABLE 10.3 Forms of Trainer*/Participant Interaction Used During Shaping and Task Practice

Interaction Type	Definition	Used in Shaping	Used in Task Practice
Feedback	Providing specific knowledge of results about a participant's performance on a shaping trial or task practice session (e.g., the number of repetitions in a set period of time or time required to perform a task or specific number of repetitions)	Provided immediately after each trial	Provided as global knowledge of results at the end of the entire task practice activity
Coaching	Providing specific suggestions to improve movements; aspects of this procedure are described in the behavioral literature as cueing and prompting	Provided liberally throughout all shaping trials	Provided throughout the entire task practice session, though not as often as in shaping
Modeling	When a trainer physically demonstrates a task	Provided at the beginning of the shaping activity; repeated between trials as needed	Provided at the beginning of a task practice activity
Encouragement	Providing enthusiastic verbal reward to participants to increase motivation and promote maximal effort (e.g., "That's excellent, that's good, keep trying")	Provided liberally throughout all shaping trials	Provided throughout the entire task practice session, though not as often as in shaping

* Trainer: Physical therapist or physical therapist assistant.

To achieve this goal, a set of techniques termed a *transfer package* is employed, which has the effect of making the patient accountable for adherence to the requirements of the therapy. In this way the patient becomes responsible for his or her own improvement. In the life situation, the participant must be actively engaged in and adhere to the intervention without constant supervision. Attention to adherence is directed to using the more impaired UE during functional tasks and obtaining appropriate assistance from caregivers, if present (i.e., assistance to prevent patients from struggling excessively, but allowing them to try as many tasks by themselves as is feasible), and to wearing the mitt as much as possible (when it is safe to do so).

Potential solutions to these adherence challenges have been used to increase adherence to exercise in older adults—the population most commonly experiencing stroke and subsequently most likely to receive CI therapy.[34] Two psychological factors, self-efficacy and perceived barriers, have been identified as the strongest and most consistent predictors of adherence to physical activity in older adults. *Self-efficacy* is defined as an individual's confidence in his or her ability to engage in the activity on a regular basis; it is related to both the adoption and maintenance of a target behavior.[35-38] Studies have demonstrated that self-efficacy can be enhanced through training and feedback.[39-41] *Perceived barriers* may incorporate both objective and subjective components.[35-37] *Objective obstacles* can be reduced through environmental and task adaptation. *Subjective barriers* may be reduced by such interventions as confidence-building, problem-solving, and refuting the beliefs that hinder activity.

Intervention Principles

A number of individual intervention principles have been successfully applied to enhance adherence to exercise and physical function-oriented behaviors. Four are most relevant to and are utilized in the adherence-enhancing behavioral components of CI therapy: *monitoring, problem-solving, behavioral contracting,* and *social support.*

Monitoring

Monitoring is one of the most commonly used strategies and involves asking participants to observe and document their performance of target behaviors (see the section on the home diary later in the chapter).[34] Patients may be asked to record a variety of aspects of these behaviors, including *mode of activity, duration, frequency, perceived exertion,* and *psychological response.* Patients should be asked to submit their monitoring records to facilitate consistency and completeness of records, but most importantly to promote adherence to the self-monitoring strategy.

Problem-Solving

Interventions to promote problem-solving involve partnerships between the therapist and patient that ultimately teach individuals to identify obstacles that hinder them, generate potential solutions, select a solution for implementation, evaluate the outcome, and choose another solution if needed.[36]

Behavioral Contracting

Behavioral contracting involves asking participants to write down the specific behaviors they normally carry out during the course of a day, and then entering into an agreement with the therapist as to which behaviors the patients will carry out and in what way they will be carried out. Verification of the execution of the contract occurs as part of the monitoring aspects of the procedure.

Social Support

Educating and enlisting the caregiver to provide the optimal amount of support (e.g., encouraging the patient's independence with tasks as much as possible but also assisting the patient when absolutely necessary to prevent frustration on the part of the patient) are important to successfully using the mitt restraint and more involved UE in the home and community setting.[42] This social support is optimized by reviewing the terms of the behavioral contract and administering a *caregiver contract* with anyone who spends a significant amount of time with the patient.

Monitoring, problem-solving, contracting, and social support interventions have been used successfully, alone or in combination, to enhance adherence to physical activity in a variety of participant groups with a variety of activity limitations.

Adherence-Enhancing Behavioral Subcomponents

The full range of adherence-enhancing behavioral subcomponents currently employed in the CI therapy protocol include daily administration of the *Motor Activity Log (MAL),* a structured, scripted interview that elicits information on how well and how often the more affected UE was used in 30 important activities of daily life.[1,43-46] Also included is a patient-kept home diary, problem-solving procedures, individual behavioral contracts with both the patient and the caregiver independently, a daily schedule constructed by the therapist, a home skill assignment, a home practice schedule, and a post-treatment contact. Table 10.4 lists each transfer package component and categorizes each according to the adherence-enhancing intervention principle(s) employed. Each transfer package subcomponent is described below, in the order in which they are encountered by the patient during a typical intervention period.

Motor Activity Log (MAL)

Scoring on the MAL is carried out with respect to two six-point rating scales: the *Amount of Use Scale* (Table 10.5) and the *How Well Scale* (Table 10.6). Using the MAL, respondents are asked to rate how much (i.e., amount of use [AOU]) and how well (HW) they use their more affected UE for 30 important activities of daily living (ADL) in the home over a specified period using the two rating scales.[1,43-46] The 30 ADL tered independently to the patient in the research or clinical

TABLE 10.4 Adherence-Enhancing Intervention Principles Emphasized in Each CI Therapy Transfer Package Component

Transfer Package Component	Monitoring	Problem-Solving	Behavioral Contracting	Social Support
Motor Activity Log	X	X	X	
Behavioral contract		X	X	X
Caregiver contract			X	
Home diary	X	X		
Home skill assignment		X	X	
Daily schedule	X			X
Home practice	X		X	
Contact post-treatment	X	X	X	

TABLE 10.5 Motor Activity Log Amount of Use Scale

0 = Did not use my weaker arm (not used)

1 = Occasionally tried to use my weaker arm (very rarely)

2 = Sometimes used my weaker arm but did most of the activity with my stronger arm (rarely)

3 = Used my weaker arm about half as much as before the stroke (1/2 prestroke)

4 = Used my weaker arm almost as much as before the stroke (3/4 prestroke)

5 = Used my weaker arm as normal as before the stroke (same as prestroke)

setting, or to an informant when available. This provides a quantified record of patient progress during treatment and can be used as a supplement to a therapist's clinical notes. The tasks include such activities as brushing teeth, buttoning a shirt or blouse, and eating with a fork or spoon. As part of our research, this information is gathered about the use of the more affected UE in the week and year prior to the participant's enrollment in the project, the day before and after the episode of care begins and ends, on each day of the intervention (i.e., the whole MAL on the first day of each week and alternate halves of the instrument on each of the other weekdays), weekly by phone for the 4 weeks after the end of treatment, and at several times during the 2-year follow-up period. In the clinic, the MAL is administered before training on the first treatment day,

TABLE 10.6 Motor Activity Log How Well Scale

0 = The weaker arm was not used at all for that activity (never).

1 = The weaker arm was moved during that activity but was not helpful (very poor).

2 = The weaker arm was of some use during that activity but needed some help from the stronger arm or moved very slowly or with difficulty (poor).

3 = The weaker arm was used for the purpose indicated, but movements were slow or were made only with some effort (fair).

4 = The movements made by the weaker arm were almost normal but not quite as fast or accurate as normal (almost normal).

5 = The ability to use the weaker arm for that activity was as good as before the injury (normal).

TABLE 10.7 Activities Included on the 30-Item Motor Activity Log

1. Turn on a light with a light switch
2. Open a drawer
3. Remove an item of clothing from a drawer
4. Pick up a phone
5. Wipe off a kitchen counter or other surface
6. Get out of a car
7. Open a refrigerator
8. Open a door by turning a doorknob
9. Use a TV remote control
10. Wash your hands
11. Turning the water on/off with knob or lever on the faucet
12. Dry your hands
13. Put on your socks
14. Take off your socks
15. Put on your shoes
16. Take off your shoes
17. Get up from a chair
18. Pull a chair away from the table before sitting down
19. Pull a chair toward the table after sitting down
20. Pick up a glass, bottle, drinking cup, or can
21. Brush your teeth
22. Put makeup base, lotion, or shaving cream on face
23. Use a key to unlock a door
24. Write on paper
25. Carry an object in hand
26. Use a fork or spoon for eating
27. Comb hair
28. Pick up a cup by the handle
29. Button a shirt
30. Eat half a sandwich or finger foods

on each day during treatment, immediately after treatment, and once a week for the first month after treatment. Several studies concerning the clinimetric properties of the MAL have shown the measure to be reliable and valid.[43-46] Moreover, the MAL does not produce a treatment effect when administered to persons receiving a placebo treatment who are on the same treatment schedule as those receiving CI therapy.[20] Preliminary results from an ongoing experiment at the UAB suggest that this self-monitoring instrument is a very important means of producing a transfer of improved performance from the laboratory/clinic to the life situation when used in conjunction with other aspects of the CI therapy protocol, particularly concentrated training.

Behavioral Contract

The *behavioral contract (BC)* is a formal, written agreement between the therapist and patient stipulating that the patient will use the more affected UE for specific activities in the life situation. In addition, to increase the use of a restraint device (a protective safety mitt worn on the less involved UE [see Fig. 10.1]) outside of the clinic or laboratory, the BC is helpful in increasing safety in use of the mitt, engaging the participant in active problem-solving to increase adherence, and emphasizing patient accountability for adherence. The BC is completed at the end of the first day of treatment, when the therapist has examined the patient's functional motor capacity and the participant has experienced using the mitt. The BC is signed by the therapist, the patient, and a witness; this formality emphasizes the importance of the agreement.

Before administering the BC, the therapist emphasizes the following points:

- Use of the weaker UE outside of the clinical setting is just as important as using it in the clinic, if not more so.
- The purpose of the BC is to induce the patient to use the more affected UE as much as possible.
- Safety is always the most important consideration, even more than maximal use of the more affected UE.
- At times, patients will be asked to perform activities in ways that they would not normally carry them out (e.g., use their nondominant UE to brush their teeth). It is not suggested that they adopt this approach permanently. Instead, they are asked to just perform the tasks in this way for the 2- or 3-week treatment period to encourage recovery of use of the more affected UE. It is usually at this point that the therapist briefly explains use-dependent neural reorganization. It may be helpful to use language that evokes images, such as *"Every time you use your weaker arm, you send nerve impulses to your brain that help to strengthen it, so that it is better able to move your arm."*
- Patients will be frequently asked whether they performed the activities listed in the BC, and the BC may be modified (e.g., items added or deleted) from time to time based on their performance.
- With some activities on the BC, participants may need assistance from a caregiver. In many cases, receiving this assistance is preferred to removing the mitt and using the less affected UE to complete the task because it maximizes use of the more affected UE. Activities where it is acceptable for a caregiver to assist will be discussed, agreed upon by all parties, and identified in the BC by a check in the caregiver assistance column for those tasks.
- The BC is a formal agreement between the participant and the therapy team and, as such, it should be taken very seriously. It is important to note that the therapy team also takes this agreement very seriously.

The first step in administering the BC is listing the ADL encountered by the patient on typical weekdays and on Saturdays and Sundays. The times that the patient usually carries out these activities and any distinguishing activity characteristics (e.g., equipment used and assistance provided) are also listed. Identifying the patient's typical routine is helpful for selecting items for each category of the BC that are important and meaningful to the patient. ADL are then categorized in the contract into those to be done with (1) mitt on, more affected UE only; (2) mitt off, both hands; and (3) mitt off, less affected UE. The times agreed upon for "mitt off" activities are specified and have mainly to do with safety, the use of water, and sleep; the amount of time when the mitt should be worn should also be specified.

When formulating the BC, the goal is to place as many of the patient's activities into the "mitt on, more affected UE only" category as is safe and feasible. Sometimes this means that the routine activities of the patient must be modified; adaptive equipment may be suggested or provided and/or the caregiver enlisted to assist with the task. The caregiver can participate by serving as a "second arm" or by completing components of the task that are infeasible for the patient (e.g., cutting meat for the patient during meal time). When formulating the BC, the time frame for completion must be considered. Patients may need additional time to complete their routine tasks while wearing the mitt, and the schedule should be modified to account for this. For example, a patient may need to wake up 30 minutes earlier than usual in order to complete routine activities and still arrive at the clinic at the scheduled time. The use of an assistive device when walking poses a challenge to mitt use and should be considered when formulating the BC. For example, when a patient requires the use of a straight cane for walking outside the home (e.g., in the yard or in the community), any activities performed while walking outside of the home should be placed in one of the "mitt off" categories. Also, tasks performed in social situations may pose a particular challenge for patients, as they may be embarrassed to use the mitt in public. This should be discussed frankly with the patient. The therapist should point out that the CI therapy protocol requires full participation and that failure to use the mitt whenever possible will result in a reduced outcome. Patients should be proud of their dedication to improving the use of their UE and reminded that others will view their efforts in the same way. Still, they may choose to avoid social situations that they anticipate will be uncomfortable for the short 2-week intervention period. That is acceptable if it cannot be avoided. When the patient's routine includes long periods of inactivity (e.g., many hours spent watching television), the therapist can add activities to the routine to assure that the patient is moving the more affected UE as much as possible, thereby maximizing use-dependent plastic brain reorganization.

To promote safety, therapists must point out situations in which the patient should avoid using the mitt. The "mitt off, both hands" category is for activities in which the patient should not use the mitt but could still safely incorporate use of the more affected UE into the task. Bathing and showering are included in this category. Although the mitt should be removed to avoid getting it wet and to allow use of the less affected UE for maintaining balance, the more affected UE should still be used as much as possible during the bathing process (e.g., lathering body parts and manipulating a bar of soap). Dressing is also commonly included in this category, as it is difficult to place the mitt through a shirt or blouse sleeve. Nevertheless, patients should be encouraged to use their more affected UE to manipulate buttons, fasten straps, and buckle belts whenever possible.

Therapists unfamiliar with the CI therapy protocol may have the tendency to include all bimanual tasks in this category. We believe that many bimanual tasks can be modified for inclusion into the "mitt on, more affected UE only" category by enlisting the caregiver to serve as a second UE during these tasks. For example, a jar cannot usually be opened effectively with one hand. Instead of including this task in the "mitt off, both hands" category, we believe it is preferable to ask the caregiver to stabilize the jar while the patient unscrews the lid and to include this task in the "mitt on, more affected UE only" category. Activities that typically belong in the "mitt off, less affected UE" category include those in which it is advisable for a handrail to be used, such as when ascending or descending stairs, when shaving, and while cooking. Clumsiness with these tasks could result in injury and should not be risked. Once the mitt is removed, it can be difficult to get the patient to put the mitt back on the less affected UE. For that reason, the BC specifies the time the mitt should be removed and then placed back on, reemphasizing the importance of wearing the mitt. The document is often modified during treatment as the patient gains new movement skills. An example of a completed BC is provided for Case Study 9 (Part III) online at Davis*Plus* (http://www.fadavis.com). The BC employs the adherence-enhancing intervention principles of monitoring and problem-solving to transfer treatment into the home and community environment. Since the BC specifies activities with which caregiver assistance should be provided, it also employs a social support strategy.

Caregiver Contract
The *caregiver contract* is a formal written agreement between the therapist and the patient's caregiver. It stipulates that the caregiver will be present and available while the patient is wearing the mitt and will aid in the at-home program as well as generally help to increase use of the more affected UE. It is completed after the terms of the BC with the patient are shared with the caregiver. The caregiver contract improves caregivers' understanding of the treatment program, guides caregivers to assist appropriately, and increases patient safety. The caregiver contract is signed by the therapist, patient, caregiver, and a witness, which, again, formally emphasizes the importance of the agreement. As such, it employs social support to enhance adherence to the treatment protocol.

Home Diary
The *home diary* is maintained on a daily basis. Patients list their activities outside the research laboratory or clinical setting and report whether or not they have used their more affected extremity while performing different tasks, especially those listed on the BC. The home diary and daily review of the MAL constitute the main monitoring aspects of the CI therapy protocol. They heighten patients' awareness of their use of the more affected UE and emphasize adherence to the BC and patients' accountability for their own improvement.

Problem-Solving
Discussion of the MAL and home diary also provides a structured opportunity for talking about why the weaker extremity was not used for specific activities and for problem-solving on how to use it more. For example, the patient may state that he or she was unable to pick up a sandwich with one hand and therefore removed the mitt and used the less impaired UE to assist. The therapist may then suggest that the sandwich be cut into quarters so that it is more easily manipulated with the weaker extremity. As another example, the patient might report that he or she is unable to open a door in the home because the doorknob is small and difficult to grip. The therapist may provide the individual with a doorknob build-up and suggest that it be used so that the door can be opened with the more affected UE.

Home Skill Assignment
Wearing the mitt while away from the clinic or laboratory does not assure that patients will use the more impaired UE to carry out ADL that had been accomplished exclusively with the less impaired UE, or not at all, since the stroke. The *home skill assignment* process encourages patients to try ADL that they may not otherwise have tried with the more impaired UE. The therapist first reviews a list of common ADL tasks carried out in the home. The tasks are categorized according to the rooms in which they are usually performed (e.g., kitchen, bathroom, bedroom, office, and so forth). Starting on the second day of the intervention period, patients are asked to select 10 ADL tasks from the list that they agree to try after they leave the laboratory or clinic and before they return for the next day of treatment. Tasks not on the list may be selected if desired by the patient. These tasks are to be carried out while wearing the mitt when it is possible and safe to do so. Therapists guide the patient to select five tasks that the patient believes will be relatively easy to accomplish and five tasks he or she believes will be more challenging. The 10 items selected are recorded on an assignment sheet and given to patients when they leave the laboratory or clinic for the day. The goal is for approximately 30 minutes to be devoted to trying the specified ADL tasks at home each day. The home skill assignment sheet is reviewed during the first part of the next treatment day, and then 10 additional ADL tasks are selected for home skill assignment for that evening. This process is repeated throughout the intervention period, with efforts made to encourage the use of the more impaired UE during as many different ADL tasks in as many different rooms of the patient's home as possible.

Home Practice

During treatment, as an alternative to the home skill assignment, patients are asked to spend 15 to 30 minutes at home each day performing specific UE tasks repetitively with their more affected UE; this is referred to as *home practice—during (HP-D)* [as in *during* the episode of care]. The tasks typically employ materials that are commonly available (e.g., stacking cups). This strategy is particularly helpful for individuals who are typically relatively inactive while in their home setting (e.g., spending long periods watching television) and provides more structure to using the more impaired UE than the home skill assignment. Care must be taken not to overload the patient with too many assignments while away from the laboratory or clinic, as this could prove demotivating. For this reason, therapists usually select either the home skill assignment or HP-D to encourage more real-world use of the more affected UE; rarely are both used simultaneously. Toward the end of treatment, an individualized post-treatment home practice program is drawn up, consisting of tasks that are similar to those assigned in HP-D; this is referred to as *home practice—after (HP-A)* [*after* completion of the episode of care]. For each patient, 8 to 10 activities are selected based on the patient's remaining movement deficits. Patients are asked to demonstrate understanding and proficiency with all tasks before discharge. These tasks usually employ commonly available items to increase the likelihood that they will be implemented. Patients are encouraged to select one or two tasks per day and to perform these tasks for 30 minutes daily. On the next day, patients are asked to select one or two different tasks from the HP-A assignment sheet. Patients are instructed to carry out these exercises indefinitely.

Daily Schedule

The physical therapist documents a detailed schedule of all activities carried out in the clinic on each day of the intervention. This includes the time devoted to each activity listed. The schedule specifically notes the times when the mitt is taken off and put back on the less impaired hand. The time and length of rest periods are also included. Specific shaping and task practice activities are listed, including use of only the more affected UE during lunch whenever patient function is high enough for this to be feasible. The daily schedule includes not only the length of time devoted to eating lunch, but also what foods were eaten and how this was accomplished. Information recorded on the daily schedule is particularly helpful for demonstrating improvements in daily activities to the patient; this often has the effect of motivating him or her to try harder.

Constraining (Encouraging) Participant to Use the Less Affected UE

The most commonly applied CI therapy treatment protocol has incorporated the use of a restraint (either a sling or a protective safety mitt) on the less affected UE to prevent patients from succumbing to the strong urge to use that UE during most or all functional activities, even when the therapist is present. Over the last decade, the protective safety mitt, which eliminates the patient's ability to use the fingers, has been the preferred approach for restraint. The mitt prevents functional use of the less affected UE for most purposes while still allowing protective extension of that UE in case of falling as well as permits arm swing during ambulation and to help maintain balance. Patients are taught to put on and take off the mitt (or sling) independently, and decisions are made about when its use is feasible and safe. The goal for patients with mild or moderate motor deficits is mitt use during 90 percent of waking hours. This so-called "forced use" is arguably the most visible element of the intervention to the rehabilitation community, and it is frequently and mistakenly described as synonymous with "CI therapy." However, Taub and coworkers have stated "there is . . . nothing talismanic about use of a sling, protective safety mitt or other restraining device on the less-affected UE"[2,p3] as long as the more affected UE is exclusively engaged in repeated practice. *Constraint,* as used in the name of the therapy, was intended not only to refer to the application of a physical restraint, such as a mitt, but also to indicate a *constraint* to use the more affected UE for functional activities.[2] As such, any strategy that encourages exclusive use of the more affected UE is viewed as a "constraining" component of the treatment package. For example, shaping was meant to be considered as constituting a very important constraint on behavior; the participant either succeeds at the task or is not rewarded (e.g., by praise or knowledge of improvement).

Preliminary findings by Sterr and colleagues indicate a significant treatment effect using CI therapy without the physical restraint component.[27] Likewise, our laboratory has obtained similar findings with a small group of participants ($n = 9$) when a CI therapy protocol without physical restraint was employed.[2,6] However, our study suggested that this group experienced a larger decrement at the 2-year follow-up testing than groups where physical restraint was employed. If other treatment package elements, developed in our laboratory, are not used, our clinical experience suggests that routine reminders to not use the less affected UE alone, without physical restraint, would not be as effective as using the mitt. Consequently, we use the mitt to minimize the need for the therapist or caregiver to keep reminding the patient to limit use of the less affected UE during the intervention period.

Unique Aspects of CI Therapy as a Rehabilitation Approach

Various approaches are used to improve motor function after stroke.[47] A *compensation approach* involves substitution; that is, alternate behavioral strategies are utilized to complete ADL. In traditional compensation, the activities are performed primarily with the less affected extremities.

The more affected extremities would, at most, be used as a prop or assist. This approach is believed to be particularly useful when spontaneous recovery of function has plateaued and further recovery seems doubtful.

A more optimistic view of recovery places emphasis on regaining movement on the more affected side of the body. Postinjury rehabilitation training may focus on promoting functional recovery using the concept of *true recovery*. A specific function is considered "recovered" if it is performed in the same manner and with the same efficiency and effectiveness as before the stroke. Current CI therapy promotes a newer *substitution approach.* The more affected extremities may be used in a new way, compared to before the neurological insult, to perform a functional task. The question regarding which rehabilitation strategies are most effective has been an ongoing debate in the neurorehabilitation field for many years. In a sense, the CI therapy approach cuts through these long-standing discussions about optimal treatment interventions. The CI therapy approach to stroke rehabilitation bypasses this compartmentalization of rehabilitation entirely and is not concerned with the requirement that the recovery induced by therapy involves the exact replacement of normal or prestroke coordination to produce improved motor function and functional independence or whether compensation is permitted. The objective is to enable a participant to accomplish a functional objective with the best movement of which he or she is capable as long as the more affected UE is involved. Further, due mainly to reimbursement policies, most intervention is delivered in short treatment periods, relative to CI therapy, and in a distributed manner. If applied clinically, the CI therapy approach, as used in the UAB Research Laboratory, represents a substantial paradigm shift for physical rehabilitation. The CI therapy approach is different in a variety of ways from the more traditional compensation and functional recovery approaches used, as discussed below.

Use of the More Affected Extremity

Use of the protective safety mitt prevents participants from performing ADL and training activities with the less affected extremity unless using the less affected UE is absolutely necessary for safety or to avoid having the restraining device from becoming wet with water, even if the less affected UE would normally be used for that function. For example, if the less affected UE was the dominant UE before the stroke and the task was typically performed by the dominant UE (e.g., writing or brushing the teeth), the CI therapy protocol still requires the participant to perform the task with the more affected, nondominant UE. This remains true for tasks that are bilateral in nature (e.g., folding clothing). Instead of removing the mitt and performing the task with both UEs, the participants perform the task, in a modified fashion, with the more affected UE exclusively, or they enlist the assistance of a caregiver to serve as a "second UE." Many of the CI therapy participants' ADL are modified during the training period. In this way, the

CI therapy protocol does not allow traditional compensation and deviates from a functional recovery approach where all ADL would be attempted in the "typical" manner they were performed before the stroke. The purpose of the strict adherence to using the protective safety mitt is not to encourage a permanent change in the way the participant performs ADL. Rather, use of the protective safety mitt requires the concentrated and repetitive use of the more affected UE, which leads both to overcoming the strongly learned habit of nonuse and to use-dependent cortical plasticity. Once the treatment period (i.e., 2 or 3 weeks) has ended, participants return the protective safety mitt and perform ADL in the most effective manner possible with enhanced use of the more affected UE. Interestingly, anecdotal observations suggest that after treatment many participants with more affected, nondominant UEs begin using the more affected, nondominant UE for tasks previously performed with the dominant, less affected UE. Such observations warrant further investigation.

Importance of Concentrated Practice

Although the CI therapy protocol used most often includes some sort of restraint on the less affected UE, variations in this approach (i.e., shaping only and intensive physical rehabilitation) do not.[2,8] As mentioned earlier, there is thus nothing talismanic about using a restraining device on the less affected UE. The common factor among all the interventions in the CI therapy protocol, producing an equivalently large treatment effect, appears to be repeated practice using the more affected UE and use of the transfer package. Any intervention that induces a patient to use a more affected UE many hours a day in the clinic or laboratory and at home (e.g., by the use of the transfer package) for a period of consecutive weeks should be therapeutically efficacious. These factors are likely to produce the use-dependent cortical plasticity found to result from CI therapy and are presumed to be the basis for the long-term increase in the amount of use of the more affected limb.

Conventional physical rehabilitation, regardless of the setting (i.e., inpatient or outpatient) or stage of rehabilitation (i.e., acute, subacute, or chronic), does not provide a sufficient concentration of practice. The conventional schedule falls short not only in the absolute time that using the more affected UE is required, but also in the administration of the practice periods on consecutive days (e.g., 3 hours per day of total therapy time). Clinical application of CI therapy will likely require a change in the typical scheduling pattern for rehabilitation. Episodes of care will likely need to be modified from short treatment sessions held several times a week for several months to up to 3-hour sessions carried out daily for consecutive days over a 2- or 3-week period (depending on the severity of the deficit). Increasing the amount of use by means of prescribed home practice exercises monitored by phone calls at the time of initiating and then finishing the home exercises and monitored home diaries is highly desirable, especially for weekends during treatment. Financial feasibility of this type of approach requires changes in payment structures and policies within reimbursement agencies.

Shaping as a Training Technique

CI therapy studies have used predominately either task practice or shaping for training activities. Preliminary data suggest that a predominance of shaping in the training procedures is more effective for lower functioning participants than a predominance of task practice. Use of either technique for higher functioning participants appears to be beneficial, though even here, use of shaping appears to confer a therapeutic advantage. Thus, shaping seems to be an effective training procedure for enhancing the use of the more affected UE in the life situation.

While there are many similarities between shaping and the conventional training techniques used by therapists, important differences also exist. Shaping procedures use a highly standardized and systematic approach to progress the difficulty level of motor tasks attempted. Also, feedback provided in shaping is immediate, specific, and quantitative and emphasizes only positive aspects of the participants' performance.[33] In this way, the therapist's input and continuous encouragement motivate the participant to put forth continued and maximal effort. Tasks are used that emphasize movements in need of improvement yet are within the capability of the participant. Excessive effort is avoided, as it may be demotivating for the participant. The influence of shaping is primarily behavioral in nature and directed at keeping participants motivated, fully informed of their progress in performance of a task, and focused on increasing the amount and quality of use of their UE during training. The main objective is to get the patient to use the more affected UE repeatedly in a concentrated, massed-practice fashion to overcome learned nonuse and induce use-dependent cortical plasticity. Skill acquisition regarding the specific shaping task practiced is not the primary purpose of shaping. Instead, skill attained during the practice of a shaping task is a very beneficial by-product that should be generalized into motor performance in the real-world environment. Specific skill acquisition with functional tasks is probably also encouraged during the independent trial and error that occurs outside of the clinic setting with use of the protective safety mitt and focused attention on increasing the use of the more affected UE during ADL in the participants' home environment.

Use of a Transfer Package

It is our belief that most patients (and therapy professionals) view rehabilitation as occurring primarily under the direct observation and supervision of the rehabilitation professional. We believe that continued use and practice, for many hours daily, away from the rehabilitation facility is critical to achieving permanent changes in brain plasticity and function. Another unique aspect of the CI therapy approach is its emphasis on the use of adherence-enhancing behavioral techniques (i.e., the transfer package) to facilitate the use of the more affected UE. While the use of similar behavioral techniques has been described in the physical rehabilitation literature, their use in combination and with the intensity with which they are used in the CI therapy protocol is different. The use of the transfer package provides multiple opportunities for systematically increasing attention to the use of the more affected UE, promoting participants' accountability for adhering to the CI therapy protocol, and providing structured problem-solving between therapists and participants. Intensive contact with the therapist establishes an important rapport between therapist and patient, which helps the patient view the take-home practice and mitt-wearing requirements of the therapy very seriously. Taken together, the behavioral techniques result in improved adherence to the required CI therapy procedures.

Evidence from our research suggests that this transfer package may be the most important component of the CI therapy protocol.[19] Also, studies investigating a CI therapy protocol with a reduced training component (i.e., $3\frac{1}{2}$ hours instead of 7 hours) suggest that the reduced time may produce similar results. A possible explanation for this could be successful carryover of the behavioral techniques used during the treatment period to promote adherence, even when at home and not in contact with the physical therapist. These findings highlight the importance of the "out of the clinic or laboratory" activities and the behavioral techniques needed to assure participants' adherence to use of the more affected UE.

Main Effect of CI Therapy: Increased Use

Since a true recovery approach promotes the performance of specific functional tasks in a manner that is similar to before the stroke, quality of movement is an important, if not primary, indicator of successful rehabilitation. Results from CI therapy research, as evidenced by the performance of participants after treatment on the Wolf Motor Function Test (WMFT),[48-50] suggest that participants do significantly improve their quality and skill of movement. Figure 10.5 shows a participant performing a task on the WMFT. A more powerful change, however, has been demonstrated with increased use of the more affected UE in the life situation, as indexed by results on the Motor Activity Log. Participants may well be developing new movement strategies to accomplish functional tasks. If so, this would be acceptable within the context of CI therapy and further distinguish it from more true recovery-oriented therapies.

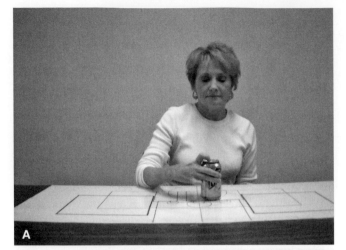

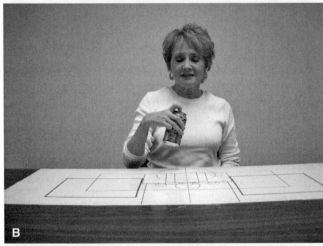

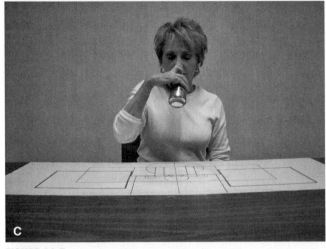

FIGURE 10.5 Participant is completing the "Lift a can" item in the Wolf Motor Function Test.

SUMMARY

Over the last 20 years, a large body of evidence has accumulated in support of using CI therapy for hemiparesis following chronic stroke (longer than 1 year). CI therapy is believed to produce these effects through two separate but linked mechanisms: *overcoming learned nonuse* and *use-dependent cortical plasticity*. These mechanisms are different from those

attributed to more conventional rehabilitation approaches that seek to achieve compensation, true recovery, and/or substitution. As a result, the CI therapy approach represents a significant paradigm shift in physical rehabilitation. With continued investigation, elaboration, and application to clinical settings, CI therapy holds substantial promise for the field of physical rehabilitation.

REFERENCES

1. Taub, E, Miller, NE, Novack, TA, et al. Technique to improve chronic motor deficit after stroke. Arch Phys Med Rehabil 74:347, 1993.
2. Taub, E, Uswatte, G, and Pidikiti, R. Constraint-induced movement therapy: A new family of techniques with broad application to physical rehabilitation: A clinical review. J Rehabil Res Dev 36:237, 1999.
3. Taub, E, Uswatte, G, and Elbert, T. New treatments in neurorehabilitation founded on basic research. Nat Rev Neurosci 3:228, 2002.
4. Taub, E. Harnessing brain plasticity through behavioral techniques to produce new treatments in neurorehabilitation. Am Psychol 59:692, 2004.
5. Morris, DM, and Taub, E. Constraint-induced therapy approach to restoring function after neurological injury. Top Stroke Rehabil 8:16, 2001.
6. Morris, DM, Crago, JE, DeLuca, SC, et al. Constraint-induced (CI) movement therapy for motor recovery after stroke. Neurorehabil 9:29, 1997.
7. Morris, DM, Taub, E, and Mark, VW. Constraint-induced movement therapy: Characterizing the intervention protocol. Eura Medicophys 42:257, 2007.
8. Taub, E, and Uswatte, G. Constraint-induced movment therapy: Answers and questions after two decades of research. Neurorehabil 21(2):93, 2006.
9. Mark, VM, and Taub, E. Constraint-induced movement therapy for chronic stroke hemiparesis and other disabilities. Res Neurol Neurosci 22:317, 2004.
10. Taub, E: Movement in nonhuman primates deprived of somatosensory feedback. Exerc Sports Sci Rev 4:335, 1977.
11. Taub, E. Somatosensory deafferentation research with monkeys: Implications for rehabilitation medicine. In Ince, LP (ed): Behavioral Psychology in Rehabilitation Medicine: Clinical Applications. Williams & Wilkins, New York, 1980, p 371.
12. Liepert, J, Miltner, WH, Bauder, H, et al. Motor cortex plasticity during constraint-induced movement therapy in stroke patients. Neurosci Lett 250:5, 1998.
13. Liepert, J, Bauder, H, Wolfgang, HR, et al. Treatment-induced cortical reorganization after stroke in humans. Stroke 31:1210, 2000.
14. Kopp, B, Kunkel, A, Muhlnickel, W, et al. Plasticity in the motor system related to therapy-induced improvement of movement after stroke. Neurorep 10:807, 1999.
15. Bauder, H, Sommer, M, Taub, E, et al. Effect of CI therapy on movement-related brain potentials. Psychophysiol 36:S31 (Abstract), 1999.
16. Wittenberg, GF, Chen, R, Ishii, K, et al. Constraint-induced therapy in stroke: Magnetic-stimulation motor maps and cerebral activation. Neurorehabil Neural Repair 17:48, 2003.
17. Levy, CE, Nichols, DS, Schmalbrock, PM, et al. Functional MRI evidence of cortical reorganization in upper-limb stroke hemiplegia treated with constraint-induced movement therapy. Am J Phys Med Rehabil 80:4, 2001.
18. Mark, VW, Taub, E, and Morris, DM. Neural plasticity and constraint-induced movement therapy. Eura Medicophys 42:269, 2006.
19. Gauthier, LV, Taub, E, Perkins, C, et al. Remodeling the brain: Plastic structural changes produced by different motor therapies after stroke. Stroke 39:1520, 2008.
20. Uswatte, G, and Taub, E. Implications of the learned nonuse formulation for measuring rehabilitation outcomes: Lessons from constraint-induced movement therapy. Rehabil Psychol 50:34, 2005.
21. Taub, E, Uswatte, G, King, DK, et al. A placebo controlled trial of constraint-induced movement therapy for upper extremity after stroke. Stroke 37:1045, 2006.
22. Winstein, CJ, Miller, JP, Blanton, S, et al. Methods for a multi-site randomized trial to investigate the effect of constraint-induced

movement therapy in improving upper extremity function among adults recovering from a cerebrovascular stroke. Neurorehabil Neural Repair 17:137, 2003.

23. Wolf, SL, Winstein, CJ, Miller, JP, et al. Effect of constraint-induced movement therapy on upper extremity function 3 to 9 months after stroke: The EXCITE randomized clinical trial. JAMA 296:2095, 2006.

24. Wolf, SL, Winstein, CJ, Miller, JP, et al. Retention of upper limb function in stroke survivors who have received constraint-induced movement therapy: The EXCITE randomized trail. Lancet Neurol 7:33, 2007.

25. Miltner, WH, Bauder, H, Sommer, M, et al. Effects of constraint-induced movement therapy on patients with chronic motor deficits after stroke: A replication. Stroke 30:586, 1999.

26. Kunkel, A, Kopp, B, Muller, G, et al. Constraint-induced movement therapy for motor recovery in chronic stroke patients. Arch Phys Med Rehabil 80:624, 1999.

27. Sterr, A, Elbert, T, Berthold, I, et al. CI therapy in chronic hemiparesis: The more the better? Arch Phys Med Rehabil 83:1374, 2002.

28. Dettmers, C, Teske, U, Hamzei, F, et al. Distributed form of constraint-induced movement therapy improves functional outcome and quality of life after stroke. Arch Phys Med Rehabil 86:204, 2005.

29. Duncan, PW, Zorowitz, R, Bates, B, et al. Management of adult stroke rehabilitation care: A clinical practice guideline. Stroke 36: 100, 2005.

30. Skinner, BF. The Behavior of Organisms. Appleton-Century-Crofts, New York, 1938.

31. Skinner, BF. The Technology of Teaching. Appleton-Century-Crofts, New York, 1968.

32. Panyan, MV. How to Use Shaping. HH Enterprises, Lawrence, KS, 1980.

33. Taub, E, Crago, JE, Burgio, LD, et al. An operant approach to rehabilitation medicine: Overcoming learned nonuse by shaping. J Exp Anal Behav 61:281, 1994.

34. Dominick, KL, and Morey, M. Adherence to physical activity. In Bosworth, HB, Oddone, EZ, and Weinberger, M (eds): Patient Treatment Adherence: Concepts, Interventions, and Measurement. Lawrence Erlbaum Assoc, Mahwah, NJ, 2006.

35. Trost, SG, Owen, N, Bauman, AE, et al. Correlates of adults' participation in physical activity: Review and update. Med Sci Sports Exerc 34:1996, 2002.

36. Dishman, RK. Determinants of participation in physical activity. In Bourchard, C, Shephard, RJ, Stephens, T, Sutton, JR, and McPherson, BD (eds): Physical Activity, Fitness and Health: International Proceedings and Consensus Statement. Human Kinetics, Champaign, IL, 1994, p 214.

37. Sallis, JF, and Owen, N. Physical Activity and Behavioral Medicine. Sage, Thousand Oaks, CA, 1999.

38. King, AC, Blair, SN, and Bild, DE. Determination of physical activity and interventions in adults. Med Sci Sports Exerc 24:S221, 1992.

39. McAuley, E. The role of efficacy cognitions in the prediction of exercise behavior in middle-aged adults. J Behav Med 15:65, 1992.

40. Rejeski, WJ, Brawley, LR, and Ambrosius, WT. Older adults with chronic disease: Benefits of group-mediated counseling in promotion of physical active lifestyles. Health Psychol 22:414, 2003.

41. McAuley, E, Jerome, GJ, Marquez, DX, et al. Exercise self-efficacy in older adults: Social, affective, and behavioral influences. Ann Behav Med 25:1, 2003.

42. DiMatteo, MR. Social support and patient adherence to medical treatment: A meta-analysis. Health Psychol 23(2):207, 2004.

43. Uswatte, G, Taub, E, Morris, D, et al. Contribution of the shaping and restraint components of constraint-induced movement therapy to treatment outcome. Neurorehabil 21(2):147, 2006.

44. Uswatte, G, Taub, E, Morris, DM et al. Reliability and validity of the upper-extremity motor activity log-14 for measuring real-world arm use. Stroke 36:2493, 2006.

45. Uswatte, G, Taub, E, Morris, D, et al. The Motor Activity Log-28: Assessing daily use of the hemiparetic arm after stroke. Neurology 67:1189, 2006.

46. Van der Lee, JH, Beckerman, H, Knol, DL, et al. Clinimetric properties of the motor activity log for the assessment of arm use in hemiparetic patients. Stroke 35:1410, 2004.

47. Shumway-Cook, A, & Woollacott, M. Motor Control: Theory and Practical Applications, ed 3. Lippincott Williams & Wilkins, Philadelphia, 2007.

48. Morris, DM, Uswatte, G, Crago, JE, et al. The reliability of the Wolf Motor Function Test for assessing upper extremity function after stroke. Arch Phys Med Rehabil 82:750, 2001.

49. Wolf, SL, Catlin, PA, Ellis, M, et al. Assessing the Wolf Motor Function Test as an outcome measure for research with patients after stroke. Stroke 32:1635, 2001.

50. Wolf, SL, Thompson, PA, Morris, DM, et al. The EXCITE Trial: Attributes of the Wolf Motor Function Test in patients with subacute stroke. Neurorehabil Neural Repair 19:194, 2005.

Case Studies

In Part III, we are privileged to bring together a group of outstanding clinicians from across the country to contribute case studies in both written (Part III) and visual (DVD) format. The contributing therapists demonstrated enormous enthusiasm for the project and an exceptional commitment to student learning. Their collective expertise is reflected in the presentation of the cases, the guiding questions posed, and critical decisions required as students progress through the cases.

The overriding goals of Part III are to provide the student an opportunity to interact with the content and to promote clinical decision-making skills through an evaluation of examination data to determine *diagnosis*, *prognosis*, and *plan of care*. The case studies focus on diagnoses familiar to the rehabilitation setting, with an overriding emphasis on improving activities, and skills that are meaningful to the individual patient and typically contribute to improved functional outcomes and quality of life. The cases are guided by the conceptual framework and practice patterns presented in the *Guide to Physical Therapist Practice*.

There are 10 case studies. Each case includes both a written (Part III) and a visual (DVD) component. The written case content is further divided into two sections: (1) *Examination* and (2) *Evaluation, Diagnosis and Prognosis, and Plan of Care*. Student evaluation of the physical therapy examination data (history, systems review, and specific tests and measures) provides the needed information on which to base decisions in determining the diagnosis, predicting the optimal levels of recovery and the timeframe in which this will occur, and developing the plan of care. Challenges to student decision-making are introduced through guiding questions addressing specific considerations of the case example.

The DVD accompanying the text includes the visual case content. For each case, there is a 6-minute visual segment distributed among sample components of the initial *examination*, sample *interventions*, and functional *outcomes*. The three segments include a planned time-lapse between episodes of filming to depict patient progress toward, or achievement of, functional

(text continues on page 248)

P A R T

III

outcomes. The majority of case studies included filming over a 4- to 6-week period. Following is a brief description of each visual segment.

- **Examination** (Video Clip 1): The first video segment focuses on elements of the physical therapy examination. Content varies based on patient presentation. The intention is to provide a more complete understanding of the patient's impairments and activity limitations as well as how they affect function.
- **Intervention** (Video Clip 2): Based on the contributing therapists' intervention strategies selected to improve functional outcomes, the second video segment presents elements of a physical therapy treatment session.
- **Outcomes** (Video Clip 3): The third video segment depicts functional outcomes toward the end of the episode of care (i.e., the efficacy of interventions on the resolution of impairments and activity limitations). Some case studies depict activities similar to those presented in the first video clip (examination) to provide a *before* and *after* comparison of the impact of intervention.

During each visual segment, the accompanying narration directs the viewer to the specific elements depicted or calls attention to unique aspects of the case. A text version of each narration is included with the written case content.

The following is a recommended sequence for using the case studies. However, based on desired learning strategies, goals, and objectives, the sequence may vary considerably. A collaborative learning environment with small groups of students working on a single case will likely optimize learning. Although not specifically indicated in the series of case study activities listed below, *each component of the sequence should include discussion among group members.* This will provide an opportunity to compare your thoughts and ideas with those of classmates, instructors, or colleagues.

1. **Consider the text case content.** Begin with the written case content. Assume you are the physical therapist managing the case and you have just completed the initial examination. Analyze and organize data from the history, systems review, and tests and measures.
2. **View Examination.** View the clip several times while observing the impairments or activity limitations (examination data) presented.
3. **Answer the text guiding questions.** With information gained from the examination data and observing the patient's motor performance, progress to the case study guiding questions. These questions are designed to promote clinical decision-making skills through evaluating the examination data, determining the physical therapy diagnosis, establishing the prognosis, and developing the plan of care.
4. **View Intervention.** The second video clip presents segments of a patient/therapist treatment session. It provides a unique opportunity to observe a sample intervention selected by the contributing therapist to

improve functional outcomes. While viewing this segment, compare and contrast the interventions presented with those you selected.

5. **View Outcomes.** Finally, the third video clip depicts functional outcomes at the end of the episode of care as well as the impact of training on the resolution of impairments and functional limitations. While viewing this segment, compare and contrast the goals and expected outcomes you identified with the functional outcomes achieved.

6. **View Answers to the Case Study Questions.** (This activity should be completed in student groups.) The therapists presenting the cases have shared their perspectives by providing answers to the guiding questions. These are available online at Davis*Plus* (www.fadavis.com). While reviewing the answers provided:

   • Compare and contrast your responses with those presented.

   • Develop a rationale for the answers provided. Does the rationale match the one you based your response on?

   • Be aware that your answers will not concisely match those provided. Remember that this *does not necessarily mean your answers are incorrect*. Often there is more than one acceptable response to the questions. Determining the efficacy of your response requires careful reflection about the rationale for your clinical decisions. It may also require one or more of the following: discussion with peers, returning to text content (or other resources) to confirm or refute your response, and/or consultation with a physical therapy faculty member or colleague.

   Outcome Measures A variety of outcome measures are incorporated into the case studies. Some are general measures of function applicable to a broad spectrum of patients, while others are diagnosis-specific. These standardized instruments provide important information about a patient's activity limitations and participation restrictions. In clinical practice, outcome measures have a range of applications, including providing baseline patient data on which to base function-oriented goals and outcomes at the start of an episode of care, as a measure of patient progress toward goals and outcomes, as indicators of patient safety, and as evidence to support the effectiveness of a specific intervention. Appendix A, "Outcome Measures Organized by the *International Classification of Functioning, Disability, and Health (ICF)* Categories," provides key references to guide exploration of specific outcome measures.

   The clinical reasoning process that leads to sound clinical decision-making is a course of action involving a range of cognitive skills that physical therapists use to process information, reach decisions, and determine actions. In a health-care environment that demands efficiency and cost-effectiveness, physical therapists are required to make complex decisions under significant practice restraints. Owing to the importance of this critical phase of physical therapy intervention, clinical decision-making requires continual practice and feedback throughout professional preparation. The intent of Part III is to offer an opportunity to guide and facilitate development of this important process.

Traumatic Brain Injury

TEMPLE T. COWDEN, PT, MPT, RANCHO LOS AMIGOS
NATIONAL REHABILITATION CENTER, DOWNEY,
CALIFORNIA

Examination

History

- Demographic Information:
Patient is a 41-year-old, Filipino-Caucasian male. He is English speaking and right-hand dominant. He was admitted to the adult brain injury service for inpatient rehabilitation following a motorcycle accident.

- Social History:
Patient is an ex-Marine; he has one son and is divorced from his wife. He lives with his fiancée in a single-story home. His fiancée has three children who live with them, ages 12, 13, and 15. The patient's fiancée does not work outside of the home but is responsible for the cooking, laundry, cleaning, and upkeep of the home, as well as taking care of the children.

- Employment:
Patient worked as an inspector for a fire safety company. His job involved driving to various locations where he inspected and tested various fire safety equipment (such as fire alarms, fire extinguishers, and so forth), which involved a moderate amount of physical activity.

- Living Environment:
Patient resides in a single-story home, which is split level, with one step to enter the home's main living room area. There are three steps to enter the home, with no handrails or ramp in place.

- General Health Status:
Patient is medically stable and able to participate in a rehabilitation program. Prior to this injury, patient was believed to be in good general health.

- Social and Health Habits:
Patient enjoys playing basketball and softball with his friends. Prior to injury, he was not involved in a formal exercise program but remained active playing sports, spending time with the children and through work activities. Patient states his favorite activities are riding motorcycles and "hanging out at the bars." While it is unclear how much, the patient has a history of alcohol use; his use of other drugs is unknown.

- Medical/Surgical History:
Medical history is unknown due to incomplete medical records from previous facility. Patient is agitated and unable to consistently and appropriately answer questions. Surgical history prior to this injury is unknown.

- History of Present Illness:
This is a 41-year-old male, status post motorcycle accident while intoxicated on June 28. The patient was reportedly found approximately 70 feet (21 m) from the site of impact. He was brought in by ambulance to an acute hospital with a Glasgow Coma Scale (GCS) score of 1-1-1; blood pressure was 90 systolic (diastolic not documented), with a heart rate of 160 beats per minute and an oxygen saturation measurement (SpO$_2$) of 80 percent using pulse oximetry. Owing to the low GCS score and decreased oxygenation, the patient was immediately intubated and ventilated. He was noted to have 2-mm pupils bilaterally, was nonreactive with motor function evident on only the left side. There were multiple skin abrasions on the right shoulder, chest, and hip. Upon admission to the acute facility, the patient underwent computed tomography (CT) scan and was diagnosed with the following: flailed chest with multiple rib fractures, lung contusions, pneumothorax, contusion and laceration of the right lobe of the liver with hemoperitoneum (presence of blood in the peritoneal cavity), fracture subluxation of the right acromioclavicular joint, and fractures of the bases of the right fourth and fifth metacarpals. A CT of the brain showed blood in the fourth ventricle, brain stem, upper cervical spinal cord, and subarachnoid space (subarachnoid hemorrhage and intracranial hemorrhage). The patient was transferred to the intensive care unit (ICU), where consultations were done by neurosurgery, infectious disease, and orthopedics. A triple lumen catheter and gastrostomy tube were inserted. No further operative intervention was planned at that time. The patient remained in critical condition in the ICU with full ventilatory support for approximately 2 weeks. On July 3, the patient had a tracheotomy. The patient underwent drainage and débridement of the right hip wound and a vacuum-assisted closure (VAC) device placement on July 23. On July 24, due to deteriorating renal function, the patient was diagnosed with acute renal failure caused by sepsis and contrast toxicity. On July 31, the patient underwent irrigation, drainage and open reduction, and internal fixation of the carpometacarpal joint of the right fourth and fifth metacarpals, with plans for immobilization for 6 weeks. On August 4, the patient experienced

an episode of asystole after the removal of a triple lumen catheter, which required cardiopulmonary resuscitation (CPR) and atropine to resolve. Due to closure of the right hip wound and suspicion of necrotizing fasciitis, he underwent further wound débridement and irrigation of the subcutaneous tissue and muscle on August 13. It was then discovered that the patient had bilateral common femoral popliteal and left peroneal deep venous thromboses (DVTs), and an inferior vena cava filter was placed. By early September, the patient was considered medically stable. He was able to tolerate a tracheostomy collar; he was more alert and able to respond to questions and communicate his basic wants and needs at times. However, he frequently became agitated. Patient was decannulated (removal of tracheostomy) prior to transfer to the rehabilitation facility, but the exact date was not indicated.

Admission to Rehabilitation Facility

- Chief Complaints:
  At the time of the initial examination (September 10), patient appears to be very agitated, restless, and impulsive. He complains of stomach and back pain. He also repeatedly yells out for his girlfriend and "Doc" (doctor). Patient appears to have hypersensitivity to touch and pain throughout right upper extremity (UE). Patient appears to be diaphoretic, with blood pressure of 150/110 mm Hg and a heart rate of 132 beats per minute.
- Functional Status:
  Prior to injury, patient was independent with all basic activities of daily living (BADL) and instrumental activities of daily living (IADL).
- Medications:
  Upon admission, patient was taking the following medications: Colace, Dulcolax, Buspirone, Clotiapine, Metoprolol, Omeprazole, Ranitidine (changed to Prevacid upon admission), Levetiracetam, Lovenox, Sertraline, and Olanzapine. The patient was also taking Vicodin and Keppra for prophylactic use (patient has no history of seizures). Upon admission, this was changed to Neurontin because Keppra (Levetiracetam) has been found to increase agitation in some patients.

Systems Review

- Cardiovascular/Pulmonary System:
  - Heart rate: 132 beats per minute seated at edge of bed with regular rhythm
  - Respiratory rate: 18 breaths per minute
  - Blood pressure: 150/110 mm Hg
  - Oxygen saturation: 98 percent on room air
  - Temperature: 98.2 degrees Fahrenheit (36.8°C)
  - Edema: Mild bilateral pitting edema of legs and feet; right foot 2+, left foot 1+
- Integumentary System:
  - Scar(s): Right hip with well-healed scar. Upper abdominal midline scar (from gastrostomy tube placement). Right hand has sutures in place on fourth and fifth fingers.
  - Skin color: Black, necrotic tissue of left second and third toes. Face is pale, sweaty, and warm to the touch.
  - Skin integrity: Healing tracheostomy scar. Excessive dryness and flaking of both feet. Excessively thick and long toenails bilaterally. Left UE excoriation.
- Musculoskeletal System:
  - Gross symmetry: Obvious right shoulder deformity due to separation. Patient maintains right elbow flexed at about 90 degrees. Patient does not have normal midline orientation. He requires some assistance to maintain upright sitting balance without back support.
  - Gross range of motion (ROM): Right UE limitations noted at shoulder (flexion, abduction, and external rotation), elbow, and wrist. Left UE ROM within functional limits (WFL). Decreased ROM evident at both knees (Fig. CS1.1).
  - Gross strength of right extremities: Right UE demonstrates significant weakness and is typically maintained in a flexed position (Fig. CS1.2). The patient is able to actively move the right lower extremity (LE) against gravity (Fig. CS1.3).
  - Height: 6 ft 4 in. (2.9 m)
  - Weight: 198 lb (89.9 kg)
- Neuromuscular System:
  - Gross coordinated movement: Patient is able to move from supine-to-sitting at the edge of the bed without assistance. However, he requires supervision when sitting without a back support for prolonged periods, owing to poor balance and forwardly flexed posture with decreased trunk control. When sitting, he is unable to reach outside of his base of support (BOS) without loss of balance. He is unable to perform sit-to-stand transfers, even with the bed elevated, without maximal assistance from the therapist due to difficulty with task planning and diminished LE strength (Fig. CS1.4). Patient requires maximal assistance to move from bed-to-wheelchair due to

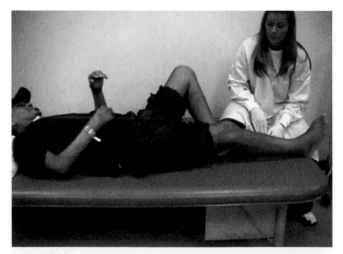

FIGURE CS1.1 ROM limitations are evident in the right knee (lacks full extension). *Not shown:* Limitations also exist in the left knee.

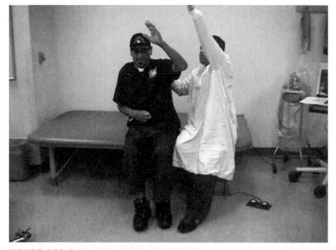

FIGURE CS1.2 In sitting, significant weakness is evident in the right UE (unable to move against gravity). The right UE is flexed and adducted with the hand tightly fisted. The left UE is able to move against gravity (shoulder abducts, externally rotates with elbow flexion).

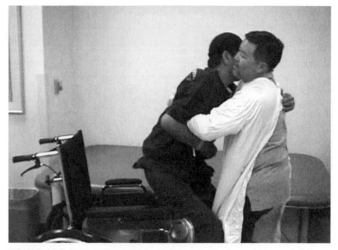

FIGURE CS1.4 Patient requires maximal assistance to transfer from wheelchair-to-platform mat. The patient lacks extension control at both hips and knees. Right UE remains flexed and adducted with hand tightly fisted.

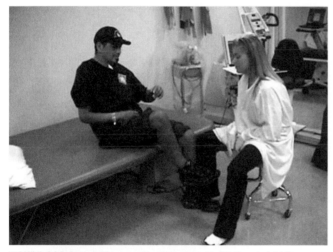

FIGURE CS1.3 In sitting, patient is able to lift the right LE against gravity (hip flexes with knee flexion). Note posterior shift of the trunk that accompanies the lift; patient moves into a sacral sitting position.

impulsivity, decreased strength, and impaired balance. Ambulation ability could not be examined initially due to safety concerns as well as patient agitation.
• Motor function (motor control and motor learning): Patient is able to voluntarily move all four extremities. Weakness of right UE is greater distally than proximally. He is able to follow simple commands for movement, but with poor consistency, which appears to be a result of restless, agitated behavior. No ankle clonus is present.
• Communication and cognition: The patient is alert and oriented to person and place. Voice is slightly dysarthric, but patient is generally understandable. At previous facility, patient had participated minimally in a speech-language

program; he had not received any previous physical therapy services. Patient is very restless, demonstrating continual writhing and movement from supine-to-sitting up in bed. Patient demonstrates impulsive behavior; he attempts to climb over bedrails and lies down without regard to his position in bed or the presence of bedrails. He answers simple personal questions appropriately, but is highly distractible and has only about 60 percent accuracy for known personal information.

Tests and Measures

• Sensory Integrity:
Light touch and superficial pain sensations appear grossly intact for both LEs and the left UE. Unable to perform even a general light touch examination of right UE secondary to patient guarding. Unable to formally test light touch and superficial pain sensations because of patient's inability to follow testing instructions (secondary to cognitive impairments and decreased attention).
• Strength:
Unable to accurately examine strength, secondary to difficulty following testing instructions. (*Note:* Approximately 2 days after the initial consult, the therapist was able to complete the Manual Muscle Test [MMT].) Right LE is weak; patient is unable to move all joints through complete range against gravity. See Table 1.1. Patient is unwilling to even attempt movement of right UE due to complaints of pain and weakness. Atrophy of right deltoid is noted. Left UE demonstrates functional strength throughout.
• Range of Motion: See Table CS1.2.
• Cranial Nerve Function:
Visual fields are grossly intact (CN II). Pupils are equal, round, and reactive to light and accommodation; extra ocular muscles are intact (CN III, IV, V). Face is symmetrical (CN VII). Hearing is grossly intact (CN VIII).

TABLE CS1.1 Lower Extremity Manual Muscle Test

Joint	Motion	Left	Right
Hip	Flexion	3/5	3/5
	Extension	2/5	2/5
	Abduction	2/5	2/5
Knee	Flexion	3/5	3/5
	Extension	3/5	3/5
Ankle	Dorsiflexion	3/5	2/5
	Plantarflexion (tested supine)	2/5	2/5

All scores are based on a 0 to 5 scale: 5, normal; 4, good; 3, fair; 2, poor; 1, trace; 0, no contraction.

TABLE CS1.2 Passive Range of Motion Examination (in degrees)

Joint	Motion	Left	Right
Shoulder	Flexion	WFL	0–90*
	Extension	WFL	WFL
	Abduction	WFL	0–80*
	Internal rotation	WFL	WFL
	External rotation	WFL	0–30*
Elbow	Flexion	WFL	15–150
Wrist	Flexion	WFL	0–60
	Extension	WFL	0–30
Hip	Flexion	WFL	WFL
	Extension	WFL	WFL
	Abduction	WFL	WFL
Knee	Flexion	5–110	3–110
	Extension	Unable to achieve full knee extension	
Ankle	Dorsiflexion	WFL*	WFL*
	Plantar flexion	WFL	WFL

*Indicates movement was accompanied by pain.
Abbreviation: WFL, within functional limits.

Palate is symmetrical in elevation; phonation is clear (CN IX, X). Tongue is midline with protrusion and limited ROM (CN XII).

- Deep Tendon Reflexes:
LUE 1+, right LE 2+, bilateral patellar reflex 2+, bilateral Achilles tendon reflex 1+. Key to grading:
  - 0, no response
  - 1+, present but depressed, low normal
  - 2+, average, normal
  - 3+, increased, brisker than average possibly but not necessarily abnormal
  - 4+, very brisk, hyperactive with clonus, abnormal
- Balance:
Patient demonstrates poor seated balance, although he is able to sit upright independently using a back support. He is unable to reach outside of his BOS for functional activities without loss of balance or fall. He typically demonstrates a kyphotic posture. Patient has poor standing balance, as he is unable to achieve or maintain full standing without maximal assistance from the therapist. He is unable to perform dynamic movements during standing without loss of balance.
- Gait:
Unable to examine
- Activities of Daily Living (ADL):
  - Basic Activities of Daily Living (BADL): Patient requires moderate to maximal assistance or total dependence for execution of all ADL.
  - Instrumental Activities of Daily Living (IADL): Dependent

Evaluation, Diagnosis and Prognosis, and Plan of Care

Note: Prior to considering the guiding questions below, view the Case Study 1 Examination segment of the DVD to enhance understanding of the patient's impairments and activity limitations. Following *completion of the guiding questions*, view the Case Study 1 Intervention segment of the DVD to compare and contrast the interventions presented with those you selected. Last, progress to the Case Study 1 Outcomes segment of the DVD to compare and contrast the goals and expected outcomes you identified with the functional outcomes achieved.

Guiding Questions

1. Describe this patient's clinical presentation in terms of:
   a. Impairments
   b. Activity limitations
   c. Participation restrictions
2. Identify three impairments you would address initially to improve this patient's activity limitations and participation restrictions.

3. Identify three goals to address the impairments you identified above and the expected outcomes to improve the patient's activity limitations and participation restrictions.

4. Describe three treatment interventions focused on functional outcomes that could be used during the first 2 weeks of therapy. Indicate how you could progress each intervention, and include a brief rationale that justifies your choices.

5. What important safety precautions should be observed during treatment of this patient?

6. Identify factors, both positive (assets) and negative, that play a part in determining the patient's prognosis for recovery.

7. Describe strategies that can be used to develop self-management skills and promote self-efficacy in achieving goals and outcomes.

8. How can the physical therapist facilitate interdisciplinary teamwork to assist in reaching identified goals and functional outcomes?

Reminder: Answers to the Case Study Guiding Questions are available online at Davis*Plus* (www.fadavis.com).

VIEWING THE CASE: PATIENT WITH TRAUMATIC BRAIN INJURY

As students learn in different ways, the DVD case presentation (examination, intervention, and outcomes) is designed to promote engagement with the content, allow progression at an individual (or group) pace, and use of the medium or combination of media (*written*, *visual*, and *auditory*) best suited to the learner(s). The DVD includes both *visual* and *auditory* modes. Following is the case study summary and *written* DVD narration.

Video Summary
Patient is a 41-year-old male with traumatic brain injury undergoing active rehabilitation. The video shows examination and intervention segments for both inpatient and outpatient rehabilitation episodes of care. Outcomes are filmed at 3 and 7 weeks after the initial examination.

Complete Video Narration
Examination:
- The patient performs a squat pivot transfer with assistance. He requires both verbal and tactile cues to shift his weight forward in preparation to stand. He is able to initiate pushing with his lower extremities; however, he is unable to maintain his forward head and body position and does not have the strength to come to a complete standing position. He is unable to effectively contribute to the pivot portion of the transfer and requires complete assistance.
- When moving from sitting-to-supine, the patient has difficulty controlling the momentum of his body and rolls to the left side before lying supine. Due to bilateral lower extremity tightness and discomfort, he must be given verbal cues to lie with his legs as straight as possible.
- When moving from supine-to-sitting, he uses momentum by flexing his body forward and rocking.
- The patient sits with impaired sitting posture; he consistently leans toward the right side and back into sacral sitting. With verbal and visual cues, he is able to move back into a more correct sitting alignment by pulling with his left hand.
- The patient performs a sit-to-stand transfer using a specialized lift and walker system that provides trunk and upper extremity support. Once in standing, the patient is unable to achieve an erect posture, even with tactile and verbal cues. He demonstrates significant bilateral hip and knee flexion and falls backward into sitting.

Intervention:
- It is now 1 week later. The patient performs a sit-to-stand transfer with minimal assistance and verbal cues. However, he is unable to maintain standing and falls backward.
- During a stand pivot transfer, the patient relies upon the therapist for support and balance.
- The patient ambulates using a walker system for trunk and upper extremity support, a right ankle-foot orthosis, and two-person assist.
- After a week of gait training, the patient is able to ambulate with a front-wheeled walker that has been modified with a right forearm trough attachment. The patient has difficulty steering the walker, so the therapist has put a sand weight on the front of the walker to slow the progression. He no longer requires an ankle-foot orthosis. Balance can safely be maintained with the help of only one therapist.
- During stair training, the patient requires left upper extremity use and maximal assistance to prevent backward loss of balance. Verbal cues are given for proper task sequencing. He maintains a forward flexed body position and uses a step-to pattern when ascending and descending stairs. Without therapist assistance, the patient would be unable to complete the task.
- It is now 3 weeks later. The patient is being evaluated during his first outpatient visit. He ambulates using a

front-wheeled walker without the forearm trough attachment. While he is no longer in need of assistance, he reports that he does not walk without someone close by, as he is fearful of falling.
- The therapist asks the patient to walk without the walker, which he has never done before. The therapist provides contact guard supervision. Note the decreased step length and speed, wide base of support, and upper extremity high guard position, all in an effort to achieve greater stability.
- The patient demonstrates significant improvement in his ability to ascend and descend stairs. He requires only contact guard supervision. He practices step-ups in the parallel bars. The therapist provides verbal and manual cues to maintain an upright body position and activate his extensors.

Outcomes:
- It is now 1 month later. The patient demonstrates increased control and can independently perform sit-to-stand transfers and standing without upper extremity support.
- The patient stands on a foam mat with only occasional upper extremity support. The therapist maintains contact from behind for safety. Note his left ankle instability.
- The patient marches in place on the foam, with left upper extremity support. The therapist maintains contact from behind for safety.

Traumatic Brain Injury: Balance and Locomotor Training

HEIDI ROTH, PT, MSPT, NCS, AND
JASON BARBAS, PT, MPT, NCS, REHABILITATION
INSTITUTE OF CHICAGO, CHICAGO, ILLINOIS

Examination

History

- Demographic Information:
  Patient is a 47-year-old, right-handed, Caucasian male.
- Social History:
  Patient is single; patient's mother lives in the area.
- Employment:
  Patient has not been employed since his injury 2 years ago, but he previously worked for a garage manufacturing company.
- Education:
  Patient has a college degree.
- Living Environment:
  Patient currently resides in an assisted living apartment.
- General Health Status:
  Patient is in generally good health, mildly overweight, with decreased activity tolerance.
- Social and Health Habits:
  Patient leads a primarily sedentary lifestyle, is a cigarette smoker, and reports drinking five to six alcoholic beverages per week. His social network is limited to visiting his mother and other residents at the assisted living facility. He reports using a local gym occasionally.
- Family History:
  Patient does not report any significant family history of major medical conditions.
- Medical/Surgical History:
  Patient suffered a traumatic brain injury approximately 2 years ago during a motor vehicle collision.
- Current Condition/Chief Complaint:
  The patient presents for outpatient physical therapy services. He reports a decline in endurance and difficulty moving his left leg. He also reports a worsening of balance with falls at home (two falls in the past 2 months).
- Activity Level:
  Patient is independent in the home environment in all basic activities of daily living (BADL) and requires assistance in the community and for instrumental activities of daily living (IADL) (e.g., managing his finances and medications). He reports walking with a cane at times, but he also uses a rolling walker. He recently purchased a motorized scooter and reports a decrease in activity level since buying the scooter. Prior to his injury, patient was independent with all BADL and IADL.
- Medications:
  Upon admission to outpatient services, the patient was taking the following medications: Metformin, 500 mg twice a day; Metoprolol, 50 mg twice a day; Trazadone, 50 mg once a day; Zanaflex, 2 mg four times a day; Hydrochlorothiazide, 25 mg once a day; Vitamin B_1, 100 mg once a day; Prilosec, 20 mg once a day; Reglan, 10 mg three times a day; Dicyclomine, 20 mg twice a day; Amantad (Amantadine), 100 mg once a day; Tramadol, 50 mg every 6 hours as needed; Folic Acid, 1 mg once a day; Ibuprofen, 800 mg three times a day as needed; multivitamin, once a day; Buspar HCL 5 mg twice a day.

Systems Review

- Communication/Cognition:
  - Rancho Los Amigos Levels of Cognitive Functioning (RLA LOCF), Scale: Level 7.
  - Although the patient is independent with verbal communication, he demonstrates concrete thinking, decreased short-term memory, increased time for new learning, and decreased safety awareness.
- Learning:
  - Patient requires multiple demonstrations of new activities, with both written and verbal reinforcement.
- Cardiovascular/Pulmonary System:
  - Resting heart rate (HR) = 72; Exercise HR = 90; Five minutes postexercise HR = 82
  - Resting blood pressure (BP) = 130/76; Exercise BP = 146/92; Five minutes postexercise BP = 138/80
  - 6-Minute Walk Test = 418 feet with straight cane
  - Edema = absent
- Integumentary System:
  - No skin abnormalities are noted.
- Musculoskeletal System:
  - Height: 5 ft 10 in. (1.77 m)
  - Weight: 220 lb (99.8 kg)
  - Gross strength: Bilateral upper extremities (UEs) within functional limits (WFL); decreased strength noted in bilateral lower extremities (LEs), with left lower extremity (LE) weaker than right LE (Table CS2.1).

TABLE CS2.1 Manual Muscle Test: Lower Extremities

Lower Extremity Motions Tested	Initial Examination		Discharge*	
	Left	Right	Left	Right
Hip extension	2/5	3/5	3-/5	4/5
Hip flexion	4/5	5/5	5/5	5/5
Hip adduction	3/5	3/5	4/5	5/5
Hip abduction	2/5	3/5	4/5	5/5
Knee flexion	4/5	4/5	4/5	5/5
Knee extension	4/5	5/5	5/5	5/5
Ankle DF	3/5	4/5	3/5	4/5
Ankle PF	3/5	3/5	3/5	3/5

*Discharge occurred 8 weeks after initial examination.

All scores are based on a 0 to 5 scale: 5, normal; 4, good; 3, fair; 2, poor; 1, trace; 0, no contraction.

Abbreviations: DF, dorsiflexion; PF, plantarflexion.

TABLE CS2.2 Modified Ashworth Scale for Grading Spasticity

LE Muscle Groups	Left LE	Right LE
Hip extensors	1+	0
Hip flexors	1+	0
Hip adductors	1+	0
Hip abductors	0	0
Knee extensors	2	0
Knee flexors	3	0
Ankle dorsiflexors	1	0
Ankle plantarflexors	1+	0

Key: 0, no increase in tone; 1, slight increase in tone, manifested by a catch and release, or by minimal resistance at the end of the ROM when the affected part(s) is(are) moved into flexion or extension; 1+, slight increase in muscle tone manifested by a catch, followed by minimal resistance throughout the remainder (less than half) of the ROM; 2, more marked increase in muscle tone through most of the ROM, but the affected part(s) is(are) easily moved; 3, considerable increase in muscle tone; passive movement is difficult; 4, affected part(s) is(are) rigid in flexion or extension.

- Gross range of motion (ROM): WFL throughout bilateral UEs and LEs.
- Neuromuscular System:
  - Gross coordinated movement: Decreased coordination and speed of movement bilaterally, more exaggerated in left upper extremity (UE) and left LE.
  - Spasticity: Increased spasticity noted throughout left LE (Table CS2.2).
  - Sitting balance: Independent with static and dynamic sitting balance with eyes open (EO) and eyes closed (EC); able to reach outside base of support (BOS) without compensatory movements of opposite UE or LEs.
  - Standing static balance: Able to maintain static standing balance on level surface without UE support. Demonstrates increased postural sway and loss of balance with EC, with decreased BOS, and when standing on soft (compliant) surfaces. Delayed balance reactions noted in all planes.
  - Standing dynamic balance: Demonstrates loss of balance during all dual-task activities, such as turning the head during forward walking (up/down/right/left), changing speed and direction, and stepping over and around obstacles.
- Functional Status:
  - Transfers: Able to perform all transfers and bed mobility with modified independence (requires assistive device); however, extra time is needed to accomplish the transfers. He has difficulty transitioning from sit-to-stand from low or soft surfaces.
  - Gait analysis: Patient ambulates with a straight cane in the home and community. He demonstrates significantly decreased gait speed. He ambulates with a decreased step length (right > left), decreased left weight shift, decreased left knee extension during stance, and decreased left terminal knee extension (Fig CS2.1). He also exhibits a wide BOS, decreased left push-off at terminal stance, decreased left heel strike (initial contact), and

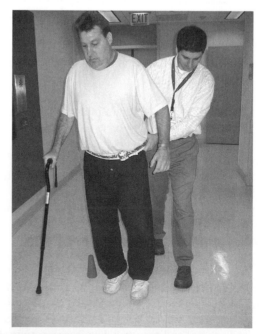

FIGURE CS2.1 Patient ambulates with a straight cane with decreased step length, decreased left weight shift, and decreased left knee extension. He also exhibits decreased arm swing on the left.

diminished arm swing bilaterally. During swing phase of the left LE, spasticity is increased and inadequate dorsiflexion is noted. Decreased left hip extension is evident during terminal stance. Although the patient typically demonstrated a wide walking BOS, when asked to negotiate an obstacle course placed on the floor (requiring heightened cognitive monitoring), his BOS tended to decrease (Figure CS2.2).

- Community mobility: Prior to purchase of motorized scooter, the patient ambulated with a cane and reports experiencing frequent loss of balance with curbs, ramps, uneven surfaces, and busy environments. Primary means of community mobility is now the scooter (past 5 months).

Tests and Measures

- Sensation:
  - Diminished light touch distal to left knee.
  - Proprioception: Intact at right ankle, knee, and hip; left hip and knee intact, left ankle decreased joint position sense (4/10 accuracy).
- Strength:
  - Manual muscle test (MMT) scores at initial examination and at discharge (8 weeks later) are reported for both LEs in Table CS2.1.
- Spasticity:
  - Modified Ashworth Scale scores for both LEs are reported in Table CS2.2. Scores were unchanged from initial exam to discharge (8 weeks later).
- Endurance, Balance, and Gait:
  - The results of standardized tests for endurance, balance, and gait are reported at initial exam, at 4 weeks, and at 8 weeks (discharge) in Table CS2.3.

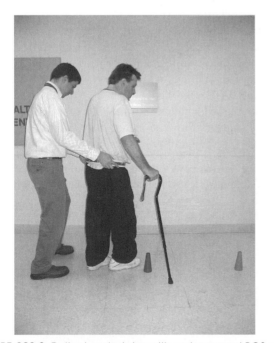

FIGURE CS2.2 Patient ambulates with a decreased BOS while walking through an obstacle course.

- Among the data reported in Table CS2.3 are scores from the Functional Reach Test. This is a practical, easily administered screen for balance problems originally developed for use with older adults. It is the maximal distance one can reach forward beyond arm's length as measured by a yardstick attached to a wall. The patient stands sideward next to a wall with the shoulder flexed to 90 degrees, the elbow extended, and the hand fisted (Fig. CS2.3). Using the yardstick, an initial measurement is taken of the position of the third metacarpal. The patient is then asked to lean as far forward as possible without losing balance or taking a step (Fig. CS2.4). A second measure is then taken and subtracted from the first to obtain a final measure in inches.

TABLE CS2.3 Standardized Tests for Endurance, Balance, and Gait			
Test Performed	Initial Examination	4 Weeks	8 Weeks
6-Minute Walk (ft)	413 (126 m)	518 (158 m)	602 (183 m)
10-Meter Walk (sec)	22	20	15
Gait Speed (m/sec)	0.45 (1.5 ft/sec)	0.50 (1.6 ft/sec)	0.67 (2.1 ft/sec)
Timed Up and Go (sec)	24	21	20
Dynamic Gait Index	7/24	11/24	17/24
Berg Balance Test	30/56	30/56	40/56
Rhomberg (EO) (sec)	5	10	30
Rhomberg (EC) (sec)	0	3	10
Tandem Stance (right or left LE front) (sec)	0	0	0
Semitandem Stance (sec)	7	10	30
Functional Reach (in.)	4 (10 cm)	6 (15 cm)	>10 (25 cm)
Assistive Device	Straight cane	Straight cane	Straight cane

Abbreviations: EO, eyes open; EC, eyes closed.

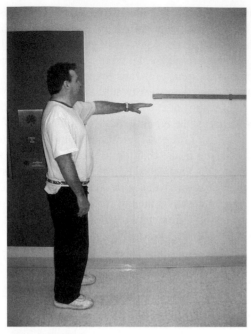

FIGURE CS2.3 Patient is standing sideward next to a wall with the left shoulder flexed to 90 degrees and the elbow extended (start of the Functional Reach Test). Note the relatively wide stance. Typically, this test is performed with a fisted hand. Owing to the patient's decreased short-term memory and increased time required for new learning, difficulty was experienced understanding the directions for keeping the hand in a fisted position. Based on this limitation, the test was modified and measures taken from the tip of the middle phalanx.

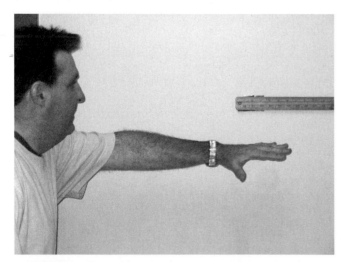

FIGURE CS2.4 Patient is instructed to reach forward as far as possible without raising the heels from the floor (end of the Functional Reach Test).

Evaluation, Diagnosis and Prognosis, and Plan of Care

Note: Prior to considering the guiding questions below, view the Case Study 2 Examination segment of the DVD to enhance understanding of the patient's impairments and activity limitations. Following *completion of the guiding questions,* view the Case Study 2 Intervention segment of the DVD to compare and contrast the interventions presented with those you selected. Last, progress to the Case Study 2 Outcomes segment of the DVD to compare and contrast the goals and expected outcomes you identified with the functional outcomes achieved.

Guiding Questions

1. Describe this patient's clinical presentation in terms of:
   a. Impairments
   b. Activity limitations
   c. Participation restrictions
2. Identify five patient assets from the history and examination that would positively influence his physical therapy outcomes.
3. Identify five factors from the patient's history and examination that might negatively influence his physical therapy outcomes.
4. What impairments would you focus on during the physical therapy episode of care to address the patient's activity limitations and participation restrictions?
5. Identify anticipated goals (8 weeks) for balance and gait and the expected functional outcomes.
6. Describe three interventions focused on improving balance and gait that you would implement during the first 1 or 2 weeks of therapy. Indicate how you could progress each intervention, and include a brief rationale for your choice.
7. What strategies would you utilize to optimize motor learning within a therapy session as well as for carry-over (retention) of learned activities?
8. Identify appropriate goals for the home exercise program (HEP).
9. Describe the elements and activities of a HEP.
10. What strategies can you include in your plan of care (POC) regarding fall prevention in the home?

Reminder: Answers to the Case Study Guiding Questions are available online at Davis*Plus* (www.fadavis.com).

⊙ VIEWING THE CASE: PATIENT WITH TRAUMATIC BRAIN INJURY

As students learn in different ways, the DVD case presentation (examination, intervention, and outcomes) is designed to promote engagement with the content, allow progression at an individual (or group) pace, and use of the medium or combination of media (*written*, *visual*, and *auditory*) best suited to the learner(s). The DVD includes both *visual* and *auditory* modes. Following is the case study summary and *written* DVD narration.

Video Summary

Patient is a 47-year-old male with traumatic brain injury undergoing active rehabilitation. The video shows examination and intervention segments during outpatient rehabilitation, with an emphasis on locomotor and balance training. Outcomes are filmed 8 weeks after the initial examination.

Complete Video Narration

Examination:

- The patient is admitted for outpatient therapy with complaints of difficulty moving his left lower extremity, worsening balance, and history of recent falls at home. When walking at home, he uses a straight cane. Note decreased step length, left weight shift, and hip and knee extension. He also exhibits a wide base of support with decreased push-off and heel strike.
- When walking without a cane, the patient demonstrates increased difficulty moving his left lower extremity and increased lateral tilt of the trunk to the right. Note decreased step length and decreased arm swing.
- When asked to stand in a tandem heel-toe position, his balance control is poor. Note increased sway and stepping with high guard arm position.
- When asked to stand on one limb, the patient is unable to maintain the position and demonstrates lateral touchdown of his foot with high guard arm position.
- When asked to stand with feet together, the patient exhibits impaired balance with increased sway and frequent use of high guard arm position.
- When asked to stand with feet together and eyes closed, the patient reveals worsening balance control. Note increased sway and hip and knee flexion.

Intervention:

- The patient is walking on a motorized treadmill using a harness for safety but with no body weight support. He begins with bilateral upper extremity support and progresses to unilateral and then no upper extremity support.
- The patient is asked to walk while counting backward from 100.
- The patient practices turning and side-step walking to the right, side-step walking to the left, and backward walking on the treadmill.
- The patient practices walking on the treadmill using faster speeds and alternating hand supports.
- The patient practices walking, stepping over and around obstacles. The therapist provides verbal cues and contact guarding.
- The patient practices stepping up on a low 4-inch step. Note poor balance control requiring minimal assistance of the therapist. The patient then steps up and down the other side of the step.
- The patient practices standing on foam and swinging a golf club. Contact guarding is required.

Outcomes:

- It is now 8 weeks later. The patient is able to maintain standing balance with feet together. Tandem stance is more problematic, but the patient eventually stabilizes. Use of high guard arm position is still evident.
- The patient walks independently using a straight cane. Note increased speed and turning control.
- When walking without the cane, both speed and control are improved. Lateral lean to the right is still evident.

3

Spinal Cord Injury: Locomotor Training

ELIZABETH ARDOLINO, PT, MS,[1] ELIZABETH WATSON, PT, DPT, NCS,[1] ANDREA L. BEHRMAN, PT, PHD,[2] SUSAN HARKEMA, PHD,[3] AND MARY SCHMIDT-READ, PT, DPT, MS[1]

Examination

History

The patient presents with incomplete paraplegia, secondary to an anterior spinal cord infarction that occurred while he was snowboarding. The patient was admitted to a pediatric acute trauma center and then completed a 4-week stay in an acute rehabilitation facility. He was referred to a locomotor training clinic for outpatient therapy and initiated this therapy 4 months after his injury.

- Demographic Information:
  The patient is a 17-year-old white male.
- Past Medical History:
  Patient history is unremarkable except for occasional migraine headaches and delayed sleep phase syndrome (dissociation between the patient's circadian rhythm and the external environment).
- Social History:
  The patient is a junior in high school. Prior to his injury, he ran cross-country and played lacrosse. He is an honors student and is active in his church youth group. At the time of the initial outpatient locomotor training evaluation, the patient was being home-schooled.
- Living Environment:
  The patient lives with his parents and three older siblings in a two-story house with a stair glide to the second floor. There is a ramp at the main entrance to the house. The patient has a Quickie TNT ("Takes No Tools") manual wheelchair, as well as a tub bench and a commode at home.
- Current Medications:
  Baclofen, 10 mg twice a day; Gabapertin/Neurontin, 600 mg twice a day; aspirin, 80 mg daily; and Detrol LA twice a day.
- Patient Goals:
  Patient has identified the following goals for the physical therapy episode of care:
  - Ambulate independently with or without an assistive device.
  - Return to high school at an ambulatory level.

---

[1]Magee Rehabilitation Hospital, Philadelphia, Pennsylvania

[2]College of Public Health and Health Professions, University of Florida, Gainesville

[3]Department of Neurological Surgery, University of Kentucky, Louisville

Systems Review

- Cardiovascular/Pulmonary System:
  Heart rate (HR):
  - Sitting at rest in manual wheelchair, HR = 82 beats per minute.
  - Supine on flat mat, HR = 71 beats per minute
  Blood pressure (BP): Sitting at rest in manual wheelchair, BP = 108/65
  Orthostatic testing:
  - BP resting in supine = 105/61
  - Immediately upon passive return to upright supported sitting, BP = 66/42
  - After 2 minutes of upright supported sitting, BP = 90/60
  - After 5 minutes of upright supported sitting, BP = 99/58
  - After 10 minutes of upright supported sitting, BP = 101/63
- Musculoskeletal System:
  - Gross range of motion (ROM): Within normal limits (WNL) in both upper extremities (UEs) and lower extremities (LEs).
  - Gross strength testing: Both UEs are symmetrical and strength is WNL. The left LE has good to fair voluntary movement, and the right LE has trace to absent voluntary movement.
  - Height: 5.75 ft (1.75 m).
  - Weight: 138 lb (62.6 kg).
- Integumentary System:
  Skin is intact with no open lacerations, abrasions, or pressure ulcers. There is no history of pressure ulcers.
- Neuromuscular System:
  Balance: The patient is able to sit unsupported in a chair but is unable to stand without support.
  - Sitting posture: In a relaxed seated position with UEs resting on thighs, the patient demonstrates increased thoracic and lumbar kyphosis (Fig. CS3.1). When asked to sit fully upright, the patient presents with an increased lumbar lordosis. He uses minimal UE support with his hands on his thighs to attain an upright sitting posture (Fig. CS3.2).
  - Standing posture: In supported standing, the patient presents with a severely increased lumbar lordosis, hyperextension of the thoracic spine, and genu recurvatum of the right knee (Fig. CS3.3).
- Functional Status:
  - Transfers: The patient is independent, with squat pivot transfers to even and uneven surfaces.

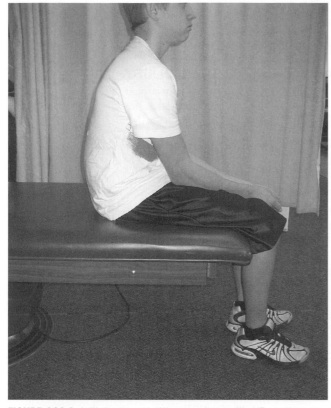

FIGURE CS3.1 Initial relaxed sitting posture with UEs resting on thighs. Note the increased thoracic and lumbar kyphosis.

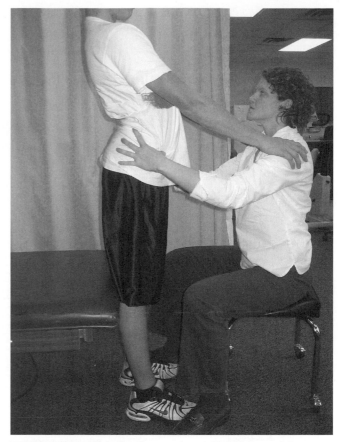

FIGURE CS3.3 Initial standing posture with UE support from hands placed on therapist's shoulders. Note the increased lumbar lordosis and hyperextension of the thoracic spine. Although obscured in the image, genu recurvatum of the right knee is also present.

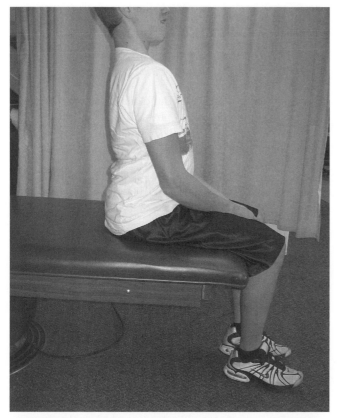

FIGURE CS3.2 Initial upright sitting posture achieved using UE support from hands placed on thighs. Note the increased lumbar lordosis.

- Locomotion: The patient is primarily a manual wheelchair user; he requires maximum assistance from two therapists to ambulate 5 ft (1.52 m) with a rolling walker.
- Communication/Cognition:
  The patient is alert and oriented to person, place, and time. He is able to answer questions appropriately regarding his needs and goals for therapy. He prefers to learn through demonstration.

Tests and Measures

- Sensory/Motor Function:
  The American Spinal Injury Association's (ASIA) *Standard Neurological Classification of Spinal Cord Injury* form was used to document sensory and motor function (Fig. CS3.4)
- Muscle Tone:
  The Modified Ashworth Scale was used to grade spasticity (Table CS3.1).
- Balance:
  - The Modified Functional Reach Test was used to examine sitting balance (Table CS3.2).
  - The purpose of the Modified Functional Reach Test is to determine how far the patient can reach outside of his

Patient Name_____ Date of Exam_____

Examiner Name_____ Comments_____

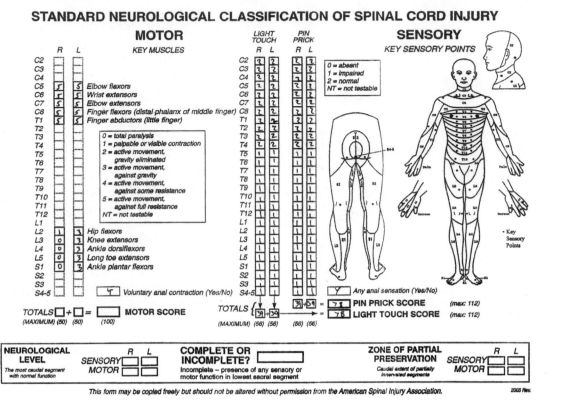

FIGURE CS3.4 The patient's sensory and motor scores using the American Spinal Injury Association (ASIA) Examination Form: *Standard Neurological Classification of Spinal Cord Injury.* (American Spinal Injury Association. International Standards for Neurological Classification of Spinal Cord Injury. American Spinal Injury Association, Chicago, 2006.)

base of support (BOS) while positioned in short-sitting. The patient begins with his back resting against the chair backrest and then raises one UE to 90 degrees of shoulder flexion, parallel to a yardstick positioned on the wall next to him. The examiner notes the patient's starting point; the patient reaches forward with a fisted hand as far as possible without losing his balance. The examiner notes the farthest point that the patient reaches (measure taken at third metacarpal), and then the patient returns to the starting position. The test is performed three times, and the results are averaged.

- The Berg Balance Scale was used to examine standing balance (Table CS3.3). The patient scored a 9/56, with difficulty performing any standing tasks that required standing without UE support, indicating a 100 percent risk of falls at an ambulatory level.
- Fall Risk:
 The patient's fall risk was determined using the Performance-Oriented Mobility Assessment (POMA) (Table CS3.4). The patient scored a total of 6/28, with difficulty performing any standing tasks that required standing without an assistive device, indicating 100 percent risk of falls at an ambulatory level.

- Ambulation:
 - The 10-Meter Walk Test: The patient was unable to complete this test without physical assistance.
 - The 6-Minute Walk Test: The patient was unable to complete this test without physical assistance.

Step Training With Body Weight Support System and a Treadmill

Four main elements comprise the examination in the step training environment: *stand retraining, stand adaptability, step retraining,* and *step adaptability.*

1. Stand retraining:
 The test begins with the patient standing on the treadmill (TM) with 75 percent of body weight supported. The amount of body weight supported is then lowered until the patient can no longer maintain an upright standing posture, even with maximal assistance from the trainers. Each trainer (physical therapist or physical therapist assistant) then states the amount of assistance being provided at each body segment (e.g., foot/ankle, knee, and hip/pelvis) (Table CS3.5).

TABLE CS3.1 Modified Ashworth Scale for Grading Spasticity[a]

Muscle Group	Right LE	Left LE
Hip Flexors	0	0
Hip Extensors	1+	1+
Hip Adductors	1	1
Knee Flexors	0	1
Knee Extensors	1	1
Plantarflexors	1	1+
Invertors	0	0
Evertors	0	1

Key: 0, no increase in tone; 1, slight increase in tone, manifested by a catch and release, or by minimal resistance at the end of the ROM when the affected part(s) is(are) moved into flexion or extension; 1+, slight increase in muscle tone manifested by a catch, followed by minimal resistance throughout the remainder (less than half) of the ROM; 2, more marked increase in muscle tone through most of the ROM, but the affected part(s) is(are) easily moved; 3, considerable increase in muscle tone; passive movement is difficult; 4, affected part(s) is(are) rigid in flexion or extension.

[a]Bohannon, R, and Smith, M. Interrater reliability of a modified Ashworth scale of muscle spasticity. Phys Ther 67:206, 1987.

2. Stand adaptability:

The purpose of this test is to examine the body weight parameters needed to maintain independence at different body segments. Stand adaptability includes: *static standing, lateral weight shifts,* and *step weight shifts.*

• Static standing: The therapist examines the amount of body weight support (BWS) necessary for each body segment to attain independence. The test begins at the lowest BWS achieved during the stand retraining portion. The BWS is then slowly raised. As the

TABLE CS3.2 Modified Functional Reach Test[a]

Forward Reaches	Length, in. (cm)
Reach #1	21.0 (53.34)
Reach #2	20.5 (52.07)
Reach #3	22.5 (57.15)
Mean	21.3 (54.10)

[a]Lynch, SM, Leahy, P and Barker, SP. Reliability of measurements obtained with a modified functional reach test in subjects with spinal cord injury. Phys Ther 78(2):128, 1998.

amount of BWS increases, the trainers are able to decrease the amount of assistance provided/required at each segment. Each trainer verbally identifies when assistance is no longer needed and the body segment becomes independent (Table CS3.6).

• Lateral weight shifts: Starting with the patient in a stance position, the therapist determines the amount of BWS and assistance necessary for the patient to perform lateral weight shifts in both directions. The trainers verbally identify the amount of assistance required at each body segment (Table CS3.7). The body weight supported is the amount that allows the majority of the body segments to be independent during the weight shifts.

• Step weight shifts: The trainers determine the amount of BWS and assistance necessary for the patient to perform an anterior weight shift when one LE is in a forward step position. The test begins at the same amount of BWS used during the lateral weight shifts, starting with the right LE forward. The test is repeated with the left LE in a forward step position. Each trainer identifies the amount of assistance required at each segment (Tables CS3.8 and CS3.9).

3. Step retraining:

The purpose of this test is to determine the optimal BWS and TM speed parameters to establish a kinematically correct stepping pattern. The test begins using the amount of BWS established during the stand adaptability weight shifting. The speed on the TM is gradually increased until a normal walking speed is reached (~2.4 mph [3.9 km/hr]). The amount of trainer assistance necessary to achieve an optimal stepping pattern is reported and documented (Table CS3.10).

4. Step adaptability:

The purpose of this test is to determine the amount of BWS and TM speed parameters necessary to maintain independence (no trainer assistance) at each body segment. The test begins at the parameters established during step retraining. The amount of BWS is slowly increased and the speed is slowly decreased until independence is reached at each segment of the body. If independence is not reached with 75 percent of the patient's body weight supported at a speed of 0.6 mph, then the level of assistance required at the given body segment is reported and documented (Table CS3.11).

Evaluation, Diagnosis and Prognosis, and Plan of Care

Note: Prior to considering the guiding questions below, view the Case Study 3 Examination segment of the DVD to enhance understanding of the patient's impairments and activity limitations. Following *completion of the guiding questions*, view the Case Study 3 Intervention segment of the DVD to

(text continues on page 269)

TABLE CS3.3 Berg Balance Scale[a,b,c]

Item	Score
1. Sitting to standing	1—needs minimal aid to stand or stabilize
2. Standing unsupported	0—unable to stand 30 seconds without support
3. Sitting with back unsupported but feet supported on floor or on a stool	4—able to sit safely and securely for 2 minutes
4. Standing to sit	1—sits independently but has uncontrolled descent
5. Transfers	3—able to transfer safely with definite need of hands
6. Standing unsupported with eyes closed	0—needs help to keep from falling
7. Standing unsupported with feet together	0—needs help to assume position and unable to stand for 15 seconds
8. Reaching forward with outstretched arm while standing	0—loses balance while trying, requires external support
9. Picking up object from the floor from a standing position	0—is unable to try/needs assistance to keep from losing balance/falling
10. Turning to look behind over your left and right shoulders while standing	0—needs assistance while turning
11. Turn 360 degrees	0—needs assistance while turning
12. Place alternate foot on step or stool while standing unsupported	0—needs assistance to keep from falling/unable to try
13. Standing unsupported one foot in front	0—loses balance while stepping or standing
14. Standing on one leg	0—is unable to try or needs assist to prevent fall
	Total Score: 9/56

[a]Berg, K, et al. Measuring balance in the elderly: Preliminary development of an instrument. Physiotherapy Canada 41:304, 1989.

[b]Berg, K, et al. A comparison of clinical and laboratory measures of postural balance in an elderly population. Arch Phys Med Rehabil 73:1073, 1992.

[c]Berg, K, et al. Measuring balance in the elderly: Validation of an instrument. Can J Public Health 83 (suppl 2):S7, 1992.

TABLE CS3.4 Performance-Oriented Mobility Assessment (POMA)[a]

	Balance Portion		
Task	Description of Balance	Possible	Score
Sitting Balance	Leans or slides in chair Steady, safe	= 0 = 1	1
Arises	Unable without help	= 0	1
	Able, uses arms to help	= 1	
	Able without using arms	= 2	

TABLE CS3.4 Performance-Oriented Mobility Assessment (POMA)ᵃ *(continued)*

Balance Portion

Task	Description of Balance	Possible	Score
Attempts to arise	Unable without help	= 0	1
	Able requires more than one attempt	= 1	
	Able to rise on one attempt	= 2	
Immediate standing balance (first 5 seconds)	Unsteady (swaggers, moves feet, trunk sway)	= 0	1
	Steady but uses walker or other support	= 1	
	Steady without walker or other support	= 2	
Standing Balance	Unsteady	= 0	1
	Steady but wide stance (medial heels more than 4 inches apart) and uses cane or other support	= 1	
	Narrow stance without support	= 2	
Nudged	Begins to fall	= 0	0
	Staggers, grabs, catches self	= 1	
	Steady	= 2	
Eyes closed	Unsteady	= 0	0
	Steady	= 1	
Turning 360 degrees	Discontinuous steps	= 0	0
	Continuous steps	= 1	
	Unsteady	= 0	0
	Steady	= 1	
Sitting Down	Unsafe (falls into chair)	= 0	1
	Uses arms or not a smooth motion	= 1	
	Safe, smooth motion	= 2	
Balance Score			**6/16**

Gait Portion

Task	Description of Gait	Possible	Score
Initiation of Gait	Any hesitancy	= 0	0
	No hesitancy	= 1	
Step Length and Height	a. Right swing foot does not pass left stance foot with step	= 0	0
	b. Right foot passes left stance foot	= 1	0

(table continues on page 268)

TABLE CS3.4 Performance-Oriented Mobility Assessment (POMA)[a] *(continued)*

Gait Portion

Task	Description of Gait	Possible	Score
	c. Right foot does not clear floor completely with step	= 0	0
	d. Right foot completely clears floor	= 1	
	e. Left swing foot does not pass right stance foot with step	= 0	0
	f. Left foot passes right stance foot	= 1	
	g. Left foot does not clear floor completely with step	= 0	0
	h. Left foot completely clears floor	= 1	
Step Symmetry	Right and left step length not equal	= 0	0
	Right and left step appear equal	= 1	
Step Continuity	Stopping or discontinuing between between steps	= 0	0
	Steps appear continuous	= 1	
Path	Marked deviation	= 0	0
	Mild/moderate deviation or uses walking aid	= 1	
	Straight without walking aid	= 2	
Trunk	Marked sway or uses walking aid	= 0	0
	No sway but flexion of knees or back, or spreads arms out while walking	= 1	
	No sway, no flexion, no use of arms, and no use of walking aid	= 2	
Step Width	Heels apart	= 0	0
	Heels almost touching while walking	= 1	
Gait Score			**0/12**
Balance + Gait Score			**6/28**

[a]Tinetti, ME. Performance-oriented assessment of mobility problems in elderly patients. J Am Geriatr Soc 34:119–126, 1986.

TABLE CS3.5 Stand Retraining

Body Segment	Level of Assistance	Percent of BWS
Right Knee	Minimal	10
Right Ankle	Independent	10
Left Knee	Independent	10
Left Ankle	Independent	10
Trunk	Moderate	10
Hips/Pelvis	Moderate	10

Abbreviation: BWS, body weight support.

TABLE CS3.8 Stand Adaptability: Step Weight Shifting (Right Foot Forward)

Body Segment	Level of Assistance	Percent of BWS
Right Knee	Moderate	50
Right Ankle	Independent	50
Left Knee	Minimal	50
Left Ankle	Independent	50
Trunk	Independent	50
Hips/Pelvis	Maximal	50

TABLE CS3.6 Stand Adaptability: Static Standing

Body Segment	Level of Assistance	Percent of BWS
Right Knee	Minimal	75
Right Ankle	Independent	10
Left Knee	Independent	10
Left Ankle	Independent	10
Trunk	Independent	25
Hips/Pelvis	Minimal	75

TABLE CS3.9 Stand Adaptability: Step Weight Shifting (Left Foot Forward)

Body Segment	Level of Assistance	Percent of BWS
Right Knee	Moderate	50
Right Ankle	Independent	50
Left Knee	Minimal	50
Left Ankle	Independent	50
Trunk	Independent	50
Hips/Pelvis	Moderate	50

TABLE CS3.7 Stand Adaptability: Lateral Weight Shifting

Body Segment	Level of Assistance	Percent of BWS
Right Knee	Minimal	50
Right Ankle	Independent	50
Left Knee	Minimal	50
Left Ankle	Independent	50
Trunk	Independent	50
Hips/Pelvis	Minimal	50

compare and contrast the interventions presented with those you selected. Last, progress to the Case Study 3 Outcomes segment of the DVD to compare and contrast the goals and expected outcomes you identified with the functional outcomes achieved.

Guiding Questions

1. Based on the ASIA examination data presented in Figure CS3.4, what is the patient's LE motor score?
2. Based on the ASIA examination data presented in Figure CS3.4, what is the patient's neurological level? Using Box CS3.1 below, what is the patient's impairment classification?
3. Using the *Guide to Physical Therapist Practice*, identify the patient's physical therapy diagnosis.

TABLE CS3.10 Step Retraining

Body Segment	Level of Assistance	Percent of BWS	TM Speed, mph (km/hr)
Right Knee	Maximal	35	2.4 (3.9)
Right Ankle	Maximal	35	2.4 (3.9)
Left Knee	Moderate	35	2.4 (3.9)
Left Ankle	Moderate	35	2.4 (3.9)
Trunk	Independent	35	2.4 (3.9)
Hips/Pelvis	Moderate	35	2.4 (3.9)

TABLE CS3.11 Step Adaptability

Body Segment	Level of Assistance	Percent of BWS[a]	TM Speed, mph (km/hr)
Right Knee	Maximal	55	0.6 (1)
Right Ankle	Maximal	55	0.6 (1)
Left Knee	Moderate	55	0.6 (1)
Left Ankle	Moderate	55	0.6 (1)
Trunk	Independent	35	2.4 (3.9)
Hips/Pelvis	Moderate	55	0.6 (1)

[a]Unable to raise BWS to greater than 55 percent because patient no longer able to achieve foot flat (loading response) during stepping at greater BWS.
Abbreviations: BWS, body weight support; TM, treadmill.

4. Formulate a physical therapy problem list for the patient. For each problem identified, indicate whether it is a *direct impairment*, *indirect impairment*, *composite impairment*, or *activity limitation*.

5. For patients with spinal cord injury (SCI), the LE motor score (LEMS) from the ASIA examination as well as the ASIA Impairment Scale classification has been used to predict ambulation ability. Based on the patient's LEMS and Impairment Scale classification, what is your prediction for this patient's ambulatory potential? Consider whether the patient has the potential to be either a household or community ambulator or whether he will be primarily a wheelchair user. What assistive or orthotic devices might be used to improve this patient's function?

6. *Activity-based therapy*, including the use of locomotor training (LT), offers another perspective on predicting ambulation ability. Activity-based therapy focuses on the use of task-specific training to provide appropriate sensory and kinematic cues to the nervous system in order to foster neurological recovery. Again, consider the patient's ambulatory potential. Before making a

BOX CS3.1 ASIA Impairment Scale[a]

A = Complete: No motor or sensory function is preserved in the sacral segments S4 to S5.
B = Incomplete: Sensory but not motor function is preserved below the neurological level and includes the sacral segments S4 to S5.
C = Incomplete: Motor function is preserved below the neurological level, and more than half of key muscles below the neurological level have a muscle grade less than 3.
D = Incomplete: Motor function is preserved below the neurological level, and at least half of key muscles below the neurological level have a muscle grade of 3 or more.
E = Normal: motor and sensory function is normal.

[a]American Spinal Injury Association. International Standards for Neurological Classification of Spinal Cord Injury. American Spinal Injury Association, Chicago, 2006.

decision about ambulatory potential, consider: (a) the patient's performance during the step retraining portion of the initial examination (see Table CS3.10), and (b) the principles of LT (weightbearing is maximized, kinematics and sensory cues are optimized with emphasis placed on motor recovery while minimizing compensatory strategies). Consider also the patient's LE motor score identified in question 1 and the patient's impairment scale classification identified in question 2.

7. Identify the duration of the episode of care needed to achieve the level of ambulation identified in question 5 (e.g., household or community ambulator or primarily a wheelchair user).

8. Identify the duration of the episode of care needed to achieve the level of ambulatory potential identified in question 6 using activity-based therapy, including the use of locomotor training (LT).

9. Table CS3.12 identifies a series of assistive devices and one entry labeled orthotic intervention. In the spaces provided in the table, state how these devices are, and are not, consistent with the following LT principles.

   * *Maximize LE weightbearing:* Patients are encouraged to stand as often as possible, using the UEs as little as possible.
   * *Provide appropriate sensory cues:* These cues include providing the correct tactile information during stepping on the treadmill and while walking at as close to normal walking speed (2.0 to 2.6 mph [3.2 to 4.2 km/hr]) as possible.
   * *Provide appropriate kinematics:* Patients are encouraged to attain an upright trunk with a neutral pelvis throughout the entire gait cycle, hip extension during terminal stance, and heel strike at initial contact.
   * *Maximize independence and minimize compensation:* Patients attempt to use the least restrictive assistive device possible and minimize the use of bracing.

10. Box CS3.2 identifies the *focus of progression for LT* using (A) BWS and a TM and (B) using overground walking; as well as (C) a sample progression of LT for the patient using sessions 1 and 20 as examples. Examine the focus of progression for both BWS and TM training and the overground progression. Next, examine the sample progression of LT for the case study patient (sessions 1 and 20). Based on each example, list two goals for progression during the next treatment sessions (2 and 21) in each of the following areas:
    * Step training on the BWS system
    * Sit-to-stand transfers
    * Standing balance
    * Overground ambulation

Reminder: Answers to the Case Study Guiding Questions are available online at Davis*Plus* (www.fadavis.com).

TABLE CS3.12 Assistive Device/Orthoses: Consistency/Inconsistency With Locomotor Training Principles		
Assistive Device/ Orthoses	Consistent Aspects	Inconsistent Aspects
Rolling Walker		
Bilateral Lofstrand Crutches		
Bilateral Single-Point Canes		
Unilateral Single-Point Cane		
Orthotic Intervention		

BOX CS3.2 Focus of Progression for LT Using BWS and a TM, Focus of Progression for LT Overground, and Sample Progression of LT for the Case Study Patient.

A. Focus of Progression: LT Using BWS and a TM
- Decreasing the amount of body weight supported (i.e., increase LE weightbearing)
- Achieving a normal walking speed (2.0 to 2.6 mph [3.2 to 4.2 km/hr])
- Improving endurance (the goal is to maintain 60 minutes of weightbearing on a TM with at least 20 minutes of stepping)
- Promoting independence of body segments (initial focus on the trunk and pelvis)

B. Focus of Progression: LT Overground
- Achieving proper kinematics during functional mobility (e.g., sit-to-stand transfers, standing, and ambulation)
- Minimizing the use of compensatory strategies
- Minimizing the use of assistive devices

C. Sample Progression of LT for Case Study Patient
Session 1 Example: During session 1 using the BWS system and a TM, the patient completed a total of 49 minutes of weightbearing, with 22 minutes of stepping at a TM speed of 2.4 mph (3.9 km/hr) with an average of 37 percent BWS. He required moderate assistance at his pelvis, maximal assistance at his right knee and ankle, and moderate assistance at his left knee and ankle. In the overground environment, he performed sit-to-stand transfers from a standard-height mat table with UE support from a rolling walker; he required minimal assistance at pelvis and right knee.

Once standing, he required increased UE support to maintain standing balance and minimal assistance at the right LE to prevent knee buckling. He ambulated 10 feet (3 m) with a rolling walker, with minimal assistance of one physical therapist at his pelvis and minimal assistance of two physical therapists (one at each LE) to advance the limb during swing and to maintain hip and knee extension during stance. Increased lumbar lordosis was noted during all standing and ambulation activities.

Session 20 Example: During session 20 using the BWS system and a TM, the patient completed a total of 60 minutes of weightbearing, with 30 minutes of step retraining at a TM speed of 2.6 mph (4.2 km/hr), with an average of 33 percent BWS. He required minimal assistance at the pelvis to attain proper alignment, moderate assistance at the right knee and ankle, and minimal assistance at the left knee and ankle. In the overground environment, he performed sit-to-stand transfers from a standard-height mat, with minimal assistance at the pelvis without UE support. Using a wide BOS, he was able to maintain standing balance with supervision without UE support for 30 seconds. He ambulated 250 ft (76.2 m) using bilateral Lofstrand crutches with contact guard at pelvis for balance and alignment. The patient was independent in advancing each LE. He continued to present with increased lumbar lordosis, although it is slightly diminished compared to session 1.

VIEWING THE CASE: PATIENT WITH SPINAL CORD INJURY

As students learn in different ways, the DVD case presentation (examination, intervention, and outcomes) is designed to promote engagement with the content, allow progression at an individual (or group) pace, and use of the medium or combination of media (*written*, *visual*, and *auditory*) best suited to the learner(s). The DVD includes both *visual* and *auditory* modes. Following is the case study summary and *written* DVD narration.

Video Summary
Patient is a 17-year-old male with an incomplete spinal cord injury (T4, ASIA C) referred to a locomotor training clinic for outpatient rehabilitation, initiated 4 months post injury. The video shows examination and intervention segments with an emphasis on locomotor and balance training. Outcomes are filmed after 75 treatment sessions.

Complete Video Narration
Examination:
- The step training begins with an examination of the patient's standing posture and need for assistance to maintain a standing position.

- Stand adaptability examines the patient's ability to complete both lateral and stride weight shifts. The patient is first asked to shift weight laterally from side to side with assistance as needed. The patient completed lateral weight shifts with 50 percent body weight support and minimal assistance at pelvis and lower extremities.
- The patient is assisted into stance position and shifts weight forward and back. Assistance is provided as needed. Stride weight shifts were completed at 50 percent body weight support with maximum assistance. Note that the top hand of the therapist assists at the hamstring tendons to facilitate knee flexion or at the patellar tendon to facilitate knee extension. The bottom hand facilitates the anterior tibialis tendon to promote ankle dorsiflexion or the Achilles tendon to promote ankle plantarflexion and a foot flat position during stance.
- The patient requires minimal assistance to achieve standing and cannot maintain standing without upper extremity support.
- The patient is able to perform a squat pivot transfer independently.

- Short-sitting balance is maintained for 2 minutes without support. Note excessive lordosis and increased thoracic extension.
- The patient stands with an assistive device. He maintains standing with upper extremity support. As in sitting, standing posture is characterized by excessive lordosis and increased thoracic extension.

Intervention:
- This is the 55th treatment session. The patient requires 25 percent body weight support, at a speed of 2.6 miles per hour. On the left, tactile cues are only at the knee, as the ankle is now independent.
- During the treatment session, the first 5 minutes focus on step adaptability to promote independent stepping.
- Here, the patient practices moving from sit-to-stand without upper extremity support while minimizing compensatory strategies. The patient also practices tandem stance, which requires minimal assistance.
- The patient practices walking overground without an assistive device.
- The patient practices side-stepping to improve balance and hip abductor control.
- Gait is observed with bilateral canes and then with the trekking poles.
- Here, sit-to-stand transfers are again practiced.
- The patient then practices slowly lowering his trunk to the mat with a return to sitting. Limitations include decreased abdominal activation with resulting lordosis. Continued abdominal strengthening is important and will be included in the home exercise program.

Outcomes:
- This outcomes segment was filmed after 75 treatment sessions and 20 sessions after the intervention video.
- Shown here is the ability to independently place feet together and maintain standing for more than 1 minute.
- The patient attempts to stand without upper extremity support. This activity is challenged by decreased voluntary gluteal activation.
- The patient demonstrates good ability to weight shift laterally onto lower extremity while turning to look over right shoulder.
- A lateral view of standing posture illustrates improvements in postural alignment.
- The patient attempts to stand without upper extremity support but uses right hand to assist.
- The patient is able to turn 360 degrees but requires increased time with loss of balance upon completion.
- Demonstrated here is the ability to independently stand with one foot in front; however, he is unable to maintain this position for a full 30 seconds.
- Shown here is preparation for another 360-degree turn to right, which is accomplished independently.
- The patient attempts to alternately place each foot on an 8-inch step. Note that right lower extremity extensor tone impairs lifting ability.
- The patient attempts to lift his right lower extremity to complete unilateral stance. Increased extensor tone and decreased hip flexor activation impair ability to raise the right foot. He is able to maintain left unilateral stance for 3 seconds.

Spinal Cord Injury

DARRELL MUSICK, PT, AND
LAURA S. WEHRLI, PT, DPT, ATP
CRAIG HOSPITAL, DENVER, COLORADO

Examination

History

- Demographic Information:
  The patient is a 43-year-old, Caucasian, English-speaking male with a postgraduate education.
- Social History:
  The patient is married with two teenage children. He recently moved to the state of Washington with the military and participates in social athletics, including baseball, basketball, and ice hockey.
- Employment:
  Patient is a member of the executive staff in a military medical group as a nurse practitioner and chief of nursing.
- Living Environment:
  Patient lives in a one-story private home with one 6-inch (15 cm) step to enter.
- General Health Status:
  Patient is an active, healthy individual.
- Past Medical History:
  Hypertension (controlled with Lisinopril), bradycardia, basal cell carcinoma (removed without complication), kidney stone several years ago, hyperlipidemia (controlled with Zocor), allergic rhinitis (controlled with Singulair). No known drug allergies.
- Current Condition/Chief Complaints:
  On November 21, patient was driving a borrowed all terrain vehicle (ATV) when he lost control. He was thrown from the vehicle and hit his head/helmet on a pipe in a gully. He felt immediate pain in his back. He reports that he had difficulty breathing owing to rib pain and immediately had no feeling in his legs ("I couldn't feel or move my legs"). He was transported by helicopter to a hospital in Reno, Nevada. The patient also reported he was able to contract his quadriceps slightly until just prior to reaching the hospital. He was found to have:
- L1 burst fracture
- Left 1st through 10th rib fractures with left pulmonary contusion
- Left hemopneumothorax requiring chest tube placement
- Left T1 transverse process fracture
- T2 to T7 spinous process fractures
- T10 to T12 right posterior medial rib fractures
- Left scapular body fracture
On November 24, the patient underwent surgery for a T11–L3 laminectomy and posterior lateral fixation. He was immobilized in a custom thoracolumbosacral orthosis (TLSO); weightbearing as tolerated (WBAT) on left upper extremity (UE).

Systems Review

- Cardiovascular/Pulmonary System:
  - Heart rate: 79 beats per minute
  - Blood pressure: 104/67 mm Hg
  - Respiratory rate: 16 breaths per minute
- Musculoskeletal System:
  - Gross symmetry: Visible rib deformities on left thorax; left lower extremity (LE) swelling
  - Gross range of motion (ROM): LE ROM generally within functional limits (WFL), with the exception of moderately tight hamstrings and hip rotation bilaterally; contracted left plantarflexors. UE ROM is also generally WFL, with the exception of tightness in bilateral shoulder flexion, abduction, and rotation (greater on left).
  - Gross strength: Grossly normal strength throughout UEs; 0/5 strength in bilateral LEs
  - Height: 6 ft 2 in (1.9 m)
  - Weight: 170 lb (77 kg)
- Integumentary System:
  - Multiple ecchymoses on all four extremities
  - Prominent ecchymoses on right lateral chest wall and left chest wall
  - Small open wounds on right posterior upper arm and anterior forearm
  - No pressure ulcers
- Neuromuscular System:
  - Normal reflexes on bilateral UEs
  - Diminished reflexes on bilateral LEs
  - Normal sensation to the level of T10 on the left trunk and to T12 on the right trunk
  - Diminished rectal tone and no voluntary anal contraction
  - Balance impaired in short- and long-sitting
- Functional Status:
  - Functional mobility skills require dependent assistance at this time

Tests and Measures

- Arousal, Attention, and Cognition:
  - No signs or symptoms of traumatic brain injury (TBI) noted by psychologist
  - Oriented to time, place, and person
  - Arousal, attention, cognition, and recall appear to be within normal limits (WNL)
- Sensory Integrity:
  - American Spinal Injury Association (ASIA) sensory test (Fig. CS4.1)
  - Pinprick sensation normal C2–T12 bilaterally
  - Light touch sensation normal C2–T10 left; C2–L1 right
  - No sensation at S4–5 or deep anal sensation
- Muscle Performance:
  - ASIA motor test (Fig. CS4.1)
  - 5/5 strength: C5–T1 bilaterally
  - 0/5 strength: L2–S1 bilaterally
  - No voluntary anal contraction
  - Trunk and upper abdominal muscles present but unable to test owing to TLSO
- Pain:
  - Left shoulder pain at rest without pain medication 2/10
  - Left shoulder pain with activity without pain medication 6/10
- Posture:
  - Examined in short-sitting with UE support
  - Forward head posture
  - Trunk stabilized in TLSO
  - Neutral pelvic tilt
  - LEs in neutral alignment
- Range of Motion (ROM):
  - Goniometric measures of the LEs indicated bilateral tightness in hip flexion, hip internal and external rotation, straight leg raises, ankle dorsiflexion; contracted left plantarflexors (right plantarflexion WNL) (Table CS4.1).
  - UE ROM limitations included shoulder flexion, abduction, and internal and external rotation. Greater limitations noted at left shoulder secondary to left scapular body fracture and associated pain.
- Environmental, Home, and Work Barriers:
  Review of house floor plans and discussion with patient and family provided the following information:
  - The one-story private home has one 6-inch (15-cm) step to enter. The bedroom, kitchen, and living areas are wheelchair accessible from the main entrance. The

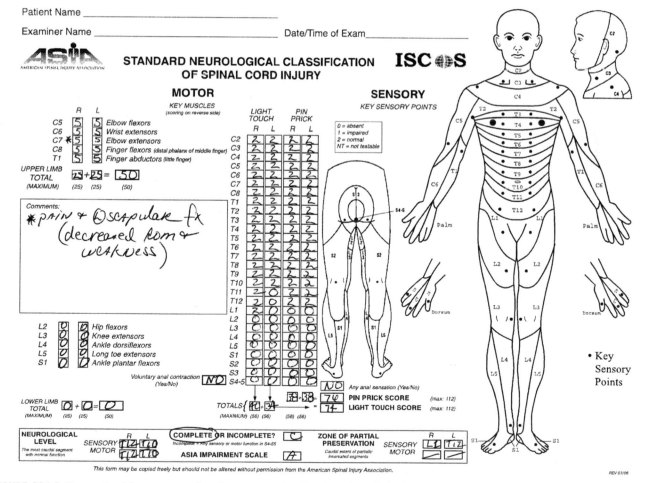

FIGURE CS4.1 The patients' sensory and motor scores using the American Spinal Injury Association (ASIA) Examination Form: *Standard Neurological Classification of Spinal Cord Injury.* (American Spinal Injury Association. International Standards for Neurological Classification of Spinal Cord Injury. American Spinal Injury Association, Chicago, 2006.)

TABLE CS4.1	Range of Motion Values (in degrees) Indicating Areas of Joint Motion Limitations[a]		
Joint	**Motion**	**Right**	**Left**
Shoulder	Flexion	0–160	0–150
	Abduction	0–130	0–105
	Internal Rotation	0–65	0–50
	External Rotation	0–70	0–65
Hip	Flexion	0–112	0–110
	Internal Rotation	0–23	0–30
	External Rotation	0–35	0–30
	Straight Leg Raise	0–70	0–70
Ankle	Dorsiflexion	0–3	None[b]
	Plantarflexion	0–55	13–50

[a]All other ROM values WNL.

[b]Unable to achieve neutral starting position for measurement.

master bathroom doorway is 30 inches (76 cm) wide. The toilet is in a separated area of the bathroom with a 28-inch (71-cm) wide entry and privacy wall. The shower stall is 60 × 60 inches (1.5 × 1.5 m) with a 1.5-inch (3.8-cm) lip at the entrance.
- At work, administrative areas, office, and desk are accessible. The patient must give presentations and speeches frequently and would like to stand at lectern in bilateral knee-ankle-foot orthoses (KAFO).

Evaluation, Diagnosis and Prognosis, and Plan of Care

Note: Prior to considering the guiding questions below, view the Case Study 4 Examination segment of the DVD to enhance understanding of the patient's impairments and activity limitations. Following *completion of the guiding questions*, view the Case Study 4 Intervention segment of the DVD to compare and contrast the interventions presented with those you selected. Last, progress to the Case Study 4 Outcomes segment of the DVD to compare and contrast the goals and expected outcomes you identified with the functional outcomes achieved.

Guiding Questions

1. Review Figure CS4.1. What is the patient's physical therapy diagnosis? More specifically, what is the neurological level of injury and where does the patient place on the ASIA Impairment Scale (Box CS4.1)?

BOX CS4.1 ASIA Impairment Scale[a]

A = Complete: No motor or sensory function is preserved in the sacral segments S4 to S5
B = Incomplete: Sensory but not motor function is preserved below the neurological level and includes the sacral segments S4 to S5.
C = Incomplete: Motor function is preserved below the neurological level, and more than half of key muscles below the neurological level have a muscle grade less than 3.
D = Incomplete: Motor function is preserved below the neurological level, and at least half of key muscles below the neurological level have a muscle grade of 3 or more.
E = Normal: motor and sensory function is normal.

[a]American Spinal Injury Association. International Standards for Neurological Classification of Spinal Cord Injury. American Spinal Injury Association, Chicago, 2006.

2. What Preferred Practice Pattern from the *Guide to Physical Therapist Practice* should be used?
3. How many weeks of treatment would you anticipate will be needed for inpatient rehabilitation?
4. Identify the patient's impairments and the resulting activity limitations.
5. From the information gathered during the examination, what impairments do you anticipate will affect the patient's prognosis?
6. List the interventions that you would include in the plan of care (POC).
7. What will the patient need to consider to ensure home accessibility?
8. Identify three pieces of equipment the patient will require at discharge.
9. What is the patient's prognosis with respect to functional outcomes at the end of his rehabilitation stay? How would you describe his anticipated activity limitations and participation restrictions at 1 year after discharge?

Reminder: Answers to the Case Study Guiding Questions are available online at Davis*Plus* (www.fadavis.com).

VIEWING THE CASE: PATIENT WITH SPINAL CORD INJURY

As students learn in different ways, the DVD case presentation (examination, intervention, and outcomes) is designed to promote engagement with the content, allow progression at an individual (or group) pace, and use of the medium or combination of media (*written*, *visual*, and *auditory*) best suited to the learner(s). The DVD includes both *visual* and *auditory* modes. Following is the case study summary and *written* DVD narration.

Video Summary

Patient is a 43-year-old male with a complete spinal cord injury (T10, ASIA A) and multiple fractures undergoing active rehabilitation. The video shows examination and intervention segments during inpatient rehabilitation. Outcomes are filmed 9 weeks after initial examination.

Complete Video Narration

Examination:

- Sitting balance is an important functional skill. Leaning forward and balancing with and without hand support are examined. Movements are slow, suggesting the presence of pain and decreased confidence. Note the exaggerated compensatory arm motions during unsupported sitting.
- Hesitance to touch the floor can be a sign of musculoskeletal pain but may also indicate a fear of falling. This fear prevents forward lean and transfer ability. The patient moves slowly, touches the floor briefly, and requires moderate assistance to return to upright.
- The ability to use a transfer board is examined. Assistance is required with placement of the board due to impaired dynamic sitting balance. He demonstrates slow, inefficient, small movements of hips during the transfer. His head remains relatively upright, and he leans his head and shoulders toward the wheelchair. A more efficient technique would be to use the *head-hips principle*, which requires the head and shoulders to lean opposite of the desired direction of the hips.
- Maximum assistance is required to move from supine to long-sitting. Diminished hamstring length prevents long-sitting without upper extremity support. Hamstring stretching will become a high-priority intervention to improve mat mobility and leg management skills.

Intervention:

- During balance training, the patient learns and practices his limits of stability and reaching abilities. Dynamic sitting balance is the foundation for success in performing transfers and bed mobility skills. Here, the patient practices unsupported sitting while reaching in all directions.
- Adding the ball toss increases the challenge to dynamic sitting balance.

- Intervention includes overcoming the fear of leaning forward. Here, the patient answers "No" to the question, "Are you in pain?" The purpose of this intervention is to demonstrate to the patient that he will not fall from the mat in this forward flexed position as long as his feet are directly beneath his knees.
- Improving transfers is dependent on the patient's understanding of the head-hips principle. Here, the patient is instructed in the importance of moving the head and shoulders down and away from the direction of transfer, resulting in an unweighting of the opposite hip.
- The patient continues to require assistance with transfers. A key point in teaching the head-hips principle is to cue the patient to move the head and shoulders closer to the "pushing" hand.
- The patient now places the transfer board independently. Note that movements remain inefficient and redundant.
- Hamstring tightness is addressed before further sit-to-supine activities.
- When moving from short- to long-sit, it is important for the patient to use the right arm when moving legs to the left. This allows using the entire upper body movement to drive moving the legs. He uses his left hand for balance and pulls his upper body back and onto his left elbow.
- Moving from supine-to-sit, the patient tucks the chin and pulls up with his hands partially under the hips. From on-elbows, he weight shifts to one elbow to straighten the opposite arm.
- Instruction in performing wheelies is critical to use of wheelchair on outdoor terrain.

Outcomes:

- Short-sitting balance and ability to touch the floor have significantly improved. He is less hesitant to touch the floor and able to maintain dynamic sitting balance easily. He appears slightly unstable here, but was just permitted to remove the spinal orthosis 1 day prior to this session. Given his level of injury and duration of intervention, his balance skill is appropriate and will continue to improve as he adjusts to the lack of exterior support.
- The transfer board continues to be used for mat-to-wheelchair transfers. He demonstrates a good head-hips relationship and improved efficiency.
- The patient has improved with all mat activities and moves easily between supine and long-sitting. Further intervention will focus on movement speed and efficiency.
- Patient is able to maintain a static wheelie for greater than 30 seconds. He negotiates an obstacle quickly and smoothly. He is progressing to more difficult obstacles such as curbs.

Peripheral Vestibular Dysfunction

JoAnn Moriarty-Baron, PT, DPT
Southern New Hampshire Rehabilitation
Center, Nashua, New Hampshire

Examination

History

- Demographic Information:
  Patient is a 65-year-old female who presents for evaluation and treatment owing to complaints of dizziness that began 4 to 6 weeks ago. She is ambidextrous and wears glasses and contact lenses.
- Employment, Living Environment, and Social History:
  Patient is a retired high school guidance counselor but works as part-time summer help in a perennial garden nursery. She lives alone but has a busy social life and travels frequently.
- Past Medical History:
  She states she is in excellent health but has a history of cervical and lumbar arthritis, thyroid disease, high blood pressure, and elevated cholesterol levels. She also reveals that she had a lumpectomy more than 30 years ago for a benign tumor and underwent surgery for trigger finger (stenosing tenosynovitis) 3 years ago. She reports a "bout of viral meningitis" over 20 years ago and experienced an isolated episode of atrial fibrillation approximately 1 year ago. She is scheduled for left foot neuroma removal surgery in 2 weeks. She exercises four or five times per week for 20 to 60 minutes and enjoys walking and going to the gym.
- Current Condition/Chief Complaints:
  Patient reports that when she awoke dizzy one morning 4 to 6 weeks ago, she experienced nausea and difficulty walking that lasted for a few days. She went to her primary care physician, who put her on Meclizine for 10 days. She notes gradual improvement in her symptoms and describes her current condition as "stable." She denies falling. She states that, at this time, looking up and turning to the right continue to cause increased symptoms. She experiences occasional spinning dizziness with quick head movements and states that sometimes she does not spin but also does not feel normal. She states she frequently feels off balance. She denies tinnitus, hearing loss, or fullness or pressure in her ears.

Systems Review

- Musculoskeletal System:
  No formal examination was performed given the nature of the patient's complaints and lack of observable physical impairments.

Tests and Measures

- Rating of Symptom Severity:
  At the start of today's examination, the patient rates her symptoms as a "1 to 2" on a scale of 0 to 10.
- Dizziness Handicap Index:
  Her score on the Dizziness Handicap Index (DHI)[1] is a 26 on a scale of 0 to 100.
- Balance and Visual Testing:
  - Modified Clinical Test for Sensory Integration in Balance (mCTSIB)[2]: Results from the mCTSIB are presented in Table CS5.1.
  - Walking With Quick Head Turns to Left and Right: When performing this activity, the patient demonstrates minor disruption in gait.
  - Oculomotor Testing in Room Light: The patient's gaze and nystagmus are normal in room light. She was able to perform smooth pursuits in horizontal, vertical, and diagonal planes without interruption. Tests for saccadic control in the horizontal and vertical planes were also normal but more difficult to perform to the right.
  - Head Thrust Test: The patient's head thrust test was positive to the right. The patient performed a saccadic eye movement to return her gaze to the target following a quick head movement to the right.
  - Dynamic Visual Acuity Testing: This test was performed in the standing position using a Lighthouse ETDRS™ (Early Treatment Diabetic Retinopathy Study) wall chart. It was negative, as there was a one-line discrepancy between what the patient could read with her head still (no movement) compared to when her head was moving at a rate of approximately two repetitions per second (2 Hz). However, she reported an increase in symptoms from "1 to 2" to "3 to 4" on a 0 to 10 scale with this activity.
  - Observation for Nystagmus Using the Infrared Video Goggles Without a Visual Reference: Under observation in the video goggles, the patient demonstrated a consistent, left beating nystagmus with forward, left, and right gaze.
  - The Head Shaking Induced Nystagmus Test[3] Using the Infrared Video Goggles: This test provoked a slightly left-beating nystagmus. The patient reported feeling "woozy" with a symptom intensity of "2 to 3" on a 0 to 10 scale.

TABLE CS5.1 Modified Clinical Test for Sensory Integration and Balance (mCTSIB)

Standing Position	Time (sec)	Postural Sway	Loss of Balance
EO, FT, SS	30	WNL	No
EO, FT, CS	30	Min increased sway	No
EO, FT, on foam	30	WNL	No
EC, FT, on foam	25	Min-mod increased sway	No
EO, tandem, SS sharpened Romberg	5	Increased sway to right	To the right
EC, tandem, SS sharpened Romberg	Immediate fall	N/A	To the left

Abbreviations: CS, compliant surface; EO, eyes open; EC, eyes closed; FT, feet together; min, minimal, min-mod, minimal to moderate, N/A, not applicable; SS, solid surface; WNL, within normal limits.

- The Right Hallpike-Dix Test[4] Using the Infrared Video Goggles: The right Hallpike-Dix Test was positive for an up beating, counterclockwise nystagmus of short duration. The patient complained of feeling dizzy while in the test position and reported that she was "slightly" dizzy upon returning to the sitting position.
- The Left Hallpike-Dix Test Using the Infrared Video Goggles: The patient denied symptoms with the left Hallpike-Dix Test but demonstrated a consistent left beating nystagmus.
- The Right Roll Test Using the Infrared Video Goggles: This test revealed a left beating nystagmus.
- The Left Roll Test Using the Infrared Video Goggles: This test also revealed a left beating nystagmus.

Evaluation, Diagnosis and Prognosis, and Plan of Care

Note: Prior to considering the guiding questions, view the Case Study 5 Examination segment of the DVD to enhance understanding of the patient's clinical presentation. Following *completion of the guiding questions,* view the Case Study 5 Intervention segment of the DVD to compare and contrast the interventions presented with those you selected. Last, progress to the Case Study 5 Outcomes segment of the DVD to compare and contrast the goals and expected outcomes you identified with the functional outcomes achieved.

Guiding Questions

1. Given this patient's report at the initial examination, identify the most likely cause(s) of her complaints of dizziness, disequilibrium, and motion sensitivity.
2. Which clinical examination findings reveal abnormality in the vestibular system? Analyze and interpret these results.
3. Determine a working diagnosis (diagnostic hypothesis) for this patient.
4. Describe this patient's clinical presentation in terms of:
   a. Impairments
   b. Activity limitations
   c. Participation restrictions
5. Using the *Guide to Physical Therapist Practice,* identify the appropriate practice pattern for the patient.
6. Describe the plan of care (therapeutic interventions) you will use to address the impairments.
7. What are your anticipated goals and expected outcomes for the patient? State the time frame in which you expect to meet these expectations.
8. Explain how your working diagnosis would change if a positive Hallpike-Dix test was your only abnormal finding.
9. Describe the therapeutic intervention you will employ to address impairments associated with a positive Hallpike-Dix test.

Reminder: Answers to the Case Study Guiding Questions are available online at Davis*Plus* (www.fadavis.com).

REFERENCES

1. Jacobsen, GP, and Newman, CW. The development of the dizziness handicap inventory. Arch Otolaryngol Head Neck Surg 116:424, 1990.
2. Rose, DJ. Fallproof!: A Comprehensive Balance and Mobility Training Program. Human Kinetics, Champaign, IL, 2003.
3. Hain, TC, Fetter, M, and Zee, D. Head-shaking nystagmus in patients with unilateral peripheral vestibular lesions. Am J Otolaryngol 8:36, 1987.
4. Dix, R, and Hallpike, CS. The pathology, symptomatology and diagnosis of certain common disorders of the vestibular system. Ann Otol Rhinol Laryngol 6:987, 1952.

VIEWING THE CASE: PATIENT WITH PERIPHERAL VESTIBULAR DYSFUNCTION

As students learn in different ways, the DVD case presentation (examination, intervention, and outcomes) is designed to promote engagement with the content, allow progression at an individual (or group) pace, and use of the medium or combination of media (*written*, *visual*, and *auditory*) best suited to the learner(s). The DVD includes both *visual* and *auditory* modes. Following is the case study summary and *written* DVD narration.

Video Summary

Patient is a 65-year-old female referred to a vestibular clinic with peripheral vestibular dysfunction. The video shows examination and intervention segments during outpatient rehabilitation, with an emphasis on oculomotor, balance, and locomotor training. Outcomes are filmed after seven treatment sessions within 10 weeks.

Complete Video Narration

Examination:

- The following segments contain the examination findings obtained using the infrared video goggles: with forward gaze, one sees a left beating nystagmus; left gaze causes an intensified left beating nystagmus; and with right gaze, one notes a mild left beating nystagmus.
- The Head Shaking Induced Nystagmus Test results in a left beating nystagmus and the patient complains of feeling "woozy." View this once the side-to-side motion of the eye stops.
- The left Hallpike-Dix Test does not elicit a rotary nystagmus, and the patient denies symptoms. The left beating nystagmus remains.
- With the right Hallpike-Dix Test, one clearly observes a brief, counterclockwise, and up beating nystagmus. The patient reports feeling dizzy.
- The following segments depict the initial examination findings on the Clinical Test for Sensory Integration and Balance. The patient demonstrates normal postural stability under the first condition.
- She is able to maintain the second condition with a minimal increase in postural sway. It is essential to utilize appropriate guarding techniques with this testing.
- The patient is able to maintain the fourth condition with normal postural sway.
- Under the fifth condition, she demonstrates increased ankle strategies with moderately increased postural sway.
- In the Sharpened Romberg position with eyes open, our patient demonstrates considerable difficulty.
- With eyes closed, she demonstrates an immediate loss of balance to the left.

Intervention:

- In order to address deficits in gaze stability, the patient is instructed to perform times one (×1) viewing horizontally and vertically.
- To progress this exercise, the patient walks a few steps toward and away from the letter chart while performing times one viewing.
- For a more dynamic progression of gaze stability, she holds a target at arm's length, then performs the activity while walking. Note the postural disturbance that occurs with all of these tasks.
- The final progression of this activity reduces the inputs from the periphery.
- In order to improve the somatosensory inputs, the patient receives instruction on how to practice at home. She is told to place a folded exercise mat in front of her kitchen sink to maintain safety during practice.
- She is directed to include tandem standing with her eyes open as part of the home program to improve postural control when the base of support is reduced.
- She receives special instructions to maintain her center of mass over her back heel for improved stability. In addition, she must practice with visual feedback removed.
- In order to address the functional impairment of unsteady gait and to promote adaptation of the vestibular system, she must practice walking with varied inputs from the right and left sides.

Outcomes:

- The following segments depict the final assessment of the patient in the goggles.
- With forward, right, and left gaze, one notes that a slight left beating nystagmus remains.
- This Head Shaking Induced Nystagmus Test leaves the eye stable and without lateral eye movement. The patient denies any symptoms or dizziness. View this once the eyelid opens.
- With the right Hallpike-Dix Test, one notes the absence of rotary nystagmus, and the patient denies symptoms.
- Upon discharge assessment, one observes the improvement in postural stability under the fourth condition of the Clinical Test for Sensory Integration and Balance.
- Under the fifth condition, she is now able to maintain control following a few seconds of increased sway.
- She is able to perform the Sharpened Romberg position with eyes open with normal postural sway.
- At discharge, her Sharpened Romberg with eyes closed remains abnormal but has improved.

Parkinson's Disease

EDWARD WILLIAM BEZKOR, PT, DPT, MTC
RUSK INSTITUTE OF REHABILITATION MEDICINE,
NEW YORK CITY, NEW YORK

Examination

History

- Demographic Information:
  Patient is an 84-year-old male with a 9-year history of Parkinson's disease.
- History of Present Illness:
  The patient has experienced a recent deterioration of balance, gait, endurance, and strength. He was hospitalized for 12 days to monitor the deterioration and adjust medications accordingly. The patient was then transferred to an inpatient rehabilitation facility for 2 weeks, has received home physical therapy for 4 weeks, and now has been referred for outpatient physical therapy.
- Past Medical History:
  Patient reports prostate cancer, left upper extremity (UE) adhesive capsulitis (status post trauma from a motor vehicle accident), and depression.
- Past Surgical History:
  Patient reports right total knee arthroplasty (status post 8 years), left total knee arthroplasty (status post 4 years), and left total hip arthroplasty (status post 3 years).
- Medications:
  Sinemet, Miropex, Lexapro, Iron, and Zocor.
- Social History:
  Patient is retired and lives with his wife. She is also retired and able to provide limited assistance during the day secondary to her history of cardiac disease. A recently hired aide provides 4 hours of assistance per day.
- Living Environment:
  The patient lives in an apartment with no steps. He has the following durable medical equipment: straight cane, tripod rollator, shower chair, commode, and two grab bars installed in the bathroom.
- General Health Status:
  Fair.
- Prior Level of Function:
  Prior to last hospitalization, the patient ambulated independently with a straight cane.
- Current Level of Function:
  The patient ambulates using a straight cane at home for short distances and ambulates outside with a rollator and contact guard assistance secondary to imbalance and fall risk. The patient reports an average of three falls per month. He uses a motorized scooter when traveling farther than four blocks. He reports difficulty with rolling in bed in both directions, transferring from supine-to-sit and sit-to-stand, donning and doffing clothes, and eating.

Systems Review

- Cardiovascular/Pulmonary System:
  - Heart rate: 70 beats per minute
  - Respiratory rate: 24 breaths per minute
  - Blood pressure: 128/76 mm Hg
- Musculoskeletal System:
  - Height: 5 ft 8 in. (1.7 m)
  - Weight: 185 lb (84 kg)
  - Gross symmetry: Patient presents with decreased lumbar lordosis, rounded shoulders, increased thoracic kyphosis, and forward head posture.
  - Gross range of motion (ROM): Patient presents with gross limitations in active ROM in both UEs and both lower extremities (LEs), with greater limitations in the left UE and, LE.
  - Gross strength: Patient presents with gross limitations in the strength of both UEs and both LEs, with greater limitations in the left UE and LE.
- Neuromuscular System:
  - Gait: The patient ambulates 400 feet (122 m) with a rollator and contact guard assistance secondary to imbalance and fall risk. He ambulates up and down four steps with bilateral handrails and minimal assistance to maintain balance and encourage weight shift. The patient uses a step-to gait pattern on stairs.
  - Balance: The patient presents with good static sitting balance and fair dynamic sitting balance. He presents with poor static and dynamic standing balance.
- Functional Status:
  - Functional mobility: The patient performs bed mobility with contact guard assistance for rolling in both directions and minimal assistance for scooting in bed. He transfers supine-to-sit with contact guard assistance. Transfers from sit-to-stand require minimal assistance to initiate motion and encourage anterior progression of the torso.
  - Self-care and home management: The patient requires minimal assistance when donning and doffing clothes. He requires supervision to minimal assistance when eating secondary to tremors and decreased fine motor control.

- Motor function (motor control, motor learning): The patient's impaired motor control is apparent; increased difficulty is noted during initiation of bed mobility, transfers, and ambulation. The patient presents with daily freezing episodes (inability to continue an activity). When he is asked to perform functional activities, including transfers, ambulation, and fine motor tasks with increased speed or with additional task demands, the quality and safety of movement deteriorate.
- Tone: Moderate cogwheel rigidity is present in both UEs and LEs and is particularly apparent during elbow and knee extension. The left UE and LE are more impaired than the right.

Tests and Measures

- Posture:
  Reedco Posture Score Sheet: 40/100. The patient presents with deficits in all planes, with the most pronounced postural abnormalities being increased thoracic kyphosis, rounded shoulders, forward head, and anteriorly inclined torso.
- Aerobic Capacity/Endurance:
  Results of the 6-Minute Walk Test[1] are presented in Table CS6.1. Patient ambulates with a rollator and minimal assistance.
- Sensory Integrity:
  - Impaired response to light touch on bilateral plantar surfaces (no response to light touch during 4 of 10 trials on right foot and during 6 of 10 trials on left foot).
  - Impaired ability to discriminate between sharp and dull sensations on bilateral plantar surfaces (inability to discriminate during 5 of 10 trials on feet bilaterally).
  - Impaired proprioceptive awareness on great toe bilaterally (incorrect response 4 of 10 trials on right foot and 6 of 10 trials on left foot). Intact proprioceptive awareness at ankles bilaterally.
- Strength:
  Results of the Manual Muscle Test and grip strength values (dynamometer) are presented in Table CS6.2.
- Range of Motion:
  - Results of the active ROM (AROM) examination for the cervical and lumbar spine are presented in Table CS6.3.

- AROM values for the hips, ankles, and shoulders are presented in Table CS6.4.
- Passive ROM (PROM) values for the hips, ankles, and shoulders are presented in Table CS6.5.
- Deep Tendon Reflexes:
  Patient presents with bilateral 1+ (present but depressed, low normal) triceps response and 0 (no response) for bilateral bicep, hamstring, patellar, and ankle responses.
- Tone:
  - On the Modified Ashworth Scale[2] bilateral hamstrings present with minimal resistance through range and moderate resistance at end range (3/4)
  - Bilateral quadriceps present with minimal resistance through the entire range (2/4).
- Coordination:
  Results of coordination tests are presented in Table CS6.6.
- Pain:
  Patient reports 3/10 left shoulder pain at rest and 9/10 left shoulder pain with activity (0 = no pain and 10 = worst possible pain).
- Balance:
  - Berg Balance Scale[3-5] (with use of rollator): 26/56, indicating a 100 percent risk for falls.
  - Functional Reach Test[6-8]: 4 inches (10 cm), indicating a high risk for falls.
  - Dynamic Gait Index[9] (with use of rollator): 10/24, indicating an increased risk of falls with dynamic activities.
  - EquiTest Balance Analysis (NeuroCom® International, Inc., Clackamas, Oregon)
    - Sensory Organization Test (SOT) composite score = 39. The patient presents with below-normal balance for his age group in conditions 3, 4, 5, and 6. The patient fell on every trial in conditions 5 and 6. Sensory analysis indicates moderate deficits in the visual system and maximal deficits in the vestibular system.
    - Strategy analysis: Results show a reliance on ankle strategies and decreased hip strategies.
    - Center of gravity analysis: Results indicate decreased weightbearing on the right LE in neutral and in squat positions at different angles of knee flexion. Most significant was a 13 percent decrease in weightbearing on the right LE with a 60-degree squat.
    - Adaptation test: Patient presents with minimal reflexive response to rotary toe up/down perturbations.
    - Rhythmic weight shift: Directional control composite scores were 79 percent in the frontal plane and 64 percent in the sagittal plane. The patient demonstrated deficits in directional control that were most apparent in the sagittal plane at faster speeds.
- Gait:
  Timed Up and Go Test[10] (patient performed test with rollator and contact guard assist): 26 seconds, indicating high risk for falls.
- Functional Independence Measure (FIM):[11]
  Results of the FIM are presented in Table CS6.7.

TABLE CS6.1 6-Minute Walk Test

Test	HR	BP	RR	SaO$_2$
Pre-Test	63	128/76	24	90
Post-Test	66	138/79	24	96

Note: Lowest O$_2$ saturation during walking: 86; total distance covered: 528 feet (177 m).

Patient required two rest intervals during the test.

Abbreviations: BP, blood pressure; HR, heart rate; RR, respiratory rate; SaO$_2$, oxygen saturation.

TABLE CS6.2 Manual Muscle Test and Grip Strength Values[a]

Joint	Motion	Right	Left
Hip	Flexion	4/5	4/5
	Extension	3/5	3/5
	Abduction	4−/5	4−/5
	Adduction	4−/5	4−/5
Knee	Flexion	4+/5	4+/5
	Extension	5/5	5/5
Ankle	Plantarflexion	3+/5	4+/5
	Dorsiflexion	3+/5	4+/5
Shoulder	Flexion	4−/5	3/5
	Extension	4/5	3/5
	Abduction	3+/5	3−/5
	Internal rotation	4/5	3/5
	External rotation	4/5	3/5
Hand	Grip strength	55 lb (25 kg)	20 lb (9 kg)

[a] With the exception of grip strength, all scores are based on a 0 to 5 scale: 5, normal; 4, good; 3, fair; 2, poor; 1, trace; 0, no contraction. Strength tested within available ROM.

TABLE CS6.3 Active Range of Motion: Cervical and Lumbar Spine

Body Segment	Motion	Range (degrees)
Cervical spine	Flexion	0–30
	Extension	0–18
	Rotation right	0–52
	Rotation left	0–38
	Sidebend right	0–10
	Sidebend left	0–30
Lumbar spine	Flexion	0–15
	Extension	0–5
	Rotation right	0–6
	Rotation left	0–4
	Sidebend right	0–10
	Sidebend left	0–20

TABLE CS6.4 Active Range of Motion: Hips, Ankles, and Shoulders

Joint	Motion	Right (degrees)	Left (degrees)
Hip	Straight leg raise	0–35	0–25
	Flexion	0–100	5–90
	Extension	0–0	Lacks 5° to full extension
	Abduction	0–20	0–10
Ankle	Plantarflexion	0–10	0–10
	Dorsiflexion	0–5	0–5
Shoulder	Flexion	0–110	0–70 (painful)
	Extension	0–20	0–20
	Abduction	0–120	0–60 (painful)
	Internal rotation	0–18	0–10 (painful)
	External rotation	0–40	0–36 (painful)

TABLE CS6.5 Passive Range of Motion: Hips, Ankles, and Shoulders

Joint	Motion	Right (degrees)	Left (degrees)
Hip	Straight leg raise	0–40	0–30
	Flexion	0–110	5–90
	Extension	0–0	Lacks 5° to full extension
	Abduction	0–25	0–10
Ankle	Plantarflexion	0–10	0–10
	Dorsiflexion	0–5	0–5
Shoulder	Flexion	0–120	0–100 (painful)
	Extension	0–20	0–20
	Abduction	0–120	0–80 (painful)
	Internal rotation	0–20	0–10 (painful)
	External rotation	0–45	0–45 (painful)

TABLE CS6.6 Coordination Tests

Coordination Test	Grade Right	Grade Left
Finger-to-nose	4	3
Finger-to-therapist's finger	3	3
Pronation/supination	4	4
Heel-on-shin	4	3
Tapping (foot)	4	4

Scoring: 5, normal performance; 4, minimal impairment; 3, moderate impairment; 2, severe impairment; 1, activity impossible.

TABLE CS6.7 Components of Functional Independence Measure (FIM): Transfers and Locomotion

Activity	FIM Score[a]
Transfers: Bed/Chair/Wheelchair	4
Transfers: Toilet	6
Locomotion: Walk	4
Locomotion: Wheelchair	7
Locomotion: Stairs	2

[a]Scoring: 7 = Complete independence (timely, safety); 6 = Modified independence (device); 5 = Supervision (subject = 100%); 4 = Minimal assistance (subject = 75% or more); 3 = Moderate assistance (subject = 50% or more); 2 = Maximal assistance (subject = 25% or more); 1 = Total assistance or not testable (subject less than 25%).

- Disease-Specific Measures:
  - The Parkinson's Disease Quality of Life (PDQL)[12] questionnaire:
    - Parkinsonian symptoms: 37
    - Systemic symptoms: 23
    - Social functioning: 22
    - Emotional functioning: 28
    - **Total: 110/185**
    Note: The PDQL is a self-administered measure that contains 37 items in four subscales: *Parkinsonian symptoms*, *systemic symptoms*, *social functioning*, and *emotional functioning*. An overall score can be derived, with a higher score indicating better perceived quality of life.
  - The Unified Parkinson's Disease Rating Scale (UPDRS)[13]:
    - Mentation, behavior, and mood: 4
    - ADL: 19
    - Motor: 23
    - **Total: 46/199**

Note: The UPDRS is a rating tool designed to follow the longitudinal course of Parkinson's disease. It is made up of several sections including: *Mentation, Behavior, and Mood*; *Activities of Daily Living* (ADL); and *Motor Examination*. Items are evaluated by interview. Some sections require multiple grades assigned to each extremity. A total of 199 points are possible; 199 represents the worst [total] disability, and 0 represents no disability. The UPDRS also includes the *Modified Hoehn and Yahr Staging* (disease severity is divided over five stages into unilateral or bilateral signs; higher numbered stages represent progressively more difficulty with mobility and balance) and the *Schwab and England Activities of Daily Living Scale* (estimates are made of the percentage of impairment ranging from 0% = vegetative functions [bedridden] to 100% = completely independent).

- The Modified Hoehn and Yahr Staging: The results place the patient in Stage 3 and indicates significant slowing of body movements, early impairment of equilibrium while walking or standing, and generalized dysfunction that is moderately severe.
- The Schwab and England Activities of Daily Living Scale: Score is 70 percent, which indicates that the patient is not completely independent, has greater difficulty with some chores, takes twice as long to accomplish, and is conscious of difficulty and slowness.

Evaluation, Diagnosis and Prognosis, and Plan of Care

Note: Prior to considering the guiding questions below, view the Case Study 6 Examination segment of the DVD to enhance understanding of the patient's impairments and activity limitations. Following *completion of the guiding questions*, view the Case Study 6 Intervention segment of the DVD to compare and contrast the interventions presented with those you selected. Last, progress to the Case Study 6 Outcomes segment of the DVD to compare and contrast the goals and expected outcomes you identified with the functional outcomes achieved.

Guiding Questions

1. Identify or categorize this patient's clinical presentation in terms of the following:
   a. Direct impairments
   b. Indirect impairments
   c. Composite impairments
   d. Actvity limitations and participation restrictions
2. Identify anticipated goals (remediation of impairments) and expected outcomes (remediation of activity limitations/participation restrictions) that address the attainment of functional outcomes.
3. Formulate three treatment interventions focused on functional outcomes that could be used during the first 2 or 3 weeks of therapy. Indicate a progression for each

selected intervention. Provide a brief rationale for your choices.

4. For each of the three phases of motor learning (cognitive, associated, and autonomous) describe what strategies can be used to enhance achievement of the stated goals and outcomes.

5. What strategies can be used to develop self-management skills and promote self-efficacy to enhance the achievement of stated goals and outcomes?

Reminder: Answers to the Case Study Guiding Questions are available online at Davis*Plus* (www.fadavis.com).

REFERENCES

1. Schenkman, M, Cutson, T, Kuchibhatla, M, et al. Reliability of impairment and physical performance measures for persons with Parkinson's disease. Phys Ther 77:19, 1997.
2. Bohannon, R, and Smith, M. Interrater reliability of a modified Ashworth scale of muscle spasticity. Phys Ther 67:206, 1987.
3. Berg, K, et al. Measuring balance in the elderly: Preliminary development of an instrument. Physiother Can 41:304, 1989.
4. Berg, K, et al. A comparison of clinical and laboratory measures of postural balance in an elderly population. Arch Phys Med Rehabil 73:1073, 1992.
5. Berg, K, Wood-Dauphinee, S, Williams, J, et al. Measuring balance in the elderly: Validation of an instrument. Can J Public Health 83 (suppl 2):S7, 1992.
6. Duncan, P, Weiner, D, Chandler, J, et al. Functional reach: A new clinical measure of balance. J Gerontol 45:M192, 1990.
7. Duncan, P, Studenski, S, Chandler, J, et al. Functional reach: Predictive validity in a sample of elderly male veterans. J Gerontol 47:M93, 1992.
8. Weiner, D, Duncan, P, Chandler, J, et al. Functional reach: A marker of physical frailty. J Am Geriatr Soc 40:203, 1992.
9. Shumway-Cook, A, and Woollacott, M. Motor Control Translating research into Clinical Practice Lippincott Williams & Wilkins Baltimore, MD, 2007, pp 395–396.
10. Podsiadlo, D, and Richardson, S. The timed "up and go": A test of basic functional mobility for frail elderly patients. J Am Geriatr Soc 39:142, 1991.
11. Guide for the Uniform Data Set for Medical Rehabilitation (including the FIM instrument), Version 5.0. State University of New York, Buffalo, 1996.
12. Hobson, P, Holden, A, and Meara, J. Measuring the impact of Parkinson's disease with the Parkinson's Disease Quality of Life questionnaire. Age and Ageing 28:341, 1999.
13. Fahn, S, and Elton, R. Unified Parkinson's Disease Rating Scale. In Fahn, S, et al (eds): Recent Developments in Parkinson's Disease, vol 2. Macmillan Health Care Information, Florham Park, NJ, 1987, pp 153–163.

VIEWING THE CASE: PATIENT WITH PARKINSON'S DISEASE

As students learn in different ways, the DVD case presentation (examination, intervention, and outcomes) is designed to promote engagement with the content, allow progression at an individual (or group) pace, and use of the medium or combination of media (*written*, *visual*, and *auditory*) best suited to the learner(s). The DVD includes both *visual* and *auditory* modes. Following is the case study summary and *written* DVD narration.

Video Summary

Patient is an 84-year-old male with a 9-year history of Parkinson's disease. The video shows examination and intervention segments during outpatient rehabilitation following episodes of inpatient rehabilitation (2 weeks) and home physical therapy (4 weeks). Outcomes are filmed after 6 weeks of intervention.

Complete Video Narration

Examination:

• The patient required assistance to roll, owing to decreased thoracolumbar flexion and rotation, and an inability to dissociate the pelvis from trunk.

• The patient was unable to scoot to the head of the mat secondary to decreased hamstring and gluteal strength and decreased hip extension range.

• During transition from supine-to-sit, rigidity of the lower quarter and deficits in core and upper extremity strength are apparent. Moderate assistance is required. Note the patient's facial masking.

• During sit-to-stand transfers, anterior weight shift is impaired by diminished strength and trunk mobility. The extension phase is slow and labored.

• In moving to quadruped, impaired tricep and iliopsoas strength limit required elbow extension and posterior pelvic translation. Assistance is required to shift weight posteriorly and extend elbows.

• Sitting on a ball makes evident core stability weakness, decreased proprioception, and diminished balance control.

• The patient was able to override involuntary facial masking while performing specific facial expressions such as frowning or pursing the lips. Facial animation was also apparent when he told a funny story.

• Maintaining an upright posture was difficult owing to impaired core stability. Additional testing indicated vestibular deficits and poor anticipatory and reactionary balance reactions.

Intervention:

• This treatment segment occurred 3 weeks after the examination. Here, upper extremity flexion patterns are used to promote improved posture and costal expansion.

• Lower trunk rotation was used to decrease tone and promote relaxation prior to stretching. The contract-relax stretching technique was chosen, as it promotes autogenic inhibition while avoiding isometric contractions that may increase rigidity.

- To avoid flexion contractures of the trunk and limbs, the patient often exercised in prone. Contract-relax stretching of the restricted iliopsoas and rectus femoris increased the patient's hip extensibility.
- Here pelvic anterior elevation and posterior depression were initially taught followed by distal resistance to the femur.
- Mass trunk patterns were used to improve mobility. Emphasis was on improved motor recruitment, timing, and strength during rolling to the left.
- The Smart Balance Master was effective in strengthening the vestibular system, increasing limits of stability, and improving righting reactions.
- Braiding is an important activity because it emphasizes lower trunk rotation with stepping and side-stepping movements.
- Group classes provide opportunities for socialization, camaraderie, and support. The patient attended a Tai Chi class for patients with Parkinson's disease. He enjoyed the class and verbalized a sense of accomplishment with successful performance of each new sequence. The benefits of Tai Chi include relaxation, improved confidence, balance, flexibility, and increased strength and endurance.

Outcomes:
- This outcomes video was filmed 6 weeks after the treatment video. Note that the patient is now able to roll to both the left and right independently with improved speed.
- The patient is also able to scoot independently. Note that wearing sneakers increases traction and improves efficiency of movement.
- The patient was successful in transferring from supine-to-sitting but uses an inefficient movement pattern.
- Rocking is no longer required to transfer from sit-to-stand.
- Gait and dynamic balance improved over the episode of care. However, inadequate trunk rotation persisted. Three hundred sixty-degree turns required increased time and several steps to complete.
- Success was achieved in reaching the goal of independently climbing 20 steps with one handrail using a step-over-step gait pattern.

CASE STUDY 7

Spinal Cord Injury

PAULA ACKERMAN, MS, OTR/L, MYRTICE ATRICE, PT, BS, TERESA FOY, BS, OTR/L, SARAH MORRISON, PT, BS, POLLY HOPKINS, MOTR/L, AND SHARI McDOWELL, PT, BS
SHEPHERD CENTER, ATLANTA, GEORGIA

Examination

History

The patient is a 21-year-old female involved in a motor vehicle accident on January 4. She was a restrained passenger in a reclined position when the car hydroplaned head-on into a guard rail. The patient denied loss of consciousness (Glasgow Coma Scale = 15). She was taken to a local medical center, where she presented with immediate loss of movement and sensation in her lower extremities (LEs).

Imaging revealed a burst fracture of the L1 vertebral body and lamina, an L2–3 right transverse process fracture, and bony fragments were noted to have extended into the spinal canal. There was a 40 percent lateral displacement of the spinal cord in relation to the vertebral bodies. In addition to the spinal cord injury (SCI), she sustained a right pneumothorax, right pulmonary contusion, and multiple rib fractures on the right. The methylprednisolone (a high-dose steroid aimed at reducing the swelling) protocol was initiated in the emergency room. A T11–L3 posterior spinal stabilization was performed on January 5. Postoperatively she remained paraplegic and had sensation to her abdominal area. A computed tomography (CT) scan of the head was negative. A prophylactic vena cava filter was placed during the surgery on January 5.

- Demographic Information:
  - Height: 5 ft 5 in. (1.7 m)
  - Weight: 114 lb (52 kg); previously 125 lb (57 kg) at the time of her accident
- Social History:
  Patient lives with her mother and grandmother. Her parents are divorced. She denies tobacco or alcohol use.
- Employment:
  Patient is a full-time student at a local community college and is interested in obtaining her degree in early childhood education. She also worked part-time as a dance instructor at a local dance studio.
- Living Environment:
  The family lives in a one-story rental home. There are two steps leading up to the front door. They do not have plans to move or the financial means to purchase a home at this time.

- General Health Status:
  Prior to her injury, the patient was in very good health. She is an accomplished dancer, having won multiple state and national dance competitions. She had asthma as a child; however, she has had no difficulties with asthma in adulthood.
- History of Present Illness:
  The patient was admitted to a SCI Model System of Care for rehabilitation on January 16. The initial examination indicated a T9 SCI with an American Spinal Injury Association (ASIA) Impairment Scale designation of A: complete injury (no motor or sensory function is preserved in the sacral segments S4 to S5).[1] Initial radiological films revealed a stable T11 to L3 fusion (Fig. CS7.1). She arrived in a thoracolumbosacral orthosis (TLSO), which was replaced with a less-restrictive Jewett™ brace to decrease the risk of skin breakdown in areas of no sensation and to allow ease of forward flexion at the hips during transfers. The brace was discontinued on February 11. The admission motor and sensory screening examinations revealed right upper extremity (UE) paresthesias and weakness, which were monitored and eventually resolved without specific intervention. The patient presented with a chest tube for a residual pneumothorax. The pneumothorax resolved over the course of 10 days, at which time the chest tube was removed without complications.

  The patient presented with a neurogenic bladder and bowel upon admission. A Foley catheter had been placed to manage her bladder at the previous medical center. This was discontinued, and intermittent catheterizations were initiated, which she eventually learned to manage independently. Manual evacuation of the rectal vault and suppositories were initiated to establish a program to manage her neurogenic bowel. Her hospital course was complicated by a urinary tract infection (UTI), multiple episodes of insufficient rectal vault evacuation, and intermittent abdominal discomfort. The clinical examination of the lower abdomen was negative. A kidney ureter and bladder (KUB) x-ray revealed constipation, which remained unresolved despite adherence to a routine bowel program. Results of an abdominal and pelvic CT scan revealed moderate to marked stool in the colon. This resolved prior to discharge.

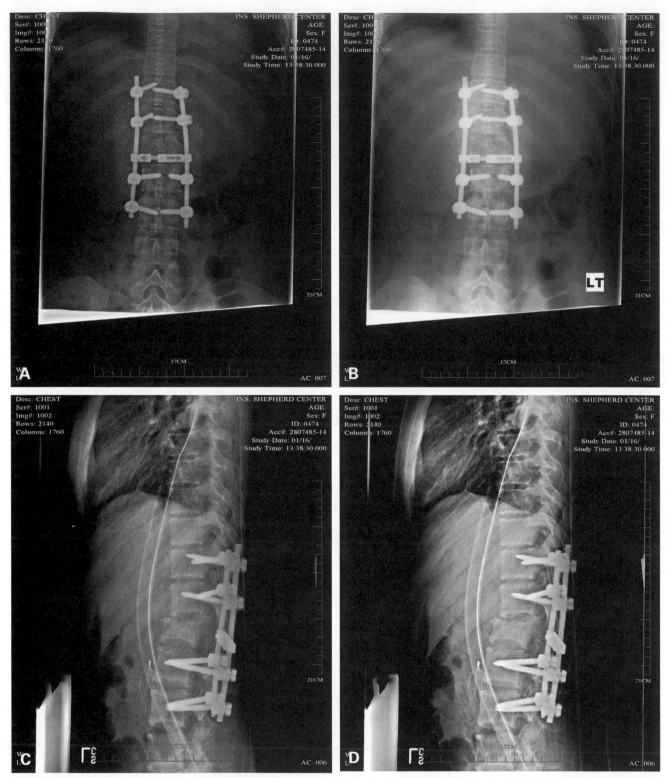

FIGURE CS7.1 Thoracolumbar x-rays of T11–L3 posterior spinal stabilization using cross-linking devices (**A** and **B**: posterior views; **C** and **D**: lateral views).

However, the patient had a poor appetite throughout her stay, and supplemental nutritional support was provided. Her prealbumin level (indicator of visceral protein status) was within normal limits (24.6 mg/dL).

- Medications:
  Macrobid, Fragmin, and Pepcid.

Systems Review

- Cardiovascular/Pulmonary System:
  Lungs were clear to auscultation with a chest tube in place on the right. The patient denied chest pain (other than the chest tube site), shortness of breath, nausea, or

vomiting. She had pneumonia and asthma as a small child but has had no problems as an adult.

- Heart rate: Normal (regular) heart rate and rhythm without murmurs
- Respiratory rate: 15 breaths per minute (deep breaths were painful)
- Vital capacity: 1 liter
- Blood pressure: 110/68 mm Hg

Tests and Measures

- American Spinal Injury Association (ASIA) Impairment Scale:[1]
  - The patient is classified as a complete spinal cord injury (ASIA designation: A [Box CS7.1]).
  - Sensory and motor neurological level is T9 bilaterally (Fig. CS7.2).
- Functional Independence Measure (FIM):[2]
  Results from the FIM are presented in Table CS7.1.
- Strength:
  Results from the Manual Muscle Test (admission data) are presented in Table CS7.2.
- Range of Motion (ROM):
  - Left UE ROM was within normal limits (WNL).

BOX CS7.1 ASIA Impairment Scale[1]

A = Complete: No motor or sensory function is preserved in the sacral segments S4 to S5.
B = Incomplete: Sensory but not motor function is preserved below the neurological level and includes the sacral segments S4 to S5.
C = Incomplete: Motor function is preserved below the neurological level, and more than half of key muscles below the neurological level have a muscle grade less than 3.
D = Incomplete: Motor function is preserved below the neurological level, and at least half of key muscles below the neurological level have a muscle grade of 3 or more.
E = Normal: Motor and sensory function is normal.

- At admission, right shoulder ROM was limited to 90 degrees of flexion and 90 degrees of abduction. Pain noted as 9/10 on numeric pain scale (10 = worst pain; 0 = no pain); described as a sharp pain. An empty end-feel was noted.
- Balance:
  - On admission Modified Functional Reach Test[3] = 10.5 in. (26.67 cm)

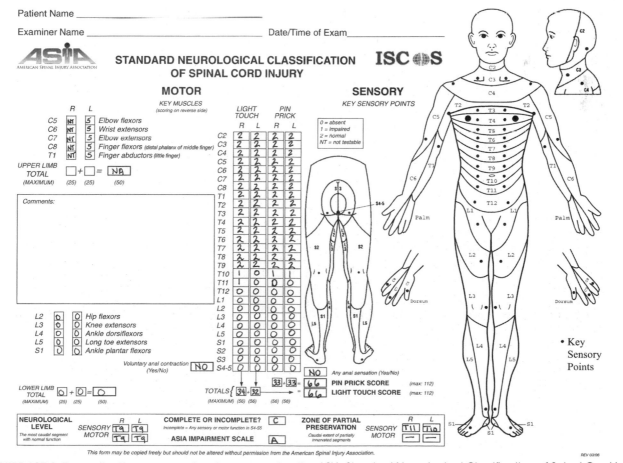

FIGURE CS7.2 The patient's sensory and motor scores using the ASIA *Standard Neurological Classification of Spinal Cord Injury.*

TABLE CS7.1 Functional Independence Measure (FIM)[2]

	FIM Scores[a]: Admission January 16	FIM Scores[a]: Discharge February 29
Self-Care		
Eating	7	7
Grooming	7	7
Bathing	1	7
Dressing, upper	2	7
Dressing, lower	1	7
Toileting	1	6
Sphincter Control		
Bladder	1	6
Bowel	1	5
Transfers		
Transfer, bed	1	5
Transfer, toilet	1	5
Transfer, tub	1	5
Locomotion		
Wheelchair	3	6
Stairs	1	1
Communication		
Comprehension	7	7
Expression	7	7
Social Cognition		
Social interaction	7	7
Problem-solving	7	7
Memory	7	7

[a]Scoring is as follows: 7 = Complete independence (timely, safety); 6 = Modified independence (device); 5 = Supervision (subject = 100%); 4 = Minimal assistance (subject = 75% or more); 3 = Moderate assistance (subject = 50% or more); 2 = Maximal assistance (subject = 25% or more); 1 = Total assistance or not testable (subject less than 25%).

TABLE CS7.2 Manual Muscle Test Scores (January 18)[a]

Joint	Muscle	Right	Left
Shoulder	Medial rotators	3/5	5/5
	Lateral rotators	3/5	5/5
	Flexion	3/5	5/5
	Abduction	3/5	5/5
	Extension	3/5	5/5
Elbow	Flexion	3/5	5/5
	Extension	4/5	5/5
Wrist	Flexion	3/5	5/5
	Extension	3/5	5/5
Fingers	Flexion	4/5	5/5
	Extension	4/5	5/5
Hip	Flexion	0/5	0/5
	Extension	0/5	0/5
Knee	Flexion	0/5	0/5
	Extension	0/5	0/5
Ankle	Dorsiflexion	0/5	0/5
	Plantarflexion	0/5	0/5
Toes	Flexion	0/5	0/5
	Extension	0/5	0/5

[a]All scores are based on a 0 to 5 scale: 5, normal; 4, good; 3, fair; 2, poor; 1, trace; 0, no contraction.

Note: At the time of discharge, strength in the right UE improved to 5 out of 5 throughout.

- At discharge Modified Functional Reach Test = 27.5 in. (70 cm)
- Tone and Reflexes:
  - Deep tendon reflexes (DTR) for bilateral quadriceps tendons: 0/4 (no response)
  - Babinski sign: Positive
  - Hypotonic
- Pain:
  - The patient reported 8/10 pain in the area of the chest tube and rib fractures (10 = worst pain; 0 = no pain).
  - A Fentanyl patch and Dilaudid (as needed) were initiated to manage pain.
  - All pain medication was discontinued by the time of discharge.
  - See the ROM section above for shoulder pain information.

Evaluation, Diagnosis and Prognosis, and Plan of Care

Note: Prior to considering the guiding questions below, view the Case Study 7 Examination segment of the DVD to enhance understanding of the patient's impairments and activity limitations. Following *completion of the guiding questions*, view the Case Study 7 Intervention segment of the DVD to compare and contrast the interventions presented with those you selected. Last, progress to the Case Study 7 Outcomes segment of the DVD to compare and contrast the goals and expected outcomes you identified with the functional outcomes achieved.

Guiding Questions

1. In addition to those mentioned in the case, what other examination tools could you perform to measure the patient's activity level?
2. Organize and analyze the available data to develop a problem list. Identify:
   a. Impairments, direct
   b. Impairments, indirect
   c. Activity limitations
   d. Participation restrictions
3. What are the concerns with the patient losing 11 pounds since the injury?
4. This patient presents with T9 paraplegia with an ASIA designation of A. What classification is this (see Box CS7.1)?
5. Describe components of transfer training for this patient. What modifications are necessary? Progression? What additional wheelchair skills should be included in her POC?
6. How might your treatment plan for mobility skills and transfers differ if the patient had presented with an ASIA designation of B, C, or D (as described in Box CS7.1)?
7. Based on her history of being a dancer and dance teacher, what are the patient assets that can be used to her advantage during rehabilitation?
8. What additional goals would you develop for the patient's post acute rehabilitation? What functional outcomes would you identify?
9. Considering that the patient lives in a rental property, what basic recommendations would you have for home modifications?
10. What durable medical equipment needs do you anticipate?

Reminder: Answers to the Case Study Guiding Questions are available online at Davis*Plus* (www.fadavis.com).

REFERENCES

1. American Spinal Injury Association (ASIA) Examination Form. *Standard Neurological Classification of Spinal Cord Injury.* American Spinal Injury Association. International Standards for Neurological Classification of Spinal Cord Injury. American Spinal Injury Association, Chicago, 2006.
2. Guide for the Uniform Data Set for Medical Rehabilitation (including the FIM instrument), Version 5.0. State University of New York, Buffalo, 1996.
3. Lynch, SM, Leahy, P, and Barker, SP: Reliability of measurements obtained with a modified functional reach test in subjects with spinal cord injury. Phys Ther 78(2):128, 1998.

VIEWING THE CASE: PATIENT WITH SPINAL CORD INJURY

As students learn in different ways, the DVD case presentation (examination, intervention, and outcomes) is designed to promote engagement with the content, allow progression at an individual (or group) pace, and use of the medium or combination of media (*written*, *visual*, and *auditory*) best suited to the learner(s). The DVD includes both *visual* and *auditory* modes. Following is the case study summary and *written* DVD narration.

Video Summary

Patient is a 21-year-old female with a complete spinal cord injury (T9, ASIA A) undergoing active rehabilitation. The video shows examination and intervention segments during inpatient rehabilitation, with an emphasis on transfer and wheelchair mobility skills training. Outcomes are filmed 4 weeks after the initial examination.

Complete Video Narration

Examination:
- Here, *forced expiratory volumes* are measured. Absence of nose clips is due to anxiety.
- Using the American Spinal Injury Association's examination form, 28 key sensory points were tested along the dermatomes on each side of the body. These points are tested and scored separately for light touch and sharp/dull discrimination.
- A gross examination of range of motion and muscle tone is performed.
- Here the therapist lifts the lower extremity to test the right quadriceps reflex.
- A gross examination of active upper extremity range of motion is performed. Note the presence of the Jewett brace.
- A gross examination of upper extremity strength is performed. Note the apparent weakness on the right.
- Using momentum, the patient practices rolling. Note therapist's hand placements to assist.
- Here a forward supine-to-sit maneuver is performed. Note the initial lift is obtained by placing hands under hips.
- At this early point in the episode of care, transfers require maximal assistance for lower extremity management. The therapist provides assistance in moving forward in the

chair and with placement of the sliding board. The Jewett brace impacts transfer ability, as it limits forward rotation of the trunk and head. The transfer is accomplished using slow, inefficient movements. The head and trunk remain relatively upright. The orthosis also limits use of the head-hips principle, which requires the head and shoulders to lean opposite the desired direction of the hips.

Intervention:

- This intervention segment was filmed 2 weeks after the examination. It focuses on transfers and wheelchair mobility skills. The patients is progressed to performing the sliding board transfer upward a softer surface.
- The patient practices assuming a long-sitting position from prone on elbows. In addition to its direct functional implications, this activity is also an important strengthening exercise for shoulder extensors and scapular adductors.
- Lower extremity management is a skill with important functional carryover for bed mobility, dressing, personal hygiene, and movement transitions. Using the upper extremities, weight shift, and momentum, the patient practices moving the lower extremities up onto the mat. Minimal assistance is required from the therapist. Here the patient transfers from wheelchair to a tub seat using a sliding board. The patient is practicing sliding board placement, forward rotation of the upper body at the hips, lifting the body along the sliding board surface, and lower extremity management. Moderate assistance is required from the therapist. Note that the spinal orthosis is no longer worn.

- Here the patient practices transferring from commode seat to wheelchair using a sliding board. The block under the patient's feet provides a pivot point to improve balance as she prepares to transfer into the wheelchair. It also provides a stable surface to assist balance during her bowel program. Once in the wheelchair, the patient places feet on footrests and removes the sliding board.
- Finding a balance point is an important precursor to performing wheelies. Note how the patient's hands interact with the wheel to maintain balance.
- Here, a small wheelie is used to progress up a 2-inch curb.

Outcomes:

- The patient performs a depression transfer from bed to wheelchair with contact guarding. She is able to independently reposition herself in the wheelchair.
- Following discharge, intervention for lower extremity management will continue in the outpatient setting. Independence in this area is anticipated with continued improvements in strength, dynamic balance, and awareness of her new center of mass. Her bed mobility skills are now independent for rolling, supine-to-sit, and scooting in all directions.
- Here the patient practices ascending and descending a 4-inch curb. Note improvements in using her head for balance; however, she continues to exhibit decreased trunk flexion.
- Note head position while practicing curb descent.

Patient With Stroke: Home Care Rehabilitation

LYNN WONG, PT, MS, DPT, GCS
CARITAS HOME CARE, METHUEN, MASSACHUSETTS

Examination

History

- Demographic Information:
  The patient is an 86-year-old widowed female, status post mild ischemic cerebrovascular accident (CVA) with left hemiparesis. She is receiving skilled nursing care, physical therapy (PT), occupational therapy (OT), and home health aide services through a home health agency. The patient was born in Austria and is a Holocaust survivor.
- Living Environment/General Health Status:
  The patient is currently living with her son and daughter-in-law in their small two-story home. The family room is used as her bedroom, which is one step down from the main level of the home (the guest bedroom is up 10 steep steps from the main level). She is using a hospital bed. The patient previously lived alone in a one-level condominium and was independent and active in the community, although she did not drive. She previously ambulated without an assistive device and enjoyed reading, crocheting, cooking, and baking. She also enjoyed playing Scrabble (a word game in which words are formed from individual lettered tiles on a game board) and participated in exercise classes through the local recreation department 2 or 3 days per week (Tai Chi, water walking in season, and general exercise classes). Her son, daughter-in-law, and the patient state that their collective goal is for her to return to her own home, with added services if necessary.
- Past Medical History:
  CVA sustained 3 weeks ago, hypertension (HTN), depression after her husband's death, urinary incontinence, and bilateral tibia/fibula fracture secondary to a motor vehicle accident (MVA) approximately 15 years ago.
- Medications:
  Sertraline, 25 mg daily; Metoprolol, 50 mg daily; Aggrenox, 1 tablet twice a day; hydrochlorothiazide, 12.5 mg twice a day; Valsartan, 160 mg twice a day; Acidophilus, 2 tablets three times a day; Zofran, 4 mg as needed; milk of magnesia, as needed; bisacodyl, as needed; acetaminophen, 650 mg as needed; Pepcid, 20 mg twice a day; Ambien, 5 mg at bedtime; Detrol LA, 2 mg twice a day; Colace, 100 mg twice a day.

- History of Present Illness:
  Patient presented to her local hospital with left-sided weakness and inability to ambulate. Initial computed tomography (CT) scan was negative. She was seen by a physical therapist and a speech and language pathologist. She was placed on nectar thick liquids secondary to dysphagia. After 5 days, she was transferred to an acute rehab hospital. She received PT, OT, and speech therapy there for approximately 2 weeks, with steady improvements in left-sided return and function. Patient experienced an episode of near syncope and was transferred back to an acute care hospital. She was diagnosed with near syncope, dehydration, and a urinary tract infection (UTI). Her UTI was treated with ciprofloxacin, 250 mg twice a day for 7 days, and her dehydration was treated with intravenous (IV) hydration. Physical therapy was resumed, and a swallowing evaluation was requested. The evaluation noted adequate improvement in swallowing to discontinue the thickened liquids. After 7 days in the acute care hospital, the patient was discharged to her son and daughter-in-law's home with 24-hour supervision and assistance from family and companions as well as home care as mentioned above (skilled nursing, PT, OT, and home health aide services).

Systems Review

- Mental Status:
  - Alert, oriented to person, place, and time, and cooperative and motivated.
- Neuromuscular System:
  - Mild left hemiparesis
  - No synergy influence noted
  - Tone normal
- Cardiopulmonary System:
  - Resting heart rate: 80 beats per minute; heart rate after ambulation: 80 beats per minute
  - Resting blood pressure: 168/62 mm Hg; blood pressure after ambulation: 200/82 mm Hg
  - Resting respiratory rate: 18 breaths per minute; 26 breaths per minute after ambulation
  - SpO_2: 99 percent on room air at rest
  - Edema: none present

- Integumentary System:
  - Skin integrity is intact.
  - Skin color is slightly pale.
  - No scars are noted, and her skin is normally mobile.
- Musculoskeletal System:
  - Height: 5 ft 2 in. (1.6 m)
  - Weight: 132 lb (60 kg)
  - No complaints of pain
  - Range of motion (ROM): All joints within normal limits (WNL) except the left lower extremity (LE) presents with 0 degrees of dorsiflexion.
  - Strength: Manual Muscle Test (MMT) grades are presented in Table CS8.1.

Tests and Measures

- Sensation:
  - Light touch: Intact
  - Proprioception: Decreased in left upper extremity (UE)
- Functional Status:
  - Bed mobility
    - Rolling: Modified independence; pulls on rail of hospital bed with right UE to assist
    - Scooting: Supervision (minimal verbal cues required for technique and foot placement)
    - Sit-to-supine: Supervision for LE placement
    - Supine-to-sit: Independent; requires increased time and effort

TABLE CS 8.1 Manual Muscle Test[a]

Motion Tested	Left	Right
Shoulder flexion	4+/5	4+/5
Shoulder abduction	4+/5	4+/5
Elbow flexion	4–/5	4+/5
Elbow extension	4–/5	4+/5
Mass grasp	4/5	4+/5
Hip flexion	4/5	4/5
Hip extension	3/5	4–/5
Hip abduction	3/5	4–/5
Knee extension	4+/5	4+/5
Knee flexion	4+/5	4+/5
Dorsiflexion	4/5	5/5
Plantarflexion	4/5	5/5

[a]All scores are based on a 0 to 5 scale: 5, normal; 4, good; 3, fair; 2, poor; 1, trace; 0, no contraction.

- Transfers
  - Sit-to-stand: Modified independence; once standing, requires standard straight cane to maintain initial balance
  - Stand-to-sit: Supervision; lowers self using right UE to control descent
  - Symmetry: Asymmetrical, with increased weightbearing on the right
- Gait/locomotion
  - Ambulated 75 feet (23.6 m) with standard straight cane and supervision
  - Gait deviations include decreased step length bilaterally, decreased left stance time and weightbearing, and minimally decreased left toe clearance during swing
- Balance
  - Static sitting: Able to withstand minimal challenges (perturbations) in all directions
  - Dynamic sitting: Able to reach minimal distances outside her base of support (BOS) in all directions
  - Static standing: Able to maintain static standing without an assistive device or assistance; unable to withstand any challenges (perturbations)
  - Dynamic standing: Requires supervision and use of a standard straight cane at all times for balance and safety
- Activities of daily living (ADL):
  - Able to dress self while sitting in a chair once clothing is laid out on an adjoining table
  - Requires increased time to don and doff socks and tie and untie shoes secondary to decreased fine motor coordination of left distal UE
  - Requires minimum assist for sponge bathing (for back and feet)
  - Requires minimum to moderate assist to shower using a handheld shower nozzle and a tub seat without a back

Evaluation, Diagnosis and Prognosis, and Plan of Care

Note: Prior to considering the guiding questions below, view the Case Study 8 Examination segment of the DVD to enhance understanding of the patient's impairments and activity limitations. Following *completion of the guiding questions*, view the Case Study 8 Intervention/Outcomes segment of the DVD to compare and contrast the interventions and functional outcomes presented with those you identified.

Guiding Questions

1. Develop a problem list for this patient, including:
   a. Impairments
   b. Activity limitations
   c. Participation restrictions

2. Using the *Guide to Physical Therapist Practice*, determine the physical therapy diagnosis for this patient. Provide justification for your decision.

3. Identify five goals and outcomes for this patient that could be accomplished within the next 4 weeks.

4. Using three goals and outcomes identified in question 3, describe the interventions you would use to achieve each. If appropriate, indicate a progression for each intervention. Provide a brief rationale for the interventions you selected.

5. What activities should be included in the patient's home exercise program (HEP)? Provide a brief rationale for each activity selected.

6. What motor learning strategies would enhance this patient's ability to achieve the stated goals and outcomes?

7. The patient and her family express a desire for her to return to her one-level condominium and live alone. How realistic is this goal? Provide a rationale for your decision.

8. What do you think is an appropriate discharge plan for this patient? Provide justification for your response.

Reminder: Answers to the Case Study Guiding Questions are available online at Davis*Plus* (www.fadavis.com).

VIEWING THE CASE: PATIENT WITH STROKE

As students learn in different ways, the DVD case presentation (examination, intervention, and outcomes) is designed to promote engagement with the content, allow progression at an individual (or group) pace, and use of the medium or combination of media (*written*, *visual*, and *auditory*) best suited to the learner(s). The DVD includes both *visual* and *auditory* modes. Following is the case study summary and *written* DVD narration.

Video Summary

Patient is an 86-year-old female with stroke and left hemiparesis. The video shows examination and intervention/outcomes segments during two sessions of home care physical therapy following inpatient rehabilitation (2 weeks). Emphasis is on balance and locomotor training. The intervention/outcomes segment was filmed after eight visits over 4 weeks.

Complete Video Narration
Examination:
- The patient practices moving from one side of the bed to the other using bridge and place.
- The patient practices rolling supine to sidelying using a left lower extremity D1 flexion pattern.
- The patient moves from sidelying to sitting on the side of the bed.
- In sitting, the patient demonstrates mild coordination deficits in the left upper extremity in rapid alternating movements.
- The left foot demonstrates mild deficits in coordination of foot tapping.
- In sitting, the patient demonstrates reaching to the left side using the left upper extremity.
- Reaching movements are slowed with increased postural demands in standing.

- The patient maintains standing in modified plantigrade position while the therapist applies light medial-lateral resistance.
- The patient practices sit-to-stand transfers, moving the hips to the left side. The therapist assists with placement of the hips and feet.
- The patient practices walking using a straight cane, down and up a single step, progressing to up and down stairs to the second floor. The therapist provides close supervision and verbal cueing.

Intervention and Outcomes:
- It is now 4 weeks later; the patient has received twice weekly physical therapy visits in the home setting. She demonstrates greater ease getting out of bed.
- Note improved sit-to-stand transfers.
- The therapist stops the therapy session to take the patient's blood pressure, given her history of hypertension.
- The patient stands at the kitchen counter using both hands for support and practices the following exercises:
  - Knee flexion with hip extension
  - Alternating hip and knee flexion (marching)
  - Heel rises and toe rises
  - Hip abduction with extension
  - Partial squats
  - Knee flexion with hip extension
  - Hip extension with knee straight
- The patient practices walking without a cane. Note absence of arm swing.
- The patient holds onto two dowels with the therapist walking behind and also holding the dowels. She practices reciprocal arm swing while walking.

Patient With Stroke: Constraint-Induced Movement Therapy

DAVID M. MORRIS, PT, PHD, SONYA L. PEARSON, PT, DPT, AND EDWARD TAUB, PHD
UNIVERSITY OF ALABAMA AT BIRMINGHAM

Examination

History

- Demographic Information:
  The patient is a 63-year-old, African American male who sustained an ischemic cerebrovascular accident (CVA) 6 months previously, resulting in right-side hemiparesis.
- Social History:
  The patient is married and lives in a single-level home with his wife and daughter. He reports a history of smoking (quit more than 40 years ago) and drinks alcohol socially on occasion. He enjoyed carpentry, fishing, and hunting prior to his stroke.
- Employment:
  Patient is a retired steel mill worker.
- Past Medical History:
  The patient reports no past surgeries or significant medical problems except for hypertension and type II diabetes; both are currently under control with lifestyle changes and medications.
- History of Present Illness:
  Patient sustained an ischemic CVA, resulting in right-side hemiparesis. Magnetic resonance imaging (MRI) revealed a left pontine infarction. Cerebral angiography revealed severe stenosis of the right vertebral artery and proximal basilar artery. Prior to the stroke, the patient was right-handed.
- Chief Complaint:
  Patient complains he is unable to use his right arm and hand effectively. His goals are to use his right arm and hand well enough to perform household chores and return to his hobbies.
- Medications:
  Current medications include aspirin, Glucotrol, Glucophage, Coumadin, and Warfarin.

Systems Review

- Communication/Language:
  - Patient exhibits mild dysarthria.
- Cognition/Affect:
  - There is no cognitive impairment as evidenced by his Mini Mental State Examination[1] score of 30.
  - No abnormalities in affect are noted.

- Cardiovascular/Pulmonary System:
  - Heart rate: 72 beats per minute and strong.
  - Blood pressure: 110/80 mm Hg (sitting).
  - Respiratory rate: 16 breaths per minute, regular and unlabored.
- Integumentary System:
  - No abnormalities are noted.
- Musculoskeletal System:
  - Height: 6 ft 1 in. (1.9 m)
  - Weight: 205 lb (93 kg)
  - Passive range of motion (PROM) is within normal limits (WNL) in all extremities, except for shoulder flexion, abduction, and external rotation in the right upper extremity (UE).
  - Gross strength is WNL in the left upper and lower extremities (LEs); patient demonstrates weak, active movement in the right upper and lower extremities.
- Neuromuscular System:
  - There is mild right facial droop (lower quadrant).
  - Hemiparesis is present in the right extremities.
  - Patient is able to actively extend his right wrist to 10 degrees past neutral and able to extend his second, third, and fourth digits (i.e., index, middle, and ring fingers, respectively) beyond 10 degrees at each finger joint. He is unable to extend his fifth digit.
- Learning Style:
  Patient reports that he likes to observe prior to learning a new movement skill.

Tests and Measures

- Tone:
  The examination results of tone in elbow flexors, forearm pronators, and wrist flexors from the Modified Ashworth Scale[2] for grading spasticity are presented in Table CS9.1.
- Range of Motion:
  UE range of motion (ROM) results are presented in Tables CS9.2 (passive ROM) and CS9.3 (active ROM).
- Balance:
  Balance was examined using the following:
  - The Established Populations for Epidemiologic Studies of the Elderly (EPESE)[3-4] short performance battery (Table CS9.4)
  - The 360-degree turn test, a brief examination of dynamic balance that is scored on qualitative characteristics in the

TABLE CS9.1 Modified Ashworth Scale for Grading Spasticity[a]

Muscle Group	Left	Right
Elbow flexors	0	2
Forearm pronators	0	1+
Wrist flexors	0	1+

[a] All movements measured in sitting position.

Key: 0, no increse in tone; 1, slight increase in tone, manifested by a catch and release, or by minimal resistance at the end of the ROM when the affected part(s) is(are) moved into flexion or extension; 1+, slight increase in muscle tone manifested by a catch, followed by minimal resistance throughout the remainder (less than half) of the ROM; 2, more marked increase in muscle tone through most of the ROM, but the affected part(s) is(are) easily moved; 3, considerable increase in muscle tone; passive movement is difficult; 4, affected part(s) is(are) rigid in flexion or extension.

TABLE CS9.2 Upper Extremity Passive Range of Motion (in degrees)

Motion	Left	Right
Shoulder flexion	0–135	0–100
Shoulder abduction	0–130	0–80
Shoulder internal rotation	0–15	0–15
Shoulder external rotation	0–85	0–75
Elbow flexion	0–155	0–155
Forearm supination	0–90	0–60
Forearm pronation	0–90	0–90
Wrist flexion	0–90	0–70
Wrist extension	0–85	0–50

TABLE CS9.3 Upper Extremity Active Range of Motion (in degrees)[a]

Joint	Left	Right
Thumb CMC abduction	0–37	0–28
Second finger MCP extension	0–5	0–40
Fifth finger MCP extension	0–5	0–37
Wrist flexion	0–80	0–50
Wrist extension	0–65	0–10
Elbow flexion	0–145	0–140
Elbow extension	90–0	90–64
Forearm supination	0–90	0–30
Shoulder flexion	0–115	0–50
Shoulder abduction	0–110	0–55

[a] All movements measured in sitting position.
Abbreviations: CMC, carpometacarpal; MCP, metacarpophalangeal.

Physical Performance Test[5] and as a timed quantitative item on the Berg Balance Scale.[6-8] Results are displayed in Table CS9.5.
- Motor Function:
Detailed examination of motor function was conducted using the following:
- The Fugl Meyer Assessment of Physical Performance (FMA)[9] is an impairment-based test of motor ability that examines sensation, ROM, pain, and quality of movement during a series of increasingly more difficult motor tasks. The pretreatment FMA recording sheet is displayed in Case Appendix A (located at the end of this case study).

- The Wolf Motor Function Test (WMFT)[10-12] is a laboratory performance test that employs 17 motor tasks; 15 are timed and 2 involve measures of strength. The testing administration is standardized and ordered sequentially from simple to complex. The 15 timed tasks are filmed and later rated by masked scorers for functional ability (FA) using a six-point rating scale (0 to 5) (Box CS9.1). The two strength tasks are: (1) forward flexion of the shoulder in a seated position to the top of a 10-inch box on a facing table using weights up to 20 lb (9 kg) strapped to the forearm, and (2) dynamometer grip strength for 3 seconds with the elbow flexed to 90 degrees. The pretreatment WMFT score sheet is displayed in Table CS9.6.
- The Motor Activity Log (MAL) is a structured interview that includes the MAL Amount of Use Scale and the MAL How Well Scale (see Chapter 10, Tables 10.5 and 10.6, respectively). Respondents are asked to rate *how much* and *how well* they use their more affected UE for 30 activities of daily living (ADL) tasks outside the clinical setting. (See Chapter 10, Table 10.7 for the activities included in the MAL and Table 10.1 for grading criteria [minimum active ROM and MAL scores].) The pretreatment MAL scores are presented in Case Appendix B.
- The Stroke Impact Scale (SIS)[13-15] is a full-spectrum health status interview that measures changes in eight impairment, function, and quality of life subdomains

TABLE CS9.4 Performance in Tests of Standing Balance (EPESE Protocol)[a]

Test	Scoring	Patient Time (sec)
Side-by-Side Stand	0 = Unable to hold position for more than 9 seconds (inability to complete test) 1 = Able to stand with feet side by side for 10 seconds, unable to hold in semitandem for 10 seconds If able to hold for 10 seconds, go to next posture.	10
Semitandem Stand	2 = Able to stand in semitandem position for 10 seconds, unable to hold a full tandem position for more than 2 seconds If able to hold for 10 seconds, go to next posture.	10
Full Tandem Stand	3 = Able to stand in full tandem position for 3 to 9 seconds 4 = Able to stand in full tandem position for 10 seconds, highest possible score	10
	Total Score: 4	

[a]The patient was asked to stand using three foot positions: side-by-side, semitandem (heel of one foot next to the great toe of the other foot), and full tandem (heel of one foot directly in front of other foot) for 10 seconds each.

TABLE CS9.5 Performance in Test of Dynamic Balance: 360-Degree Turn

Trial/Average	Turn to Right	Turn to Left
Trial 1	11.15 sec; 13 steps	13 sec; 13 steps
Trial 2	9.84 sec; 10 steps	12.56 sec; 12 steps
Average	10.5 sec; 12 steps	12.78 sec; 12.5 steps

Scoring: Total time and steps per turn.

following stroke. The pretreatment SIS score sheets are presented in Case Appendix C. Although not included for this patient, a ninth question (titled *Stroke Recovery*) asks the patient for an estimate of the amount of recovery of function he or she has experienced. The directions for this question read: *On a scale of 0 to 100, with 100 representing full recovery and 0 representing no recovery, how much have you recovered from your stroke?* The patient responds by selecting one of the following options: 100, 90, 80, 70, 60, 50, 40, 30, 20, 10, 0. The patient completes a daily activity log as presented in Figure CS9.2.

Evaluation, Diagnosis and Prognosis, and Plan of Care

Note: Prior to considering the guiding questions below, view the Case Study 9 Examination segment of the DVD to enhance understanding of the patient's impairments and activity limitations. Following *completion of the guiding questions*, view the Case Study 9 Intervention segment of the DVD to compare and contrast the interventions presented with those you selected. Last, progress to the Case Study 9 Outcomes segment of the DVD to compare and contrast the goals and expected outcomes you identified with the functional outcomes achieved.

Note: The reader is referred to Chapter 10, *Constraint-Induced Movement Therapy,* for a detailed discussion of constraint-induced movement (CI) therapy.

Note: See Case Appendix E for additional Case Study 9 materials available online at Davis*Plus* (www. fadavis.com).

Guiding Questions

1. Using the *Guide to Physical Therapist Practice*, identify the preferred practice pattern that best describes this patient's diagnosis.
2. Using the University of Alabama grading system (see Chapter 10, Table 10.1) for UE function, which category would be assigned to this patient?

BOX CS9.1 Wolf Motor Function Test Functional Ability Rating Scale

0 = Does not attempt with UE being tested.

1 = UE being tested does not participate functionally; however, an attempt is made to use the UE. In unilateral tasks, the UE not being tested may be used to move the UE being tested.

2 = Does, but requires assistance of the UE not being tested for minor readjustments or change of position, or requires more than two attempts to complete, or accomplishes very slowly. In bilateral tasks, the UE being tested may serve only as a helper.

3 = Does, but movement is influenced to some degree by synergy or is performed slowly or with effort.

4 = Does, movement is close to normal* but slightly slower; may lack precision, fine coordination, or fluidity.

5 = Does; movements appear to be normal.*

*For the determination of normal, the less involved UE can be utilized as an available index for comparison, with premorbid UE dominance taken into consideration.

Abbreviation: UE, upper extremity.

3. Identify UE movement impairments that should be considered as targets for designing shaping and task practice activities.

4. Discuss factors that will likely negatively influence this patient's participation in the CI therapy protocol.

5. Discuss factors that will likely positively influence this patient's participation in the CI therapy protocol.

6. Using the patient's typical routine (see Case Appendix D), identify activities that could be listed in the *"mitt on, more affected UE only"* category of the behavioral contract. (**Note:** Activities can be modified to allow for inclusion in this category.)

7. Using the patient's typical routine (see Case Appendix D), identify activities that for safety reasons should be placed in the *"mitt off, both hands"* and *"mitt off, less affected UE only"* categories.

8. Using MAL change scores, what are the expected outcomes of application of the CI therapy protocol?

9. Describe two shaping and two task practice activities that would be appropriate for this patient.

10. Describe the appropriate delivery schedule of the CI therapy protocol for this patient.

Reminder: Answers to the Case Study Guiding Questions are available online at Davis*Plus* (www.fadavis.com).

TABLE CS9.6 Pretreatment Wolf Motor Function Scores

Task	Performance Time (sec)	Functional Ability Rating[a]
1. Forearm to table (side)	2.40	3
2. Forearm to box (side)	11.87	2
3. Extend elbow (side)	2.59	2
4. Extend elbow (weight)	3.50	3
5. Hand to table (front)	1.40	3
6. Hand to box (front)	3.21	2
7. Reach and retrieve	0.93	3
8. Lift can	120+	1
9. Lift pencil	4.18	3
10. Lift paper clip	120+	1
11. Stack checkers	120+	1
12. Flip cards	21.56	2
13. Turn key in lock	12.34	3
14. Fold towel	50.59	2
15. Lift basket	16.34	2
Median Score	11.87	NA
Mean Score	32.73	2.2
Log Squared Mean	2.29	NA
Strength Measures		
Weight to box	0 lb (0 kg)	
Grip strength	5.14 lb (2.33 kg)	

[a] See Box CS9.1.

REFERENCES

1. Folstein, MF, Folstein, SE, and McHugh, PR. "Mini-mental state." A practical method for grading the cognitive state of patients for the clinician. J Psychiatr Res 12(3):189, 1975.

2. Bohannon, R, and Smith, M. Interrater reliability of a modified Ashworth scale of muscle spasticity. Phys Ther 67:206, 1987.

3. Guralnik, J, Ferrucci, L, Simonsick, EM, et al. Lower-extremity function in persons over the age of 70 years as a predictor of subsequent disability. N Engl J Med 332(9):556, 1995.

4. Guralnik, J, Simonsick, EM, Ferrucci, L, et al. A short physical performance battery assessing lower extremity function: Association with self-reported disability and prediction of mortality and nursing home admission. J Gerontol 49:M85–M94, 1994.

5. Reuben, DB, and Siu, AL. An objective measure of physical function of elderly outpatients: The Physical Performance Test. J Am Geriatr Soc 38:1105, 1990.
6. Berg, K, et al. Measuring balance in the elderly: Preliminary development of an instrument. Physiother Can 41:304, 1989.
7. Berg, K, et al. A comparison of clinical and laboratory measures of postural balance in an elderly population. Arch Phys Med Rehabil 73:1073, 1992.
8. Berg, K, Wood-Dauphinee, S, Williams, J, et al. Measuring balance in the elderly: Validation of an instrument. Can J Public Health 83 (suppl 2):S7, 1992.
9. Fugl-Meyer, A, Jaasko, L, Leyman, I, et al: The post stroke hemiplegic patient, 1. A method for evaluation of physical performance. Scand J Rehabil Med 7:13, 1975.
10. Wolf, SL, Lecraw, DE, Barton, LA, et al. Forced use of hemiplegic upper extremities to reverse the effect of learned nonuse among chronic stroke and head injured patients. Exp Neurol 104:125, 1989.
11. Wolf, SL, Catlin, PA, Ellis, M, et al. Assessing Wolf Motor Function Test as outcome measure for research in patients after stroke. Stroke 32:1635, 2001.
12. Morris, DM, Uswatte, G, Crago, JE, et al. The reliability of the Wolf Motor Function Test for assessing upper extremity function after stroke. Arch Phys Med Rehabil 82:750, 2001.
13. Duncan, PW, Lai, SM, Bode, RK, et al. Stroke Impact Scale-16: A brief assessment of physical function. Neurol 60(2):291, 2003.
14. Lai, SM, Perera, S, Duncan, P, et al. Physical and social functioning after stroke: Comparison of the Stroke Impact Scale and Short Form-36. Stroke 34(2):488, 2003.
15. Duncan, PW, Bode, R, Lai, SM, et al. Rasch analysis of a new stroke-specific outcome scale: The Stroke Impact Scale. Arch Phys Med Rehabil 84(7):950, 2003.

VIEWING THE CASE: PATIENT WITH STROKE

As students learn in different ways, the DVD case presentation (examination, intervention, and outcomes) is designed to promote engagement with the content, allow progression at an individual (or group) pace, and use of the medium or combination of media (*written*, *visual*, and *auditory*) best suited to the learner(s). The DVD includes both *visual* and *auditory* modes. Following is the case study summary and *written* DVD narration.

Video Summary
Patient is a 63-year-old male with stroke and right hemiparesis (6 months post-stroke). The video shows examination and interventions segments during outpatient rehabilitation receiving constraint-induced (CI) movement therapy. Outcomes are filmed at 2 weeks and 1 year post-treatment.

Complete Video Narration
Examination:
- The participant is instructed to place his arm on the table as quickly as possible.
- While the task is completed relatively quickly, his movements lack smoothness and the arm is dropped onto the table.
- Performance time is 2.40 seconds, and Functional Ability Rating is 3.
- Participant is instructed to slide his hand across the table away from the body, straightening the elbow.
- He exhibits difficulty with movements that are slowed and demonstrates compensatory movements of the trunk.
- Performance time is 3.50 seconds, and Functional Ability Rating is 2.
- The participant is instructed to lift the can to his mouth without touching his lips. He is shown how to use a cylindrical grasp instead of an overhand grasp.
- He was unable to grasp the can and therefore was unable to complete the task.
- Performance time is 120-plus seconds, and Functional Ability Rating is 1.

- The participant is instructed to pick up the pencil using his thumb and first two fingers and hold it in the air.
- He accomplished the task relatively quickly and exhibits abnormal synergistic movement, as evidenced by excessive elbow flexion and shoulder abduction in the reaching arm. He also exhibits excessive effort and appears to be holding his breath.
- Performance time is 4.18 seconds, and Functional Ability Rating is 3.
- The participant is instructed to pick up the paper clip using his thumb and index finger and hold it in the air.
- The participant was unable to grasp the paper clip and therefore was unable to complete the task.
- Performance time is 120-plus seconds, and Functional Ability Rating is 1.
- The participant is instructed to pick up the basket and place it on the table. He is then instructed to slide the basket across the table to the far edge of the table.
- He requires several attempts to complete different parts of the task.
- He also exhibits abnormal synergistic movements as evidenced by excessive shoulder abduction of the lifting arm and excessive trunk rotation. Performance time is 16.34 seconds, and Functional Ability Rating is 2.

Intervention:
- The participant is instructed to lift three blocks up onto the box as quickly as possible yet with good quality. Notice how the therapist demonstrates the task before he begins. Ten trials of the task will be performed before moving onto the next shaping task. The therapist provides encouragement throughout the trial along with coaching tips for improving skill. Feedback is also provided, consisting of how many seconds were required to lift all four blocks onto the box.
- Elements of the participant's performance are reviewed and recorded on the shaping data sheet after completing all 10 trials of the task.

- While not visible on this video, the participant is wearing a mitt restraint on his less affected arm and has been instructed to rest that arm in his lap.
- The therapist determined that the participant would be successful with a more difficult version of the task and shapes the task for greater challenge. An additional block is added for task completion. The therapist could also have selected other task elements to shape the task, including using a higher box, moving the box farther away, or using blocks of larger sizes.
- At the end of the 10 trials, the therapist provides summary feedback about the participant's performance by providing the average and best trial scores. The therapist also creates a graph depicting all 10 trial scores and reviews the graph with the participant.

Outcomes:
- The task is slightly slower yet smoother and with better control.
- Performance time is 2.48 seconds, and Functional Ability Rating is 3.
- The participant performs the task much quicker and with slightly less difficulty.
- Performance time is 1.01 seconds, and Functional Ability Rating is 2.
- Although the participant is able to grasp and lift the can, he does so with great difficulty.
- Performance time is 22.41 seconds, and Functional Ability Rating is 2.
- The participant accomplished the task slightly quicker, yet he showed excessive effort and abnormal synergistic movement.
- Performance time is 4.06 seconds, and Functional Ability Rating is 3.
- Although the participant is able to grasp and lift the paper clip, he does so with some difficulty.
- Performance time is 4.25 seconds, and Functional Ability Rating is 3.
- The participant completes the task much quicker and with less effort.

- Performance time is 6.26 seconds, and Functional Ability Rating is 3.
- The participant has maintained his improvements with this task as evidenced by the smoothness of his movements.
- Performance time is 2.12 seconds, and Functional Ability Rating is 3.
- The participant performed the task more quickly than immediately posttreatment and with greater ease.
- Performance time is 0.81 second, and Functional Ability Rating is 3.
- One year after treatment, the participant has not maintained his ability to grasp and lift the can.
- Performance time is 120-plus seconds, and Functional Ability Rating is 1.
- The participant is still able to lift the pencil yet does so more slowly and requires more attempts to complete the task.
- Performance time is 8.03 seconds, and Functional Ability Rating is 2.
- The participant is still able to complete the task yet does so more slowly and requires more attempts to complete the task.
- Performance time is 10.18 seconds, and Functional Ability Rating is 2.
- The participant completes the task much more slowly than immediately posttreatment and with slightly more difficulty.
- Performance time is 10.59 seconds, and Functional Ability Rating is 2.
- The test scores suggest that the participant did improve and maintain this improvement on many of the skills. Real-world improvements on actual use of the more affected extremity in the participant's home and community environment can be found in the results of the Motor Activity Log. As with most research with participants receiving the constraint-induced therapy intervention, this participant showed greater improvements on the Motor Activity Log than with the Wolf Motor Function Test.

Components of the Fugl-Meyer Evaluation of Physical Performance Used to Examine Patient

TABLE	Components of the Fugl-Meyer Evaluation of Physical Performance Used to Examine Patient

RANGE OF MOTION

Joint	Movement	Score	Scoring Criteria
Shoulder	Flexion	1	0 = Only a few degrees of motion
	Abduction to 90°	1	1 = Decreased passive range of motion
	External rotation	1	2 = Normal passive range of motion
	Internal rotation	1	
Elbow	Flexion	2	
	Extension	2	
Wrist	Flexion	1	
	Extension	1	
Fingers	Flexion	1	
	Extension	2	
Forearm	Pronation	2	
	Supination	1	
Total ROM Score:		**16**	

PAIN

Joint	Movement	Pain Score	Scoring Criteria
Shoulder	Flexion	1	0 = Marked pain at end of range or pain through range
	Abduction to 90°	1	
	External rotation	1	1 = Some pain
	Internal rotation	1	2 = No pain
Elbow	Flexion	2	
	Extension	2	
Wrist	Flexion	2	
	Extension	2	

(table continues on page 304)

TABLE	Components of the Fugl-Meyer Evaluation of Physical Performance Used to Examine Patient *(continued)*

PAIN (CONTINUED)

Joint	Movement	Pain Score	Scoring Criteria
Fingers	Flexion	2	
	Extension	2	
Forearm	Pronation	2	
	Supination	2	
	Total Pain Score:	**20**	

SENSATION

Type of Sensation	Area	Score	Scoring Criteria
Light touch	Upper arm	1	0 = Anesthesia
	Palm of hand	1	1 = Hyperesthesia/dysesthesia
			2 = Normal
Proprioception	Shoulder	2	0 = No sensation
	Elbow	2	1 = Three-quarters of answers are correct, but considerable difference in sensation compared with unaffected side
	Wrist	2	
	Thumb	2	2 = All answers correct, little or no difference
	Total Sensation Score:	**10**	

MOTOR FUNCTION (IN SITTING)

	Item	Score	Scoring Criteria
Reflexes	Biceps	2	0 = No reflex activity can be elicited
	Triceps	2	2 = Reflex activity can be elicited
Flexor synergy	Elevation	1	0 = Cannot be performed at all
	Shoulder retraction	1	1 = Performed partly
	Abduction (at least 90°)	1	2 = Performed faultlessly
	External rotation	1	
	Elbow flexion	1	
	Forearm supination	1	
Extensor synergy	Shoulder adduction/ internal rotation	1	0 = Cannot be performed at all
	Elbow extension	1	1 = Performed partly
	Forearm pronation	1	2 = Performed faultlessly

TABLE Components of the Fugl-Meyer Evaluation of Physical Performance Used to Examine Patient *(continued)*

MOTOR FUNCTION (IN SITTING, CONTINUED)

	Item	Score	Scoring Criteria
Movement combining synergies	Hand to lumbar spine	1	0 = No specific action performed
			1 = Hand must pass anterior superior iliac spine
			2 = Performed faultlessly
	Shoulder flexion to 90°; elbow at 0°	0	0 = Arm is immediately abducted, or elbow flexes at start of motion
			1 = Abduction or elbow flexion occurs in later phase of motion
			2 = Performed faultlessly
	Pronation/supination of forearm with elbow at 90° and shoulder at 0°	1	0 = Correct position of shoulder and elbow cannot be attained, and/or pronation or supination cannot be performed at all
			1 = Active pronation or supination can be performed even within a limited range of motion, and at the same time the shoulder and elbow are correctly positioned
			2 = Complete pronation and supination with correct positions at elbow and shoulder
Movement out of synergy	Shoulder abduction to 90°, elbow at 0°, and forearm pronated	0	0 = Initial elbow flexion occurs or any deviation from pronated forearm occurs
			1 = Motion can be performed partly, or, if during motion, elbow is flexed or forearm cannot be kept in pronation
			2 = Faultless motion
	Shoulder flexion 90°—180°, elbow at 0°, and forearm in midposition	0	0 = Initial flexion of elbow or shoulder abduction occurs
			1 = Elbow flexion or shoulder abduction occurs during shoulder flexion
			2 = Faultless motion
	Pronation/supination of forearm, elbow at 0°, and shoulder between 30° and 90° of flexion	0	0 = Supination and pronation cannot be performed at all or elbow and shoulder positions cannot be attained
			1 = Elbow and shoulder properly positioned, and pronation and supination performed in a limited range
			2 = Faultless motion

(table continues on page 306)

TABLE	Components of the Fugl-Meyer Evaluation of Physical Performance Used to Examine Patient *(continued)*

MOTOR FUNCTION (IN SITTING, CONTINUED)

	Item	Score	Scoring Criteria
Normal reflex activity (This stage is included only if the patient attains a score of 6 in stage above: *Movement out of synergy.*)	Biceps and/or finger flexors and triceps	0	0 = At least two of the three phasic reflexes are markedly hyperactive 1 = One reflex is markedly hyperactive, or at least two reflexes are lively 2 = No more than one reflex is lively, and none are hyperactive
Wrist	Stability, elbow at 90° and shoulder at 0°	0	0 = Patient cannot dorsiflex (extend) wrist to required 15° 1 = Dorsiflexion (extension) is accomplished, but no resistance is taken 2 = Position can be maintained with some (slight) resistance
	Flexion/extension, elbow at 90° and shoulder at 0°	1	0 = Volitional movement does not occur 1 = Patient cannot actively move the wrist joint throughout the total range of motion 2 = Faultless, smooth movement
	Stability, elbow at 0° and shoulder at 30°	0	0 = Patient cannot dorsiflex (extend) wrist to required 15° 1 = Dorsiflexion (extension) is accomplished, but no resistance is taken 2 = Position can be maintained with some (slight) resistance
	Flexion/extension, elbow at 0° and shoulder at 30°	1	0 = Volitional movement does not occur 1 = Patient cannot actively move the wrist joint throughout the total range of motion 2 = Faultless, smooth movement
	Circumduction	1	0 = Cannot be performed 1 = Jerky motion or incomplete circumduction 2 = Complete motion with smoothness
Hand	Finger mass flexion	1	0 = No flexion occurs 1 = Some flexion, but not full motion 2 = Complete active flexion (compared with unaffected hand)

TABLE	Components of the Fugl-Meyer Evaluation of Physical Performance Used to Examine Patient *(continued)*

MOTOR FUNCTION (IN SITTING, CONTINUED)

	Item	Score	Scoring Criteria
	Finger mass extension	1	0 = No extension occurs
			1 = Patient can release an active mass flexion grasp
			2 = Full active extension
	Grasp #1: MCP joints are extended and proximal and distal IP joints are flexed; grasp is tested against resistance	0	0 = Required position cannot be acquired
			1 = Grasp is weak
			2 = Grasp can be maintained against relatively great resistance
	Grasp #2: Patient is instructed to adduct thumb, with a scrap of paper interposed; all other joints at 0°	0	0 = Function cannot be performed
			1 = Scrap of paper interposed between the thumb and index finger can be kept in place, but not against a slight tug
			2 = Paper is held firmly against a tug
	Grasp #3: Patient opposes thumb pad against the pad of index finger, with a pencil interposed	1	0 = Function cannot be performed
			1 = Pencil interposed between the thumb and index finger can be kept in place, but not against a slight tug
			2 = Pencil is held firmly against a tug
	Grasp #4: The patient should grasp a small can by opposing the volar surfaces of the first and second fingers against each other	1	0 = Function cannot be performed
			1 = A can interposed between the thumb and index finger can be kept in place, but not against a slight tug
			2 = A can is held firmly against a tug
	Grasp #5: The patient grasps a tennis ball with a spherical grip or is instructed to place his/her hand in a position of thumb abduction with abduction and flexion of the second, third, fourth, and fifth fingers	1	0 = Function cannot be performed
			1 = A tennis ball can be kept in place with a spherical grasp, but not against a slight tug
			2 = A tennis ball is held firmly against a tug
Coordination/ Speed: finger to nose (five repetitions in rapid succession while patient is blindfolded)	Tremor	2	0 = Marked tremor
			1 = Slight tremor
			2 = No tremor

(table continues on page 308)

TABLE	Components of the Fugl-Meyer Evaluation of Physical Performance Used to Examine Patient *(continued)*

MOTOR FUNCTION (IN SITTING, CONTINUED)

Item	Score	Scoring Criteria
Dysmetria	1	0 = Pronounced or unsystematic dysmetria 1 = Slight or systematic dysmetria 2 = No dysmetria
Speed	1	0 = Activity is more than 6 seconds longer than unaffected hand 1 = Activity is 2 to 5 seconds longer than unaffected hand 2 = Less than 2 seconds difference
Total Motor Score:	27	

Abbreviations: MCP, metacarpophalangeal; IP, interphalangeal.

Pretreatment Motor Activity Log (MAL) Scores

TABLE Pretreatment Motor Activity Log (MAL) Scores			
Task Number	Task	Amount of Use[a]	How Well[b]
1	Turn on a light with a light switch	1	1
2	Open a drawer	1	2
3	Remove an item of clothing from a drawer	1	2.5
4	Pick up the phone	0	0
5	Wipe off a kitchen counter or other surface	0	0
6	Get out of a car (includes only the movement needed to get the body from sitting to standing outside of the car, once the door is open)	2	2
7	Open the refrigerator	1	3
8	Open a door by turning a doorknob	1	1
9	Use a TV remote control	1	1
10	Wash hands (includes lathering and rinsing; does not include turning water on and off with a faucet handle)	5	1
11	Turn water on and off with knob or lever on the faucet	0	0
12	Dry hands	5	1
13	Put on socks	2	1.5
14	Take off socks	0	0
15	Put on shoes (includes tying shoestrings and fastening straps)	1	1.5
16	Take off shoes (includes untying shoestrings and unfastening straps)	0	0
17	Get up from a chair with armrests	0	0
18	Pull a chair away from the table before sitting down	0	0
19	Pull chair toward the table after sitting down	0	0
20	Pick up a glass, bottle, drinking cup, or can (does not need to include drinking)	1	1.5

(table continues on page 310)

TABLE Pretreatment Motor Activity Log (MAL) Scores *(continued)*

Task Number	Task	Amount of Use[a]	How Well[b]
21	Brush teeth (does not include preparing toothbrush or brushing dentures)	0	0
22	Put makeup, lotion, or shaving cream on face	0	0
23	Use a key to unlock a door	0	0
24	Write on paper (if dominant arm was most affected, "Do you see it to write?"; if nondominant arm was most affected, drop the item and assign "NA")	1	0.5
25	Carry an object in hand (draping an item over the arm is not acceptable)	1	2
26	Use a fork or spoon for eating (refers to the action of bringing food to the mouth with a fork or spoon)	0	0
27	Comb hair	0	0
28	Pick up a cup by a handle	0	0
29	Button a shirt	4	2
30	Eat half a sandwich or finger foods	0	0
	Mean Score:	**0.7**	**0.8**

[a]*Amount of Use Scale:* 0 = did not use my weaker arm (not used); 1 = occasionally tried to use my weaker arm (very rarely); 2 = sometimes used my weaker arm but did most of the activity with my stronger arm (rarely); 3 = used my weaker arm about half as much as before the stroke (half pre-stroke); 4 = used my weaker arm almost as much as before the stroke (3/4 pre-stroke); 5 = used my weaker arm as normal as before the stroke (same as pre-stroke).

[b]*How Well Scale:* 0 = the weaker arm was not used at all for that activity (never); 1 = the weaker arm was moved during that activity but was not helpful (very poor); 2 = the weaker arm was of some use during that activity but needed some help from the stronger arm or moved very slowly or with difficulty (poor); 3 = the weaker arm was used for the purpose indicated but movements were slow or were made with only some effort (fair); 4 = the movements made by the weaker arm were almost normal but not quite as fast or accurate as normal (almost normal); 5 = the ability to use the weaker arm for that activity was as well as before the injury (normal).

Stroke Impact Scale (SIS): Pretreatment Scores

1. In the past week, how would you rate the strength of your . . .	A lot of strength	Quite a bit of strength	Some strength	A little strength	No strength at all
a. arm that was most affected by your stroke?	5	4	3	②	1
b. grip of your hand that was most affected by your stroke?	5	4	3	②	1
c. leg that was most affected by your stroke?	5	4	③	2	1
d. foot/ankle that was most affected by your stroke?	5	4	③	2	1

2. In the past week, how difficult was it for you to . . .	Not difficult at all	A little difficult	Somewhat difficult	Very difficult	Extremely difficult
a. remember things that people just told you?	⑤	4	3	2	1
b. remember things that happened the day before?	⑤	4	3	2	1
c. remember to do things (e.g., keep scheduled appointments or take medication)?	⑤	4	3	2	1
d. remember the day of the week?	⑤	4	3	2	1
e. concentrate?	⑤	4	3	2	1
f. think quickly?	⑤	4	3	2	1
g. solve problems?	⑤	4	3	2	1

3. In the past week, how often did you . . .	None of the time	A little of the time	Some of the time	Most of the time	All of the time
a. feel sad?	⑤	4	3	2	1
b. feel that there is nobody you are close to?	⑤	4	3	2	1

c. feel that you are a burden to others?	⑤	4	3	2	1
d. feel that you have nothing to look forward to?	⑤	4	3	2	1
e. blame yourself for mistakes that you made?	⑤	4	3	2	1
f. enjoy things as much as ever?	5	4	3	2	①
g. feel quite nervous?	⑤	4	3	2	1
h. feel that life is worth living?	5	4	3	②	1
i. smile and laugh at least once a day?	5	4	3	2	①

4. In the past week, how difficult was it to ...	Not difficult at all	A little difficult	Somewhat difficult	Very difficult	Extremely difficult
a. say the name of someone who was in front of you?	⑤	4	3	2	1
b. understand what was being said to you in a conversation?	⑤	4	3	2	1
c. reply to questions?	⑤	4	3	2	1
d. correctly name objects?	⑤	4	3	2	1
e. participate in a conversation with a group of people?	⑤	4	3	2	1
f. have a conversation on the telephone?	⑤	4	3	2	1
g. call another person on the telephone, including selecting the correct phone number and dialing?	⑤	4	3	2	1

5. In the past 2 weeks, how difficult was it to ...	Not difficult at all	A little difficult	Somewhat difficult	Very difficult	Could not do at all
a. cut your food with a knife and fork?	5	4	3	②	1
b. dress the top part of your body?	5	4	③	2	1
c. bathe yourself?	5	4	3	②	1
d. clip your toenails?	5	4	3	②	1
e. get to the toilet on time?	⑤	4	3	2	1
f. control you bladder (not have an accident)?	5	④	3	2	1

g. control your bowels (not have an accident)?	⑤	4	3	2	1
h. do light household tasks/chores (e.g., dust, make a bed, take out garbage, do the dishes)?	5	4	③	2	1
i. go shopping?	5	4	3	2	①
j. do heavy household chores (e.g., vacuum, laundry, or yard work)?	5	4	③	2	1

6. In the past 2 weeks, how difficult was it to . . .	Not difficult at all	A little difficult	Somewhat difficult	Very difficult	Could not do at all
a. stay sitting without losing your balance?	⑤	4	3	2	1
b. stay standing without losing your balance?	⑤	4	3	2	1
c. walk without losing your balance?	5	④	3	2	1
d. move from a bed to a chair?	5	④	3	2	1
e. walk one block?	5	4	③	2	1
f. walk fast?	5	4	③	2	1
g. climb one flight of stairs?	5	4	③	2	1
h. climb several flights of stairs?	5	4	3	②	1
i. get in and out of a car?	5	4	③	2	1

7. In the past 2 weeks, how difficult was it to use your hand that was most affected by your stroke to . . .	Not difficult at all	A little difficult	Somewhat difficult	Very difficult	Could not do at all
a. carry heavy objects (e.g., bag of groceries)?	5	4	3	2	①
b. turn a doorknob?	5	4	3	2	①
c. open a can or jar?	5	4	3	2	①
d. tie a shoe lace?	5	4	3	2	①
e. pick up a dime?	5	4	3	2	①

8. During the past 4 weeks, how much of the time have you been limited in . . .	**None of the time**	**A little of the time**	**Some of the time**	**Most of the time**	**All of the time**
a. your work (paid, voluntary, or other)?	5	④	3	2	1
b. your social activities?	5	④	3	2	1
c. quiet recreation (crafts, reading)?	5	4	3	②	1
d. active recreation (sports, outings, travel)?	5	④	3	2	1
e. your role as a family member and/or friend?	5	4	③	2	1
f. your participation in spiritual or religious activities?	5	4	3	②	1
g. your ability to control your life as you wish?	5	④	3	2	1
h. your ability to help others?	5	④	3	2	1

The Patient's Typical Daily Activity Log

Daily Activity Schedule
Weekdays:

Time	Activity	Details (if needed)
6:00 am	Wake up	
6:05 am	Make coffee	Automatic coffeemaker
6:15 am	Let dogs out/feed dogs	Dry dog food
6:30 am	Drink coffee/watch news on TV	
6:45 am	Eat breakfast	Cereal, toast, juice
7:00 am	Shower	
7:15 am	Shave	Disposable safety razor
7:20 am	Brush teeth	Electric toothbrush
7:30 am	Get dressed	
8:00 am	Leave home for clinic	
12 noon	Leave clinic for home	
12:30 pm	Eat lunch	Sandwich, chips, fruit, iced tea
1:30 pm	Walk dogs	Two small dogs on sidewalk
2:30 pm	Read mail/newspaper; check e-mails	
4:00 pm	Yard work/housework	
5:00 pm	Watch news on TV	
6:00 pm	Eat dinner	Meat, veg., salad, bread, iced tea
7:00 pm	Watch TV	
9:30 pm	Wash face/brush teeth	
9:45 pm	Put on pajamas	
10:00 pm	Go to bed	

Daily Activity Schedule
Saturdays:

Time	Activity	Details (if needed)
8:00 am	Wake up	
8:05 am	Make coffee	Automatic coffeemaker
8:15 am	Let dogs out/feed dogs	Dry dog food
8:30 am	Drink coffee/watch news on TV	
8:45 am	Eat breakfast	Waffles, bacon, juice
9:00 am	Shower	
9:15 am	Shave	Disposable safety razor
9:20 am	Brush teeth	Electric toothbrush
9:30 am	Get dressed	
10:00 am	Grocery shopping with wife	
12 noon	Lunch out with wife	
1:00 pm	Movies, park, or mall with wife	
3:30 pm	Laundry	

4:30 pm	Read mail/newspaper; check e-mails	
6:00 pm	Eat dinner	Meat, veg., salad, bread, iced tea
7:00 pm	Play cards/board games with neighbors	
9:30 pm	Wash face/brush teeth	
9:45 pm	Put on pajamas	
10:00 pm	Go to bed	

Daily Activity Schedule
Sundays:

Time	Activity	Details (if needed)
8:00 am	Wake up	
8:05 am	Make coffee	Automatic coffeemaker
8:15 am	Let dogs out/feed dogs	Dry dog food
8:30 am	Drink coffee/watch news on TV	
8:45 am	Eat breakfast	Omelet, sausage, juice
9:00 am	Shower	
9:15 am	Shave	Disposable safety razor
9:20 am	Brush teeth	Electric toothbrush
9:30 am	Get dressed	
10:00 am	Church with wife	
12:00 noon	Lunch out with family at brother's home	Meat, veg., salad, bread, iced tea
2:30 pm	Watch sports on TV with brother	
4:30 pm	Read mail/newspaper; check e-mails	
6:00 pm	Eat light dinner	Sandwiches, chips, iced tea
7:00 pm	Watch TV	
9:30 pm	Wash face/brush teeth	
9:45 pm	Put on pajamas	
10:00 pm	Go to bed	

The following additional Case Study 9 materials are available for review online at Davis*Plus* (www.fadavis.com).

Note: The following additional Case Study 9 materials are ordered based on their relevance to the case and the progression the materials would be used with or by the patient.

Box ACS9.1:   Overview: Repetitive, Task-Oriented Training Program

Box ACS9.2:   Patient's Behavioral Contract

Table ACS9.1: Activity Modifications to Allow Tasks to Be Placed in the "Mitt On, More Affected UE Only" Category of the Behavioral Contract

Box ACS9.3:   Shaping Task: Blocks to Box

Box ACS9.4:   Shaping Task: Flipping Dominoes

Box ACS9.5:   Task Practice Activity: Screwing in a Light Bulb/Tightening Nuts and Bolts

Box ACS9.6:   Task Practice Activity: Sanding/Painting

Table ACS9.2: Bank of Shaping and Task Practice Activities Used for Repetitive, Task-Oriented Training in the Clinic

Table ACS9.3:   Shaping Data Recording Sheet

Table ACS9.4:   Task Practice Activity Data Recording Sheet

Table ACS9.5:   Daily How Well Ratings During the Intervention Period

Box ACS9.7:   Participant/Caregiver Agreement

Table ACS9.6:   Home Skill Assignment Sheet

Box ACS9.8:   Daily Schedule for Treatment Day 3

Box ACS9.9:   Home Practice (After)

Box ACS9.10:   Overview: Outcomes

Table ACS9.8:   Results of Wolf Motor Function Test (Performance Time [Seconds])

Table ACS9.9:   Results of Wolf Motor Function Test (Functional Ability Rating)

Table ACS9.10: Results of Motor Activity Log (Amount of Use)

Table ACS9.11: Results of Stroke Impact Scale (SIS)

Examination

History

- Demographic Information:
  The patient is a 55-year-old, African American male presenting to inpatient rehabilitation status post left basal ganglia hemorrhage with right hemiparesis.
- Past Medical History:
  The patient has a medical history significant for hypertension, hyperlipidemia, and chronic renal insufficiency.
- History of Present Illness:
  The patient presented to the emergency room 1 week ago with a complaint of right-sided weakness and was noted to be hypertensive. During his acute hospital stay, he was found to be positive for right posterior tibial vein deep vein thrombosis (DVT), with resultant inferior vena cava (IVC) filter placement. His acute hospital course was otherwise uncomplicated, and he was transferred to inpatient rehabilitation to address the chief complaints of gait and balance deficits and difficulties with activities of daily living (ADL).
- Diagnostic and Laboratory Findings:
  - A computed axial tomography (CAT) scan of the brain revealed left basal ganglia hemorrhage with minimal mass effect (midline displacement) and no intraventricular hemorrhage. Magnetic resonance imaging (MRI) showed a 0.59-in. (1.5-cm) intracranial hemorrhage in the left basal ganglia region, left lateral thalamus, and left internal capsule. No neurosurgical intervention was recommended (the IVC filter was placed, as anticoagulation was contraindicated).
  - White blood cell count = 5.2, hemoglobin = 11.4, hematocrit = 34.7, platelets = 221.
- Medications:
  - Prior to admission: Zocor, Coreg, Lopressor
  - Admission medications: Labetalol, Hydrochlorothiazide, Lotrel, Nexium, Singulair, Ambien
- Social History:
  Prior to admission, the patient was independent in ambulation without an assistive device and independent in all ADL. He lived alone in a two-level house with three steps to enter with one right-side railing. Inside the home, 12 steps lead to the second floor with a right-side railing,

where the bedroom and bathroom are located. Both of his parents are alive and healthy, and the patient denies a family history of diabetes, hypertension, or stroke. The patient denies tobacco use and notes minimal use of alcohol for social occasions.
- Employment:
  Patient was employed full time as a registered nurse in a rehabilitation hospital, working a 12-hour overnight shift 3 or 4 days per week.

Systems Review

- Cardiovascular/Respiratory:
  - Heart rate: 68 beats per minute
  - Blood pressure: 108/76 mm Hg
  - Respiratory rate: 18 breaths per minute
- Cognition and Communication:
  - Alert and oriented times three and able to follow multistep commands.
  - Independent for basic and social communication; speech is fluent, with biographical naming intact.
  - Pleasant and cooperative throughout the examination process, with a mildly flat affect noted.
  - Mild difficulty with short- and long-term recall, number skills, concentration, and auditory comprehension/processing time.
- Vision:
  - Slight ptosis of right eye noted.
  - Extraocular motions intact, with pupils equally round and reactive to light and accommodation.
  - Reports no loss of vision, blurred vision, or double vision; wears glasses for distance.
- Musculoskeletal System:
  - Gross range of motion (ROM): Right lower extremity (LE) shows mild limitations, with greatest limitations in hip extension and ankle dorsiflexion (Table CS10.1).
  - Gross strength: Right LE shows mild losses in hip and knee strength, with greatest loss in ankle dorsiflexion (Table CS10.2).
  - Height: 6 ft 5 in. (196 cm)
  - Weight: 230 lb (104 kg)
- Neuromuscular System:
  - Patient presents with decreased initiation of movement, decreased smooth coordinated movements, and diminished speed (velocity) of movement.

TABLE CS10.1 Lower Extremity Range of Motion (in degrees)

Joint	Motion	Right	Left
Hip	Flexion	0–100	0–110
	Extension	0–5	0–10
	Internal rotation	0–20	0–30
	External rotation	0–50	0–40
	Abduction	0–45	0–45
	Adduction	0–20	0–20
	Straight leg raise	0–70	0–85
Knee	Flexion	0–125	0–125
	Extension	0–0	0–0
Ankle	Dorsiflexion	0–2	0–8
	Plantarflexion	0–45	0–45

- Tone: Hypotonia of right LE; tone within normal limits (WNL) in left LE.
- Patient is left-hand dominant.
- Other Systems:
  - No significant findings noted for integumentary, gastrointestinal, and genitourinary systems.

TABLE CS10.2 Manual Muscle Test[a]

Joint	Motion	Right	Left
Hip	Flexion	3–/5	4+/5
	Extension	3+/5	5/5
	Internal rotation	4/5	4+/5
	External rotation	4/5	5/5
	Abduction	3+/5	5/5
	Adduction	4/5	5/5
Knee	Flexion	3/5	5/5
	Extension	3–/5	5/5
Ankle	Dorsiflexion	1/5	4+/5
	Plantarflexion	3/5	5/5

[a]All scores are based on a 0 to 5 scale: 5, normal; 4, good; 3, fair; 2, poor; 1, trace; 0, no contraction.

- Patient presents with no significant complaints of depression or change in mood, and no psychiatric history.

Tests and Measures

- Edema (Circumferential Measurements):
  - Right LE: 18.7 in. (47.5 cm) at midcalf, 13.2 in. (33.5 cm) at ankle, inferior to malleoli
  - Left LE: 17.9 in. (45.5 cm) at midcalf, 13.2 in. (33.5 cm) at ankle, inferior to malleoli
- Sensory Integrity:
  - Intact to light touch and pinprick in left LE
  - Decreased to light touch and pinprick throughout distal right LE, with inconsistent responses noted for L3–L5 dermatomes
- Pain:
  - Pain of 2/10 noted in distal right LE at rest (10 = worst pain; 0 = no pain).
  - Pain of 5/10 in right hamstring with standing or elongation (10 = worst pain; 0 = no pain).
- Coordination:
  - Demonstrates a positive response for finger-to-nose test (dysmetria) using right UE.
  - Positive right pronator drift (indicative of spasticity) evident. *Note:* To test for pronator drift, the patient is asked to hold the position of 90 degrees of shoulders flexion, with the elbows extended, forearms supinated, and eyes closed. Forearm pronation indicates the patient has a pronator drift.
  - Difficulty noted with rapid alternating movements (dysdiadochokinesia) bilaterally, including forearm pronation/supination and foot tapping.
- Posture:
  - Sitting: The patient sits with a forward head, rounded shoulders, increased thoracic kyphosis, reduced lumbar lordosis, and excessive posterior pelvic tilt (Fig. CS10.1); he also demonstrates a sloped right shoulder position with shortening of right side trunk musculature (Fig. CS10.2). In sitting, the patient typically demonstrates excessive left lateral lean and increased weightbearing on the left ischial tuberosity.
  - Standing: The patient demonstrates decreased right knee (Fig. CS10.3) and hip extension in stance. When standing without an assistive device, the patient maintains a forwardly flexed posture (Fig. CS10.4) and requires minimal assistance.
- Functional Status:
  - Wheelchair mobility: Moderate assistance is required to propel a wheelchair 10 ft (3 m).
  - Rolling: Supervision is required for rolling toward both left and right. Decreased initiation of movement is noted when rolling toward left side. Movement transitions for supine-to/from-prone require supervision.
  - Supine-to-sidelying-to-sitting: Close supervision is required from supine-to-sidelying on left. Minimal assistance is required from supine-to-sidelying on right, with use of bilateral UEs to assist in right LE management. Minimal

assistance is required for moving from sidelying-to-sitting.

- Sit-to-supine: Close supervision is required. The patient uses both UEs and left LE to assist with right LE placement onto mat.
- Sit-to-stand: Requires minimal assistance (Fig. CS10.5).
- Stand-to-sit: Requires minimal assistance to control descent

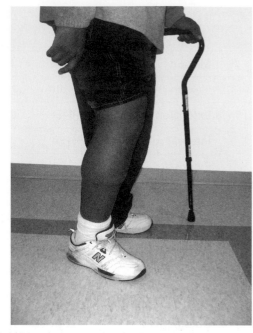

FIGURE CS10.3 Lateral view of right knee showing decreased knee extension in stance position. Although not visible here, diminished hip extension is also noted. Note swelling of right calf.

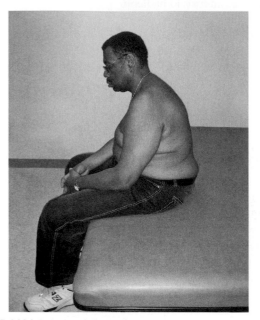

FIGURE CS10.1 Lateral view of seated posture. Note the forward head, rounded shoulders, increased thoracic kyphosis, and reduced lumbar lordosis.

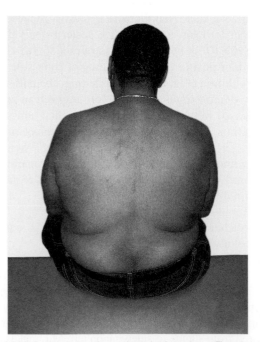

FIGURE CS10.2 Posterior view of seated posture. The right shoulder is slightly lower than the left with shortening of right side trunk musculature.

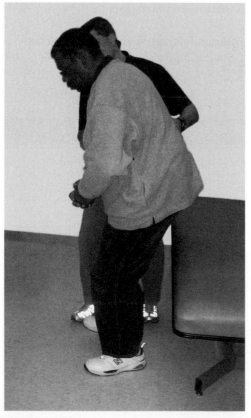

FIGURE CS10.4 Lateral view of standing posture without use of an assistive device. The patient assumes a forwardly flexed posture of head, neck, and trunk with increased hip and knee flexion. Minimal assistance from the therapist is required.

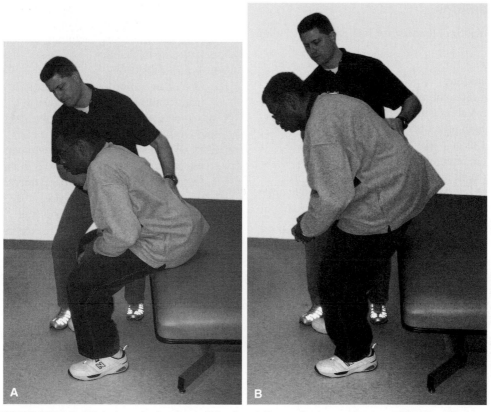

FIGURE CS10.5 **(A)** In transferring from sit-to-stand, the patient experiences difficulty with forward translation of the upper body over the feet. As the patient typically sits with a posterior pelvic tilt and increased thoracic kyphosis, he attempted to bring body weight forward by increasing thoracic kyphosis as he flexed the hips (body weight too far posterior). This brings the head forward but does not effectively translate the body mass horizontally. In addition, limitations in ankle ROM reduced the ability to position the feet behind the knees to allow the lower leg to rotate effectively over the foot. **(B)** Attempts to achieve upright standing posture and balance following sit-to-stand transfer. Note that the patient maintains a downward gaze toward the floor and keeps the upper trunk flexed (instead of extended) when weight is shifted forward. This posturing impairs his sense of postural alignment and vertical orientation.

- Sit-pivot transfer from wheelchair to mat: Requires contact guard assistance
- Sit-pivot transfer from mat to wheelchair: Requires contact guard assistance
- Balance:
  - Static sitting balance: Supervision
  - Dynamic sitting balance: Supervision
  - Static standing balance: Contact guard to minimal assistance
  - Dynamic standing balance: Minimal assistance
- Ambulation:
  - Walks 5 ft (1.5 m) on level surfaces with minimal to moderate assistance using a narrow base quadruped (quad) cane held in left hand.
  - Demonstrates decreased thoracic trunk extension, excessive left lateral lean, and greater weightbearing through the less involved left LE. During swing, there is insufficient right hip and knee flexion and ankle dorsiflexion (decreased foot clearance). During stance, there is decreased right hip and knee extension. Decreased step length noted bilaterally.

- Decreased endurance for upright standing and ambulation.
- Stairs: Unable to examine secondary to impairments in strength, balance, and tolerance for upright position.
- Patient's Goal:
  "To walk and do things by myself at home and work."

Evaluation, Diagnosis and Prognosis, and Plan of Care

Note: Prior to considering the guiding questions below, view the Case Study 10 Examination segment of the DVD to enhance understanding of the patient's impairments and activity limitations. Following *completion of the guiding questions*, view the Case Study 10 Intervention segment of the DVD to compare and contrast the interventions presented with those you selected. Last, progress to the Case Study 10 Outcomes segment of the DVD to compare and contrast the goals and expected outcomes you identified with the functional outcomes achieved.

Guiding Questions

1. Develop a clinical problem list for this patient, including the following:
   a. Impairments
   b. Activity limitations
   c. Participation restrictions
2. How might the patient's impairments in right ankle ROM and strength affect his gait?
   a. What phases of gait will be affected?
   b. Describe three interventions to address the impairments at the right ankle.
   c. If therapeutic interventions do not improve right ankle function, what compensatory strategies/devices might you consider?
3. In the inpatient rehabilitation setting, the patient receives 3 hours of therapy per day, 5 days a week. Establish one goal and a logical time frame for goal achievement for the following activity limitations:
   a. Sit-to/from-stand transfers
   b. Sit-pivot (lateral) transfers
   c. Ambulation
   d. Stair climbing

4. Based on the patient's clinical presentation, develop a plan of care (POC) for motor learning and describe appropriate strategies, including the following:
   a. Schedule of practice
   b. Types of feedback
   c. One other motor learning strategy to enhance achievement of this patient's outcomes
5. Based on the patient's goal of returning to home and work:
   a. Describe two task-specific treatments that will address the goal of *returning to work* as a nurse.
   b. Describe two task-specific treatments that will address the goal of *returning to home*.
6. The patient is unable to perform stair climbing.
   a. From a therapeutic exercise perspective, identify three muscle groups critical to the patient's ability to climb stairs and one exercise for each group identified.
   b. Describe one *part-task* and one *whole-task* practice strategy with a progression of each that could be used to improve the patient's ability to climb stairs.

Reminder: Answers to the Case Study Guiding Questions are available online at Davis*Plus* (www.fadavis.com).

VIEWING THE CASE: PATIENT WITH STROKE

As students learn in different ways, the DVD case presentation (examination, intervention, and outcomes) is designed to promote engagement with the content, allow progression at an individual (or group) pace, and use of the medium or combination of media (*written*, *visual*, and *auditory*) best suited to the learner(s). The DVD includes both *visual* and *auditory* modes. Following is the case study summary and *written* DVD narration.

Video Summary

Patient is a 55-year-old male with stroke and right hemiparesis. The video shows examination and intervention segments during inpatient rehabilitation. Outcomes are filmed after 4 weeks.

Complete Video Narration

Examination:
- The patient stands up and sits down from an elevated platform mat. He demonstrates poor posture and control with uneven foot placement. He sits down with excessive speed.
- The patient performs a lateral transfer to his uninvolved left side with close supervision.
- The patient stands asymmetrically with excessive weight-bearing on the left side and requires minimal assistance.
- When instructed to walk, he has difficulty initiating the movement. The therapist provides minimal assistance and verbal cues to sequence the task. Note his kyphotic posture and excessive hip and knee flexion.

Intervention:
- It is now 2 weeks later. The patient practices sit-to-stand from a mat that has been progressively lowered. The therapist provides verbal cues to emphasize the forward weight shift in standing up and sitting down slowly.
- The patient practices walking using a small-based quad cane. A dorsiflexion assist wrap has been applied to the right ankle. The therapist provides contact guard and verbal cues to sequence the task and to increase speed.
- The patient practices standing while pouring from a pitcher into a glass and then reaching with the left hand across midline and placing the cup to the right side. A blocked practice schedule was used at first, progressing to a variable schedule of tasks. The therapist provides verbal cues and contact guarding.
- The patient practices stepping up with the left foot onto a 2-inch step. The activity is progressed to higher steps and then to stair climbing.

Outcomes:
- It is now 26 days following the initial examination. The patient is able to independently perform sit-to-stand transfers with improved control.
- The patient shows similar improvements in speed and ease of lateral transfers, performing the task to his involved right side.

• The patient's gait shows improvement in alignment, weight shifting, right knee control, step length, and reciprocal pattern. A dorsiflexor wrap is still used due to continuing limitations in dorsiflexor strength.

• The patient demonstrates improved standing balance control with practice of upper extremity tasks required for his job as a rehabilitation nurse. The therapist provides supervision only, no hands-on assistance or cues.

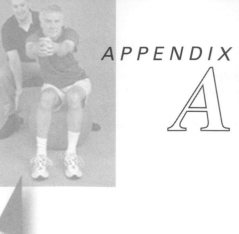

Outcome Measures Organized by the *International Classification of Functioning, Disability, and Health (ICF)* Categories

Body Structure and Function Measures	References
Manual Muscle Test (MMT)	Hislop, HJ, and Montgomery, J. Daniels and Worthingham's Muscle Testing: Techniques of Manual Examination, ed 8. Saunders (Elsevier), Philadelphia, 2007. Kendall, F, McCreary, E, Provance, P, et al. Muscles: Testing and Function with Posture and Pain, ed 5. Lippincott Williams & Wilkins, Baltimore, 2005.
Goniometry	Norkin, C, and White, J. Measurement of Joint Function, ed 4. FA Davis, Philadelphia, 2009.
Modified Ashworth Scale	Bohannon, RW, and Smith, MB. Interrater reliability of a modified Ashworth scale of muscle spasticity. Phys Ther 67:206, 1987. Blackburn, M, van Vliet, P, and Mockett, SP. Reliability of measurements obtained with the Modified Ashworth Scale in the lower extremities of people with stroke. Phys Ther 82:25, 2002. Haas, BM, Bergstrom, E, Jamous A, et al. The interrater reliability of the original and the modified Ashworth scale for the assessment of spasticity in patients with spinal cord injury. Spinal Cord 34:560, 1996.
Glasgow Coma Scale (GCS)	Jennett, B, and Teasdale, G. Management of Head Injuries. FA Davis, Philadelphia, 1981.
Rancho Levels of Cognitive Function (LOCF) [TBI]	Hagen, C, Malkmus, D, and Durham, P. Levels of cognitive functioning. In Rehabilitation of the Head Injured Adult: Comprehensive Physical Management. Downey, CA: Professional Staff Association of Ranchos Los Amigos Hospital, 1979.
ASIA Impairment Scale—Standard Neurological Classification of Spinal Cord Injury	American Spinal Injury Association. International Standards for Neurological Classification of Spinal Cord Injury. American Spinal Injury Association, Chicago, 2006.
Mini Mental State Exam (MMSE)	Folstein, MF, Folstein, SE, and McHugh, PR. "Mini-mental state." A practical method for grading the cognitive state of patients for the clinician. J Psychiatr Res 12(3):189, 1975.
Fugl-Meyer [CVA]	Fugl-Meyer, AR, Jaasko, L, Leyman, I, et al. The post-stroke hemiplegic patient: A method for evaluation and performance. Scand J Rehabil Med 7:13, 1975. Fugl-Meyer, AR. Post-stroke hemiplegia assessment of physical properties. Scand J Rehabil Med 63:85, 1980. Gladstone, DJ, Danells, CJ, and Black, S. The Fugl-Myer assessment of motor recovery after stroke: A critical review of its measurement properties. Neurorehabil and Neural Repair 16:232, 2002.

Body Structure and Function Measures	References
The National Institutes of Health (NIH) Stroke Scale [CVA]	Brott, T, Adams, HP, Olinger, CP, et al. Measurements of acute cerebral infarction: A clinical examination scale. Stroke 20:864, 1989. Goldstein, LB, Bertels, C, and Davis, JN. Interrater reliability of the NIH stroke scale. Arch Neurol 46:660, 1989. Heinemann, A, Harvey, R, McGuire, JR, et al. Measurement properties of the NIH stroke scale during acute rehabilitation. Stroke 28:1174, 1997. The NIH Stroke Scale is available online at http://www.ninds.nih.gov/doctors/NIH_Stroke_Scale.pdf.
Postural Assessment Scale for Stroke Patients (PASS) [CVA]	Benaim, C, Perennou, DA, Villy, J, et al. Validation of a standardized assessment of postural control in stroke patients: The Postural Assessment Scale for Stroke Patients (PASS). Stroke 30:1862, 1999. Pyoria, O, TaLvitie, U, Nyrkko, H, et al. Validity of the Postural Control and Balance for Stroke Test. Physiother Res Int 12(3):162, 2007.
Unified Parkinson's Disease Rating Scale (UPDRS)	Fahn, S, and Elton, R. Unified Parkinson's Disease Rating Scale. In Fahn, S, et al (eds): Recent Developments in Parkinson's Disease, vol 2. Macmillan Health Care Information, Florham Park, NJ, 1987, pp 153–163. Unified Parkinson's Disease Rating Scale is available online at http://www.mdva.org/library/ratingscales/pd/updrs.pdf.

Abbreviations: CVA, cerebrovascular accident; TBI, traumatic brain injury.

Activity Measures	References
Functional Independence Measure (FIM)	Guide for the Uniform Data Set for Medical Rehabilitation (Adult FIM), version 5.0. State University of New York at Buffalo, 1996. Dodds, TA, Martin, DP, Stolov, WC, et al. A validation of the functional independence measurement and its performance among rehabilitation in-patients. Arch Phys Med Rehabil 74:531, 1993. Linacre, JM, Heinemann, AW, Wright, BD, et al. The structure and stability of the Functional Independence Measure. Arch Phys Med Rehabil 75:127, 1994. Long, WB, Sacco, WJ, Coombes, SS, et al. Determining normative standards for Functional Independence Measure transitions in rehabilitation. Arch Phys Med Rehabil 75:144, 1994. Hamilton, BB, Laughlin, JA, Fielder, RC, et al. Interrater reliability of the 7-level Functional Independence Measure (FIM). Scand J Rehabil Med 26:115, 1994. The FIM is available online at email: info@udsmr.org, or website: http://www.udsmr.org.
Functional Assessment Measure (FIM/FAM)	Linn, RT, Blair, RS, Granger, CV, et al. Does the Functional Assessment Measure (FAM) extend the Functional Independence Measure (FIM™) Instrument? A Rasch analysis of stroke patients. J Outcome Measure 3:339, 1999. Hall, KM. The Functional Assessment Measure (FAM). J Rehabil Outcomes 1(3):63, 1997. Hall, KM, Mann, N, High, WM, et al. Functional measures after traumatic brain injury: Ceiling effects of FIM, FIM+FAM, DRS, and CIQ. J Head Trauma Rehabil 11(5):27, 1996. The FIM/FAM is available online at http://www.brif.info/pdf/tools/famform.pdf.

(table continues on page 326)

Activity Measures	References
Disabilities of the Arm, Shoulder, and Hand Outcome Measure (DASH)	Beaton, DE, Davis, AM, Hudak P, and McConnell, S. The DASH (Disabilities of the Arm, Shoulder, and Hand) Outcome Measure: What do we know about it now? Br J of Hand Ther 6(4):109, 2001. Beaton, DE, Katz, JN, Fossel AH, et al. Measuring the whole or the parts? Validity, reliability & responsiveness of the Disabilities of the Arm, Shoulder, and Hand Outcome Measure in different regions of the upper extremity. J Hand Ther 14(2):128, 2001. Bot, SDM, Terwee, CB, van der Windt, DAWM, et al. Clinimetric evaluation of shoulder disability questionnaires: A systematic review of the literature. Ann Rheum Dis 63(4):335, 2004. The DASH is available online at http://www.dash.iwh.on.ca/.
Lower Extremity Functional Scale (LEFS)	Wang, Y-C, Hart, DL, Stratford, PW, and Mioduski, JE. Clinical interpretation of a Lower-Extremity Functional Scale-derived computerized adaptive test. Phys Ther 89(9):957, 2009. Lin, C-W, Moseley, AM, Refshauge, KM, and Bundy, AC. The Lower Extremity Functional Scale has good clinimetric properties in people with ankle fracture. Phys Ther 89(6):580, 2009. Binkley, JM, Stratford, PW, Lott, SA, and Riddle, DL. The Lower Extremity Functional Scale (LEFS): Scale development, measurement properties, and clinical application. Phys Ther 79(4):371, 1999. The LEFS is available online at http://www.tac.vic.gov.au/upload/LE.pdf.
Barthel Index (BI)	Granger, CV, Devis, LS, Peters, MC, et al. Stroke rehabilitation analysis of repeated Barthel Index measures. Arch Phys Med Rehabil 60:14, 1979. Mahoney, FI, and Barthel, DW. Functional evaluation: The Barthel Index. Maryland State Med J 14:61, 1965.
The Physical Performance Test	Reuben, DB, and Siu, AL. An objective measure of physical function of elderly populations: The Physical Performance Test. J Am Geriatr Soc 38:1105, 1990.
High Level Mobility Assessment Tool (HiMat) [TBI]	Williams, GP, Robertson, V, Greenwood, KM, et al. The high-level mobility assessment tool (HiMAT) for traumatic brain injury. Part 1: Item Generation. Brain Injury 19(11):925, 2005. Williams, GP, Robertson, V, Greenwood, KM, et al. The High-Level Mobility Assessment Tool (HiMAT) for traumatic brain injury. Part 2: Content validity and discriminability. Brain Injury 19(10):833, 2005. Williams GP, Greenwood KM, Robertson VJ, et al. High-Level Mobility Assessment Tool (Hi-MAT): Inter-rater reliability, retest reliability, and internal consistency. Phy Ther 86:395, 2006. The HiMat is available online at http://www.tbims.org/combi/himat/index.html.
Wheelchair Skills Test (WST) [SCI]	Kirby, RL, Dupuis, DJ, MacPhee, AH, et al. The Wheelchair Skills Test (version 2.4): Measurement properties. Arch Phys Med Rehabil 85:794, 2004. *Videotapes for Wheelchair Users and Wheelchair Skills Program (WSP) Version 4.1 Manual* available online at http://www.wheelchairskillsprogram.ca/eng/overview.htm. Additional online resoures: *The Powered Wheelchair Training Guide* http://www.wheelchairnet.org/WCN_Prodserv/Docs/PWTG/WCN_PWTG.html *The Manual Wheelchair Training Guide* http://www.wheelchairnet.org/wcn_prodserv/Docs/WCN_MWTG.html *A Guide to Wheelchair Selection* http://www.wheelchairnet.org/WCN_Prodserv/Docs/WCN_PVAguide.html

Activity Measures	References
Wolf Motor Function Test (WMFT) [CVA]	Wolf, SL, Catlin, PA, Ellis, M, et al. Assessing Wolf Motor Function Test as outcome measure for research in patients after stroke. Stroke 32:1635, 2001. Morris, DM, Uswatte, G, Crago, JE, et al. The reliability of the Wolf Motor Function Test for assessing upper extremity function after stroke. Arch Phys Med Rehabil 82:750, 2001.
Motor Activity Log (MAL) [CVA]	Wolf, SL, Thompson, PA, Morris, DM, et al. The EXCITE trial: Attributes of the Wolf Motor Function Test in patients with subacute stroke. Neurorehabil Neural Repair 19:194, 2005. Uswatte, G, Taub, E, Morris, D, et al. The Motor Activity Log-28: Assessing daily use of the hemiparetic arm after stroke. Neurology 67:1189, 2006. Van der Lee, JH, Beckerman, H, Knol, DI, et al. Clinimetric properties of the Motor Activity Log for the assessment of arm use in hemiparetic patients. Stroke 35:1410, 2004.
Berg Balance Scale (BBS)	Berg, K, Wood-Dauphinee, S, Williams, J, et al. Measuring balance in the elderly: Preliminary development of an instrument. Physiother Can 41:304, 1989. Berg, KO, Maki, B, Williams, JI, et al. Clinical and laboratory measures of postural balance in an elderly Population. Arch Phys Med Rehabil 73:1073, 1992. Berg, KO, Wood-Dauphinee, SL, Williams, JI, et al. Measuring balance in the elderly: Validation of an instrument. Can J Public Health 83:S7, 1992. Berg, KO, Wood-Dauphinee, S, and Williams, JI. The balance scale: Reliability assessment with elderly residents and patients with an acute stroke. Scand J Rehabil Med 27:27, 1995.
Functional Reach (FR)	Duncan, P, et al. Functional Reach: A new clinical measure of balance. J Gerontol 45:M192, 1990. Duncan, P, et al. Functional Reach: Predictive validity in a sample of elderly male veterans. J Gerontol 47 M93, 1992. Weiner, D, et al. Functional Reach: A marker of physical frailty. J Am Geriatr Soc 40:2, 1992.
Multidirectional Reach	Newton, R. Validity of the Multi-directional Reach test: A practical measure for limits of stability in older adults. J Gerontol Med Sci 56(4):M248, 2001.
Modified Functional Reach (seated)	Lynch, SM, Leahy, P, and Barker, S. Reliability of measurements obtained with a modified functional reach test in subjects with spinal cord injury. Phys Ther 78(2):128, 1998.
Stops Walking When Talking (SWWT)	Lundin-Olsson L, et al. Stops Walking When Talking as a predictor of falls in elderly people. Lancet 348:617, 1997.
Timed Up & Go (TUG)	Ng, SS, and Hui-Chan, CW. The Timed Up & Go test: Its reliability and association with lower-limb impairments and locomotor capabilities in people with chronic stroke. Arch Phys Med Rehabil 86:1641, 2005. Podsiadlo, D, et al. The timed "Up & Go": A test of basic functional mobility for frail elderly persons. J Am Geriatr Soc 39:142, 1992.
Performance Oriented Mobility Assessment (POMA)	Tinetti, M. Performance-oriented assessment of mobility problems in elderly patients. J Am Geriatr Soc 34:119, 1986.
Clinical Test for Sensory Integration in Balance (CTSIB)	Shumway-Cook, A, and Horak, F. Assessing the influence of sensory interaction on balance. Phys Ther 66(10):1548, 1986.

(table continues on page 328)

Activity Measures	References
Modified Clinical Test for Sensory Integration in Balance (mCTSIB)	Rose, DJ. Fallproof!: A Comprehensive Balance and Mobility Training Program. Human Kinetics, Champaign, IL, 2003.
Functional Gait Assessment (FGA)	Wrisley, DM, et al. Reliability, internal consistency, and validity of data obtained with the Functional Gait Assessment. Phys Ther 84:906, 2004.
Modified Emory Functional Ambulation Profile (mEFAP)	Baer, HR, and Wolf, SL. Modified Emory Functional Ambulation Profile: An outcome measure for rehabilitation for post stroke gait dysfunction. Stroke 32:973, 2001. Wolf, SL, Catlin, PA, and Gage, K. Establishing the reliability and validity of measurements using the Emory Functional Ambulation Profile. Phys Ther 79:1122, 1999. Nelson, AJ. Functional ambulation profile. Phys Ther 54:1059, 1974.
10-m Walk Test	Collen, FM, Wade, DT, and Bradshaw, CM. Mobility after stroke: Reliability of measures of impairment and disability. Int Disabil Studies 12:6, 1990. Bohannon, RW, Andrews, AW, and Thomas, MW. Walking speed: Reference values and correlates for older adults. J Orthop Sports Phys Ther 77:86, 1996.
6-Minute Walk Test	Enright, PL, and Sherrill, DL. Reference equations for the six-minute walk in healthy adults. Am J Respir Crit Care Med 158:1384, 1998. Liu, J, Drutz, C, Kumar, R, et al. Use of six minute walk test post stroke. Is there a practice effect? Arch Phys Med Rehabil 89:1686, 2008. Fulk, G, Echternach, J, Nof, L, and O'Sullivan, S. Clinometric properties of the six-minute walk test in individuals undergoing rehabilitation poststroke. Physiother Theory and Pract 24:195, 2008.
Dynamic Gait Index (DGI)	Shumway-Cook, A, and Woollacott, M. Motor Control: Translating Research into Clinical Practice, ed 3. Lippincott Williams & Wilkins, 2007, pp 395–396. Jonsdottir, J, and Cattaneo, D. Reliability and validity of the Dynamic Gait Index in persons with chronic stroke. Arch of Phys Med and Rehabil 88(11):1410, 2007. Walker, ML, Austin, AG, Banke, GM, et al. Reference group data for the Functional Gait Assessment. Phys Ther 87(11):1468, 2007. Wrisley, D, Marchetti, GF, Kuharsky, DK, and Whitney, SL. Reliability, internal consistency, and validity of data obtained with the Functional Gait Assessment. Phys Ther 84(10):906, 2004.
Observational Gait Analysis (OGA)	Norkin, C. Examination of gait. In O'Sullivan, S, and Schmitz, T: Physical Rehabilitation, ed 5. FA Davis, Philadelphia, 2007, pp 320–334. Pathokinesiology Service and Physical Therapy Department. Observational Gait Analysis Handbook. Los Amigos Research and Education Institute, Downey, CA, 2001. Perry, JP. Gait Analysis: Normal and Pathological Function. Thorofare, NJ: SLACK, Inc, 1992.

Abbreviations: CVA, cerebrovascular accident; SCI, spinal cord injury; TBI, traumatic brain injury.

Participation Measures	References
The MOS SF-36	Anderson, C, Laubscher, S, and Burns, R. Validation of the short-form (SF-36) health survey questionnaire among stroke patients. Stroke 27:1812, 1996. Ware, JE, and Sherbourne, CD. The MOS 36-Item Short-Form Health Survey (SF-36). I. Conceptual framework and item selection. Med Care 30:473, 1992. The SF-36 Health Survey is available online at http://www.rand.org/health/surveys/sf36item/.
Participation Objective, Participation Subjective (POPS)	Brown, M, Dijkers, MPJ, Gordon, W, et al. Participation Objective, Participation Subjective: A measure of participation combining outsider and insider perspectives. J Head Trauma Rehabil 19(6):459, 2004. Mascialino, G, Hirshson, C, Egan, M, et al. Objective and subjective assessment of long-term community integration in minority groups following traumatic brain injury. NeuroRehabilitation 24(1):29, 2009. The POPS is available online at http://www.tbims.org/combi/pops/Appendix%201.doc
Impact of Participation and Autonomy (IPA)	Cardol, M, de Haan, RJ, de Jong, BA, et al. Psychometric properties of the impact on participation and autonomy questionnaire. Arch Phys Med Rehabil 82(2):210, 2001. The IPA is available online at http://nivel.nl/pdf/INT-IPA-E.pdf.
Activities and Balance Confidence Scales (ABC)	Lajoie, Y, and Gallagher, SP. Predicting falls within the elderly community: Comparison of postural sway, reaction time, the Berg Balance Scale, and the Activity-Specific Balance Confidence scale for comparing fallers and non-fallers. Arch Gerontol Geriatr 38:11, 2004. Myers, AM, Fletcher, PC, Myers, AN, et al. Discriminative and evaluative properties of the ABC Scale. J Gerontol A Biol Med 53A:M287, 1998. Powell, LE, and Myers, AM. Activities-Specific Balance Confidence (ABC) Scale. J Gerontol 50A:M28, 1995. The ABC Scale is available online at http://www.pacificbalancecenter.com/forms/abc_scale.pdf.
Tinetti Falls Efficacy Scale (FES)	Harada, N, Chiu, V, and Damon-Rodriquez, J. Screening balance and mobility impairment in elderly individuals living in a residential care facility. Phys Ther 75:462, 1995.
Dizziness Handicap Inventory (DHI)	Jacobson, GP, and Newman, CW. The development of the dizziness handicap inventory. Arch Otolaryngol Head Neck Surg 16:424, 1990.
Modified Fatigue Impact Scale (mFIS)	Fisk, JD, et al. The impact of fatigue on patients with multiple sclerosis. Can J Neurol Sci 21(1):9, 1994. Fisk, JD, et al. Measuring the functional impact of fatigue: Initial validation of the Fatigue Impact Scale. Clin Infect Dis 1(Suppl):S79, 1994.
Outpatient Physical Therapy Improvement in Movement Assessment Log (OPTIMAL)	Guccione, AA, Mielenz, TJ, Devellis, RF, et al. Development and testing of a self-report instrument to measure actions: Outpatient Physical Therapy Improvement in Movement Assessment Log (OPTIMAL). Phys Ther 85(6):515, 2005. OPTIMAL is available online at http://www.apta.org.

(table continues on page 330)

Participation Measures	References
The Craig Handicap Assessment and Reporting Technique (CHART)	Walker, N, Mellick, D, Brooks, CA, and Whiteneck, GG. Measuring participation across impairment groups using the Craig Handicap Assessment Reporting Technique. Am J Phys Med Rehabil 82(12):936, 2003. Hall, KM, Dijkers, M, Whiteneck, G, et al. The Craig Handicap Assessment and Reporting Technique (CHART): Metric properties and scoring. J Rehabil Outcomes Meas 2(5):39, 1998. CHART is available online at http://www.tbims.org/combi/chart/index.html.
Stroke Impact Scale (SIS)	Duncan, PW, Lai, SM, Bode, RK, et al. Stroke Impact Scale-16: A brief assessment of physical function. Neurol 60 (2):291, 2003. Lai, SM, Perera, S, Duncan, PW, et al. Physical and social functioning after stroke: Comparison of the Stroke Impact Scale and Short Form-36. Stroke 34 (2):488, 2003. Duncan, PW, Bode, R, Lai, SM, et al. Rasch analysis of a new stroke-specific outcome scale: The Stroke Impact Scale. Arch Phys Med Rehabil 84(7):950, 2003. The *Guide for Stroke Impact Scale Administration* is available online at http://www.chrp.org/pdf/HSR082103_SIS_Handout.pdf.

Note: All websites referenced in tables accessed September 30, 2009.

INDEX

Page numbers followed by *b* indicate boxes; *f*, figures; *t*, tables.

A

Ability(ies)
definition of, 7*b*
Activation, definition of, 36
Activity(ies)
categories of, 13
complex, 9
of daily living
basic, 9, 13
instrumental, 9, 13
definition of, 3*b*
lead-up, in motor learning, 22
Activity-based task analysis, 12–13
Activity-based, task-oriented intervention(s),
13–17, 14*b*
Activity demands, 13
of self-feeding, 219–220, 219*f*, 220*f*
Activity limitations, definition of, 3*b*
Activity log, for unsupervised practice, 22
Adaptability, of skills, as measure of motor
learning, 18, 18*b*
Adaptation, 7
Adaptive balance control, in standing, 164
Agonist reversals, as PNF technique, 35*b*
Alternate tapping, as NDT treatment technique,
38*b*
American Spinal Injury Association (ASIA),
*Standard Neurological Classification of
Spinal Cord Injury* of, 263, 264*f*, 289*f*
Amount of Use Scale, 237, 238*t*
Ankle strategy, in standing, 164, 165*f*
promoting, 182, 183*f*
Antagonist reversals of, as PNF technique, 34–35*b*
Antalgic gait, 197*b*
Anticipation timing, 9
definition of, 10*b*
Anticipatory motor control, for balance
definition of, 5*b*
in kneeling, 130
in quadruped, 81
in standing, 164
Approximation, for facilitation, 34*b*
ASIA. *See* American Spinal Injury Association),
*Standard Neurological Classification of
Spinal Cord Injury* of
Asset list, in clinical decision-making, 9
Associative stage, of motor learning, 19, 23–24*t*
Asymmetrical tonic neck reflex (ATNR),
functional rolling and, 46*b*
ATNR. *See* Asymmetrical tonic neck reflex
(ATNR)

Attitudinal factors, rehabilitation and, 10
Autonomous stage, of motor learning, 19, 24*t*

B

BADL (basic activities of daily living), 9, 13
Balance
definition of, 110
Balance training strategies
in kneeling, 130–132, 130*f*, 131*f*, 132*f*
in prone on elbows, 69
in quadruped, 81–82
in sitting, 110–116
adaptive, 116
on ball
dynamic activities as, 113–116, 114*f*,
115*f*, 116*f*
static activities as, 113, 113*f*
with manual perturbations, 111–112
on moveable surface, 112–113, 112*f*, 113*f*
student practice activity in, 118–119*b*
in standing
adaptive, activities and strategies for
improving, 188–189, 189*b*
compensatory training for, 190, 191*b*
equipment sources for, 193
interventions to improve, 182–190
promoting ankle strategies for, 182, 183*f*
promoting hip strategies for, 182–183,
183*f*, 184*f*
promoting stepping strategies for, 183, 184*f*
sensory, interventions to improve, 190
student practice activity on, 191–192*b*
using force-platform biofeedback, 188, 188*f*
using manual perturbations, 183, 185
using mobile and compliant surfaces,
185–188, 185*f*, 186*f*, 187*f*, 188*f*
Balance training, in traumatic brain injury, case
study on, 257–261
Ball activities
for balance strategies
in kneeling, 131–132, 132*f*
in sitting
dynamic activities on, 113–116, 114*f*,
115*f*, 116*f*
size of, guidelines for, 113*b*
static activities on, 113, 113*f*
in standing, 187–188, 188*f*
half-sitting/half-kneeling on, 134–135, 134*f*
passing, catching, and throwing, sitting on
ball, 115–116, 116*f*

Bandwidth feedback, 20*b*
Barriers, perceived, as predictors of adherence to
physical activity, 236
Base of support (BOS), for sitting, 99*b*
Basic activities of daily living (BADL), 9, 13
Bed skills
interventions to improve control of, 45–70
prone extension as, 60–61, 61*f*
prone on elbows as, 61–70. *See also* Prone,
on elbows
rolling as, 45–55. *See also* Rolling
sidelying as, 56–60. *See also* Sidelying
Behavioral contract, in constraint-induced
movement therapy, 237–240, 238*t*
Behavioral methods, adherence-enhancing, to
increase transfer to life situation, 234–241.
See also Transfer package in constraint-
induced movement therapy
Behavioral shaping techniques, in motor
learning, 14
Berg Balance Scale, 264, 266*t*, 326
Bilateral transfer, in motor learning, 22
Biofeedback, force-platform, in standing balance
control, 188, 188*f*
Blocked practice, in motor learning, 21, 22*b*
Body functions, definition of, 3*b*
Body structures, definition of, 3*b*
Body weight support (BWS) system, in improving
locomotor skills, 209–211, 210*b*, 211*b*
Braiding, 202–204, 203*f*, 204*f*
Bridging, 15*b*, 87–95
student practice activity on, 92*b*, 95*b*

C

Caregiver contract, in constraint-induced
movement therapy, 240
Change of support strategies, in standing, 164, 165*f*
Chop pattern, PNF 31*b*
resisted, in sitting, 107, 108*f*
reverse, 31*b*, 32*b*
Closed environment, in motor learning, 22
Closed-loop system, 5
Closed motor skill, definition of, 7*b*, 10*b*
Coaching, in shaping and task practice, 236*t*
Cognitive stage, of motor learning, 18–19, 23*t*
Community integration, of locomotor training, 215
Compensation, definition of, 6
Compensatory intervention
for balance control in standing, 190, 191*b*
for motor learning, 40, 40*b*

for upper extremity skill development, 224–226, 225f, 226f
  student practice activity on, 227b
Complex motor skills, definition of, 7b, 9
Concentrated practice, in constraint-induced movement therapy, 242–243
Concurrent feedback, in motor learning, 20
Constant feedback, in motor learning, 20b
Constraint-induced movement therapy (CIMT), 232–245
  adherence-enhancing behavioral methods to increase transfer to life situation in, 234–241. *See also* Transfer package in constraint-induced movement therapy
  Amount of Use Scale, 237, 238t
  How Well Scale, 237, 238t
  modified, in upper extremity skill development, 228–230, 230b
Context-specific learning, in motor learning, 22
Contextual factors, definition of, 3b
Continuous motor skills, definition of, 7b
Contract
  behavioral, in constraint-induced movement therapy, 237–240, 238t
  caregiver, in constraint-induced movement therapy, 240
Contract-relax (CR), PNF technique, 35b
Controlled mobility, 6–7, 8t
Creeping, in quadruped, 80–81, 80f, 81f
Criterion skill, 8
Cross-stepping, 202, 202f
Curbs, ascending and descending, in wheelchair using wheelies, 158–161, 159f, 160f, 161f

D

Decision-making
  clinical, framework for, 3–11
  in motor learning, 24–25, 24b
Degrees of freedom, definition of, 5b
Delayed feedback, 20b
Developmental sequence skills, 5
Disability(ies)
  definition of, 4b
  risk factors for, environmental, 9
  terminology on, 3–4b
Disc, inflated, for balance strategies
  in kneeling, 131, 131f
  in sitting, 112, 112f
  in standing, 187, 187f
Discrete motor skills, definition of, 7b
Distributed practice, in motor learning, 21, 22b
Dual-task skills, definition of, 7b
  to enhance motor learning, 19
  in testing level of control, in standing, 166, 170
  in varying locomotor task demands, 205, 208f, 209
Dynamic postural control, 6–7, 8t
Dynamic reversals, PNF technique, 34b, 49–50, 50f

E

Environment, 9–10
  closed, in motor learning, 22
  factors, 3b
  open, in motor learning, 22
  structuring of
    in motor learning, 22

Environmental demands, 13
  of locomotor tasks, varying, strategies for, 207b
EquiTest Balance Analysis, 282
Expert models, to enhance motor learning, 18–19
Externally paced skills, definition of, 10b
Extrinsic feedback, in motor learning, 20

F

Facilitation
  definition of, 36
  neuromuscular
    in motor learning, 36, 38
    proprioceptive. *See* Proprioceptive neuromuscular facilitation (PNF)
Feedback, in motor learning, 20
  bandwidth, 20b
  constant, 20b
  delayed, 20b
  faded feedback, 20b
  extrinsic (augmented), 20
  intrinsic, 20
  knowledge of performance (KP), in motor learning, 20
  knowledge of results (KR), in motor learning, 20
  schedules of, 20
  in shaping and task practice, 236t
  summed, 20b
Fine motor skill, definition of, 7b
Finger manipulation, for self-feeding, 218, 219f
Flexibility exercises, in improving standing control, 166, 167f, 167t
Flexion-adduction-external rotation pattern, PNF
  lower extremity, 27b, 28b, 29b
  upper extremity, 26b
Floor, transfers from
  to standing, 181–182, 182f
  to wheelchair, 153–155, 154f, 155f
Foam rollers, in promoting balance control in standing, 185, 186f, 187
Force platform, standing balancing on, 188, 188f
  limits of stability, 188f
  postural stability, 188f
Fugl-Meyer Assessment of Physical Performance, 299–303t, 325
Function, promoting, 1–41
Function-induced recovery, 6
Functional activity analysis, worksheet for, 13b
Functional Independence Measure (FIM), 284t, 290t, 325
Functional limitation, definition of, 4b
Functional mobility skills (FMS), 13
Functional Reach Test, 260f, 326
Functional Reach Test, Modified, 263

G

Gait
  antalgic, 197b
  circumducted, 198b
  deviations in, common, 197–198b
  steppage, 198b
  terminology for, 194, 195–196t
  Trendelenburg, 197b
Gait cycle, 194
Generalizability, of skills, as measure of motor learning, 18, 18b

Grasp
  gross, for self-feeding, 218, 218f
  promoting
    compensatory training in, 225–226, 225f
    motor learning in, 227
    neuromuscular facilitation in, 221–222
Gross motor skill, definition of, 7b
Guided movement, in activity-based, task-oriented intervention, 16–17, 17b

H

Half-kneeling, 16b, 120f, 132–136
  general characteristics of, 132
  student practice activity on, 136–137b
Health condition, definition of, 3b
Health status, definition of, 4b
Heel-sitting position, 75–77, 76f, 77f, 125–128, 126f, 127
Helplessness, learned, counteracting, 22
High organization, definition of, 5b
Hip strategy, in standing, 164, 165f
  promoting, 182–183, 183f, 184f
Hold-relax-active contraction (HRAC), as PNF technique, 35b
Hold-relax-active motion, as PNF technique, 35b
Hold-relax (HR), as PNF technique, 35b
Home diary, in constraint-induced movement therapy, 240
Home practice, in constraint-induced movement therapy, 241
Home skill assignment, in constraint-induced movement therapy, 240
Hooklying position, 82–87
  general characteristics of, 82–83
  student practice activity on, 88b
How Well Scale, 237, 238t
HR. *See* Hold-relax (HR)
HRAC. *See* Hold-relax-active contraction (HRAC)

I

Impairments
  definition of, 3b
  identification and correction of, in motor learning, 15–16
Inhibition, definition of, 36
Inhibitory pressure, 39–40b
Inhibitory tapping, as NDT treatment strategy, 38b
Instrumental activities of daily living (IADL), 9, 13
International Classification of Functioning, Disability, and Health (ICF), World Health Organization, 3, 3b
Interventions, to improve control in
  bed skills, 45–70
  bridging, 87–96. *See also* Bridging
  hooklying, 82–87. *See also* Hooklying
  kneeling and half-kneeling control, 120–137. *See also* Kneeling
  locomotor skills, 194–215. *See also* Locomotor skills
  quadruped, 70–82. *See also* Quadruped
  sitting and sitting balance skills, 97–119. *See also* Sitting
  standing and standing balance skills, 163–193. *See also* Standing
  transfers, 138–156. *See also* Transfer(s)

upper extremity skills, 216–231. *See also* Upper extremity skills
Interventions to improve motor control and learning, 12–41
Intrinsic feedback, in motor learning, 20
Irradiation, for facilitation, 33*b*

J

Joint approximation, 39*b*
Joint traction, 39*b*

K

Kneel-walking, 129–130, 130*f*
Kneeling, 16*b*, 120–132, 120*f*
  general characteristics of, 121
  prerequisite requirements for, 121
  student practice activity on, 136–137*b*
Knowledge of performance (KP), in motor learning, 20
Knowledge of results (KR), in motor learning, 20

L

Lead-up activities, in motor learning, 22
Lead-up skills, 8
Learned nonuse, 6, 232
Learning
  context-specific, in motor learning, 22
  motor. *See* Motor learning
  negative, practice in, 20–21
  transfer of, in motor learning, 22
Life span, motor skills across, 5–6
Lift, upper extremity pattern, PNF, 31*b*, 32*b*
  in kneeling, 128–129, 129*f*
  in sitting, 107, 109*f*
Limits of stability (LOS)
  in sitting, 103
  in standing, 163
  standing on force platform, 188*f*
Locomotor skills
  demands of, varying, strategies for, 205, 206–207*b*, 208*f*, 209
  improving
    body weight support in, 209–211, 210*b*, 211*b*
    interventions for, 194–215
    treadmill training in, 209–211, 210*b*, 211*b*
  student practice activities on, 211, 212–213*b*
  training in
    overview of, 214–215
Logrolling, from sidelying, 48–49, 49*f*
Long-sitting
  active holding in, 101, 101*f*
  scooting in, 116–117
  for transfer skills practice, 151, 151*f*
Lower extremity patterns, PNF, 28–31*b*
  D1 F and E, 28–29*b*
  D2 F and E, 29–31*b*
Lunges, from standing, 181, 181*f*, 182*f*

M

Manual contacts, for facilitation, 33*b*
Massed practice, in motor learning, 21, 22*b*
Mental practice, in motor learning, 21, 22*b*
Mobility, 6, 8*t*, 9
Modeling, in shaping and task practice, 236*t*

Modified Ashworth Scale, 259*t*, 262, 297, 324
Modified Clinical Test for Sensory Integration in Balance (mCTSIB), 279*t*, 327
Modified constraint-induced movement therapy (mCIMT), in upper extremity skill development, 228–230, 230*b*
Modified plantigrade, 16*b*, 170–174. *See also* Plantigrade, modified
Motor ability, 7
Motor Activity Log (MAL), in constraint-induced movement therapy, 237, 238*t*, 239*t*, 297, 305–306*t*, 309–310*t*
Motor control, 4, 5
  definition of, 5*b*
  terminology on, 5*b*
Motor learning
  definition of, 4, 5*b*, 18
  feedback in, 32–33
  interventions for, 12–41
  measures of, 18, 18*b*
  practice in, 20–22
  stages of, 18–19
    associative, 10, 19, 23–24*t*
    autonomous, 19, 24*t*
    cognitive, 18–19, 23*t*
  strategies for, 18–25
  structuring environment in, 22
  transfer of learning in, 22
Motor milestones, 5
Motor program, 4
  definition of, 5*b*
Motor recovery, 6
  definition of, 5*b*
Motor skill(s)
  across life span, 5–6
  definition of, 7*b*
Movement(s)
  facilitated, 36, 38
  guided, 16–17, 17*b*
Movement time, 7–8

N

NDT. *See* Neuro-developmental treatment (NDT)
Negative learning, 20–21
Neuro-developmental treatment (NDT), 36, 37–38*b*
Neuromotor training approaches, to motor learning, 25–40
Neuromuscular facilitation techniques, 25–40
Nonuse, learned, 6, 232

O

Open environment, in motor learning, 22
Open-loop system, 4
Open motor skill, definition of, 7*b*, 10*b*
Overflow, for facilitation, 33*b*
Overground examination, in locomotor training, 214–215

P

Parkinson's disease, case study on, 281–286
Participation, definition of, 3*b*
Participation restrictions, definition of, 3*b*
Pathology, definition of, 4*b*
Pathophysiology, definition of, 4*b*
Perceived barriers, as predictors of adherence to physical activity, 236

Performance, definition of, 4*b*
Performance-Oriented Mobility Assessment (POMA), 264, 266–268*t*, 327
Performance test, as measure of motor learning, 18, 18*b*
Peripheral vestibular dysfunction, case study on, 278–280
Personal factors, definition of, 3*b*
Placing, as NDT treatment strategy, 38*b*
Plantigrade, modified, 16*b*, 170–174. *See also* modified plantigrade
Plasticity, brain, use-dependent, 232
PNF. *See* Proprioceptive neuromuscular facilitation (PNF)
Postural alignment
  impairments in
    sitting, 98
    standing, 164–166
  normal
    sitting, 97
    standing, 163*f*, 164*f*
Postural control
  dynamic, 6–7, 8*t*
  static, 6, 8*t*
Postural fixation
  in sitting, 111
  in standing, 164
Postural synergies, normal, in standing, 164
Practice, in motor learning, 20–22
  blocked, 21, 22*b*
  concentrated, in constraint-induced movement therapy, 242–243
  distributed, 21, 22*b*
  home, in constraint-induced movement therapy, 241
  massed, 21, 22*b*
  mental, 21, 22*b*
  parts-to-whole, 8–9, 17
  random, 21, 22*b*
  serial, 21, 22*b*
  trial-and-error, 18
Prehension, promoting
  compensatory training in, 225–226, 225*f*
  motor learning in, 227
  neuromuscular facilitation in, 221–222
Prehension patterns, for self-feeding, 218, 218*f*
Pressure, inhibitory, 39–40*b*
Pressure tapping, as NDT treatment strategy, 38*b*
Proactive motor control, definition of, 5*b*
Problem-solving, in constraint-induced movement therapy, 237, 240
Prone on elbows, 15*b*, 61–70
  general characteristics of, 61
  student practice activity on, 69–70*b*
Prone extension, 60–61, 61*t*
  general characteristics of, 60
Proprioception, visual, 9–10
  definition of, 10*b*
Proprioceptive neuromuscular facilitation (PNF)
  foundation procedures for, 33–34*b*
  in motor learning, 25, 26–36*b*, 36
  patterns of, 25
    head and trunk, 31–33*b*
    lower extremity, 27–31*b*
    upper extremity, 26–27*b*

techniques of, 34–36b
  terminology of, 36t
  in upper extremity skills development, 222–224, 223f, 224f
Propulsion, of wheelchair, 156, 156f
  on inclines, 156
Psychosocial factors, rehabilitation and, 10

Q

Quadruped, 15b, 70–83
  assist-to-position
    from prone on elbows, 70–71, 71f
    from side-sitting, 71–72, 71f
  balance strategies in, 81–82
  creeping in, 80–81, 80f, 81f
  general characteristics of, 70
  improving control in, interventions for, 70–82
  movement transitions from
    to bilateral heel-sitting position, 75–76, 76f
    to heel-sitting on one side, 76–77, 77f
    to side-sitting, 77, 77f
  student practice activity on, 82–83b

R

Random practice, in motor learning, 21, 22b
Reach, upper extremity
  compensatory training for, 224–225
  facilitating, 221, 221f
  motor learning in, 226–227
Reaction time, 7
Reactive balance control
  in kneeling, 130–131
  in quadruped, 81–82
  in standing, 164
Reactive motor control, definition of, 5b
Recall schema, definition of, 5b
Reciprocal trunk patterns, outcomes and indications for, 59
Recognition schema, definition of, 5b
Recovery
  function-induced, 6
  motor, 6
    definition of, 5b
  spontaneous, 6
  true, 242
Reference of correctness
  to enhance motor learning, 18
Reflex hierarchical theory, 5
Reflexes, tonic, functional rolling and, 46b
Regulatory conditions, definition of, 10b
Repeated contractions, (repeated stretch) as PNF technique, 35b
Repeated stimulation, temporal summation from, 38
Repetitive, task-oriented training, in constraint-induced movement therapy, 232, 234
Replication, 50–51, 51f
Resistance, 39b
  to contextual change in locomotor tasks, 205
  for facilitation, 33b
Resisted progression (RP), as PNF technique, 35–36b
  for creeping in quadruped, 80–81, 80f, 81f
  for kneel-walking, 129–130, 130f

for walking
  braiding, 204
  forward and backward, 199–200, 199f, 200f
  side-stepping, 200, 201f, 202, 202f
Response time, 8
Retention, as measure of motor learning, 18, 18b
Retention interval, in motor learning, 18
Retention test, as measure of motor learning, 18, 18b
Reversals
  of antagonists, as PNF technique, 34–35b
  dynamic, 49–50, 50f. See also Dynamic reversals
  stabilizing. See also Stabilizing reversals
Reverse chop, 31b, 32b
Reverse lift, 31b, 32b
Rhythmic initiation (RI), 49, 49f
  as PNF technique, 34b
Rhythmic rotation (RRo)
  as NDT treatment strategy, 38b
  as PNF technique, 35b
Rhythmic stabilization (RS), as PNF technique, 35b
RI. See Rhythmic initiation (RI)
Risk factors, for disability, environmental, 9
Rolling, 45–54
  application of PNF extremity patterns to, 51–55
  characteristics of, 45
  interventions for, 48–49
  student practice activity on, 55b
  task analysis for
    components of, 47b
    guidelines for, 47–48
    student practice activity on, 48b
  techniques and verbal cues for, 49–54
Rotation
  rhythmic. See Rhythmic rotation (RRo)
  trunk. See Trunk, rotation of
RP. See Resisted progression (RP)
RRo. See Rhythmic rotation (RRo)
RS. See Rhythmic stabilization (RS)

S

Safety mitt, in constraint-induced movement therapy, 232, 233f
Schema, definition of, 5b
Scooting
  off table into modified standing, 117–118, 117f
  in sitting positions, 116–117, 117f
Segmental rolling, 57
Segmental trunk patterns, 58–59, 58f, 59f
Self-efficacy, as predictor of adherence to physical activity, 236
Self-feeding, 216–220
  activity analysis of, 216
  activity demands of, 219–220, 219f, 220f
  environmental factors for, 220
  lead-up skills for, 217–218, 217f, 218f, 219f
  musculoskeletal performance components of, 217–219
  neurological performance components of, 217–219
  treatment strategies and considerations for, 220–230

Self-paced skills, definition of, 10b
Sensory components, of standing, 164
Sensory control, of balance in standing, interventions to improve, 190
Sensory influence, on sitting, 99b
Sensory stimulation, in motor learning, 38
Serial motor skills, definition of, 7b
Serial practice, in motor learning, 21, 22b
Shaping, in constraint-induced movement therapy, 234, 235f, 236t, 243
Shoulder
  stability and mobility of, for self-feeding, 217, 217f
  stabilization of
    compensatory training in, 224, 225f
    motor learning in, 226–227
    in upper extremity skill development, 222–223, 223f, 224f
Side-sitting
  active holding in, 101, 101f
  movement transitions between kneeling and, combination of isotonics in, 126–127, 127f
  transitions from quadruped to, dynamic reversals in, 77, 77f
Side-stepping, 200, 201f, 202, 202f
Sidelying, control in, 56–60
  general characteristics of, 56, 56f
  logrolling from, 48–49, 49f
  student practice activity on, 60b
  trunk control in, improving, treatment strategies for, 56
  with trunk counterrotation, 58–59, 58f, 59f
  trunk rotation in, 57–58
Simple motor skills, definition of, 7b
Sit pivot transfer, 150–153, 150–153f
Sitting, improving control, 15b, 97–119
  adaptive balance control in, 110–116. See also Balance strategies, in sitting
  alignment in, 97–98, 97f, 98b, 98f
  long-. See Long-sitting
  scooting off table from, to modified standing, 117–118, 117f
  short-, scooting in, 117, 117f
  side-, active holding in, 101, 101f
  student practice activities in, 118–119b
Skill(s), 7–9, 8t
  adaptability of, as measure of motor learning, 18, 18b
  closed, definition of, 10b
  criterion, 8
  definition of, 7
  externally paced, definition of, 10b
  functional mobility, 13
  lead-up, 8
  open, definition of, 10b
  self-paced, definition of, 10b
  splinter, 9
Slow reversals. See Dynamic reversals
Social environment, rehabilitation and, 10
Social support, in constraint-induced movement therapy, 237
Somatosensory challenges, to improve sensory control of balance, 190
Somatosensory control, in standing, 164
Spatial summation, 38
Specificity, of training, 16
Speed-accuracy trade-off, 8

Spinal cord injury
    case studies on, 274–277, 287–292
    locomotor training in, case study on, 262–273
Splinter skills, 9
Spontaneous recovery, 6
Squats, partial wall, from standing, 179–181, 180*f*
Stability, 6, 8*t*
Stabilizing reversals, as PNF technique, 34–35*b*, 64
Stair-climbing, 204, 205*f*
Stance phase, of gait cycle, 194, 195*t*
Stand pivot transfer, 149–150
Stand retraining, in spinal cord injury, 265, 269*t*
Standard Neurological Classification of Spinal Cord Injury of American Spinal Injury Association (ASIA), 263, 264*f*, 289*f*
Standing 16*b*, 163–193
    active limb movements in, 176, 177*b*, 177*f*
    balance control in, interventions to improve, 182–190. *See also* Balance control, in standing
    general characteristics of, 163–164, 163*f*
    impairments in, common, 164, 165–166*b*
    interventions, 166–182
        to ensure safety, 170, 170*b*
        to improve flexibility, 166, 167*f*, 167*t*
        to improve strength, 166, 168–169*t*, 168*f*, 169*f*
        to vary level of difficulty, 166, 169*b*, 170
        to vary postural stabilization requirements, 166, 169*b*, 170
        verbal cueing for, 170, 170*b*
    in modified plantigrade, 170–174
    movement transitions to, from half-kneeling, 135, 135*f*
    partial wall squats from, 179–181, 180*f*
    single-limb stance in, 176
    stepping, 178–179, 178*f*, 179*f*, 180
    student practice activities in, 190, 191–192*b*
    transfers to/from floor, 181–182, 182*f*
    weight shifts, 175–176
Static-dynamic control, 7
Static postural control, 6, 8*t*
Steppage gait, 198*b*
Stepping,
    in modified plantigrade, 173
    in standing, 164 167f, 178–179, 178f, 179f, 180*f*, 183, 184*f*
Step training, 214
STLR. *See* Symmetrical tonic labyrinthine reflex (STLR)
STNR. *See* Symmetrical tonic neck reflex (STNR)
Strengthening, to improve
    sit-to/from-stand transfers, 147–148, 148*f*
    standing control, 166, 168–169*t*, 168*f*, 169*f*
    transfer skills, 155
Stretch
    for facilitation, 34*b*
    prolonged, 39*b*
    quick, 39*b*
    repeated, as PNF technique, 35*b*
Stroke
    case study on, 315–320
    constraint-induced movement therapy for, case study on, 296–314

home care rehabilitation in, case study on, 293–295
Stroke Impact Scale (SIS), 297–298, 311–314*t*, 329
Substitution approach. *See* Compensatory intervention
Summation
    spatial, in central nervous system, 38
    temporal, from repeated stimulation, 38
Summed feedback, 20*b*
Sway envelope, in standing, 163
Sweep tapping, as NDT treatment strategy, 38*b*
Swing phase, of gait cycle, 194, 195–196*t*
Symmetrical tonic labyrinthine reflex (STLR), functional rolling and, 46*b*
Symmetrical tonic neck reflex (STNR), functional rolling and, 46*b*
Systems theory, 4

T

Tapping, as NDT treatment strategy, 38*b*
Task(s)
    classification of, 8*t*
    controlled mobility, 6–7, 8*t*
    mobility, 6, 8*t*
    skill, 7–9, 8*t*
    stability, 6, 8*t*
Task analysis
    activity-based, 12–13
    definition of, 5*b*
    in gait, 194–195
    in sitting, student practice activity on, 118*b*
    in sit-to/from-stand transfers, 138–142, 140*t*
        student practice activities on, 142, 143*b*
    in standing, student practice activity on, 191*b*
    in upper extremity skills, 216–220, 216*b*, 217–220*f*
Task organization, definition of, 5*b*
Task practice, in constraint-induced movement therapy, 232, 234, 235*f*, 236*t*
Temporal summation, from repeated stimulation, 38
Terminal feedback, in motor learning, 20
Thrust, and withdrawal, PNF D1, bilateral symmetrical, in sitting, 109, 109*f*
Thumb manipulation, for self-feeding, 218, 219*f*
Tilting reactions, in standing, 164
Time
    movement, 7–8
    reaction, 7
    response, 8
Timing
    anticipation, 9
        definition of, 10*b*
    for emphasis, PNF, 33*b*
    for facilitation, 33*b*
Traction, for facilitation, 34*b*
Training
    compensatory. *See* Compensatory training
    dual-task, to enhance motor learning, 19
    locomotor, 214–215
    parts-to-whole, 8–9
    repetitive, task-oriented, in constraint-induced movement therapy, 232, 234
Transfer(s), 138–156
    ability for, outcome measures of, 155–156

floor-to-standing, 181–182, 182*f*
floor-to-wheelchair, 153–155, 154*f*, 155*f*
sit-to/from-stand, 138–149, 139*f*, 144–149*f*
    task analysis for, 138–142, 140*t*
stand-to-sit, 148
to and from wheelchair, 149–156
    sit pivot, 150–153, 150*f*, 151*f*, 152*f*, 153*f*. *See also* Sit pivot transfer
    stand pivot, 149–150
    student practice activity on, 161–162*b*
Transfer of learning, in motor learning, 22
Transfer package in constraint-induced movement therapy, 234–241
    behavioral contract in, 237–240, 238*t*
    caregiver contract in, 240
    constraining participant to use less affected UE in, 241
    daily schedule in, 241
    home diary in, 240
    home practice in, 241
    home skill assignment in, 240
    motor activity log in, 237, 238*t*, 239*t*
Transfer test, as measure of motor learning, 18, 18*b*
Traumatic brain injury
    case study on, 251–256
    case study on balance and locomotor training, 257–261
Treadmill (TM) training, in improving locomotor skills, 209–211, 210*b*, 211*b*
Treatment planning
    understanding environment in, 9–10
    understanding individual in, 9
    understanding task in, 6–9
Trendelenburg gait, 197*b*
Trial-and-error practice, in motor learning, 18
Trunk
    control of, early interventions to improve, 56–96
        bridging as, 87–96. *See also* Bridging
        hooklying as, 82–87. *See also* Hooklying position
        prone extension as, 60–61, 61*f*
        prone on elbows as, 61–70. *See also* Prone, on elbows
        quadruped as, 70–82. *See also* Quadruped
        sidelying as, 56–60. *See also* Sidelying
    counterrotation of, sidelying with, 58–59, 58*f*, 59*f*
    PNF patterns for, 31–33*b*
    postural stability of, for self-feeding, 217, 217*f*
    stabilization of, in upper extremity skill development, 222, 223*f*
Trunk rotation
    lateral, sitting on ball, 115, 115*f*
    lower, in hooklying, 83–87, 84*f*, 87*f*
    upper
        in sidelying, 57–58
        in sitting, 104, 104*f*
Turning, of wheelchair on even surfaces, 156

U

Unsupervised practice, in motor learning, 22
Upper extremity (UE)
    bilateral movement, for self-feeding, 218, 219*f*
    compensatory training for, 226
    constraint-induced movement therapy, 232, 233*t*, 241

Upper extremity patterns, PNF, 26–27b
  D1 flexion and extension, 26b
    for forearm stabilization, 223–224, 224f
      student practice activity on, 225b
    for shoulder stabilization, 222–223,
      224f
    in sitting, 106–107
  D1 thrust and reverse thrust pattern, in prone
    on elbows, 68, 68f
  D2 flexion and extension, 27b
    in kneeling, 127–128, 128f
    in quadruped, 78–79, 79f
    in sitting, 107, 107f
    in standing,modified plantigrade, 174,
      174f
Upper extremity skills
  improving, interventions for, 216–231
  for self-feeding, 216–230. *See also* Self-
    feeding
  task analysis in, 216–220, 216b, 217–220f
  treatment strategies and considerations for,
    220–230
    compensatory training as, 224–226, 225f,
      226f
    modified constraint-induced movement
      therapy as, 228–230
    motor learning as, 226–228
    neuromuscular facilitation as, 221–222
    proprioceptive neuromuscular facilitation
      as, 222–224, 223f, 224f
Use-dependent brain plasticity, 232

V

Verbal cues (VCs), in PNF, for facilitation,
  33–34b
Verbal instructions and cueing, in activity-based,
  task-oriented intervention, 17
Vestibular challenges, to improve sensory
  control of balance, 190
Vestibular system, in standing control, 164
Visual challenges, to improve sensory control of
  balance, 190
Visual guidance, for facilitation, 34b
Visual proprioception, 9–10
  in standing, 164

W

Walkie-Talkie (Walk and Talk) test, 19
Walking
  braiding, 202–204, 203f, 204f
  cross-stepping, 202, 202f
  forward and backward, 198–200, 199f, 200f,
    201f
  prerequisite requirements for, 197–198
  resisted progression, 199–200, 199f, 200f
  side-stepping, 200, 201f, 202, 202f
  stair climbing, 204, 205f
Warm-up decrement, in motor learning, 18
Weight shifting
  in bridging, 91–92, 92f
  in half-kneeling, 134
    static-dynamic control in, 134–135, 134f

  in kneeling, 124–125, 125f
  in modified plantigrade, 172-173, 172f, 173f
  in prone on elbows, 65–68, 66f, 67f
  in quadruped, 74–75, 75f
  in sitting, 103–104, 103f, 104f, 114, 114f
  in standing, 175–176
Weightbearing, common impairments in, 98b
Wheelchair
  manual, mobility skills for
    propulsion as, 156, 156f
      student practice activity on, 161–162b
    turning on even surfaces as, 156
    wheelies as, 156–158, 157f, 158f
      ascending and descending curbs using,
        158–161, 159f, 160f, 161f
    transfers to and from, 149–156. *See also*
      Transfer(s), to and from wheelchair
Wheelies, 156–158, 157f, 158f
  ascending and descending curbs using,
    158–161, 159f, 160f, 161f
Wobble board, in promoting balance control in
  standing, 185, 185f
Wolf Motor Function Test (WMFT), in stroke,
  297, 304t
Wrist, stability and mobility of, for self-feeding,
  217, 217f